Newborn Intensive Care

What Every Parent Needs to Know

Jeanette Zaichkin, RNC, MN

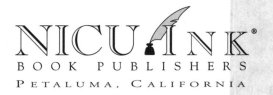
NICU Ink
BOOK PUBLISHERS
PETALUMA, CALIFORNIA

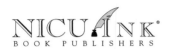

NICU INK
BOOK PUBLISHERS

1304 Southpoint Blvd., Suite 280
Petaluma, CA 94954-6861
(707) 762-2646

Editor-in-Chief:
Charles Rait, RN, MSEd, PNC

Managing Editor: *Suzanne G. Rait, RN*

Editorial Coordinator: *Tabitha Parker*

Reviewers: *Deb Blair*
G.B. Bryant, PharmD
Lucille Daudet-Mitchell
Kathleen Huggins, RN, MS
Rebecca Mullin, RN
Mr. & Mrs. John Packard
Lois Swenson-Grudt
Marsha Walker, RN, IBCLC

Editors: *Beverley DeWitt, BA*
Barbara Fuller, BA, MA
Carolyn Lund, RN, MS, FAAN
Sylvia Stein Wright, BA

Proofreader: *Jane Holly Love, MA*

Indexer: *Elinor Lindheimer*

Book Design and Composition by:
Marsha Godfrey
Sarah Waldron

LIBRARY OF CONGRESS CATALOGING-IN-PUBLICATION DATA
Newborn intensive care : what every parent needs to know / [edited by] Jeanette Zaichkin.
   p.   cm.
   Includes bibliographical references and index.
   ISBN 0-9622975-8-5
   1. Neonatal intensive care.   2. Parent and infant.   3. Hospitals—Nurs-
eries.   I. Zaichkin, Jeanette, 1956–   .
RJ253.5.N53   1996
618.92 ' 01—dc20
DNLM/DLC   96-21773
                                                              CIP

Pooh quotes from A.A. Milne, illustrated by E.H. Shepard. Copyright 1957 by E.P. Dutton, renewed 1985 by E.P. Dutton and the trustees of the Pooh Properties. Used by permission of Dutton Children's Books, a division of Penguin Books USA, Inc.

All photographs by Jeanette Zaichkin unless credited in the caption or listed below:
Ron and Sheila Harrison, Harrison's Photo Shoppe, Poplar Bluff, Missouri,
pages 1, 15, 31, 45, 65, 93, 115, 137, 163, 221, 239, 265, 281, 305, 343.

Contributed by Debbie Fraser Askin, 182; Rodney Broussard, 63, 100, 272, 334; Samantha Broussard, 340; Debra DePaul, 349 (lower); Susan Kearns, 56 (lower); the Packard family, 364; Paul White, 106; contributed by Suzanne Wilson, 178; the Wink family, 195; Dana Zaichkin, 8, 19 (lower); contributed by TrezMarie Zotkiewicz, 276, 298, 337, 338, 362; file photos, 109, 207.

ISBN: 0-9622975-8-5   Library of Congress catalog number 96-21773

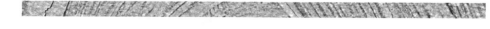

Foreword

The birth of a new baby is never easy. It is often glorified in the press and lay literature. But as a father of three wonderful children and a pediatrician for over 25 years, I am the first to say that giving birth is not easy. The pleasure and wonder of a new baby are combined with vivid moments of pain, uncertainty, bewilderment, emotional trauma, and a host of other, real experiences both physical and psychological. The outcome, in most cases, however, is well worth the ordeal. The presence of the warm, even glowing, new human being quickly allows all of the participants to make the negative parts of the event distant and vague memories and quickly make the glow of parenting the emotional context of the day.

Except if your baby is sick or premature.

With the birth of such a baby, the healing glow of parenting a new baby does not come so quickly; it may not come for weeks or even months. It will take a serious, roller coaster of a detour. The travels may move families through the high-tech world of medicine at its best and worst, hospitals at all hours of the night, people and language you never thought could or do exist. In short, the world of newborn intensive care is a world you are unprepared for.

Until now.

The book you are about to read will help untangle that new, bewildering world of your sick or premature baby. The task of the authors and editors has been to create a piece of work that adds information from the most technical to the most mundane to permit you and your family to engage this world you had no intention of entering, but have nevertheless been tossed. The material contained in this book will give you certain specific pieces of knowledge that you will find invaluable:

- It will take you through the process of your baby's new physical surroundings (the neonatal intensive care unit or NICU) from the beginning.

- It will introduce you to the people, places, language, technology, and expectations of these new surroundings.

- It will help you organize your life, now forever changed.

- It will introduce you to the possibilities for the future.

- It will help you grapple with the uncertainty you had not anticipated.

But most important, this book will help you return to having some control over your life.

The beauty of this book you are about to read is that in its presentation of clear and complete information about the world of newborn intensive care, you the parent are the focus—the person for whom the information is designed. The overall purpose is to engage you fully in this process, to allow you to enter this strange world to successfully become the ally and parent of your baby. It will give you the tools you will need to even the playing field, for your baby needs you now more than ever, and with this book you will be able to do just what your baby needs you for.

I have become a strong advocate for an emerging movement in this country that has been called family-centered care. The philosophy of this movement is that parents are the most important figures for their children, and this is especially true during times of stress, illness, or discomfort. Those of us who feel deeply about bringing parents more meaningfully into the strangest of settings, the hospitals and neonatal nurseries throughout our country, know the following facts:

- Children do better when their parents are near them during times of stress.
- The more meaningfully parents can participate in the care of their sick child, the better it will be for parents and child.
- The greater the parental involvement in all aspects of care for their child, the more likely the child will return to a state of health more quickly.
- Nurturing the positive role of parents in stressful settings will lessen the trauma and establish an even closer bond.

How does one accomplish these things? The credo for family-centered care revolves around eight key concepts:

- Respect
- Strengths
- Choice
- Flexibility

- Information
- Support
- Collaboration
- Empowerment

I strongly believe that this book embodies all these principles. Because it uses understandable language; provides the latest information; carefully employs figures, drawings, and tables; and is written in a tone of comfort, support, and understanding throughout, this book allows you to be an effective parent in this new setting. Using the material enclosed, you can regain your baby, further his or her development, and enhance both of your worlds at the same time.

There is no one more important than you for your child. You gave life to this new person, and you will need to continue to do so. What better way than in collaboration with talented and dedicated individuals in the most sophisticated of surroundings. You need them to bring a future to your baby; but just as important, they and your baby need you. If you all work together, your baby will have the best chance to be all that he or she can be, and you will have the greatest chance of emerging healthy from this artificial world of the NICU to your own real world of home and community.

Steven P. Shelov, MD, FAAP
Professor and Vice Chairman
Department of Pediatrics
Albert Einstein College of Medicine
Montefiore Medical Center
Bronx, New York

Table of Contents

Contributors

Debbie Fraser Askin, RNC, MN
Neonatal Nurse Practitioner
St. Boniface General Hospital
Winnipeg, Manitoba

Susan Tucker Blackburn, RN,C, PhD, FAAN
Professor
Department of Family and Child Nursing
University of Washington
Seattle, Washington

Ann Flandermeyer, RNC, PhD
College of Nursing and Health
University of Cincinnati
Cincinnati, Ohio

Kathleen A. Green, RNC, MSN, NNP
Neonatal Nurse Practitioner
Lenox Hill Hospital
New York, New York

Sharon Gregory, RNC, MN, CNNP
Neonatal Clinical Nurse Specialist
DeKalb Medical Center
Atlanta, Georgia

Susan M. Kearns, RNC, MN, ARNP
Neonatal Clinical Nurse Specialist
Virginia Mason Medical Center
Seattle, Washington

Carole Kenner, RNC, DNS, FAAN
Professor and Department Head of
Parent Child Health Nursing
University of Cincinnati
Cincinnati, Ohio

Cathy Livingston, MSW, LCSW-C
Perinatal Social Worker
Washington Adventist Hospital
Takoma Park, Maryland

Denise Merrill
Publisher
Neonatal and Pediatric ICU
Parenting Magazine
Irwin, Pennsylvania

Kathleen M. Pompa, RNC, MN, NNP
Neonatal Nurse Practitioner
Children's Hospital Medical Center
Cincinnati, Ohio

Ellen P. Tappero, RNC, MN, NNP
Neonatal Nurse Practitioner
Lutheran Medical Center
Wheat Ridge, Colorado

Patricia Thornburg, RN, PhD
Assistant Professor
Wright State University
Dayton, Ohio

Ginna Wall, RN, MN, IBCLC
Coordinator, Lactation Program
University of Washington Medical Center
Seattle, Washington

Jeanette Zaichkin, RNC, MN
Executive Editor,
Mother Baby Journal
Petaluma, California

TrezMarie T. Zotkiewicz, RNC, MN
Neonatal Discharge Coordinator
Ochsner Foundation Hospital
New Orleans, Louisiana

Acknowledgements

Four years of patience and teamwork have resulted in a book unlike any other for parents of special care babies. I am deeply grateful to many people who gave their time and expertise to this project.

Thanks to the authors of this book for contributing their literary talent and professional experience.

Thanks to Charles Rait—for accepting my original proposal for this book, for providing constant encouragement, and for having faith in my ability to produce a quality manuscript.

Thanks to Suzanne Rait—my friend, my mentor, my cheerleader, and editor to the editor.

Thank you to Tabitha Parker whose unending patience and sense of humor gave me hope when things looked bleak.

Thanks to the staff at NICU Ink who contributed their professional expertise and personal encouragement during the production stages of the book.

Thanks to the health care professionals and NICU families at Sacred Heart Medical Center, Spokane, Washington, for their support and assistance with photographic opportunities in the NICU.

Thanks also to my colleagues and NICU families at Madigan Army Medical Center, Ft. Lewis, Washington, for their assistance and encouragement.

I owe a debt of gratitude to my fellow colleagues who contributed to this book in so many ways:

Pamela S. Birgenheier, RN, MN; B.G. Bryant, PharmD; Susan E. Chambers, RN, BSN; Danielle DeKoker; Debra DePaul, RN, MN; Karen Harmitz, RN, BSN; Kimberly M. Horns, RN, NNP, PhD; Kathleen Huggins, RN, MS; Lorna R. Imbruglio, RNC, MSN; William Jeffries; Joyce Johnston, RN, CCRN, CCTC; Tracy Karp, RNC, MS, NNP; Dawn Knight, RNC, BAN; Karen Kuehn, RNC, MSN; Carolyn Lund, RN, MS, FAAN; Peggy Mangiaracina, RN, BSN, MA; Kristie Marbut, RN; Kathleen A. McCloskey-Downey, LPN; Margaret Miller, MS, OTR/L; Connie Mutton, RN, BSN; Nancy O'Brien-Abel, RNC, MN; Gail Peterson, RNC, BSN; Patty Port, RNC, ARNP-NNP, MSN; Ellen P. Tappero, RNC, MN, NNP; Shig Tsudaka, RN; Marsha Walker, RN, IBCLC; Todd L. Wandstrat, PharmD; Peggy L. West, RN; Karin Williamson, RN; Suzanne K. Wilson, MS, RN.

Thank you to the NICU parents who read our book prior to publication and made suggestions:

Lois Swenson-Grudt; John and Amy Packard; Deb Blair; Lucille Daudet-Mitchell.

Thank you to the many professionals whose unique contributions are much appreciated:

Ron and Sheila Harrison, The Photo Shoppe; Catherine N. Bush, Children's Medical Ventures, Inc.; Terry A. Chriswell, Corometrics Medical Systems, Inc.; Mitzi G. Cole, Wyeth-Ayerst Laboratories; Debra Kurtz, Medela, Inc.; Lita Lowry, Mead Johnson Nutritionals; Elizabeth Weadon Massari, MSMI, CMI, Medical Illustration; Ann McRedmond, RN, MSN, Ross Laboratories; Michael G. Meines, Madigan Army Medical Center, Fort Lewis, Washington; Kathleen Mignini, Ohmeda; Deborah Davis Stewart, *Safe Ride News;* Anne Taylor, American Academy of Pediatrics; Marilyn Thordarson, Sacred Heart Medical Center, Spokane, Washington; Sue Vermeulen, King County Nurses' Association, Seattle, Washington.

Thank you to the many people who contributed to the photographs and artwork for this book, and a special thanks to the hospital staff, the babies and their families who allowed us to intrude with our cameras:

Joel Austin; Cody Scott Avila; Kathleen Bares; Patrick, Kelli, and Christopher Beaulaurier; Jean Bening, RN; Lyndsay Bleeker; Patricia Bronston, LPN; James, Samantha, and Andre Broussard; Roberta Colvin, RN; Cindy Crawford; Kayla Davis-Nelson; The Drury family; Mike Dye; Catie Fluaitt; Luke and Logan Garrett; Paula Gaudet; The Grandbois family; Mary Grassi, RNC, BSN; Jeff Harmson; Karla Halsey, and Robert and Logan Hatcher; Penn, Kathy, and David Hendler; Gunnar Hendrickson; Barry January; James, Jill, and Eboni Johnson; Tyrone Johnson; Chantal Jones; The Jurrus family; Roslyn Kean, RN; Klara B. Keen; Layne Kilpatrick; Todd, Michelle, and Michael Lapeynouse; Taylor and Wendy LePiane Mewhinney; The Mazurik family; Angela Marie Martin; Kerrie and Julianne Martin; Arleen and Jared Mason; Madison May; Annie McCurdy; Vivian Victoria McGee; Rachel and Rebecca Mulgrew; Amber Marie Taylor Nunley; David Olmstead, RRT; John, Amy, and Samantha Packard; Ian Paulson; Tyler A. Pearson; Alex Joseph Peek; The Perraputo family; Angelo, Christy, Jessica, and Stephanie Pizzolatto; Andrew Pybus; Nykelas Scott Razey; Stella Reid, RN, BSN; Alexis Robirts; Rogena Brown Scrattish; Alexis and Jared Schmidt; Theresa and Ian Schwerdtfeger; Pam Sheldon, RNC, BSN; Deanna Steele, BSN, CCRN, CFRN; Stacey Stockton, RNC; Martha and Laura Strong; Brittany Strous; Robyn and Trent Thibodeaux; Michelle Vallenzuela; Margaret S. Walsh; John Thomas White; Clarence Williams IV; Kayla Wilson; the Wink family; Dana, Laura, and Stuart Zaichkin.

Introduction

The birth of a sick or premature baby is a mixed blessing. You have shared in the creation of new life, which is a miraculous accomplishment. But your baby is not perfect, which seems unfair and shatters any illusions of a traditional beginning. Parents of sick and premature babies are often torn between joy and sadness, hope and despair. For almost every parent in the neonatal intensive care unit (NICU), though, one desire remains consistently strong—and that is to be recognized as the baby's parent. In other words, NICU parents need to be included in the care of their own special babies.

The authors of this book invite you to become an important member of your baby's health care team. We believe that parents can and should play an active role in their baby's care. This book was written for parents who wish to learn about their baby's illness, how to overcome the barriers to NICU parenting, and how to prepare for and nurture their NICU graduate at home.

Some of the information in this book may seem frightening at first, but knowledge is empowering. When you understand your baby's illness and treatments, you will gain confidence and be able to communicate effectively with your baby's caregivers. You can then form the working partnership with the medical and nursing staff that is essential for your sense of control and for mutual problem solving.

Neonatal intensive care is a huge subject, and your baby will certainly not have every problem in this book. On the other hand, because your NICU experience is unique, this book cannot answer every question or prepare you for every situation. Read through the *Table of Contents* to find the sections that interest you most—and know that what interests you will change as your baby progresses through hospitalization. We hope that this information answers many of your questions, and we encourage you to ask your NICU team about what you do not understand. We hope you will feel better informed and prepared to celebrate the achievements—and manage the crises—that are an inevitable part of every family's life.

We know that you would prefer to read "he" if your baby is a boy and "she" if your baby is a girl. It is difficult to communicate with the distraction of "his/her" and "he/she," however. Therefore, the baby's gender in this book alternates by chapter. Likewise, we know that nurses come in both sexes; however, we refer to nurses as "she."

It would be unrealistic to expect a carefree journey through the NICU. Intensive care is stressful by nature and overwhelming at times. Reading this book and learning about what happens in the NICU will help you gain confidence and feel more relaxed. You will meet some incredible people to help you through the experience. You will meet other parents whose support will give you strength. You will meet health care professionals who have devoted their careers to helping babies like yours. You will discover that the NICU offers a unique blend of technology and compassion that encourages healing and growth not only for babies, but also for parents.

This is probably not the experience you have hoped or planned for, but the NICU offers opportunities you otherwise would have missed. Right from the beginning, you can learn how to communicate effectively with health care professionals and how to use community resources. You will learn to value what is unique and special about your baby and what is most important for your baby's future. And when your baby's hospital stay is over, you will probably realize that your NICU experience has made you stronger, smarter, and more aware of what is most important in your life.

We want you to have a positive NICU experience. Even though your baby has had a difficult start, it is a precious beginning just the same. Use this book to guide you through your experience, and remember that your baby's nurses and physicians are your most important sources of information. As your baby grows, you will continue to learn things about child care from teachers, coaches, health care professionals, and all the people who influence your child's life.

Learning how to be a good parent never ends. We hope you get a good start here—and enjoy learning about your very special baby.

Jeanette Zaichkin, RNC, MN

To my family.

Believe in your dreams.

Chapter 1

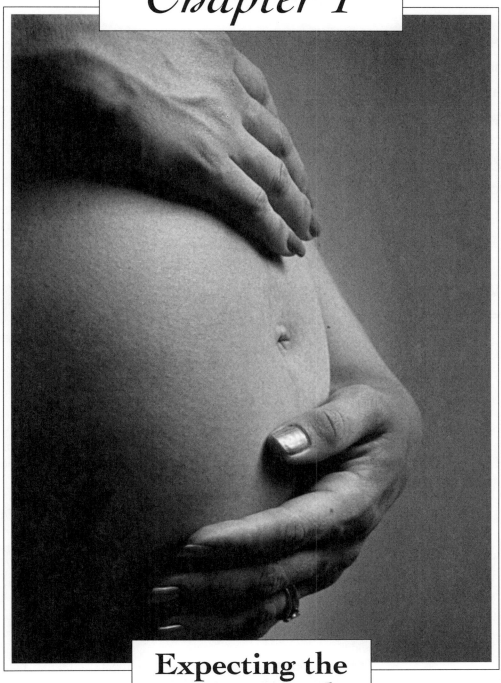

Expecting the
Unexpected

Jeanette Zaichkin, RNC, MN

❝As soon as he saw the Big Boots, Pooh knew that an Adventure was going to happen, and he brushed the honey off his nose with the back of his paw, and spruced himself up as well as he could, so as to look Ready for Anything.❞

Labor and birth are indeed an adventure unmatched by few other life experiences. Most parents anticipate the big event with a mixture of excitement and apprehension, yet few are truly prepared for complications that result in a sick newborn. A complicated labor or a sick baby changes your life in more ways than you can imagine. Finding out that pregnancy, labor, and birthing your baby may pose risks to your health or that your unborn baby may be at risk for health problems can be frightening. Understanding the basics of birthing "at risk" may help you cope with the inevitable anxiety that accompanies a different beginning.

Where Will You Give Birth?

Your baby's quality of life may depend on decisions made before his birth. By working with your perinatal team of doctors, nurses, and other health care professionals in making these decisions, you are acting as a responsible parent even before your baby is born. Your team's first recommendation may concern the hospital where your baby will be born.

Levels of Care

Hospital newborn care is classified as Level I, II, or III, depending on the services available. Although equipped to handle emergencies, many community hospitals prefer to transport pregnant women who are at risk or whose babies may be at risk to a nearby medical center where the staff is experienced and expert at managing complicated labors and sick newborns.

A hospital with a Level I nursery is equipped to handle "healthy" mothers and babies. A Level II nursery provides care for premature infants without complications and for "gaining and growing" infants who have been returned from a regional medical center for convalescence. A regional medical center (sometimes called a tertiary care center or a perinatal center) provides Level III intensive care for seriously ill babies, for those requiring technological assistance for breathing problems, and for babies requiring surgery or evaluation and stabilization of birth defects. Regional centers offer state-of-the-art equipment and highly trained specialists in medicine, nursing, and related health care fields.

The most important aspect of your community hospital may be its staff's expert ability to determine where both you and your baby will have the best outcome. If the perinatal team at your community hospital determines that your labor or your baby's birth may become complicated, its best recommendation may be that you be transported to a regional medical center before your baby is born. Even if your health care professional anticipates an uncomplicated labor, he or she may recommend maternal transport, as the process is called, so that your newborn will have the advantage of immediate admission into a neonatal intensive care unit (NICU) if he is born with complications. If you give birth in a community hospital that does not provide neonatal intensive care, your newborn faces the possibility of transport, which is stressful for the baby and may separate parents and child.

Maternal Transport

Methods of maternal transport depend on the seriousness of your condition and how close you are to the medical center. Some regional medical centers send their specially trained perinatal transport team to the community hospital; that team accompanies you as you travel by ambulance, helicopter, or other aircraft. Other community hospitals use a local ambulance company for transport, sending members of their own labor and delivery staff with you to ensure your safe arrival at and admission to the medical center.

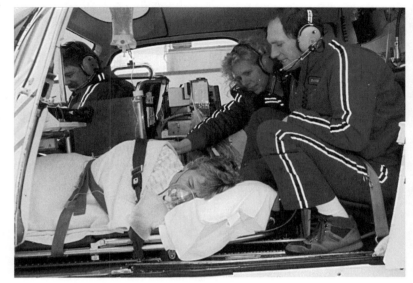

Maternal transport by helicopter.

This expectant mother prepares for transport by helicopter. The transport team provides reassurance and a safe trip.

Even though transport may be in your or your baby's best medical interest, it comes with a personal price. When you change hospitals, you usually lose the services of your own physician or midwife and your chosen pediatrician. You may be far from home, without the support of family and friends. In addition, maternal transport may mean making long-term arrangements for the care of your household and other children in your absence.

Your partner or support person may worry about your health and safety and the uncertain health of your unborn baby. Witnessing the flurry of activity that accompanies transport and sensing the urgency of the situation, your partner may feel all the responsibility for holding things together.

During this stressful time, partners need to communicate honestly with each other. Lend each other support, and be together if possible when information is given. Stress makes it difficult to hear everything that health care providers tell you. Partners may be able to clarify the facts for one another.

Your labor and delivery nurse at the community hospital or a member of the transport team should provide your partner or support person with directions to the medical center and to its perinatal unit. Your case manager should be able to tell your partner about inexpensive lodging and parking discounts at or near the medical center. You should also get important information from your nurse, social worker, or case manager for navigating this unfamiliar system.

The transport process can be frightening for parents. Not only is it an unanticipated new experience, but you can no longer deny the reality of your complications. If you are able, tell your health care team what you are feeling, and ask questions about what will happen next. The members of your perinatal team realize that you are apprehensive and will make every attempt to keep you informed and as comfortable as possible.

Your Care Providers

The personnel attending your labor and your infant's birth will depend on your circumstances. When you become sick or your labor becomes complicated, many interventions become necessary. People and machines may fill the room until you wonder if anyone remembers you are in the bed.

Following are descriptions of the care providers you may encounter during labor. Chapter 3 is devoted to helping you understand the roles of the many people involved in caring for your baby in the NICU, and how best to communicate with them.

Your Labor Nurse

Most women establish firm bonds with the nurse who guides and supports them through labor and birth. Your labor nurse will be your primary source of information, your advocate, and your link to the many people involved in your care. Your nurse's expertise will become obvious as she performs the tasks necessary to ensure a safe labor and birth. But just as important as her technical skills are her abilities to promote the natural processes of birth and to help keep you and your partner involved in the overall plan of care.

Physicians

If your labor becomes complicated, your family physician or midwife may call specialists to assist. An obstetrician is a physician who specializes in women's health care issues. A perinatologist is an expert in maternal-fetal medicine.

"We shopped for a hospital and chose the one with the nicest interior decorating. Our priorities changed when we had an emergency cesarean. Thank goodness there was also an expert staff who saved my baby's life."

In a teaching hospital, residents and interns may be interested in your progress; participation in your care is an important part of their medical education. You may wish to ask your labor nurse to help you limit the number of students and interns involved in your labor and birth, however.

Your obstetrician may administer whatever pain control you need. Some facilities use the services of anesthesiologists, physicians trained to administer medications that reduce pain and/or cause unconsciousness. Nurses with advanced practice education, called certified registered nurse anesthetists (CRNAs), can also administer anesthesia in collaboration with an anesthesiologist.

Other Hospital Personnel

In addition to your labor nurse and physician, other specialized hospital staff may participate in your care. Laboratory personnel will draw your blood,

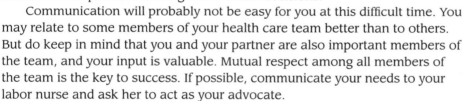

a sonographer may conduct your ultrasound, and a social worker may meet with you to discuss available resources and personal needs. Each member of the hospital team supports an important aspect of your care.

What to Expect from the Team

All members of your health care team should intro-duce themselves by name and title before examining you or asking questions about your history. You should expect courteous and respectful treatment. Even in an emergency, team members should protect your privacy by closing hallway doors and using privacy screens dur-ing caregiving.

Most hospitals make an effort to ask you the same questions only once or twice; sometimes repetition is unavoidable, however. You may feel that a multitude of caregivers whom you have never before met and who never seem to talk to one another are asking you the same questions. It may help to realize that different members of the health care team look for specific sorts of information within your answers so that they can make the best possible nursing and medical decisions.

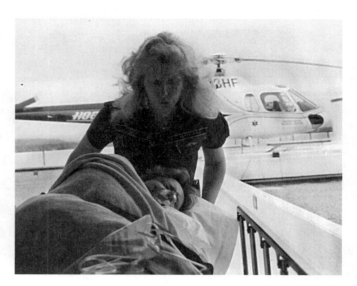

Arrival at the regional medical center.

The expertise of the transport nurse assures a safe arrival and a smooth transition to new caregivers.

Communication will probably not be easy for you at this difficult time. You may relate to some members of your health care team better than to others. But do keep in mind that you and your partner are also important members of the team, and your input is valuable. Mutual respect among all members of the team is the key to success. If possible, communicate your needs to your labor nurse and ask her to act as your advocate.

When your labor becomes complex or if your health care team antici-pates problems with your baby, you can expect basic interventions to ensure the best possible outcome. Your health care team is committed to pro-viding you with as satisfying a birth experience as possible. If complications develop, however, your safety and that of your baby become the biggest prior-ity. The goal is to deliver you and your baby in the best possible shape. Following are explanations of some of the equipment that may be used to accomplish that goal.

Intravenous Line

Your physician may limit your intake of food and beverages shortly before you give birth. This is to prevent vomiting and potential aspiration (inhalation of fluid into the lungs) if cesarean birth, and therefore anesthesia, becomes neces-sary. To provide a route for fluids and medications, an intravenous (IV) line will be inserted somewhere on your hand or arm. The IV line may be "capped off" and reconnected to the tubing only when a constant infusion of fluid or medica-

Equipment During Labor

tion is necessary. Having this "cap," called a heparin lock (or heparin well), is less cumbersome than being continuously "hooked up" to IV tubing.

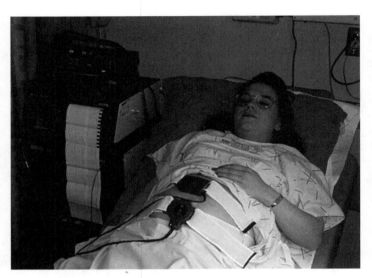

External fetal monitor.

The external fetal monitor uses two belts across the mother's abdomen. One belt holds a tocotransducer that senses the abdominal pressure changes of uterine contractions. The other belt holds an ultrasound transducer that detects fetal heart sounds.

Electronic Fetal Monitoring

Electronic fetal monitoring (EFM) is now standard practice during labor. It is used to track your baby's heart rate and monitor maternal uterine contractions. Your nurse watches for changes in the baby's heart rate to identify a baby who may be having trouble. Electronic fetal monitoring also helps the nurse evaluate the adequacy of uterine contractions and the progress of labor. The nurse uses EFM as one part of the whole clinical picture to assess how well mother and baby are progressing through labor and birth. In cases of preterm labor, basing obstetrical care on interpretation of the preterm infant's fetal heart rate tracing has been shown to significantly improve the baby's outcome.[1]

The fetal heart rate monitor gives a digital readout of the baby's heart rate, and in some systems, a wavelike pattern of the baby's heart rate and your contractions is printed on a strip of graph paper. In state-of-the-art systems, the nurse and physician use a computer or video system to review your data rather than analyzing output on graph paper. The recent advances in computer technology also allow some hospitals to modem your EFM tracing to obstetrical experts in other institutions for consultation.

Two different types of electronic fetal monitoring are available. External fetal monitoring uses two elastic belts fastened around the mother's abdomen. One belt holds an ultrasound transducer (doppler) and detects your baby's heart sounds. The second belt holds a disc called a tocotransducer that senses pressure changes on the abdomen. The tocotransducer records the frequency and duration of uterine contractions, but the actual intensity of the contractions cannot be accurately recorded using external fetal monitoring.[2] Internal fetal monitoring allows precise measurement of the strength of uterine contractions and provides beat-to-beat assessment of your baby's heart rate.[2]

An internal fetal monitor involves two pieces of monitoring equipment. The first piece is the internal scalp electrode that measures your baby's heart rate more accurately than the doppler device used for external monitoring. An internal electrode looks like spiral wire. Your nurse or doctor guides the electrode up through the birth canal and through the cervix (the opening to the uterus) and attaches it to your baby. The tip of the electrode slides just under the surface of the baby's skin nearest to the mother's cervical opening (usually the baby's head or bottom, depending on the baby's position). Care is taken to avoid your baby's face or genitals. Your baby's electrode wire leads back out of the birth canal, attaches to a small plate wrapped around the mother's thigh, and connects to the fetal monitor by a cord.[2] The wire is removed from the baby at birth. The second part of the internal fetal monitoring system is called an internal uterine pressure catheter (IUPC). This pressure-sensing catheter is guided up through the birth canal and through the cervix and is placed inside the uterus. The IUPC accurately records frequency, duration, and strength of the mother's contractions.[2]

In order to use internal monitoring, your membranes must be ruptured (your water must be broken) and your cervix must be dilated enough that the two parts of the monitoring equipment can be placed into the uterus. Internal fetal monitoring is not used as often as external fetal monitoring but is valuable if labor becomes complicated or if your baby's heart rate pattern suggests potential trouble. Internal fetal monitoring is more invasive and carries more risk than external fetal monitoring but is necessary and worthwhile if your physician requires precise information to help ensure a safe labor and birth.[2]

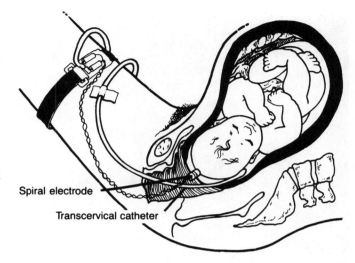

Spiral electrode

Transcervical catheter

Internal fetal monitor.

The internal fetal monitor uses a fetal scalp electrode and an internal pressure catheter. The internal monitor provides more accurate information about your contractions and fetal heart rate than the external fetal monitor. Courtesy of Childbirth Graphics, Waco, Texas.

Oxygen

An unborn baby depends on his mother for oxygen and nutrition. Oxygen supply to the baby decreases during every uterine contraction. A healthy baby tolerates this normal part of labor without problems.[3] The baby may receive an unusually low oxygen supply during contractions, however, if the placenta is not functioning at its best or if a maternal medical condition (such as high blood pressure or heart disease) is present and reduces oxygen circulation in the mother's body.[4] Your baby's oxygen supply may also be insufficient if maternal contractions come too close together or if the baby's umbilical cord becomes temporarily pinched off during contractions.[4] In any of these cases, your doctor or nurse may request that you wear an oxygen mask to help the baby receive extra oxygen during labor.

Labor and Birth Management

Once you are declared "at risk," technology and intervention replace your anticipated birth experience in the homelike atmosphere of your community hospital. The mood is more serious, the medical personnel are more numerous, and your anxiety is understandably high. Most parents feel powerless in this situation. It is true that many factors are no longer within your control. But understanding the reasons behind the decisions medical personnel are making and how those decisions affect you and your baby will help you cope with this adventure.

Negotiating

If you have reached the point in your pregnancy when you have planned your labor and birth experience but then find that you are at risk, you may be able to hold on to parts of your dream. When your physician recommends cesarean birth, for example, ask if you may play the music you planned for labor in the operating room. If you have an internal fetal monitor in place and can no longer walk around the room, ask if you may sit in the rocking chair next to the bed. Having some control over your care may reduce the intensity of your feelings of loss for the "perfect" labor and birth and may help them resolve more quickly.

Vaginal Birth or Cesarean Birth?

The members of the health care team want your birth experience to be meaningful even under difficult circumstances. Their overall goals are to ensure a safe labor and to deliver your baby to the neonatal team in the best possible condition. This can be a special challenge when the forces of labor and birth present potential hazards for you and your baby.

When spontaneous vaginal birth is deemed safe for you and your baby, this is the option of choice. Because it is a "normal" birth experience, some women find a vaginal birth more emotionally satisfying. More important, a vaginal birth eliminates the risks of operative and postoperative complications and shortens your hospital stay and recovery period.[5]

An obstetric condition such as fetal distress, acute maternal bleeding, or serious maternal illness usually makes a cesarean birth the choice for the best possible outcome for you and/or your baby.[6] Remember that your health care professionals have experience and training in this type of medical and nursing care; their clinical judgments are based on careful consideration of the risks and benefits of each birthing method.

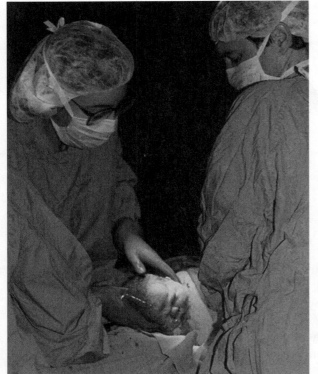

Cesarean birth.

This baby was positioned head down in the uterus. The obstetrician first guides the baby's head through the abdominal incision, then delivers the rest of the baby's body.

The safest method of delivery for a preterm infant who has no problems other than the early delivery is debatable at present.[1,6] Research suggests that there is no benefit to performing a cesarean section just because a baby is preterm. The risk of complications does increase during preterm labor, however.[6] A cesarean birth may be performed for very low birth weight infants demonstrating fetal stress, breech presentation (buttocks or feet first instead of the head), intrauterine growth retardation, when labor fails to progress, or there are maternal conditions such as high blood pressure (hypertension) or serious bleeding.[6]

If you are in preterm labor and are giving birth vaginally, you may discover that labor and birth progress quickly once things begin to happen.[6] Even though a vaginal birth is a natural process, an unusually fast birth (called a precipitous birth) can be frightening. Mothers who birth precipitously often feel out of control and as if they missed the whole thing. Because caregivers and equipment must move quickly, a precipitous birth often feels like an emergency. Your labor nurse, who acts as your advocate and primary information source during labor, will support you through the urgency of the birth. Afterward, ask her to help you review what happened, validate what you remember, and clarify details that are important to you.

Special Interventions during Labor and Birth

Induction of Labor

Under special circumstances, your labor may be induced. This means that uterine contractions are deliberately started with medication before labor begins on its own.[7]

Labor is induced when a specific obstetric or medical problem is present. Labor would not be induced for a woman whose labor should be delayed or who has a high chance for needing cesarean birth (for example, for twins or more babies, because of placental problems, or if the baby is positioned differently than head down). Induction may be indicated for a variety of conditions that complicate a pregnancy—as a response to pregnancy-induced hypertension (explained in Chapter 8), some types of diabetes, or risk of infection because of prematurely ruptured membranes (the "bag of waters" has broken prior to onset of labor). Labor may also be induced for an "overdue" baby or for a sick or compromised fetus whose chances of a healthy outcome are improved with immediate neonatal intensive care.[7]

For labor induction, a drug called oxytocin is given through an IV line to stimulate uterine contractions. Sometimes a vaginal prostaglandin gel is used before oxytocin to soften, or "ripen," the cervix.[8]

Your nurse closely monitors your condition during labor induction. Your vital signs (temperature, pulse, respirations, and blood pressure) are checked frequently. Electronic fetal monitoring is used to assess your baby's well-being and your contraction pattern. Your nurse will provide encouragement and keep you informed of your progress.

Labor Augmentation

Augmentation is used when labor has already begun but is not progressing satisfactorily or has stopped altogether.[7] Labor augmentation refers to methods used to promote more effective uterine contractions. Successful labor augmentation reduces the incidence of cesarean birth and also reduces the risk of infection sometimes seen with prolonged labor.[7]

As in labor induction, oxytocin can be used to augment labor.[7] Expert and supportive nursing care can be expected during labor augmentation. Your nurse will take your vital signs frequently and use electronic fetal monitoring to assess fetal well-being and your contraction pattern.

Another method of augmentation uses a procedure called artifical rupture of the fetal membranes (AROM), or amniotomy.[7] This means that your doctor or midwife "breaks" your bag of waters to stimulate contractions. Often, AROM brings the baby's head down onto the cervix. A combination of effective uterine contractions and pressure on the cervix helps to dilate the cervix and allows the baby to be born.[7]

"I didn't really think I was in labor. Then, suddenly, I could feel the baby coming, and my husband yelled for the nurses. I had to be moved out of my room, and the bed got wedged in the doorway. The nurses were frantic, and one yelled 'Push!' I thought she was talking to me, and I was happy to oblige. My beautiful 3-pound baby boy came out like a bullet, right there in the doorway. And that's what they called him in the NICU— 'Bullet' Bradley Anderson."

Episiotomy

You may wonder if your vaginal birth will include an episiotomy (a surgical incision to enlarge your vaginal opening). The purpose of an episiotomy is to allow easy passage of your baby's head in the final moments of birth. Although an episiotomy used to be a common procedure, it is less so now.

For the birth of a preterm baby, some perinatal experts recommend a generous episiotomy to lessen the forces on the baby's small, soft head; shorten the time to push; and allow slow, controlled delivery of the baby's head.[1,9] Other experts believe that by the time the baby's head reaches the vaginal opening, it has already endured similar or even stronger pressures as it passed through the muscular birth canal.[1] No hard-and-fast rule exists regarding the need for an episiotomy in a preterm birth. Every birth is unique, and your physician will make a decision about an episiotomy based on your individual circumstances.

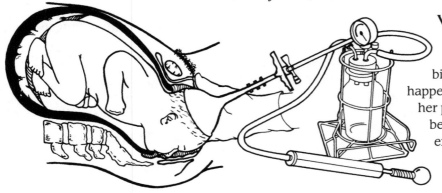
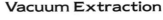

Vacuum Extraction

Sometimes a laboring woman is unable to push her baby out of the birth canal without assistance. If this happens because anesthesia has reduced her pushing power or urge to push or because of maternal exhaustion, vacuum extraction may be used to shorten the period of time the woman must push before the baby is born.[7]

In this method, a soft suction cup is applied to the top of the baby's head, and firm suction is applied. Working with the mother's contractions, the physician gently applies traction and delivers the baby's head. The vacuum extractor usually leaves a soft, temporary swelling on the baby's head, which resolves in a day or two.[7]

Vacuum extractor.

The suction cup of the vacuum extractor is applied to the top of the baby's head. Working with the mother's contractions, the physician uses traction to deliver the baby's head. Courtesy of Childbirth Graphics, Waco, Texas.

Forceps

Forceps are curved metal tongs used to shorten the pushing stage of labor and to deliver the baby's head. Forceps delivery is considered when the baby fits "tightly" in the birth canal, when the mother's power or urge to push has decreased as a result of anesthesia or exhaustion, or when a maternal medical condition (such as cardiac or circulatory disease) requires that the mother receive assistance in this pushing stage.[7] Unlike vacuum extraction, forceps can be used to accomplish a fast vaginal birth if the mother or baby develops complications late in this stage of labor. Forceps delivery is sometimes used to protect the preterm infant's fragile head from the pressures of a long stage of pushing during childbirth.[7]

Pain Management during Labor and Birth

Medications and anesthesia affect not only the mother, but the unborn baby as well. Your physician, labor nurse, and anesthesiologist or nurse anesthetist will work with you and assess your needs while bearing in mind the goal of delivering your baby in good condition.

Every labor situation is different, and no one method of pain relief is superior under all conditions.[1] Pain medication and anesthesia will depend on the many factors that contribute to the complexity of your labor and birth. Ask your physician or labor nurse what aspects of your health may influence decisions regarding pain medication and anesthesia.

If you have the opportunity, tell your labor nurse your plans for pain management. If you plan to have an unmedicated birth, she will work with you to accomplish this goal. If you change your mind and decide to use pain medication, you should feel equally supported in this decision. If your labor or birth becomes complicated and medical intervention makes medication or anesthesia necessary, your nurse will explain why and what you should expect next. When you work as a team, you can maintain a sense of control and trust your nurse's assessment of your needs.

Labor Management without Medication

Walking, if permitted, usually helps a woman cope with the early stages of labor. Sitting in a rocking chair, changing positions in bed, and using massage, visual imagery, or breathing techniques help many women cope as labor intensifies. Your labor nurse or midwife may offer more suggestions for managing discomfort.

Fear can intensify pain. For this reason, it is important to ask about anything that worries you. Education about the labor process and what to expect during labor and birth can help allay many fears and the accompanying discomfort.

A supportive partner is so important during childbirth. This person may not only respond to your requests for physical comfort through touching or providing a cool washcloth, but also provide security just by being there and sharing this experience with you. Keep communication open, and tell your partner what you expect of him or her during labor and birth. A plan may make things easier if your situation becomes complicated.

Analgesia

Pain medication that relieves pain or decreases awareness of pain is called analgesia. Medications such as meperidine hydrochloride (Demerol), butorphanol tartrate (Stadol), and nalbuphine hydrochloride (Nubain) provide good pain relief during labor. Their use during labor may be limited, however, because of the unpredictable speed of the labor and the inability of the sick or preterm baby to handle the medication.[1] Because these drugs cross the placenta and are metabolized more slowly by the fetus than by the mother, they

Forceps delivery.

Forceps are used to shorten the pushing stage of labor. Unlike the vacuum extractor, forceps can be used to accomplish a fast birth if the mother or baby experiences distress late in this stage of labor. Courtesy of Childbirth Graphics, Waco, Texas.

are rarely given if delivery is expected within three hours. Babies born with maternal pain-relief narcotics in their system may experience respiratory depression (decreased breathing effort). This further challenges the uncertain ability of immature or sick babies to breathe on their own.[1]

Anesthesia

Anesthesia refers to a method of pain control that involves partial or total loss of sensation in the affected area.[10] Anesthesia may or may not include loss of consciousness. The two major types of anesthesia are regional (including epidural and spinal) and general.

Regional anesthesia is used for moderate to severe pain or when cesarean birth is a possibility.[10] During labor, your anesthesiologist or nurse anesthetist may administer an epidural or spinal block, types of regional anesthesia that block pain sensation from the navel to the midthigh.[10] An epidural block is used for labor pain and can also be used for cesarean birth. The medication is injected through a catheter into the space outside the covering of the spinal cord. Unlike an epidural block, a spinal block is injected with a needle through the covering of the spinal cord. A spinal block can be administered more quickly than an epidural block and is also used for cesarean birth.

Epidural and spinal anesthesias do not cause drowsiness or loss of consciousness in the mother and do allow her to be awake during vaginal or cesarean birth. Regional anesthesia carries fewer risks to mother and baby than general anesthesia and does not cause respiratory depression of the baby at birth.[10]

Emergency cesarean birth may require the use of general anesthesia. This type of anesthesia is administered to the patient in the operating room through inhaled medication and/or IV medication.[10] General anesthesia produces unconsciousness. Although this type of anesthesia can be an important lifesaving tool, it carries risks for the mother and her fetus and prevents the mother from seeing her newborn in the first moments of life. It is not often used for childbirth.

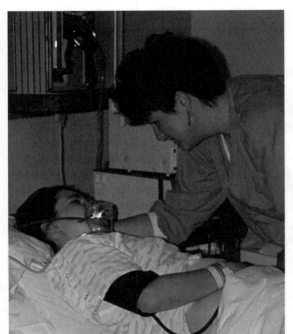

Labor and delivery expert.

Your labor nurse provides expertise and support during this very important event in your life.

Remembering What's Important

As a pregnancy progresses, the parents-to-be usually focus most of their energy and attention on labor and birth, because giving birth is the biggest and most immediate challenge. Much of your prenatal education may have focused on "planning" the birth and even on such topics as how to avoid cesarean delivery. Especially for first-time parents, imagining actually caring for the infant can be more difficult than thinking about the very real task of giving birth.

When you face a complicated labor and birth, you lose some control over the decision-making process, and when all is over, you may feel that you "didn't do it right." Most health care professionals will try to involve you in decisions when appropriate—to help you experience a satisfying and successful labor and birth. Even so, feelings of disappointment often take time to resolve. In the meantime, remember that the health care professionals involved in your care have made their best possible decisions based on what they felt was in your best interests and in the best interests of your baby.

Keep in mind that the most important part of parenting is not vaginal versus cesarean birth or pain medication versus pioneer heroism. Much more important is the quality of parenting you bring to your baby after birth and the values you teach that will influence his entire life.

Chapter 2

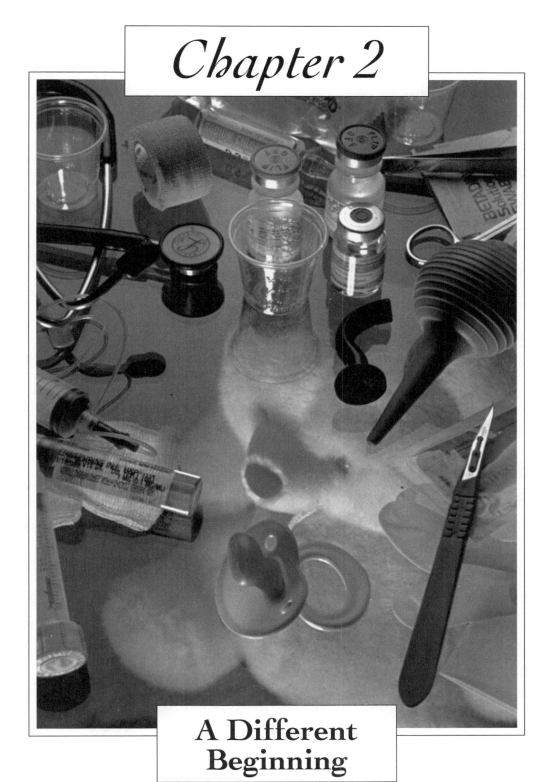

A Different Beginning

Jeanette Zaichkin, RNC, MN

"But the more
Tigger put his nose into this
and his paw into that, the more
things he found which Tiggers didn't
like. And when he had found
everything in the cupboard, and
couldn't eat any of it, he said to
Kanga, "What happens now?""

The moment of birth is usually a triumphant celebration. Not only have you made it through labor and birth, but you have produced a new little person who is very much a part of you and carries your dreams for the future.

When things don't go as expected, you face a more stressful beginning than most parents. You need to deal with the feelings of loss that accompany the birth of a sick or premature baby. You also enter a new world of medical vocabulary and technology that may, at first, seem foreign, cold, and hostile.

If you know in advance that your baby's birth may be difficult or that your newborn may need the special care of an NICU, this chapter will help you prepare. It explains what you can expect and should ease your anxiety about the sights and sounds surrounding the birth and your baby's NICU admission. If your baby has already been admitted to the NICU, this chapter will explain what you may have seen or heard in the delivery room and will acquaint you with the NICU environment.

What Can Happen at Birth

Infrequently, a baby is born sick without prior warning. Most of the time, though, the neonatal team of doctors, nurses, and other trained personnel anticipates problems and is prepared to deal with them. At every birth, members of this team work together to assess the baby's condition. Caregivers are ready to help the newborn breathe and achieve or maintain the pulse and blood pressure necessary for life.

Every birthing area is equipped to resuscitate (revive) a sick baby. Resuscitation may take place in the delivery room or in a room near the birthing area. In any case, the birth of a sick newborn brings inevitable tension into the birthing area. Equipment is checked and checked again. A physician or a nurse practitioner usually leads the neonatal resuscitation team. You may hear the team leader assigning duties and checking your baby's condition with your health care provider.

Resuscitation Equipment

Every delivery room contains equipment that the neonatal team may use to resuscitate your baby if necessary. Following are descriptions of the items found in most birthing areas.[1]

Radiant Warmer

A radiant warmer is a type of bed that consists of a mattress, usually on a mobile cart, with a heat source overhead. The mattress area is used for resuscitation and for immediate stabilization of the baby after birth, and the overhead heater helps to keep the baby warm. If your baby is placed on a radiant warmer, the staff will tell you that your newborn is "on a warmer."

Suction

Babies are often born with mucus and fluid in the mouth, nose, and throat. Suction may be needed to clear those areas and to prevent choking.

The most basic suction tool is called a bulb syringe. The caregiver first squeezes all the air out of the bulb, then gently places the pointed end in the baby's nose or mouth. When the caregiver releases her grip on the bulb, mucus and fluid are drawn into the bulb syringe, clearing the baby's breathing passages, or airway.

Wall suction is another method for clearing a baby's airway. A mechanical suction apparatus is built into the wall or radiant warmer, and a suction setup hangs on it. A thin tube (called a suction catheter) is passed into the baby's nose, mouth, throat, and perhaps, stomach. Then the fluid is "vacuumed" out at a preset, safe, suction pressure.

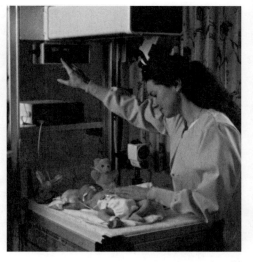

Radiant warmer.

The radiant warmer provides a mattress for the baby to lie on and overhead heat for warmth.
Courtesy of Ohmeda, Columbia, Maryland.

Oxygen

The room air we breathe contains about 21 percent oxygen. In the delivery room, nearly 100 percent oxygen is used to help a baby breathe. If your baby requires extra oxygen at birth, you may hear the NICU team say, "The baby needs some Os" (pronounced "ohs") or "The baby needs O_2" (the molecular term, pronounced oh-two). This high concentration of oxygen comes either from a portable tank on or near the radiant warmer or directly from pipes built into the wall. When the oxygen valve is open, oxygen flows through a length of flexible green tubing to your baby's location on the radiant warmer.

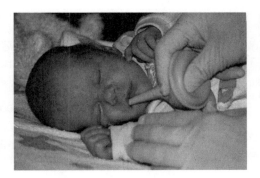

Bulb syringe.

The bulb syringe uses gentle suction to remove fluid from the baby's nose or mouth.

If your baby is breathing but does not turn pink, the stream of oxygen from the flexible green tubing will be aimed toward her nose and mouth. This is called blow-by oxygen and provides oxygen-enriched air for your baby to breathe.

Blow-by oxygen can be given instead through an oxygen bag, also called a bag and mask. An oxygen bag connects to the green

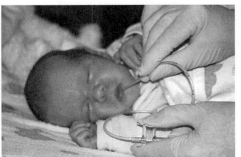

Suction catheter.

The suction catheter is attached to a wall or portable unit that uses a vacuum system to generate a preset amount of suction to clear secretions from the baby's nose, mouth, throat, or stomach.

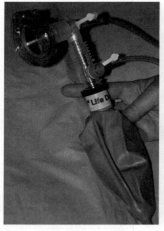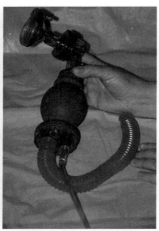

Oxygen bags.

Both types of oxygen bags pictured here are used to "bag the baby" (deliver breaths) or to give blow-by oxygen (a steady stream of oxygen held near the baby's nose and mouth). Both types have a face mask and an oxygen reservoir. The bag on the left delivers blow-by oxygen through the mask. The bag on the right delivers blow-by oxygen from the "tail" of the bag.

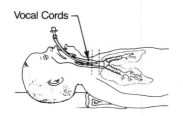

Endotracheal tube.

The endotracheal tube is positioned in the baby's trachea (windpipe) between the vocal cords. A baby with an endotracheal tube is intubated *and requires mechanical assistance to breathe. When the endotracheal tube is removed, the baby is* extubated.

Adapted from: Bloom RS, and Cropley C. 1995. *Textbook of Neonatal Resuscitation.* American Heart Association. Dallas, Texas, 5–26. Reprinted by permission.

tubing and consists of a small pouch that fills with oxygen and a soft mask that fits over the baby's nose and mouth. When oxygen flows through the bag, blow-by oxygen can be given by holding the face mask very close to the baby's mouth and nose. Some types of oxygen bags have a "tail" of flexible corrugated tubing. Oxygen also flows through this tail and out the bottom of the bag. The tail of the bag can be held near the baby's mouth and nose and provides a good source of blow-by oxygen.

An oxygen bag is primarily used to "breathe" for a baby who does not breathe without help. A member of the resuscitation team places the face mask firmly over the baby's nose and mouth and hand pumps oxygen through the bag into the baby's lungs. This is called bag-mask ventilation, or "bagging the baby."

Endotracheal Tube

An endotracheal (ET) tube is a thin plastic tube that can be placed directly into your baby's trachea (windpipe). It is then connected either to the oxygen bag or to a ventilator (also called a respirator). Placement of an endotracheal tube is called intubation. Because the ET tube is positioned between your baby's vocal cords, your baby will not be able to make crying noises while the tube is in place.

An ET tube provides a direct route to your baby's lungs and is the most effective means for delivering oxygen and the pressure necessary to help your baby breathe. When an oxygen bag is attached to the ET tube and the care-giver squeezes oxygen from the bag into your baby's lungs, the baby is being "hand-bagged." When a respirator is connected to the ET tube, the baby is being "mechanically ventilated."

Emergency Medications

In rare cases, a baby is born so seriously ill that medications must be administered to save her life. Various medications are available to stimulate the heart, increase blood pressure, and correct chemical imbalances in the baby's blood. Some medications can be administered through the ET tube, but most must be injected directly into the baby's bloodstream through a blood vessel.

Resuscitation Activities

The steps taken to resuscitate a newborn depend on the infant's condition at birth and on the baby's special needs. A full-term baby who is pink and crying but has internal organs exposed on her abdomen, for example, will require interventions different from those needed by a preterm infant who has difficulty taking that first breath. Although babies require resuscitation because of various problems, the following concerns are typical in most infant resuscitations.[1]

Warmth

When your baby is born, the delivering physician will suction her mouth and nose and cut the umbilical cord. The physician may take your baby to the radiant warmer or may hand the baby to a member of the neonatal resuscitation team. When your baby is placed under the warmer, she is immediately wiped dry to prevent chilling.

Breathing

Breathing supplies oxygen and maintains the heart rate. An eternity may seem to pass before you hear your baby's first cry, but most babies make some crying efforts in the first minute after birth. The neonatal team may provide tactile stimulation (gentle rubbing of the baby's back and flicking of the feet) to encourage breathing. If your baby does not breathe in a few moments, is too weak to breathe regularly, or has a heart rate (pulse) of less than 100 beats per minute, an oxygen bag will be used to bag her.

When a baby is bagged, some of the oxygen also goes down the baby's esophagus (food pipe) and collects in the stomach. If the baby's stomach is allowed to fill with air, it will push up on the diaphragm, leaving less room for the baby's lungs to inflate. Just as you have trouble taking a deep breath after eating a big meal, air in your baby's stomach will keep her from breathing effectively. Therefore, if your baby needs more than a minute or two of bagging or if her stomach looks bloated, her stomach will be suctioned. This not only removes the air but also cleans out any fluid that the baby could vomit and aspirate (breathe into the lungs). Then, with a suction tube functioning as an air vent, bagging can continue.

After a few breaths from the bag, most babies perk up and begin to breathe on their own. Your baby may need blow-by oxygen to keep her pink while she gets used to breathing on her own.

Heart Rate

The next priority is your baby's heart rate. If the rate is less than 100 beats per minute, bagging will continue. If your baby's heart rate is dangerously low (less than 60 beats per minute), a member of the neonatal team will begin chest compressions (pushing on your baby's chest to artificially pump your baby's heart). At this point, the situation is considered very serious, and a member of the neonatal team will prepare to intubate your baby.

Endotracheal Intubation

If the baby does not begin to breathe well on her own after a minute or two of bagging or if her heart rate is low, she will probably be intubated. Intubation is sometimes performed even before a baby is bagged. Babies at risk for meconium aspiration (explained in Chapter 10) are usually intubated and suctioned immediately. Extremely premature babies and babies who are expected to be in very serious condition at birth may be intubated as soon as possible, because this is the most effective method of ventilation. The ET tube

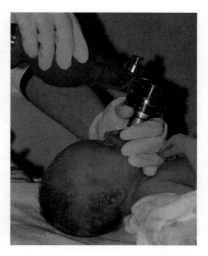

Bag-mask ventilation.

The caregiver places the oxygen bag firmly over the baby's nose and mouth and pumps oxygen into his lungs. Bagging the baby is necessary when the baby is not breathing on his own or when his heart rate is less than 100 beats per minute.

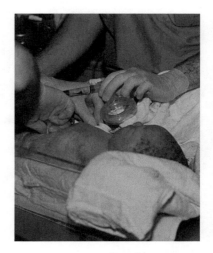

Blow-by oxygen.

A baby who is breathing but is not pink receives a steady stream of oxygen-rich air from an oxygen bag. This newly delivered infant receives blow-by oxygen from one caregiver while another caregiver monitors the baby's pulse through the umbilical cord.

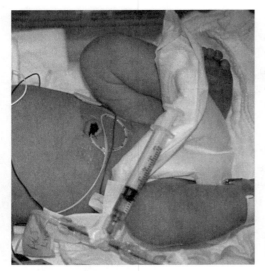

Umbilical catheter.

An umbilical catheter may be placed in one or more of the large blood vessels where the umbilical cord was connected to the placenta. When the umbilical catheter is placed in an artery, it is called an umbilical arterial catheter. When it is placed in the vein, it is called an umbilical venous catheter.

also gives the neonatal team immediate access for administration of surfactant (see Chapter 12) or emergency medications during resuscitation.

Umbilical Catheter Placement

When a baby's umbilical cord is cut, a portion of the white, jelly-like cord remains attached to the baby's abdomen. The cord contains three important blood vessels: two arteries and one large vein that provided the blood flow to and from the placenta before birth. For a while after delivery, it is possible to thread a thin tube (called a catheter) into these vessels and directly into the baby's bloodstream.

If intubation and chest compressions are in progress and the neonatal team determines that your baby needs emergency medications or fluids, an emergency umbilical venous catheter may be placed. This venous catheter is generally used only temporarily to allow medications and/or fluids to be "pushed" (given quickly and directly) into the baby's bloodstream. It is usually removed before your baby is transferred to the nursery.

Apgar Scores

At one minute of age and again at five minutes, your baby is assessed and given a number score to reflect her general condition. Apgar scores do not indicate what needs to be done during resuscitation; instead, they give the neonatal team an indication of how your baby is responding to resuscitative efforts.

To determine your baby's Apgar score, her health care team assesses five categories: heart rate, breathing, color, tone, and reflexes. Babies are assigned a score of 0, 1, or 2 in each category, with 0 indicating very depressed responses and 2 indicating very active responses. The final Apgar score is the total of the five numbers.

Few babies receive a perfect score of 10, because a baby's hands and feet usually remain blue for a while. A baby with a score of 7 to 10 is considered a "normal" newborn. An Apgar score of 4 to 6 indicates a moderately depressed newborn requiring some assistance, and an Apgar score of 0 to 3 reflects a severely depressed newborn requiring full resuscitation.[2] Keep in mind, however, that very premature babies receive lower Apgar scores than full-term infants simply because they are immature and unable to respond with loud crying and because they do not have strong muscle tone.

Apgar Scoring			
	0	**1**	**2**
Heart Rate	Absent	<100	>100
Breathing	Absent	Weak	Strong cry
Color	Blue	Body pink; arms and legs blue	Pink
Tone	Limp	Some flexion	Well flexed
Reflexes	None	Grimace	Cough or sneeze

From: Apgar V. 1953. A proposal for a new method of evaluation of the newborn infant. *Anesthesia and Analgesia* 32: 260. Reprinted by permission.

Transfer to the Nursery

Babies are usually transported to the nursery when they are breathing (either on their own or through an endotracheal tube), their heart rate is acceptable, and special problems have been stabilized. Depending on your baby's condition and on established hospital procedures, she may be carried, moved on a radiant warmer, or transferred in an incubator.

Each neonatal intensive care nursery has its own routines, but most share certain common priorities during infant stabilization. Following are explanations of the equipment found in most NICUs and of the basic procedures followed there. Chapters 10 and 12 cover serious medical problems and the equipment used in treating them.

The Admission Process

Once your baby enters the NICU, many things seem to happen at once. You probably will not be allowed into the NICU during this busy time. This is not to exclude you or to keep information from you, but rather to give the nurses and physicians time and space to stabilize your baby and to plan her care. The admission process will be more difficult and will take longer if the NICU staff must work around anxious parents and try to answer questions before anyone really knows the answers.

Priorities in the first hour include making sure your baby is warm, pink, breathing well on her own or with assistance, and maintaining an adequate blood-sugar level. Soon after birth, routine admission procedures are completed. A hospital identification bracelet is placed on your baby. At some point during admission, your baby receives an injection of vitamin K to prevent potential bleeding difficulties, and an antibiotic ointment is placed in her eyes to prevent possible infection.[3] Additional routine procedures, such as measuring and footprinting, are delayed until life-threatening conditions have been stabilized.

Staying Informed

The NICU team is very busy during your baby's first hours in the nursery. On the other hand, you are waiting and worrying, and that makes minutes seem like hours. Tell the NICU secretary where you will be, and ask to be called at the first break in the action. Check back with the NICU at least every 30 minutes. You should expect some kind of update in the first 90 minutes.

Most NICU nurses and physicians are good at keeping you informed. They will probably tell you more than you can understand at first, so don't worry if things seem unclear. Once you see your baby, you will begin to understand her problems and to learn what the staff is doing to help.

Basic NICU Tests

The most basic NICU care involves expert interpretation of x-rays and of blood and urine tests. At the same time the nurse is making sure your baby is warm and well oxygenated, other members of the neonatal team are preparing to process x-rays, blood, and urine to monitor your baby's progress.

NICU Sights and Sounds

"The nurse asked if I had any questions. I looked at all those plugs and cords and the only question I could think of was, 'What happens if the power goes out?'"

X-Rays

X-rays are an important diagnostic tool in the NICU. Although your baby is exposed to a certain amount of radiation with every x-ray, the amount is carefully controlled in relation to your baby's size and weight. Unnecessary x-rays are avoided. If the baby's genital area is in the primary x-ray beam, it is shielded with a lead cover.[4]

Blood Gases

A small amount of your baby's blood is taken for a blood gas to analyze the levels of oxygen, carbon dioxide, and other chemical components that help the practitioner assess breathing status. Results are used to determine how much or what kind of breathing assistance your baby needs. At first, as your baby's condition changes moment to moment, frequent blood gases may be necessary so that adjustments can be made in the help provided to your baby in the form of extra oxygen or mechanical ventilation. If you are interested, ask the nurse to explain the acceptable range for your baby's blood gases.

Blood for a blood gas can be taken from your baby's artery (in which case it is called an arterial blood gas, or ABG), from your baby's vein (a venous blood gas), or by pricking your baby's heel (a capillary blood gas, or CBG). Obtaining an ABG requires arterial blood, which is obtained by inserting a needle into one of the baby's arteries (usually in the wrist or ankle) or by simply withdrawing blood through the umbilical arterial catheter (this does not involve a needle stick because the catheter is already positioned in a major artery).

Arterial blood best indicates the oxygen available to the tissues; whereas capillary and venous blood have already been "used" by the body and are on the way back to the heart and lungs for a fresh oxygen supply. Therefore, an arterial blood gas provides the most precise measurement of oxygen in the blood and would be the first choice for the most accurate assessment of the baby's oxygen status.

When a baby needs a blood gas but does not have an umbilical arterial catheter, the baby's caregiver will sometimes choose to do a CBG or a venous blood gas instead of obtaining an arterial blood gas. Often, this is because obtaining a CBG or venous blood gas is easier than piercing the baby's artery, which requires special training and considerable skill. While capillary and venous blood gases are not as precise as arterial blood gases, they are still an acceptable method for assessing a baby's respiratory status. Oxygen analysis is just one component of the blood gas. With the exception of the oxygen value, all three blood gas techniques accurately measure the components needed for blood gas analysis.[5]

Many other blood tests (also called lab work or blood work) can be done, depending on the information desired. Blood may be collected to detect infection (complete blood count, or CBC, and blood culture), to assess your baby's ability to supply oxygen to her body tissues (hematocrit and hemoglobin), to determine blood sugar level (blood glucose), and to determine the balance of basic body chemicals (electrolytes, or "lytes").

A common blood test that screens your baby's blood sugar (glucose) is done right at the baby's bedside. A tiny drop of blood is placed on a chemically treated test stick. An approximation of the baby's blood glucose is displayed by a number value on a glucose meter, or a nurse visually interprets a color value. The result on the glucose test strip (for example, a Chemstrip or Dextrostix) gives the nurse a close estimation of your baby's actual blood glucose. If the test strip indicates a blood sugar outside the normal range, the nurse will draw blood for a laboratory test so she will have a precise measurement of your baby's blood sugar.[6]

Urine Tests

Kidneys are very sensitive to changes in the body. The amount of your baby's urine and what is in it can tell the NICU team much about your baby's general condition and progress after birth. Hospital laboratory technicians or an NICU nurse can do simple urine screening by placing a few drops of urine on a chemically treated "dipstick." The urine dipstick reveals color values for things such as acidity, sugar, protein, and blood.

If more than a few drops of urine are needed for laboratory testing, a specially designed plastic bag may be taped over your baby's vaginal area or penis. When the baby urinates, the urine collects in the bag. This type of urine collection is called a "clean catch."

If infection is a concern, urine may be sent to the laboratory for a "culture and sensitivity" test. This means the urine is tested for bacteria. If any are found, medical personnel determine the best antibiotic to use against the bacteria. This urine can be obtained from a clean catch, through a catheter, or the physician or NNP can perform a suprapubic tap (bladder tap). A catheterized urine sample is obtained by inserting a small sterile tube into the baby's bladder and withdrawing the urine. This type of urine collection is called a "straight cath" or an "in-and-out cath" because the catheter is removed after the urine is obtained.

A suprapubic tap (bladder tap) is performed by inserting a needle through the baby's lower abdomen and piercing the baby's bladder. The urine is then drawn up into a syringe and sent to the laboratory for analysis.

If your baby is very sick, the nurse may insert a urinary catheter into your baby's bladder and leave it in place. This is called an indwelling catheter. The catheter drains the baby's urine into a bag or syringe, where it is accurately measured or collected for testing.

Many babies in the NICU are said to be on "strict intake and output," more commonly called "strict I & O." An accurate record is kept of all fluids that go into the baby (such as IV fluids, blood products, oral fluids, and so on) and all fluids that come out (such as urine, stool, blood, and so on). The baby's fluid intake is carefully calculated and administered, usually over a 24-hour period. The baby's output is measured by weighing each diaper before and after the baby has wet or soiled it. The difference between the before and after weight of the diaper is calculated and measured as fluid output. Chapter 9 gives more information about your baby's kidneys.

"We told the family we were pregnant on Sunday. I wore my first maternity outfit on Tuesday. On Thursday, I had a crash C-section, and my daughter weighs 675 grams. We missed the entire pregnancy."

Typical NICU Equipment

Just as the delivery area is set up with basic equipment for birth, the NICU is equipped with machinery to stabilize a sick baby. Each baby's condition determines the types of technologic support she receives, but the following equipment is used in many NICU admissions.

Radiant Warmer/Incubator

In the NICU, your baby will be placed on a radiant warmer or in an incubator to stabilize her temperature. Some incubators are designed with round portholes through which you and the NICU team can touch the baby. Others are opened by pushing up the entire front covering. Even though the models differ, the priority of every radiant warmer and incubator is warmth; a baby can lose body heat quickly, and many body processes depend on maintenance of a normal temperature.[7]

Every radiant warmer and incubator is equipped with a thermostat apparatus.[7] A temperature probe is taped to your baby's body, and the preset thermostat on the heater mechanism controls heat output based on your baby's skin temperature. When your baby's skin has warmed to the preset high temperature, the heat turns down; when the infant's skin temperature cools, the heat turns back up. An incubator can use this mechanism or may maintain a constant preset temperature.

Cardiorespiratory Monitor

Most NICU babies are placed on a cardiorespiratory monitor, a device that tracks the heart rate and the rate of breathing. Three adhesive patches (leads) are placed on the baby's chest and attached by cable to the monitor. The monitor picks up the electrical activity of your baby's heart, transmits the information onto a screen, and digitally displays it as a number. The monitor also detects your baby's chest movement and displays it as respirations (breaths) per minute. The cardiorespiratory monitor is used to detect a heart rate or a respiratory rate that becomes too fast or too slow.[8]

Blood Pressure Monitor

Your baby's blood pressure may be taken in much the same way as your own. A small, plastic blood pressure cuff is wrapped around your baby's arm or leg and automatically inflates at preset time intervals to display the blood pressure reading. Your baby's blood pressure may also be continuously measured through an umbilical arterial line (discussed later in this chapter).[9]

Intravenous Line

Few babies are allowed to eat during their first hours in the NICU, and very sick or preterm babies may not take food by mouth for many days. An IV line may be placed to provide your baby with fluids, glucose, necessary body chemicals (such as sodium and potassium), and medications. Your baby's IV may be placed in her hand or lower arm, foot or lower leg, or scalp.[10]

Basic NICU equipment for initial stabilization.

This intravenous (IV) line is placed in the baby's hand. The nurse may also place the IV line in the baby's scalp or foot. The round, adhesive patches on the baby's chest are called monitor leads, or electrodes, and attach to the cardiorespiratory monitor. The shiny adhesive heart secures the thermostat probe against the baby's skin. The thermostat probe controls the heat output from the incubator or radiant warmer.

An IV line (also called a peripheral line) is positioned in a tiny vein very near the surface of the skin. It can easily be bumped out of place, allowing the IV fluid to leak out of the vein and into the surrounding tissue. This is called an infiltrated IV line. If an IV line becomes infiltrated, it must be discontinued (taken out) and restarted (placed again) at another site. Because IV placement can be stressful for your baby, your baby's nurse wants the IV line to remain at one site as long as possible. Even under the best circumstances, a peripheral IV line may last less than a day or two.

Pulse oximeter.
The pulse oximeter sensor is positioned around the baby's foot or hand...
and then secured with a type of wrapping, such as this stretchy bandage.

Umbilical Lines

Remember the two arteries and the vein in your baby's umbilical cord? An umbilical arterial catheter (UAC) may be threaded deep into a major blood vessel (the aorta) through one of the two arteries. A UAC is necessary if your baby has significant breathing problems that require frequent blood testing. Because the UAC feeds into a major blood vessel, the baby can receive fluids and medications through it, and most blood for laboratory testing can be drawn from it.[8] A UAC is pictured on page 20.

If your baby has an umbilical arterial line, the line will be connected to a transducer so that your baby's blood pressure can be displayed on the cardiac monitor. The normal range for a baby's blood pressure depends on gestational age, size, activity level, and condition.[9] If you are concerned, ask your baby's nurse what range would be considered appropriate for your baby.

Pulse Oximeter

A pulse oximeter is often used to immediately assess how well a baby is using the oxygen available to her. Although a pulse oximeter does not indicate the exact amount of oxygen in the blood, a reading above or below the accepted range alerts the nurse that the baby's oxygen level may not be acceptable. The baby's caregiver may intervene by increasing or decreasing the amount of supplemental oxygen (discussed in the next section) and/or by ordering a blood gas to determine the baby's exact respiratory status.

A pulse oximeter sensor is attached to your baby's hand or foot. It uses a light sensor to read the amount of oxygen attached to the hemoglobin molecules in the blood. For newborns, the oxygen saturation level is usually kept in a range of about 90 to 95 percent.[11]

Transcutaneous Monitor

A transcutaneous monitor (TCM) is a noninvasive system for monitoring oxygen and carbon dioxide levels in the bloodstream.[11] The TCM rests on your baby's skin and warms the area under the probe. Oxygen diffuses from the skin capillaries to the probe and a numerical value for the amount of oxygen in the blood is electronically calculated. To interpret the number, a health care provider must draw a blood sample to be analyzed for blood gases to "calibrate" the numerical reading. Respirator settings and oxygen levels can then be changed without frequent blood gases being drawn. Because of the warmth of the probe, the TCM will leave a temporary red mark on your baby's skin.

Basic Information about Oxygen

Because of prematurity or illness, your newborn may need to breathe air with a higher concentration of oxygen than is available in room air. This extra oxygen is called supplemental oxygen. The amount of oxygen delivered to your baby is expressed as a percentage. The air we breathe every day contains about 21 percent oxygen; supplemental oxygen is any amount exceeding 21 percent. All supplemental oxygen is warmed and humidified. It can be delivered in several different ways.

Oxygen in a Hood or Tent

For babies breathing independently and efficiently, supplemental oxygen can be supplied inside an oxyhood (a plastic box or hood placed over the baby's head) or, for larger infants, inside an oxygen tent (a plastic apparatus placed around the baby's upper body). If the baby is temporarily removed from the oxyhood or oxygen tent (for example, to be weighed or held for a short time), the tubing delivering the oxygen can be disconnected from the hood or tent and held in front of the baby's face.

Oxygen in an Incubator

For babies requiring low levels of supplemental oxygen (usually less than about 25 percent), some nurseries pipe the prescribed amount directly into the incubator. This method lets parents and caregivers see and care for the baby without interference from an oxyhood. Opening the incubator to care for the baby can allow the supplemental oxygen to escape and can dilute the oxygen level in the incubator with room air, but most babies receiving such low levels of supplemental oxygen are not affected by these temporary fluctuations.

Oxygen Cannula

An oxygen cannula is used to deliver supplemental oxygen to babies who require extra oxygen but are breathing well on their own. A cannula is a soft plastic tube that is placed under the baby's nose and encircles the baby's head; warm, humidified oxygen is delivered through openings in the tubing, or "prongs," under the baby's nose. Your baby may sleep with the oxygen cannula in place or in an oxygen tent placed inside the crib. An oxygen cannula is convenient for feeding, physical therapy, bathing, and other activities that are difficult to accomplish when the baby is inside a tent.

Transcutaneous monitor.

The round probe of the transcutaneous monitor sits on top of the baby's skin and monitors the oxygen and carbon dioxide levels in her blood. The warmth of this probe leaves a temporary red spot on the baby's skin. A shiny heart secures the thermostat of the radiant warmer to the baby's skin.

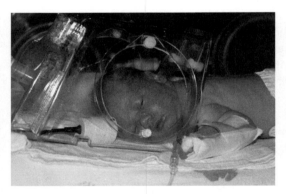

Oxygen hood.

This plastic box fits over the baby's head and encloses warm, humidified, oxygen-enriched air for the baby to breathe. An oxygen hood is also called a head box *or an* oxyhood.

Continuous Positive Airway Pressure

Continuous positive airway pressure—abbreviated CPAP and pronounced SEE-pap—is a method of assisted ventilation. With CPAP, your baby breathes on her own, but a machine keeps a steady supply of air/oxygen under pressure pushing into her lungs.[12] This helps keep the tiny air sacs in the lungs from collapsing after each breath, reducing the effort the baby must use to breathe. Continuous positive airway pressure can be delivered through your baby's nose (in which case some of the pressurized air can escape through your baby's mouth and/or down into her stomach), or your baby may be intubated so that the pressurized air is delivered directly into her lungs. (Chapters 9 and 10 provide more information about CPAP.)

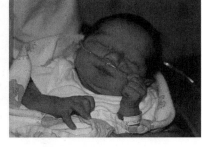

Nasal cannula.

Oxygen is delivered to this baby through a nasal cannula, a flexible hollow tube with openings, or "prongs," that fit just below the baby's nose.

Mechanical Ventilation

A ventilator (also called a respirator) is a mechanical breathing machine that delivers a controlled mixture of air and oxygen, pressure with each breath, and a certain number of breaths per minute (rate). The "stiffer" a baby's lungs, the higher the pressure must be to move the air/oxygen through the air sacs and into the bloodstream. Very sick babies require a high level of oxygen (up to 100 percent), a high pressure, and a high rate.[12]

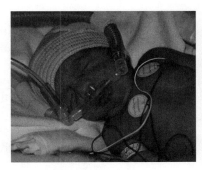

Continuous positive airway pressure.

This baby is breathing on her own while receiving oxygen under steady pressure through her nose. The CPAP makes it easier for the baby to breathe and prevents the small air sacs of the lungs from collapsing after each breath.

The ventilator is attached to your baby's ET tube. Your baby can take breaths on her own while on the ventilator. As your baby weans (needs less assistance) from the ventilator, caregivers reduce the amount of pressure supplied with each breath and the number of breaths per minute. When your baby is doing most of her own breathing, the ET tube is removed (a process called extubation), and supplemental oxygen, which is usually required at first, is delivered by oxyhood, CPAP, or nasal cannula.

Your baby can accidentally become extubated because of her own movement or because the tape or stabilizers holding the ET tube in place slip slightly. Some babies will show obvious signs of distress, such as a dropping heart rate or a color change from pink to blue, when accidentally extubated. Other babies tolerate extubation quite well for a while and may even begin to cry. A cry from your baby indicates that the ET tube has slipped out from between her vocal cords and

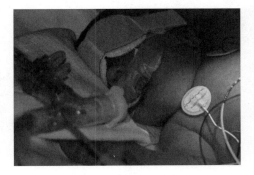

Intubated baby attached to mechanical ventilator tubing.

This endotracheal tube is secured to the baby's mouth and attached to the tubing of the ventilator. The ventilator tubing attaches to the ventilator itself, which stands on the floor near the baby's bed.

that she is extubated. Depending on her condition, a baby who accidentally extubates may be given a trial period to see if she can breathe effectively without the ventilator. If she tires or shows signs of increasing distress or if her blood gases reveal low levels of oxygen and/or high levels of carbon dioxide, CPAP or mechanical ventilation will be restarted.

Newborn Transport

If your baby is born in a community hospital but requires special care, neonatal transport is possible. Many Level II nurseries can manage babies whose care requires oxygen by hood or CPAP, and some can care for babies with umbilical arterial lines. If your baby needs a ventilator or surgery or if the neonatal team predicts that your baby's care will become complex, however, your baby will be transported to a Level III NICU.[13]

How the Transport Process Works

Your baby's physician will contact the regional medical center and arrange the transport. The medical center usually sends a transport team to assess your baby, stabilize her for the trip, and monitor needs during transport. Some community hospitals will provide a transport team of their own to take your baby to the regional center.

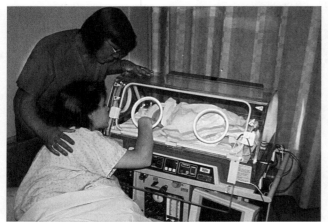

Immediately before your baby leaves your hospital, the transport team will bring her to visit with you if possible. Your baby will be inside a transport incubator, which is designed to provide warmth and carry everything that might be needed for her care. The transport team or nursery nurses will take a photograph of your baby and, if time and circumstance allow, your baby's footprints for you to keep.[13]

Saying good-bye to your baby is difficult at best. If you are still recovering from surgical anesthesia, you may not even remember seeing your baby before transport. Ask your partner or nurse to recount the events for you afterward if necessary. Even if your baby is not critically ill, separation is frightening and increases your stress.

Newborn transport.

Saying good-bye to your baby is not easy. The transport nurse will explain the process and give you a progress report when the baby arrives at the NICU.

Staying in Touch

The transport team should telephone you after arrival at the NICU and update you on your baby's condition. If you do not understand what you are told, ask your nurse to talk to your baby's NICU nurse and act as your interpreter. Be sure you have the NICU phone number and know how to call the NICU from your hospital room so that you can check on your baby's status whenever you wish.

If the Level III NICU is far from the hospital in which your baby was born, you and your partner may be faced with the additional challenge of figuring out how to be in two places at once. Long-distance transport is especially difficult if you have other children at home who need your attention.

Ask your hospital discharge planner or social worker to help you find inexpensive lodging near your baby, and try to visit early in the baby's hospitalization. If you must return home right away, figure out a system for staying in touch with the NICU. Your baby's nurse may set up a time to call you every day and tell you about your baby's progress, and you will be given the phone number to call whenever you wish. Some NICUs will send you a photograph and short note "from your baby" each week. Ask your baby's nurse about the possibility of your baby's returning to a hospital near your home for convalescence after she no longer needs intensive care. Being a "commuter parent" is not an ideal situation. The NICU should work with you to keep you informed and involved in your baby's progress.

Sorting It Out

To process and understand the birthing experience, every new parent, especially the mother, feels the need to tell and retell the story of the labor and birth. This recounting of events is especially important for parents of a sick newborn. When your baby's birth becomes a crisis, the whole experience takes on a dreamlike quality, making it hard for you to know what actually happened. Until the experience becomes real to you, coping with the challenges of NICU parenting will be difficult.

Fathers and other family members should participate in discussions of the birth events. Each person will have a different perception of what happened and feel varying levels of responsibility and powerlessness. Mothers of NICU babies may feel a sense of loss and failure. Fathers may feel torn in all directions in trying to meet the needs of other children, parents and in-laws, a sick newborn, and their partner. Nurses can be a great help as you search for answers to your questions and sort out your feelings.

Once you begin to understand what has happened and can place the events in order, you can begin to move ahead. This will not happen all at once or at the same time for everyone. Allow yourself time for personal recovery, and take advantage of supportive people who will listen to your story. You will also discover that NICU parents share many feelings. Your ability to cope will grow over time, as you learn about the resources available and gain the strength to move forward.

Chapter 3

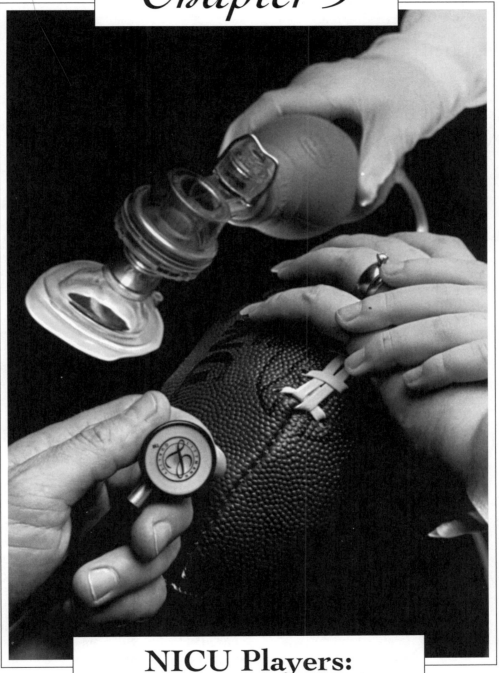

NICU Players:
Working with the Team

Susan M. Kearns, RNC, MN, ARNP

❝"Would you mind coming with me, Piglet, in case they turn out to be Hostile Animals?"❞

Winnie-the-Pooh—

The neonatal intensive care environment can be overwhelming. Not only do you find buzzing, beeping, and blinking equipment everywhere, but the crowd of people caring for your baby adds to the confusion. Often, it seems that as soon as you become familiar with all these caregivers, they disappear and a whole new group surfaces. Who are all of these people, and what are they doing for your baby? Which ones can best answer your questions? Most important, how can you communicate with this multitude to stay informed and participate in your baby's care?

Knowing who the NICU players are and what they do is the first step. Keep in mind, though, that not all NICUs are alike—some of the players described in this chapter may not be present in your hospital's nursery. Community hospitals usually have a smaller, less changeable staff, whereas medical centers employ more people for teaching and research.

The NICU Roster

You will entrust your baby to many people during his hospitalization. Each person plays an important role in the health care of your baby, and you will learn the purpose of each player by observing and asking questions when you visit the NICU. The following is a "who's who" of physicians, nurses, parent support staff, and other team members you may encounter.

Medical Staff

Is there a doctor in the house? Positively! Your baby may have more doctors than you have encountered in your entire lifetime.

Neonatologist/Attending Physician

A neonatologist is a physician who specializes in the diagnosis and treatment of sick newborns. Neonatologists have three years of specialized training beyond that required for general pediatricians, specifically to treat newborns. The neonatologist is usually the most knowledgeable and experienced member of the team treating your newborn and directs the medical care of your baby.

The neonatologist's availability varies from NICU to NICU. In some units, care is directed by a team of neonatologists. The team then shares the responsibility for providing care on a 24-hour basis; this means that each day, a different member of the team is responsible for your baby's care. In other facilities, especially those with a teaching focus, the neonatologist may be present only briefly each day for "patient rounds." During rounds, members of the health care team discuss and review your baby's current condition and medical plan. The neonatologist then makes recommendations to the other care providers based on that plan. If unexpected problems arise, the neonatologist is available to the health care team 24 hours a day.

Neonatal Fellow

A neonatal fellow is a physician who has completed medical school and three years of residency and is currently in training to become a neonatologist. Often, the fellow is more visible on the unit than is the neonatologist, but the responsibilities of a fellow vary widely. In some units, a fellow may be there all day. In other units, the fellow makes rounds in the mornings and can be called by the residents for consultation during the rest of the day.

Pediatrician

A pediatrician is a physician who has completed a pediatric residency and who provides medical care for children from birth to 18 years. Some pediatricians have training in the care of babies with special needs and will care for your baby in the NICU. Other pediatricians may not have special training in NICU care and may therefore refer your baby to a neonatologist. After your baby is discharged from the NICU, your pediatrician may assume your baby's care.

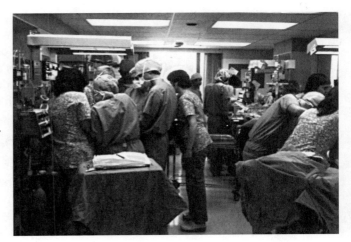

The NICU team.

The NICU is filled with nurses, physicians, and other professionals who are all expert at working with sick babies. The NICU can be incredibly busy during the admission of sick babies. Courtesy of Sacred Heart Medical Center, Spokane, Washington.

Resident

A resident is a physician who has graduated from medical school and is enrolled in a hospital-based program of specialized training called a residency program. Residency programs vary according to specialty (pediatrics, obstetrics, surgery, and so on) and in the amount of time required to complete the training. Pediatric residencies usually take three years to complete. A resident is a physician in the second or third year of the program. You may also hear a resident called an R-2 or an R-3, denoting a second- or third-year resident. Most residents in the NICU are enrolled in pediatric residencies, but residents from other specialties, such as family practice or obstetrics, are involved as well.

Residents are usually very visible on the unit. They are closely involved with your baby's daily care. The resident, along with the intern (discussed in the next section), assesses your infant daily, then plans and revises the medical care. The resident and intern perform many NICU procedures, such as intubation, placement of intravenous (IV) and arterial lines, lumbar puncture, and chest tube insertion.

Intern

An intern is a physician who has completed medical school and is in the first year of a residency program. As part of the medical team, the intern has daily involvement with your baby. Because interns are just beginning to learn about special-care infants, they work very closely with second- and third-year residents. When available, neonatal nurse practitioners also meet many of the intern's learning needs.

Neonatal Nurse Practitioner

A neonatal nurse practitioner (NNP) or advanced registered nurse practitioner (ARNP) is a registered nurse who has completed advanced education and training in the care and treatment of infants and their families. In many institutions, a nurse practitioner must have a master's degree in nursing. Working under the direction of a neonatologist or attending physician, the NNP examines, diagnoses, and designs a care plan for your baby. The NNP may also perform procedures such as intubation, line placement, chest tube insertion, and lumbar puncture. In some states, NNPs or ARNPs may prescribe medications.

Other Medical Personnel

If necessary, your baby's physician may call one or more other physicians for a consultation. These specialists may include any of the following:
- Cardiologist: specializes in diagnosis and treatment of heart problems
- Cardiac surgeon: specializes in performing surgery on the heart
- Neurologist: specializes in diagnosis and treatment of the nervous system
- Gastroenterologist: specializes in treatment of stomach and intestinal problems
- Geneticist: studies birth defects and their causes
- Hematologist: specializes in diagnosis and treatment of blood problems
- Urologist: specializes in diagnosis and treatment of the urinary tract
- Pediatric surgeon: specializes in performing surgery for newborns and children
- Pulmonologist: specializes in diagnosis and treatment of certain lung conditions
- Neurosurgeon: specializes in surgery of the brain and nervous system

Nursing Staff

Although many people think that a nurse is a nurse, nothing could be further from the truth. All nurses do have knowledge that provides the foundation for nursing practice, but most also choose an area of specialty and acquire additional skills and expertise specific to that area.

Registered Nurse

Nurses make up the nation's largest health care profession and a hospital's largest staff component. Most nurses receive their nursing education through a four-year college program (Bachelor of Science in Nursing, or BSN). Two-year community college programs (Associate Degree in Nursing, or ADN) and three-year hospital training programs (Diploma) are other educational pathways. On completing their education, nurses are required by their respective state boards of nursing to pass a written examination. Only after passing the examination can nurses use the designation Registered Nurse (RN).

Registered nurses then receive further training in their specialty from their prospective hospitals.

Nurses work collaboratively with physicians and other members of the health care team; they are not assistants. Nurses function independently, and their specific roles vary depending on the setting. A registered nurse may supervise a team of other professionals and assistants who help care for patients.

A neonatal nurse is a registered nurse who is highly educated to provide nursing care for infants and their families. The nurse caring for your baby learned NICU clinical skills through an extensive orientation program and clinical preceptorship in the NICU.

Neonatal nurses are at your baby's bedside 24 hours a day. They assess your baby's current condition and progress, carry out the physician's orders, and notify the physician or neonatal nurse practitioner (NNP) of any changes in your baby's status. The RN may make recommendations to the physician or NNP based on her assessment of your baby. The RN also plans and implements all nursing care, such as bathing, feeding, positioning, administering prescribed medications, and managing IV and arterial lines. In addition, RNs are very involved in parent education and discharge planning.

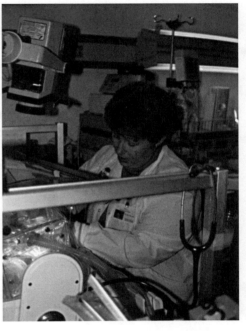

The NICU nurse.
Your baby's nurse is at the bedside more than any other professional. She is your baby's caregiver and advocate, as well as your primary source of information.

Certified Registered Nurse

A registered nurse can take a national examination that tests her knowledge in her specialty—in mother-baby nursing, NICU nursing, or critical care nursing, for example. An RN who is certified by a national testing agency will modify her RN designation to reflect this status, showing it as RNC or CCRN, for example. Some NICUs require their nurses to be certified in an NICU or related subspecialty. Other RNs take a certifying exam as part of their own professional development and a tangible sign of their commitment to excellence in their field.

Licensed Practical Nurse/Licensed Vocational Nurse

A licensed practical nurse (LPN) or licensed vocational nurse (LVN) has graduated from a state-approved technical school or community college and must pass a national written examination. The LPN/LVN provides basic bedside care and works under the direction of an RN.

Clinical Nurse Specialist

A clinical nurse specialist (CNS) is a registered nurse with a master's degree who acts as an expert and resource person for nursing staff. Clinical nurse specialists are involved in many different areas on the unit, including staff education, nursing research, consultation, direct patient care, and program development. Together with the medical team and the nursing staff, the CNS assists with the development, implementation, and evaluation of your baby's care. The CNS may make specific recommendations and offer new ideas or techniques to optimize neonatal care.

Case Manager

Some NICUs use the services of a case manager. This person is usually a nurse whose purpose is to assist the NICU team in coordinating the various components of your baby's health care needs. The case manager follows your baby's hospital course and ensures that orderly progress is being made toward discharge. The case manager may be involved in a formal manner (for example, by attending a care conference) or informally (by stopping by to visit with you when you are in the NICU).

Discharge Planner

A discharge planner does exactly what the title implies—makes the plans for your baby's discharge. Whether your baby is discharged to another facility or to home, the discharge planner makes all the necessary arrangements. If your baby will require special treatment at home (supplemental oxygen, nursing care, physical therapy, and so on), the discharge planner will make those arrangements with you. In some facilities, discharge planning may be done by someone with a different title—for example, a CNS, a case manager, or a social worker. As your baby's discharge nears, it is important to know who is responsible for discharge planning.

Parent Support Staff

Nurses and physicians provide the foundation for your baby's care. Parent support staff, who may also serve hospital patients other than NICU patients, ensure that your needs are met.

Social Worker

Parenting an infant in neonatal intensive care can be very stressful. The social worker (who has a master's degree in social work, or an MSW) is available to help you cope with that stress and manage it effectively. The social worker also knows about financial resources and discharge planning.

Lactation Consultant

If you are planning to breastfeed your baby, you probably have many questions. A lactation consultant can help you. The lactation consultant is usually a nurse, although a community hospital or community program may employ a person with lactation expertise who is not an RN. In any case, a lactation consultant has advanced education and expertise specifically related to breastfeeding. The lactation consultant can assist you with pumping your breasts and maintaining your milk supply until your baby is able to breastfeed. She can be a valuable assistant when you put your baby to the breast for the first time and make the transition to full-time breastfeeding (discussed in Chapter 5).

Financial Counselor

A financial counselor is an employee of the hospital's billing department. If you have questions concerning your hospital bill, consult the financial coun-

"At first, we laughed at the breast pump, "mooing" whenever I took it out. As the weeks went by, and my milk supply dwindled, I began to despise the pump. The lactation consultant offered help and encouragement during that stressful time. Without her, I would have stopped pumping breast milk for my baby."

selor. The financial counselor can also help you submit your bill to the appropriate agencies for payment and can set up a payment plan if you are responsible for any portion of the bill. For more information, see Chapter 7.

Parent Educator

A parent educator provides information and instruction for NICU families. This education is usually offered in a group setting, such as through scheduled classes. The parent educator is often a nurse and may function in other roles (CNS, discharge planner, primary nurse, and so on) as well.

Other Personnel

Depending on your baby's needs and the size of your hospital, you may meet additional staff members who play specialized roles in your baby's care.

Respiratory Therapist

A respiratory therapist (RT) specializes in treatments for the respiratory system. If your baby is on a ventilator, the respiratory therapist may be in charge of maintaining or adjusting ventilator settings to meet your baby's needs. The RT may set up and maintain respiratory equipment; assist with suctioning, intubation, and extubation; and, in some facilities, obtain blood gases.

Developmental Specialist

A developmental specialist is usually a nurse or an occupational or physical therapist who has advanced knowledge and expertise in infant development. In some nurseries, a developmental specialist may evaluate all infants. In other nurseries, only certain infants are referred for evaluation. The developmental specialist can offer ideas on positioning your infant and improving feeding skills and can help you and your infant's caregivers to understand your baby's cues (see Chapter 4).

Nutritionist

Many units now have a nutritionist available to evaluate infant dietary needs. Often, the nutritionist has specialized training in the nutritional needs of preterm infants and plays a key role in evaluating your baby's nutritional state. Even if your baby is not taking food by mouth, the nutritionist may recommend necessary vitamin and mineral supplements (see Chapters 5 and 9). As your baby begins to take food by mouth, the nutritionist makes recommendations regarding caloric intake to optimize weight gain and growth.

Other Support Personnel

Other personnel in the NICU may include laboratory technicians (trained to draw blood); x-ray technicians; ultrasound technicians; and others, including secretaries and housekeepers. Sometimes staff are "cross-trained"; in addition to their specialty role, they can help perform unit duties such as taking routine vital signs, administering uncomplicated feedings, and transporting patients to different areas of the hospital. Whether providing direct care or

"My husband has never been comfortable asking for directions or help of any kind. But even he has to admit that the support staff who guided us through our NICU stay were necessary and important for a good exprerience."

mopping the floor, all hospital personnel provide vital services for your baby's care.

Organized Confusion

Parents soon discover what seems to be a never-ending abundance of new faces at their baby's bedside. Even when you have sorted through all these faces and know who does what, members of the team sometimes do not seem to be available when you need them. Personnel scheduling and rotations account for much of what may seem like confusion to you. It may help to understand some general principles of hospital scheduling.

Scheduling for Physicians and Nurse Practitioners

Just a few people cannot possibly meet your baby's care needs 24 hours a day, seven days a week. Hospital staffing and scheduling is a huge job that requires constant adjustments to meet each unit's needs.

Personnel scheduling is designed to achieve around-the-clock medical and nursing care for patients. Physicians and neonatal nurse practitioners often work 24-hour shifts every three or four days. In many teaching institutions, interns and residents are on the unit Monday through Friday during the day but only stay there every third or fourth night. If you visit or have questions during the night, evening, or weekend, therefore, you may find yourself speaking with a physician you have not seen before.

Physician "rotation" is another area of confusion for parents. When physicians are in residency, they are in training within their specialty. During this time, they must learn everything there is to learn about their specialized population and its accompanying problems. To achieve the necessary training, they rotate (change assignments) through many different patient care areas. This means that about every four weeks a new resident may be assigned to care for your baby.

Other physicians (attendings, fellows, and interns) involved in your baby's care may also rotate. To provide consistent care for your baby, however, physicians rarely rotate all at the same time. Attending physicians may rotate on the first Monday of the month, fellows on the second Monday, residents on the third Monday, and so forth. It is possible—in fact, highly likely—that in a teaching institution, you may meet a new physician every week. No wonder parents feel confused and wonder who is caring for their baby!

Scheduling for NICU Nurses

Nurses in the NICU work a variety of shifts, depending on the hospital's system of care delivery. Nurses may be scheduled for 4-, 8-, 10-, or 12-hour shifts and may work just one day or as many as seven days in a row. To provide the NICU nurse with some consistency and familiarity with her patients (called patient continuity), many NICUs use a system called primary nursing. Each infant in the NICU is assigned a primary nurse from the NICU staff for each shift; the primary nurses from all of the shifts make up the primary nursing team. When the primary nurse is scheduled to work, she usually cares for your baby.

Primary nurses work closely with the medical team to plan, implement, and make recommendations for your baby's care. If a primary nurse is not on duty, an associate nurse or another member of the care team may be assigned. The associate nurse communicates closely with your baby's primary nurses to provide consistency for you and your baby. This system limits the number of caregivers, allowing a small number of nurses to become familiar with you and with your baby's individual needs.

Because of the many professionals involved in your baby's care, you may feel lost in the maze. Who will update you on your baby's progress? What questions should you ask? Who will answer your questions? How can you understand and remember what you are told?

Good communication is essential for family survival in the NICU. Without good communication, you will feel lost, frustrated, and further isolated from your baby. The following suggestions can help you open the lines of communication with your baby's health care team so that you can ask the questions you need to have answered and understand the answers.

Learn about Common NICU Problems

The more informed you are, the better you will understand what is happening to your baby. Reading this book will help. Talking with other parents who have gone through an NICU experience may help. If you like detailed information, ask your baby's nurse or physician for written material related to your baby's condition. The more you understand, the more effective an advocate you can be for your baby.

Become Familiar with the Members of Your Baby's Care Team

Because of staff rotations, parents often have difficulty identifying members of their baby's team. Until you become familiar with the system, you may need to ask, "Who is the intern?" or "Who is the resident?" Never feel shy about asking. It is your right to know who is caring for your baby!

The team members working directly with your baby are the most informed and up-to-date about your baby's progress and plan of care. Interns and residents (or, depending on the facility, NNPs or neonatologists) are usually responsible for writing orders, and the registered nurse is responsible for carrying out those orders and assessing the infant's response. Your baby's nurse should be very familiar with the care plan and should answer most of your questions in language that you can understand. The nurse spends the most time at your baby's bedside and is usually the staff member most available to you for questions and discussion. It's usually best to direct your questions to the nurse most familiar with your baby or to the physician directly managing your baby's care.

Communication as a Survival Skill

"For new parents, the NICU experience is like being dumped into one of those fancy dessert coffees. The staff members blend smoothly and work well together. But new parents just bob around on top, feeling conspicuous and vulnerable, like puffs of whipped cream."

Be Clear about How Much You Want to Know

"How are things going today?" may seem like a straightforward question to you, but NICU staff may have difficulty knowing how much and what kind of information you expect in response. Some parents want hard clinical information, such as laboratory results and ventilator settings. Other parents prefer more general information, such as how well their baby slept or whether the baby is tolerating feedings.

Communicate clearly with your baby's care providers about the type of information you expect to receive and when you want to know it. Do you want to be called immediately with test results, or can you be informed of them when you visit? Do you want to be informed only of adverse test results, or do you want to know every test result? Be honest with the NICU staff. Don't expect your baby's caregivers to read your mind.

Use Communication Openers

If you feel that members of your baby's care team are not hearing your concerns or welcoming your suggestions, you may want to try a different approach. Prefacing your questions or ideas with communication openers can help you reach your goals. These openers reflect a "we're-in-this-together" approach rather than one that demands action or raises a barrier to communication. Here are some examples:

Barriers	Openers
I want you to …	Would you think about…?
Why can't you …?	What if we tried …?
The experts say…	I read about…Do you think that might work?

Parents who use basic negotiation and diplomacy skills when communicating with the NICU team are more successful in establishing a satisfying partnership. That partnership is important as you all strive to achieve the same goal—to help your baby become well. In a healthy partnership, your ideas and concerns will receive the attention they deserve.

Ask for Clarification

Because professionals are comfortable with the topics they address often and the medical terminology they use among themselves, it is easy for them to forget that the NICU experience is an entirely new one for most parents and other family members. If you do not understand an explanation or cannot follow a discussion, do not be afraid to ask that terms be defined or that the explanation be repeated. You'll be surprised how quickly you'll pick up some of the NICU jargon, even though it may sound like a foreign language at first.

Keep Asking Questions

It is important to feel comfortable and satisfied with the answers you receive to your questions. If you are not satisfied with what you are being told or do not understand it, take your question to someone with more expertise. If the nurse is not giving you the information you need, ask to speak with the intern or NNP. If you are still not satisfied after speaking with the intern, ask to see the resident, or the fellow, or the neonatologist. Do not be afraid of offending members of the team because you are "going over their heads." Remember, this is *your* baby. You have a right to information from the most knowledgeable person available.

Keep in mind, however, that you may not get the answer you desire. Some questions have no clear answers. In other cases, too many variable factors exist to permit a specific answer. At other times, parents may be looking for an unrealistic answer to their question.

Lack of a conclusive answer can be frustrating. You may feel as if information is being kept from you, even though this is probably not the case. Acknowledging your frustration to the members of the health care team may help you deal with that feeling. Chances are that team members are also frustrated when they cannot give a conclusive answer.

Make Appointments with People You Want to See

Because of the nature of the NICU environment, it is rare for everything to happen "on schedule." Even if you have been told that the neonatologist is usually in the unit at a certain time, do not plan to "catch" the physician for a lengthy discussion during patient rounds. A more effective approach is to schedule an appointment to discuss your baby's progress. This gives the professional involved time to review and organize the most up-to-date information on your baby's case. A scheduled appointment also increases your chances for uninterrupted time to convey your questions and concerns.

Request a Care Conference

Even if you do not have specific questions about your baby's condition or plan of care, it's often helpful to meet with members of the health care team periodically for updates. Your baby's health care providers may schedule a care conference for you or you may request one. These meetings help familiarize you with team members you may not see daily. Meetings with team members can be informal, at your baby's bedside, or at a more formalized care conference. A care conference gives you the opportunity to ask questions of the appropriate person, to get updates on any significant changes in your baby's plan of care, and to learn what progress the members of the team are hoping to see your baby make.

How frequently you meet with the team depends on your baby's condition; you may meet once a day if your baby is very unstable or once every few weeks if your baby has chronic problems. Usually the members of the health care team most closely involved with your baby (for example, the neonatologist, resident, intern, nurse practitioner, and primary nurse) attend these meetings, but other personnel may be asked to attend depending on your baby's condition. You may also discover that you do not need to meet with the entire

"I was lost at first— so many people and too much information. The care conference helped me organize my thoughts and understand much of what was happening to my baby. I could breathe again."

team, that one or two key people can provide you with the information you need. Remember that these meetings are for your benefit and can be customized to meet your needs.

Ask about Your Baby's Care Plan

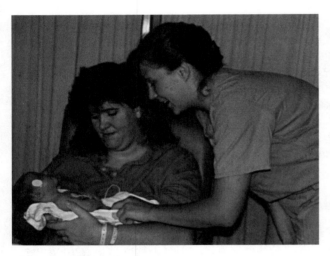

Vital communication.

The health care professionals in the NICU use every opportunity to teach you about your baby's special needs. This nurse answers the mother's questions and points out the baby's special characteristics.

Some parents want to learn as much as possible about common NICU problems, whereas others want only basic information. In any event, the care plan is what guides your baby's medical and nursing care. By understanding your baby's overall plan of care, you may better understand daily care routines and be able to recognize milestones in your baby's NICU course.

The plan of care guides how and when things are done. Its basis is your baby's individual characteristics and condition. You can learn quite a bit by asking about your baby's care plan. Depending on the level of information you want, knowing about your baby's feeding plan may be enough. Parents desiring more detailed information can ask more complex questions, such as "What is the plan for weaning my baby off the ventilator? What is the plan for dealing with my baby's heart murmur?"

It is also important to realize that care plans change. Care plans must be flexible; they depend on your baby's response to treatments as well as his overall condition. Ask frequently for an update on the plan of care. If the plan has changed, ask why: "What about my baby has changed to cause this change in care?" If the plan of care has not changed, do not be afraid to ask about that either: "Why hasn't the plan changed despite the fact that my baby hasn't [or has] gotten better?" You are not challenging anyone's expertise or knowledge. You are merely asking for clarification.

Many NICUs now utilize clinical pathways. A clinical pathway shows the expected progression of an illness or problem over a specific period of time. Clinical pathways reflect general expectations concerning a particular diagnosis; they do not incorporate your baby's individual characteristics. By reviewing the clinical pathway for your baby's condition or illness, however, you may gain insight into where your baby falls in the disease process, as well as about what to expect in the immediate future.

Ask "What If" Questions

All too often, parents do not ask the "What if?" questions, and then become frustrated because the questions have not been addressed. "What if this drug doesn't work?" "What if we decide against surgery?" "What if this treatment doesn't work?" Asking "What if?" questions should make you better informed about the treatment, procedure, or medication in question. Keep in mind that at times a definitive answer is impossible. Risks and benefits must often be weighed and decisions made without absolute answers.

Keep a Journal

Initially, you may feel too exhausted and overwhelmed to keep a journal, but try to make the effort as soon as you are able. You will be bombarded with an enormous amount of information as soon as you step into the NICU. Writing things down can help you keep your thoughts organized. Keep a record of who you spoke with and what was discussed. As you review your journal later, many of the things you jotted down may seem clearer.

Write Down Questions as You Think of Them

Families often have many questions regarding their baby, but when the opportunity arises to ask those questions, no one can remember what they were. To avoid this problem, write down your questions as they occur to you. Keep your list in your purse or wallet so that you'll have it handy when the next opportunity arises to ask your questions. You can use the same piece of paper to record the answers to your questions. When you get home, tape the piece of paper in your journal for future reference.

Taking Care of Yourself

The NICU environment can be very stressful. You will encounter many unfamiliar experiences and lots of information. You'll have a much more difficult time processing that information if you are exhausted, hungry, or sick. Try to nap during the day, or at least sit down in a quiet area and put your feet up. Try to eat regular meals or, if that is too difficult, eat frequent, healthy snacks. Allow family and friends to help out by cooking meals for you or cleaning your house. Often these people want to help but don't know how.

Because the NICU is so stressful, everyone needs an occasional break. Give yourself permission to take a day off from visiting your baby and do something for yourself. It may be difficult for you skip a daily visit, but you may find that the rest and relaxation you enjoy make the next visit even more worthwhile.

Give Yourself Some Time

Following your first NICU visit, you may feel overwhelmed by the environment and hopelessly outnumbered by the staff. In time, you will be able to identify the people who are caring for your baby and know what they do. With practice, you will learn how to communicate effectively with them and get your way at least some of the time. These are the first important steps toward active involvement in your baby's care.

Chapter 4

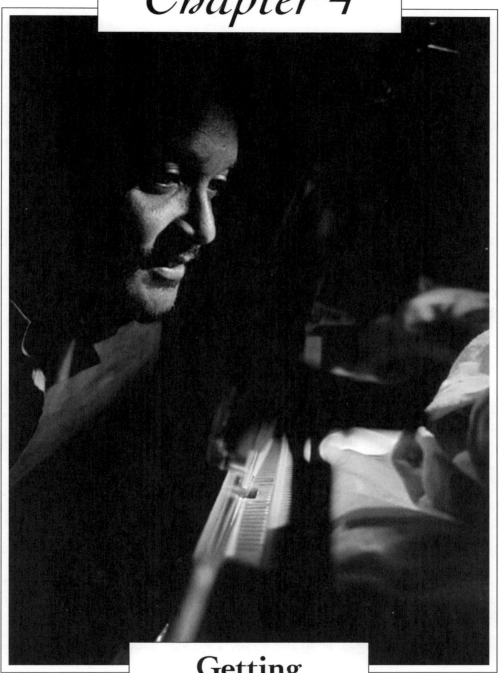

Getting Acquainted

Susan M. Kearns, RNC, MN, ARNP

"Piglet was so excited at the idea of being Useful that he forgot to be frightened any more...**"**

Getting acquainted with your baby begins with your first visit to the nursery. For many parents, that first visit involves mixed feelings. Excitement and jubilation accompany a sense of fear and loss. What will your baby look like? How will your baby act? Will you be able to hold your baby or do anything to help?

This chapter addresses your first visits to the NICU: getting ready, experiencing common reactions, and making the most of your time there. Then, to help you get acquainted with your baby, it contains an explanation of infant capabilities, states, and cues and gives you some pointers for interacting with your baby.

Your First Visit to the NICU

Depending on your baby's condition at birth, she may have been taken immediately to the NICU, without you getting as much as a glimpse of this new member of your family. During high-risk birth or emergency cesarean section, general anesthesia and the possible exclusion of the father or support person during delivery may mean that both parents feel as though they missed the whole thing. These parents see their new baby for the first time in the NICU. Most parents feel a strong desire to see and hold their baby, but these feelings are coupled with many unknowns: How did this happen? Will I feel like her mother or father? Will my baby survive?

Your first visits to the NICU lay the groundwork for later visits. If your initial visits are unpleasant experiences, subsequent visits may be even more difficult. Following are some recommendations for making your early visits positive experiences.

Be Physically Ready

If you are a mother who went through a long, hard labor or complications of illness, take a nap before you visit your baby. The more rested you are, the more information you will be able to retain. Often mothers fall asleep during their first nursery visit, especially if they have not had much sleep in the few days before the birth.

If your labor was long, you and your partner may not have eaten anything for some time. If you are able to eat, have a snack before you visit the NICU. Hypoglycemia (low blood sugar) can lead to nausea, which can cut your visit short.

Delay your visit if you are feeling faint, dizzy, or light-headed. Fainting is common for first-time NICU visitors. Just the sights and sounds of a hospital environment are enough to make some people queasy. Even if you are not bothered by the routine hospital environment, the sights, sounds, and smells of the NICU may cause you to become faint. These feelings will disappear as you grow more familiar with the environment.

Go to the bathroom before you visit. Women who have just given birth tend to urinate frequently, and the NICU may not have a bathroom for patient use. If you had a urinary catheter in place and it was recently removed, try to empty your bladder before your visit. Although your bladder may be full, you may not feel the urge until it is too late. The trip back to your room may take longer than you think.

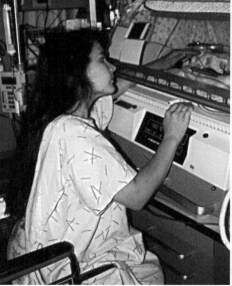

Get Updated Before You Visit

If your partner or support person has already visited the NICU, talk together about the experience. Ask your partner what you can expect to see and how your baby is doing. If this is the first visit for both of you, or if your baby's condition is changing from moment to moment, ask to speak with the NICU nurse before you visit. Knowing ahead of time what to expect will help you feel more comfortable in the NICU.

Ride to the NICU

Depending on your condition, it's generally a good idea to go to the NICU by stretcher or wheelchair. No matter how well you feel and how close the NICU is to your room, it's better to save your energy for the visit. Also, should you become faint or light-headed, you will have a place to rest until you feel better.

First visit.
Your first visit to the NICU can be overwhelming. Take advantage of a quiet moment to touch and talk to your new baby.

Take a Companion with You

If your partner or support person cannot be with you on your first visit to the NICU, ask your nurse to accompany you. You may remember little of what you are told about your baby during this visit. If someone else is with you, you will later be able to discuss forgotten details with that person.

Focus on Your Baby, Not on the Technology

Parents often remember little about their baby's appearance following their first visit to the NICU. What they do remember are the machines, tubes, and wires. This is understandable; all that NICU technology can be intimidating. Right now, though, your family and friends will want to know what your baby looks like, what color her eyes are, and whether your newborn has Uncle Joe's nose. It can be frustrating to be unable to tell them much about your baby's features after your first visit. Rest assured that with each subsequent visit, you'll notice more details about your baby and her features and behavior.

Have Realistic Expectations

Don't expect to understand everything about your baby on your first visit or to understand the purpose of each piece of equipment. You will have time for all of that later. Your first visit is a time to validate that, yes indeed, you did have a baby, and here she is. It is a first step in the process of becoming acquainted with your baby. On each subsequent visit, you will become more familiar with your baby and more knowledgeable about your baby's condition and the technology being used to help her.

Common Reactions to the First Visit

The NICU is a wealth of sensory input. On your first visit, you may be overwhelmed by the amount of equipment in the unit. Not only is the physical presence of all the equipment overwhelming, but many of the machines have their own operating noises and alarms. (Chapters 2 and 12 explain what much of that equipment is and does.) You may wonder how anyone can tell which machine is sounding an alarm. As you visit more frequently, you too will be able to distinguish between various alarm sounds and learn to "tune out" those sounds not in your baby's area.

Depending on the time of day you visit, the unit may be a flurry of activity. More people tend to be in the NICU during the day, because this is when most physicians make rounds (visit each patient) and most diagnostic testing is performed. Many different health care providers may introduce themselves to you. Don't worry during your initial visit about remembering their names or what they do—you will have time later to match names with faces and services provided. (Chapter 3 explains the roles of various NICU personnel.)

Parents report a range of reactions and emotions following their first NICU visit. How you feel may depend on whether you were expecting your infant to need NICU care after birth, your baby's condition, your own condition, and if you have any past NICU experiences.

Fear

Fear is a normal reaction to the unknown. Most parents have little previous experience with sick newborns; many are unnerved by the NICU environment and their baby's appearance. But more important, parents fear the possibility of their baby's death or disability. They may also question their own abilities to parent a child with special needs.

You may fear friends' and relatives' responses to the birth. Some mothers fear their partner will blame them for a complicated birth and fear the loss of the relationship. Fears and misgivings generally moderate over time, but most NICU parents experience some degree of fear until major issues begin to resolve.

Anger

Anger is a common reaction to the initial NICU experience. You may feel angry about your birth experience or your inability to control events in the NICU. You may feel angry at the staff ("They just don't know what they're doing"), your family and friends ("They just don't understand"), or your partner

("How can he go to work and just forget about the baby?"). You may even be angry at yourself ("Why couldn't I carry this baby to term?" or "What did I do/not do to make this happen to my baby?"). As uncomfortable as it may be to admit it, you may also feel angry at your baby ("Why couldn't you have waited for just a few more weeks?").

Most parents of NICU babies feel some anger, although they express it in different ways. Some are openly angry, demanding, and looking to blame others. Some keep their anger hidden inside. Parents may have a difficult time acknowledging the anger they feel, especially if that anger is directed toward their baby or their partner.

To cope with your anger, begin by acknowledging it to yourself, your partner, and those around you. Realize that anger is a normal, expected emotion common to most NICU parents. By discussing your feelings with NICU staff, you may begin to understand their origins. Are you upset with someone in particular, or is the situation itself the problem? By discussing your feelings, you acknowledge them. Then you can make a plan to address the problem and lessen your angry feelings.

Anger requires a tremendous amount of energy. As NICU parents, you will spend a great amount of energy just getting through each day—getting to and from the hospital, absorbing the vast amounts of information you receive, spending time with your baby, caring for yourself and your household, and coping with the unavoidable emotional ups and downs of NICU life. You'll discover that anger depletes your already-limited energy supply. Reducing your anger will give you more energy for other issues.

Guilt

Many parents express feelings of guilt after the birth of a sick baby. You may ask yourself, "What did I do to cause this?" or "What could I have done to prevent this?" And nearly every parent unnecessarily laments, "If only I hadn't..." Mothers, especially, examine their lives since the day they became pregnant—wondering if they could have changed the outcome by making different decisions or if their circumstances had been different. For many families, the reasons their baby was born sick or preterm will never be known. This situation is rarely the result of something parents did or did not do. It just happened.

Loss

As a pregnancy progresses, parents begin to envision their baby. For most parents, this mental picture resembles the babies seen in diaper and baby food advertisements. Newborn babies—even those who are born at term and perfectly healthy—do not look anything like those babies. Preterm babies, especially, do not come close to the "ideal" vision. Seeing your baby for the first time may lead to feelings of loss for that ideal.

Most mothers of term infants report that they are glad their pregnancy is over. Mothers of preterm babies, on the other hand, often mourn the loss of their pregnancy. Psychologically, you had prepared yourself for 40 weeks of

"It took us a long time to resolve our guilt. We asked the "what if" and "why us" questions for months. My wife was haunted by the TV commercials that showed the sick baby in the incubator and urged pregnant women to get prenatal care "or else." But we did nothing wrong. We had good prenatal care. What happened to us was nobody's fault—we just had really bad luck."

pregnancy. But if your baby was premature, your pregnancy probably ended before you were ready. Mothers of preterm babies frequently relate that they miss feeling the baby inside of them and were not yet ready to give birth.

If your birth didn't happen as you planned, you may also mourn the loss of that planned birth experience. Many couples today plan who will attend the birth, how the environment will look, and how they will manage pain, as well as how much medical intervention they desire. Some write detailed birth plans to convey their desires to their care provider. Unfortunately, preterm or complicated birth rarely fits those plans.

You may also feel the loss of your parenting role. Throughout pregnancy, you envisioned yourself as a parent. You pictured yourself and your partner playing with and caring for your baby. Now you must visit your baby in a foreign environment, touch your baby through a porthole, and wait for someone else to tell you when it's appropriate for you to hold or feed your baby. This certainly isn't what you anticipated!

Some parents take a long time to get over these feelings of loss. Many revisit these feelings frequently—sometimes for years—often around the time of their baby's birth. Again, this is a normal reaction for NICU families. As with anger, it often helps to discuss and acknowledge these feelings of loss. Feelings of loss may not be resolved as easily as those of anger, however.

Powerlessness

You find yourself in a strange environment, surrounded by high-tech equipment and a multitude of people telling you what you can and cannot do. Your baby cries, or her lips look dry. You want to comfort your baby, but you can't figure out how to open the incubator or where to find supplies. These feelings of powerlessness are common in the NICU.

Begin by understanding that most NICU parents feel powerless, and then acknowledge those feelings: "I feel like I can't do anything for my baby." Discuss your feelings with your baby's nurse. She can suggest ways for you to participate in your baby's care and communicate your feelings to other staff members who care for your baby so that they, too, can help involve you.

If you are not yet comfortable with your baby's nurses, you might begin by making observations and asking questions: "My baby looks uncomfortable. What can I do to help her?" or "My baby's lips are dry. What can I use to wipe them?" As you become more comfortable with the NICU environment and gain more confidence with touching and interacting with your baby, you will no longer need to ask these questions. You will know what to do and how. Feelings of confidence will begin to replace your initial feelings of powerlessness.

That "Fish-in-a-Tank" Feeling

Many parents say they feel like "fish in a tank" or "an animal at the zoo" after their early visits to the NICU. You may notice that everyone is staring at

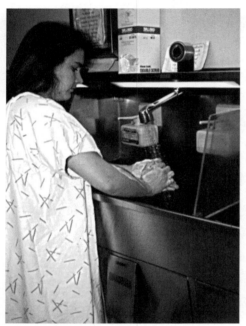

Hand washing.

Scrubbing your hands before you visit your baby is important for preventing infection. Your NICU nurse will explain the unit's "scrub and gown" policy.

you and watching your every move. The loss of privacy is marked and adds stress to your visits. The staff in the NICU are watching you—generally so that they may anticipate your needs and recognize unspoken cues that will help them assist you. In addition, other NICU parents are watching you closely, identifying you with your baby and comparing your circumstances to theirs. This initial scrutiny is part of the getting-to-know-you process. The more familiar you become with the environment, the more comfortable you will be with the NICU staff, the routines, and your ability to care for and parent your baby.

Learning the NICU Routine

Parenting a baby in the NICU is no different than learning how to do a new job. You will need time to learn what you need to know to feel comfortable. Every NICU has its own learning program for parents. This chapter provides sample orientation and learning checklists. Ask about your NICU's orientation program, and seek out the information you need to know to understand your baby's care.

Protecting Your Baby from Infection

Hand washing is the best way for you to protect your baby from infection. Each time you visit the NICU, you will be asked to scrub your hands at a sink and to cover your clothes with a clean hospital gown. Each NICU has its own "scrub and gown" policy, so ask your NICU nurse what to expect in your unit.

Some NICUs limit visitors to the baby's parents and perhaps, occasionally, grandparents. Policies for sibling visitation (by the baby's brothers and sisters) also vary from unit to unit. Siblings may be required not only to scrub and gown, but to wear a surgical mask to prevent respiratory viruses from infecting the newborn. Do not allow your other children to visit if they are experiencing fever, diarrhea, a common cold, or an ear infection or if they have recently been exposed to an illness like chickenpox. If you or your partner are experiencing any of the above symptoms, consult with your baby's nurse or health care provider before visiting your baby.

Understanding Your Baby

Your first NICU visits are the time to get comfortable with your new baby and her environment. As you become more familiar with your baby's appearance and more accustomed to the NICU environment, and as your baby grows, her capabilities will emerge little by little. What are these capabilities? What is being done to foster your baby's development? What can you do to help? How can you as a parent understand your baby's methods of communication?

Infant Capabilities

Let's begin with the sensory system—the organs your baby uses to see, hear, feel, taste, and touch. Parents are usually quite concerned with their baby's capabilities in these areas, asking such questions as "Can my baby see? Can my baby hear? Can my baby feel pain?"

Orientation Checklist for NICU Parents

General Information for Parents

Nursery telephone number

Visiting policy for parents, siblings, grandparents

Location of cafeteria, restrooms, public telephone, family waiting area

Scrub and gown policy

Infant security policy

Safekeeping place for purses, coats, briefcases, and so on, while visiting in nursery

Breast pump use; milk pumping and storing policies

Feeding schedules; how to communicate wish to perform bathing, feeding, other baby care

How to arrange consistent daily call from nursery to parent (especially if parent is far from NICU)

Policy regarding parent access to baby's chart

People Parents Need to Know

Primary Nurse

Parent contact person (nurse manager, clinical nurse specialist, case manager)

Physician managing baby's care: how to contact, who covers when managing physician is unavailable

Lactation specialist or resource person for lactation support

Social worker assigned to baby

Other caregivers (physical therapist, development therapist, and so on): when they visit, how parents can participate

Other Useful Information for Parents

Classes and support groups for parents, siblings, grandparents

Discharge criteria

Discharge planning options (rooming-in, day pass to go home briefly before discharge)

Telephone numbers for medical records, financial counselor, business office

Information Nursery Needs about Parents

Telephone numbers (best daytime phone, nighttime phone; who else to call in an emergency)

Special needs of parents (hearing or visual impairment, literacy or language barrier)

Cultural or spiritual values that will affect baby's care or parents' involvement in caregiving

Social situation that might affect protection of baby, staff, or other NICU patients (restraining order against partner or others, child custody problems, history of unstable or violent behavior on part of significant other or family members, and so on)

Learning Checklist for NICU Parents

Parents Learn About

NICU Equipment

Basic:
- gloves
- radiant warmer
- incubator
- cardiorespiratory monitor
- pulse oximeter
- transcutaneous monitor
- phototherapy equipment
- infant scales
- diaper output scale
- suction equipment
- other:

Respiratory:
- oxygen
- endotracheal tube and ventilator
- continuous positive airway pressure (CPAP)
- oxyhood
- nasal cannula
- oxygen tent
- oxygen analyzers
- chest tube
- bag and mask
- other:

Lines:
- peripheral intravenous (IV)
- umbilical catheter (arterial and venous)
- percutaneous
- other:

Feeding:
- gavage/tube
- cup/dropper
- gastrostomy tube
- pump
- infant formula (types)
- breast milk additives
- other:

NICU Medications
- intravenous (IV)
- intramuscular (IM)
- aerosol
- oral
- topical
- other:

NICU Procedures
- glucose test strip
- x-ray
- sepsis workup
- ultrasound
- computed tomography (CT) scan
- echocardiogram
- magnetic resonance imaging (MRI)
- electroencephalogram (EEG)
- other:

NICU Lab Work
- blood glucose
- complete blood count (CBC)/ hematocrit (Hct)
- arterial blood gas (ABG) capillary blood gas (CBG)
- electrolytes
- culture and sensitivity
- bilirubin
- metabolic screening
- drug level
- other:

Parents Learn To
- understand infant behavior/ developmental care
- hold and position baby correctly
- take baby's temperature
- change baby's diaper
- dress baby
- perform umbilical cord care if necessary
- perform skin care
- bathe baby
- use kangaroo care if desired/appropriate
- perform infant massage as appropriate
- use breast pump; store and use breast milk safely
- breastfeed and/or bottle feed
- perform other types of feeding (gastrostomy) if appropriate
- use bulb syringe; perform mouth care
- administer medications
- use car seat correctly
- perform infant cardiopulmonary resuscitation (CPR)
- use home monitor and equipment if necessary
- perform special care tasks
- recognize signs of illness
- immunize baby against preventable illness
- other:

Parents Know How to Access Referrals To
- support groups
- specialty medical care (cardiac, gastroenterology, and so on)
- hearing tests
- eye examinations
- occupational and/or developmental therapy
- public health nurse
- home health nurse
- Social Services
- other:

Sight

An infant's vision is the least well developed part of the sensory system at birth. Even in term infants, areas in the retina of the eye that are responsible for sharpness of vision—called visual acuity—are incompletely developed, as are the nerve fibers in the optic nerve. Therefore, infants generally have poor eyesight (20/600) and little ability to focus. The amount of color vision is not known for certain, but infants probably do not see color until two to three months of age.[1]

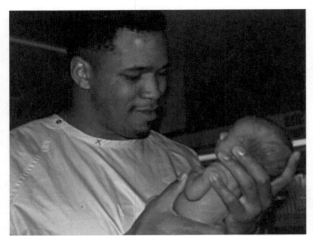

Getting acquainted.

This baby can see his father's face, feel his touch, and hear his voice. This kind of communication is important and rewarding for both father and baby.

The fetus's eyelids fuse during week 10 of gestation and remain fused until around week 26.[2] Infants born at 26 weeks gestation or earlier, therefore, may have eyelids that are still fused together. If your baby is born with fused eyelids, no special precautions or treatments are necessary. The lids will open on their own.

One of your first desires will be to see your baby with her eyes open; there is something very real, very magical, and very life-affirming about a baby with open eyes. Parents in the newborn nursery as well as in the NICU are frequently overheard saying, "Come on, open your eyes so that I know you're in there." Seeing your baby's eyes open seems to validate the person inside the body.

Visiting your baby when her eyes are open may be difficult, because your baby will sleep most of the time. But for parents whose babies are born with fused eyelids, waiting for the lids to open can be frustrating. Although this may take only a few days to happen, those few days can seem like weeks when you are anxiously waiting to make meaningful eye contact with your baby.

Initially, your baby may not be able to look at you and follow your face, but as she grows and remains awake for longer periods, her visual abilities will improve. Look at your baby face-to-face, because human faces are a baby's favorite visual stimulation. Remember that the sharpness of a baby's vision is poor, so put your face close to your baby's—about 6 to 10 inches away.

Babies also like objects with high contrast, such as bull's-eye patterns, checkerboards, and concentric circles of contrasting colors. Remember, color vision is probably poor at this time; black-and-white patterns provide the most visual interest. If your baby is able to look at things for any length of time, she may eventually become bored with the same objects. Provide a new object, and note your baby's response—very likely, new interest.

Before birth, your baby was accustomed to a dark, muted environment. To reduce environmental stress to the newborns in their care, many NICUs have substituted indirect lighting for direct fluorescent lighting or have installed dimmer switches. Blankets, placed over the incubator, can also be used to decrease the amount of light a baby receives.

Sound

Structurally, the ears begin to develop in the 4th week of gestation.[2] By week 27, the ears are functionally developed.[1] As your baby grew in your body, she was exposed to a variety of sounds, such as the maternal heart beat, sounds of digestion, blood pulsing through the vessels, and external sounds including voices. Hearing sensitivity improves with development and the term infant's response to sound is more consistent than the response of a preterm baby.[3]

Although the preterm infant can hear quite well, the auditory system is still quite vulnerable. The auditory canal continues to mature after birth, making it susceptible to noise damage. Continuous loud noises may not only harm a baby's hearing, but also produce physical stress, such as changes in heart rate, breathing patterns, blood pressure, and oxygen consumption.

Unfortunately, the NICU is a noisy place. Alarms ring. The room is filled with people having conversations. The phone rings. Charts get dropped. The intercom system never seems to stop. Potentially, all this noise can affect your baby's hearing.

Many NICUs have instituted measures to help protect your baby's hearing. Some of these include:

- Removing radios from infant areas or playing only soft, soothing music.
- Conversing softly near infants and, preferably, talking away from areas where infants are sleeping.
- Placing reminder signs near babies who are very sensitive to noise.
- Covering the top of the incubator with a blanket to muffle the sound of anything placed on top of it.
- Closing incubator portholes and doors carefully and quietly.
- Placing earmuffs over your baby's ears to help decrease noise.
- Removing telephones, or at least turning the ringer off, in patient areas.
- Providing special "quiet rooms" or areas for babies who are especially sensitive to noise. As these babies become less sensitive, they are moved back to regular patient care areas.

As your baby grows and becomes less sensitive to noise, more auditory stimulation can be introduced. How that stimulation is introduced will depend on your baby. It may mean moving your baby out of the "quiet room," removing earmuffs, or purposefully providing auditory stimulation, such as your voice, for your baby to hear. Infants can distinguish their mother's voice and focus their attention on high-pitched, rhythmic vocalizations. Therefore, it is important for you to talk to your baby.[3]

Some parents provide audiotapes of themselves reading or talking and intersperse the dialogue with soft music. The nurse who plays your recordings to your infant in your absence may tell you how your infant quiets and settles down to sleep after hearing the familiar parental voices.

Touch and Pain

The sense of touch is the first to develop in the fetus. The nerves carrying feelings to and from the extremities form during the 5th week of gestation, and

"The first time my baby looked at me it was as if a door had opened between us. I knew there was a little person in there, and I knew he was mine."

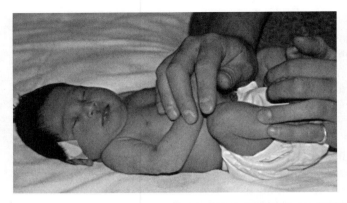

Containment.

Babies appreciate boundaries. This father can calm his baby by gently holding the baby's arms and legs securely against his body.

This bunting provides a secure "nest" for the baby. (Infant positioned in a SnuggleUp, product of Children's Medical Ventures, Inc., South Weymouth, Massachusetts.)

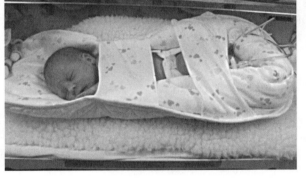

the sensory nerve endings in the skin form early in gestation.[4] Therefore, your baby has an acute sense of touch, even at 25 weeks gestational age.

Because the sense of touch is highly developed, even in preterm infants, you can easily provide your baby with this excellent type of stimulation.[5] Your baby's face, the area around the lips, and the hands are especially sensitive to your touch. You can help quiet your baby with firm, gentle stroking.[5] Tickling movements tend to make babies more agitated and are usually discouraged.

In addition to actively touching your baby, you can give a sense of security by providing boundaries. Inside your uterus, your baby was surrounded and contained by the springy uterine wall. Now, outside the uterus, she has lost that form of body containment and may be unable to bring her arms and legs in close to her body without help. Your hand placed under your infant's feet or on top of your baby's head can serve as a boundary. As your baby matures, you may find that your hand under her feet and legs is all she needs to quiet her.

Because of your baby's keen sense of touch, the surrounding surfaces are also very important. Babies prefer boundaries, or a "nest" made of soft surfaces that yield to their movements. Some units use special buntings or enclosures resembling sleeping bags to provide containment, or your NICU nurses may place a sheepskin under your baby.

For years, sheepskins have been used under patients confined to bed to decrease the formation of bedsores. In the 1960s, nurses in New Zealand began using sheepskins for special-care babies.[6] Babies on sheepskins stayed warmer and slept better. Most sheepskins used in the NICU are made of a synthetic material that can endure frequent laundering. The sheepskins provide your baby with a soft, springy boundary and an excellent surface to grab and explore.

Some NICUs no longer use sheepskins because of research that links babies who sleep on sheepskins to Sudden Infant Death Syndrome (SIDS). It is thought that babies are at risk for rebreathing their own carbon dioxide and not getting enough oxygen if placed face down on a sheepskin.[7] Many NICU staff believe that a light blanket or cloth diaper under the baby's head will take care of this concern and continue to use sheepskins, feeling that the benefits to the baby outweigh the risks. The baby is so closely monitored in the NICU that any breathing problem would be noticed quickly. Ask your baby's nurse about your NICU's current philosophy regarding sheepskins in the hospital.

When your baby comes home, she should sleep on a firm, flat mattress without a sheepskin, pillow, fluffy quilt, or plush toy underneath her.[8]

If your baby's sense of touch is well developed, does she also feel pain? Parents have asked this valid question for many years. Historically, it was believed that an infant's nervous system was too "disorganized" to recognize pain and that an infant's brain did not perceive conditions to be painful that an adult would consider to be painful. Because of this belief, painful procedures (circumcision, chest tube placement, surgery, and so forth) were performed on infants without any type of pain relief.

Current research demonstrates that infants do indeed experience pain. Studies show definite physiologic (physical) changes—such as increased heart rate, respiratory rate, and blood pressure, as well as increased oxygen use—during painful procedures. Based on these studies, neonatal pain control is now part of NICU practice.

Procedures that were once considered routine but painful are now looked at much more critically. Babies are often given local anesthesia for painful procedures, and infants are much more likely today than in the past to be given medication for general discomfort or agitation. More research is needed in the area of pain and pain control, especially in preterm infants.

Individual Temperament

Every infant is born with a unique temperament or style. Women who have been pregnant more than once may recognize these differences even before their babies are born. Mothers of twins often relate how differently the two babies acted during the pregnancy.

You may notice that your baby is more (or less) active than others in the nursery. You may observe that your baby favors a particular position. Your baby may prefer a pacifier, whereas the baby in the neighboring incubator may prefer her thumb. As you spend more time with your baby, you will become aware of her unique personality and methods for communicating likes and dislikes. To understand your baby's behavior, it helps to understand infant behavioral states and communication cues.

Behavioral States

All newborns experience six different levels of awareness. These are called behavioral states. Your baby's state influences how she responds to the environment. By learning to recognize these states, you can better understand your infant's behavior, know when to interact with your baby, and communicate effectively. Preterm babies exhibit the same behavioral states as other babies, but their behavioral states are not as clearly defined and their transitions from state to state are not as smooth or as predictable as those of term infants. The six states are deep sleep, light sleep, drowsy, quiet alert, active alert, and crying.[9,10]

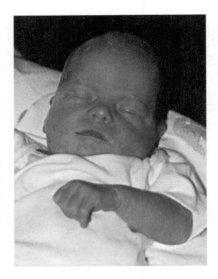

Deep sleep.

The baby is very difficult to awaken from deep sleep.

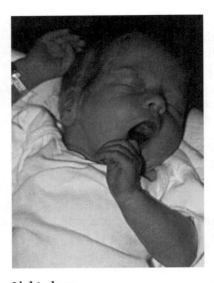

Light sleep.

The baby may move around, even fuss a little in this state, but she is not fully awake.

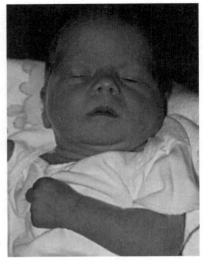

Drowsy.

The baby may open and close her eyes and move her arms and legs. By holding her upright and talking to her, you may be able to alert her. If left alone, she may go back to sleep.

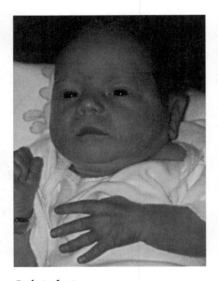

Quiet alert.

The baby "brightens" and focuses her attention on your face or voice. As your preterm baby matures, her quiet alert periods will increase.

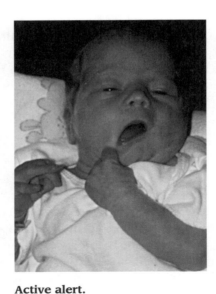

Active alert.

The baby is still alert but is easily distracted and unable to focus her attention. She may become fussy and overwhelmed. If you decrease stimulation, she may recover and return to a quiet alert state.

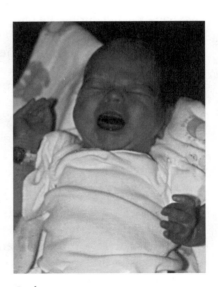

Crying.

The baby has had enough! She may calm down if held securely in quiet surroundings, given a pacifier or her fingers to suck on, or fed if she is hungry.

Deep Sleep

In deep sleep, your baby breathes regularly. The eyes are closed, with no noticeable eye movements. Your baby does not move spontaneously but may occasionally startle or jerk. While in deep sleep, your baby is difficult to arouse, is unable to respond to external stimuli, and does not participate in eating.

Light Sleep

In light sleep—also known as rapid eye movement (REM) sleep—your baby breathes irregularly. Her eyes remain closed, but eye movements can be seen beneath the lids. Some low-level activity as well as intermittent sucking movements are common in light sleep. Your baby may fuss during this state and, although not fully awake, can be awakened enough to feed. Most preterm babies spend most of their time in light sleep.

Drowsy

When in the drowsy state, your baby may open and shut her eyes, or her eyelids may flutter. She may move her arms and legs, and her breathing may become more rapid and shallow. If you speak to her or hold her in an upright position, your baby may move from drowsiness into the quiet alert state. If you leave your baby alone, she may go back to sleep.

Quiet Alert

In the quiet alert state, your baby has a "bright" look and is able to focus her attention. She does not move around much because she is paying attention to her surroundings. This is the ideal state for interacting with your baby, because she is receptive to stimulation.

Preterm babies can reach the quiet alert state, but often only for seconds. As your baby matures, her periods of quiet alertness will increase.

Active Alert

Your baby's activity increases in the active alert state. Reacting to external stimuli, she may startle and thrust her arms and legs. Her breathing is irregular, and she may or may not be fussy. During this state, your baby is unable to focus attention and has a decreased tolerance for continued stimulation. If you continue to speak to your baby or try to make eye contact, she may escalate to crying. Conversely, if you lower your voice or discontinue your interactions, she may return to the quiet alert state.

Crying

The crying state is just that—crying. Breathing is irregular, shallow, and rapid. Crying tells you that your baby can no longer cope with her surroundings.[4]

Infant Cues

Infants not only exhibit sleep-awake states, but also provide cues to help caregivers recognize their needs. For years, most infant behavior was assumed to be random and without meaning. Researchers now think that this

"I really wanted a response from my sleepy little baby! But the more we tried to get her to look at us or stay awake, the more sleepy and limp she became. Then we learned to be patient and watch for her cues—and she would slowly wake up and pay attention to us."

"random" behavior is meaningful and is an infant's means of communicating with the caregiver.

When you learn to recognize your baby's state, you will be able to choose appropriate times to interact, or "play," with your baby. Recognizing your baby's cues takes you one step further; it lets you interpret your infant's reaction to and tolerance for play. Your baby is unique and will respond to stimulation in her own way. She will be able to tell you when she has had enough and when it's time for more. Not all babies demonstrate the same behavioral cues; it is important to learn to recognize and interpret your baby's cues.

Invitation Cues

Invitation, or "ready," cues are the behaviors your baby demonstrates when she wants to interact. These cues say, in effect, "I'm ready. Let's do it!" Your baby usually shows invitation cues when in the quiet alert state.

Invitation cues include a relaxed appearance (especially of the arms and legs), a "bright" look, and regular, slow breathing. Some babies move their hands to their mouth.[11] Additional invitation cues include:[12]

- Having a stable pink color
- Moving head and limbs smoothly
- Maintaining position without squirming
- Being able to actively do things to keep self calm, such as bracing legs or feet against the bed
- Holding feet one on top of or next to the other
- Holding fingers or holding one hand in the other
- Sucking on fingers or fist
- Grasping blankets or a caregiver's fingers
- Curling up into a ball on one side
- Being able to use help offered by a caregiver to stay calm (using a pacifier, holding onto a caregiver's hands, looking at a face or an object)
- Enjoying being held; calming when held
- Focusing eyes; watching faces or objects
- Making an "ooh" face by pursing lips when looking at a face
- Trying to smile or coo
- Looking, listening, and following for sustained (but brief) periods of time

Stress Cues

Not only will babies tell you when they are ready to interact, but they will tell you when they have had enough. Infants show stress, or "take-a-break," cues when they have grown uncomfortable or are tired of stimulation. Sometimes these cues mean only that your baby needs a short break from the interaction; simply move your face or other stimulation out of view. At other times, your baby is telling you that the interaction is over, that she is ready to sleep or to be left alone. By carefully reading your baby's stress cues, you can

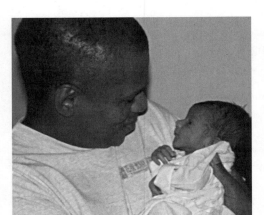

Invitation Cues.

This baby is in a quiet alert state and enjoys interaction with his father. The baby encourages his father to continue talking with him with invitation cues such as his bright expression, good eye contact, and relaxed hand position.

help her move to a lower state rather than escalate into the crying state. Stress cues include:[12]

- Changing breathing (increased rate, pauses, gasping for air)
- Changing color from pink to pale, white, or blue
- Hiccuping, gagging, or grunting
- Spitting up
- Straining as if to have a bowel movement
- Startling, tremoring, or twitching body, limbs, or face
- Coughing, sneezing, yawning, or sighing
- Squirming
- Having limp limbs, neck, face, or trunk
- Having stiff legs, arms, or fingers
- Sticking out tongue
- Arching back and neck
- Having a dull, tired, glassy-eyed appearance; staring; looking away; having a panicked or worried expression
- Crying weakly or being irritable
- Suddenly going to sleep or fussing
- Sleeping restlessly, with jerky movements or sounds, whimpering, or fussing
- Displaying frantic, ongoing, disorganized activity that your baby cannot control

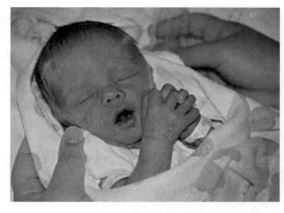

Self-comforting techniques.

By clasping his hands together and holding them near his face, this baby comforts himself and stays "organized" after feeding. When he opens his eyes, he may be able to sustain a quiet alert state and enjoy a quiet talk with his mother.

As you interact with your baby, you may begin to notice some of these stress cues. At first, after a brief rest, your infant may recover and invite more interaction. As your interaction continues, you may notice more and more stress cues, or you may see that your baby is not recovering as quickly after a break as she did earlier. At that point, your baby is telling you that it's time to stop interacting for now. If you continue stimulation, your baby may show physical signs of stress, such as apnea (breathing stops or pauses), bradycardia (low heart rate), cyanosis (blue coloring), or limpness.

Mixed Messages

Sometimes babies demonstrate a mixture of cues. For example, your baby may appear to be in the quiet alert state, ready to interact, yet at the same time be hiccuping. This mixture of cues can frustrate and confuse parents. Do you act on the invitation to interact, or do you stop what you are doing and give your baby a break?

If your baby is sending out mixed messages, look for other cues to help you decide whether to interact. For example, if your baby has sent out several invitation cues but then spits up, she may have just finished eating and needed to burp. Now that she has burped (which caused the spit-up), she is again ready for interaction. If, on the other hand, she burps and then begins to look pale and turns her gaze away from you, it's probably time for rest. It's important to look at the whole picture when interpreting cues.

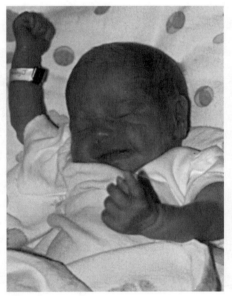

Stress cues.

This baby's closed eyes, frowning face, stiff arms, and squirming body are clear stress signals. If gently swaddled in a blanket and given a few moments of total quiet, she may settle down and recover a quieter state.

Playing with Your Baby

Now that you understand infant behavioral states and cues, it's time to put that knowledge to work. Play fosters your infant's development—it allows babies and children to learn. Although play is often seen as easy, natural, and requiring little thought, learning how to play with your baby may take some time. Initially, you may feel awkward, but as you become more familiar with your baby and see positive responses, you will look forward to your time together. Following are some pointers for a positive interaction.

Let Your Baby Take the Lead

To make the best use of your time with your baby, learn her cues by observing closely. Ask your baby's nurse to identify the cues she sees as she cares for your child. Notice what your baby is doing before any caregiving begins. Then observe your baby during and after caregiving. Discuss and compare your observations with the nurse.

Follow your baby's lead. If your baby is showing you ready signs, let her look at your face or hear your voice. *Introduce only one stimulus at a time* so your baby can concentrate and attend more effectively. Too many stimuli can overload your baby and lead to stress.

Introducing only one stimulus at a time takes practice. Speaking into a baby's face is instinctive for most of us, for example, but provides both auditory and visual stimulation. Speak to your baby first, then watch for the reaction. When your baby hears your voice, her eyes may brighten, and she may turn her head to find you. At that point, she is ready to see your face.

Positioning.

This father is trying to talk to his daughter, who is stressed and disorganized at this point. She waves her arms and has a panicked expression.

As the father gently holds the baby's arms and provides containment, she relaxes and focuses her attention on her father's face and voice.

Very premature babies or babies who are ill often cannot tolerate both seeing a face and hearing a voice or hearing a voice and being touched at the same time. They may respond rapidly with physical signs of stress. As these babies stabilize medically and grow, they learn to handle more stimulation.

In some units, each baby receives an Assessment of Preterm Infant Behavior (APIB), a formal behavioral evaluation by a specially trained nurse or developmental specialist.[13] This information, usually shared with parents, can give you a wealth of knowledge about your baby's developmental progress. An APIB evaluates how your baby reacts to stimulation and which cues she uses most often. The evaluation is usually repeated periodically to assess your baby's growing tolerance to stimulation and to identify activities that will foster development.

Use Nonnutritive Sucking

Another important developmental activity for your baby is nonnutritive sucking. This type of sucking does not provide nutrition; rather, your baby sucks on a pacifier, her finger or thumb, or your own clean finger. Nonnutritive sucking has been shown to increase weight gain, improve ability to handle feedings, and improve oxygenation. If your baby is being gavage fed (fed by tube), a pacifier may be provided during the feeding.

Help Your Baby with Positioning

Positioning is often used to help infants stay "organized" and focused. A preterm infant's muscle tone is different from that of a term infant. Term infants prefer to curl up in a flexed position. Because of their immaturity, preterm infants cannot flex their limbs and keep them flexed independently. If left to position themselves, preterm infants extend their arms and legs in a sprawling, froglike position.

Maintaining this extended posture for long periods can have serious bone, joint, and developmental consequences for a baby, such as increased neck extension with a right-sided head preference, problems with shoulder mobility, persistent arching of the neck and back, a tendency to assume a frog-leg position, and foot and ankle drop.[5] Proper positioning can help to prevent some of the problems associated with tone and posture. Flexing your baby forward and bringing her arms and legs to the center of her body makes it easier for her to focus and to discover consoling behaviors, such as finger- or hand-sucking. Body containment, by swaddling and nesting, helps your baby feel safe and secure and facilitates normal growth and development.

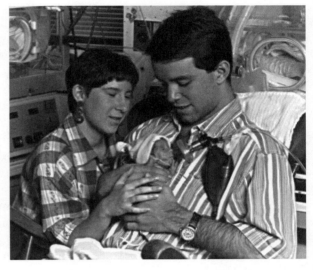

Kangaroo care.

Holding your baby skin-to-skin against your chest provides moments of closeness and belonging for parents and baby.

Ask About Kangaroo Care

You may be able to hold your special-care baby as soon as she is stable, and before she is ready to feed. If so, you may be interested in kangaroo care. Developed in South America as a way to keep premature infants warm so that they could be released early from overcrowded hospitals, kangaroo care was first described in the medical literature more than ten years ago. Mothers were instructed to hold their diaper-clad premature infants beneath their clothing, skin-to-skin, snuggled between their warm breasts.

The surprising benefits of kangaroo care for the infant include warmth, stability of heartbeat and breathing rate, increased time spent in the deep sleep and quiet alert states, decreased time spent crying, no increase in infections, increased weight gain, and increased incidence and duration of breastfeeding (see Chapter 5). Mothers who provide kangaroo care tend to have more success with lactation and a better milk supply.[14] These benefits are apparent even when kangaroo care occurs for only a few minutes each day.[15] Kangaroo care is still a new concept in many special-care nurseries, however. Talk to your baby's doctors and nurses about it.

Both mothers and fathers can give kangaroo care. Most special-care nurseries have screens that can be placed around your chair. If yours does not, simply wear a layer of clothing that opens down the front, and sit with your back to the room. Don't bother to dress your baby or wrap her in a blanket—all she needs is a diaper. You may notice that your infant tolerates these holding sessions much better when they are not preceded by undressing, diaper changing, temperature taking, dressing again, and swaddling in blankets. Snuggle your baby upright on your chest, or lay your baby with her head against your chest. What a nice pillow!

Don't be surprised if your baby roots for your nipple at the first opportunity. The rooting reflex is present around 32 weeks gestational age and gets stronger and more consistent by 36 to 37 weeks. You can see this reflex at work any time your baby's face is stroked. Her head will turn toward the stroking, and her mouth will open. You can provide a pacifier or, if you plan to breastfeed, let your baby nuzzle and lick your nipple. Even if a baby is clever enough to latch on to her mother's nipple, chances are she won't suck strongly or for very long. If you are worried that your baby may choke on your milk, you can hand-express or pump before you provide kangaroo care so that your breasts are relatively empty.

Kangaroo care is a nice way to get acquainted with your baby in the NICU. The feeling of your baby's warm skin against yours makes your baby "real" and confirms your parenthood. At a time when so many people are caring for your baby, kangaroo care provides special moments of belonging that only you can experience with your baby.

Growing With Your Baby

During your baby's stay in the NICU, you'll notice how she is growing—physically as well as developmentally. During that time, you as parents will grow as well. Each time you visit the NICU, you'll become increasingly familiar with the environment, the routine, the technology, and the staff. As your comfort level in the NICU increases, you'll become more at ease with your baby and her capabilities. Believe it or not, you'll soon be able to recognize your baby's unique language and respond appropriately to that language. During your early visits, this may seem an unreachable goal, but with patience and practice, you'll gain confidence and notice progress.

At times, you may feel extremely stressed or think that progress is at a standstill. At those times, especially, focus on the special moments you share with your baby. Celebrate accomplishments and "firsts"—the first time you hold your baby, the first bath you give, the first time you feed her. You may wish to capture these moments in a special baby book of photos and memories that mark progress during your baby's NICU stay. Those milestones are important for your baby and for you. Not only is your baby making progress, but with each milestone, you are growing as well.

Enjoy the special time you have with your baby. Although this is probably not the way you had imagined becoming acquainted, it can nevertheless be a memorable and special experience. You have come a long way, so try to relax, enjoy, and get to know this new little person you have created.

Chapter 5

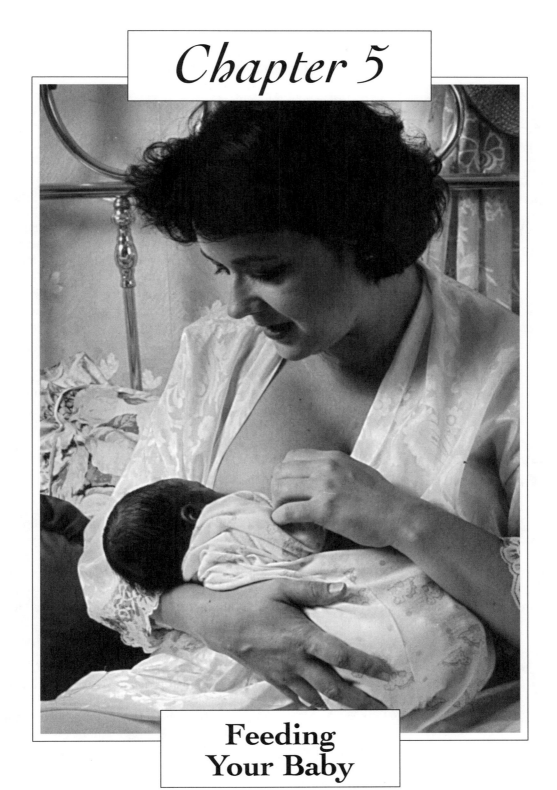

Feeding Your Baby

Ginna Wall, RN, MN, IBCLC

"Then Tigger looked up at the ceiling, and closed his eyes, and his tongue went round and round his chops, in case he had left any outside, and a peaceful smile came over his face as he said, "So *that's* what Tiggers like!""

Feeding your baby is an important parenting task and a satisfying activity you will want to share with your child. Although few NICU babies can feed directly from the breast or bottle until some time after birth, special-care infants still need nourishment. For a while they get it in different ways than healthy term infants do.

This chapter begins by explaining the special feeding approaches used early in your baby's NICU stay. It then takes a close look at a new mother's milk production and examines the differences between breast milk and formula. It goes on to teach you about techniques you can use to help your baby learn to feed—either from your breast or from a bottle.

With feeding, as with many other aspects of the NICU experience, parents need plenty of patience. But once you master the task of feeding your special-care baby, you'll find it one of the most satisfying activities you can share with your child.

Your Baby's First Feedings

You may be amazed at the strength with which your tiny newborn can suck on your finger or a pacifier shortly after birth. Your baby's ability to suck is incredible, but it doesn't mean he is ready to begin breast or bottle feedings.

Babies are able to suck long before they are able to coordinate the process of sucking, swallowing, and breathing. Babies who are born early are fed by gavage (tube) until they reach a gestational age of about 32 to 34 weeks and continue to receive supplemental gavage feedings for several weeks while they build skill at feeding from your breast or a bottle. Babies usually don't develop the strength and coordination they need to take all their feedings by suckling until they reach a gestational age of 36 or 37 weeks.

Nourishment through a Tube

For the first few hours after birth, your NICU baby will probably be kept "NPO"—that is, given nothing by mouth. Fluid and some nutrients will be fed directly into your baby's bloodstream through an IV line. After a few hours (or days, depending on your baby's status), your newborn will receive very small amounts of milk—either your breast milk or a formula. Most infants younger than 32 to 34 weeks cannot suck effectively.[1] They receive milk through a tube (called a gavage or feeding tube) inserted through the nose or mouth and advanced down into the stomach. A syringe of milk is attached to the end of the tube. The milk flows into the baby's stomach either by gravity or with the help of a small pump. Nurses watch for signs that your baby is tolerating the feedings (no vomiting, little or no milk left over in the stomach, a soft and undistended tummy, and no blood in the stools). As your baby becomes ready, he gradually gets larger amounts of milk. As the amount of milk is gradually increased, the amount of IV fluid is gradually decreased. When your baby is taking all the milk he needs for growth, he is said to be on "full feedings." At that point, he no longer needs the IV, except perhaps for medications.

Nourishment from the Breast or Bottle

Depending on your baby's gestational age and health status, he may be fed solely by gavage for several days, weeks, or even months. As he begins to develop the skills and reflexes necessary for nipple feeding, you will offer the breast or bottle for "practice." Most preterm infants are able to coordinate sucking on a nipple, swallowing milk, and remembering to breathe when they are about 32 weeks gestational age. Bottle feeding is a little trickier than breastfeeding because the milk from a bottle can flow more quickly than milk from a breast. Most preterm babies can begin to bottle feed when they are about 34 weeks gestational age.

When your baby is ready to "begin" to nipple feed, he will try the breast or bottle once, the nurse will evaluate the baby's ability to feed, and try another feeding later. Some feedings will go well; others will be more difficult. Learning to eat takes time—it doesn't happen overnight.

If you see your baby sucking on his fingers or a pacifier, you may wonder, "Why can't I just feed him? Why does he need those tube feedings?" Staff in the NICU know from experience that if you let a preterm baby less than 36 weeks gestational age try to get all his nourishment by breastfeeding or bottle feeding, he will soon become fatigued, lose weight, and have more difficulty staying warm as he uses all his energy to eat. This transition stage from gavage feeding to breast or bottle feeding is frustrating and requires patience as your baby learns and grows.

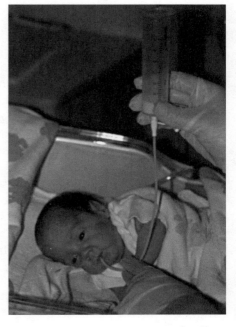

Gavage feeding.
A soft feeding tube goes through the baby's mouth and into his stomach during a gavage feeding. Ideally, the baby is given a pacifier to suck on during the feeding.

Meeting Special Nutritional Needs

Some babies are so small or sick that they cannot take in enough milk to meet their nutritional requirements. These babies need to continue to receive IV fluids with proteins, fats, and vitamins added until they are stable enough for oral feedings. This is called hyperalimentation, or total parenteral nutrition (TPN).

Preterm infants weighing less than about 1,500 grams (about 3 pounds) at birth run out of fat and carbohydrate fuel within a few days after birth and begin to use up vital body protein unless they receive adequate nutritional support.[2] For these babies, unfortified breast milk or standard infant formulas are not enough. These babies need extra nutrients to grow well, not only in weight, but in length and bone density. If you are breastfeeding, extra protein, calcium, and phosphorus will be added to your milk, either in a powder mixed into it or in equal volumes of breast milk and a liquid formula made especially for this purpose. Infants receiving formula are given specially designed preterm formulas that provide these extra nutrients. Extensive evidence shows improvement in growth and nutritional status when premature and/or sick babies receive fortified human milk, preterm infant formulas, or a combination of the two.

Glucose polymers (Polycose) and medium-chain triglyceride oil (MCT oil) may be added to breast milk or to preterm formula to provide extra energy. Glucose polymers contain sugars in a form that immature preterm newborns can easily digest and absorb. The fats in MCT oil are well absorbed and can be digested without the enzymes and bile salts these infants lack. Both provide extra calories. As your baby grows, a vitamin and mineral supplement may also be added to the diet.

Your baby's weight will probably be measured every day and plotted on a chart. To get a full nutritional picture, the NICU staff assess your baby's length, weight, head circumference, and fluid, vitamin, mineral, and protein status. Your baby's diet will change to promote optimal growth in all these areas. (Chapter 9 explains more about ways in which the nutritional needs of NICU infants are met in the early days of life.)

Breastfeeding Basics

If you have just given birth to a sick or premature baby, you may be thinking that you can't breastfeed your newborn. Take heart, because in most cases, you'll be able to feed your breast milk to your baby until he is able to suckle. In most cases, breastfeeding is the best choice for your baby and for you. Your milk is perfectly suited to nourish your baby and to provide protection from infections, allergies, and other diseases. Nothing that scientists can create in a laboratory from cow's milk or soybeans can compare with human milk. Providing breast milk to a special-care baby is a challenge, but, looking back, many NICU parents feel the advantages were worth the extra trouble.

Benefits of Breast Milk and Breastfeeding

All babies benefit from their mother's breast milk. The nutrients (protein, carbohydrates, fats, vitamins, and minerals) in human milk are present in the perfect proportions for a human baby. The proteins are made up of just the right amino acids, and the fats are a unique blend of cholesterol, omega-3 fatty acids, and other essential fats that are important for brain growth and development. All these nutrients are in forms that your baby can absorb more easily than the nutrients in breast milk substitutes made from cow's milk or soybeans.[3]

But there's more than just good nutrition in human milk. It is literally alive with cells that fight germs that can cause infections in your baby. Human milk has components in it that encourage the growth of beneficial bacteria (such as *Lactobacillus bifidus*) in your baby's stomach and intestines and inhibit the growth of harmful bacteria (such as *E. coli*). It also contains enzymes that enhance your baby's digestion and make it easier for his body to use the nutrients present in milk. Most important, breast milk contains hormones and growth factors that promote optimal growth in human infants. Scientists have isolated more than 100 of these and other beneficial components in human milk—all of which are missing from infant formulas.

Many studies show that babies who are formula fed have more ear infections, respiratory tract infections, urinary tract infections, diarrhea, and allergies than breastfed babies do.[4] Their illnesses also tend to be more severe—more likely to result in hospitalization. Breast milk confers benefits that last long after a child is weaned. Children who were breastfed as infants are less likely to have dental problems (such as decay and improper bite), juvenile-onset diabetes, certain forms of cancer, and diseases of the colon (such as ulcerative colitis).[4–8]

Another advantage of breastfeeding is that it guarantees that your baby will get the warmth and physical closeness of skin-to-skin contact when he is ready to nurse. You are probably keenly aware that the amount of time you can spend holding, rocking, and cuddling your baby is limited because he is in the intensive care nursery. As soon as your baby is ready to breastfeed, you'll get to hold your newborn against your body.[9] If you bottle feed, you can make an effort to hold your baby skin-to-skin—but when you breastfeed, you automatically have that contact at every feeding.

Advantages of Breast Milk for Preterm Infants

In the last three months of pregnancy, large protein molecules called immunoglobulins cross the placenta and are stored in the growing fetus. These immunoglobulins protect a newborn against the infections that the mother is immune to—for up to five or six months after birth. Although a premature infant misses out on some of this special protection because of the timing of birth, you can still provide your premature baby with immunoglobulins through breast milk. The milk you produce in the first few days after giving birth has the highest concentration of immunoglobulins, but you continue to give your baby extra immunoglobulins for as long as you give him your breast milk.

Human milk is important for the optimal growth and development of full-term babies, but it is even more important for babies born prematurely. If your baby is preterm, his stomach and intestines (which the NICU staff will refer to as his gastrointestinal tract, GI tract, or gut) are even smaller and less mature than the tiny, immature gut of a full-term baby.

In fact, for the first few weeks after birth, your milk will be different from the milk of a mother who gives birth at term. Your body knows that your baby came early, and it provides a milk that is better for the baby's needs. For the first two to four weeks after birth, your milk will contain more protein, fat calories, calcium, phosphorus, magnesium, zinc, sodium, and chloride than full-term milk.[10] This early milk also has a laxative effect on your baby's bowels, helping him to pass the first stools (called meconium). Stooling is an important sign that the GI tract is working; it also helps resolve jaundice (see Chapter 9). Nurses notice that babies fed their mother's milk tolerate feedings better. Human milk is easy to digest, with very little left over in the baby's

"Sticking to your decision to breastfeed is tough when your baby is in the NICU. It really helped me to talk to a mother who had been pumping for eight weeks. It can be done."

stomach. Because formula forms larger curds than breast milk, babies given formula commonly have undigested milk in their stomach two to three hours after feeding.

Researchers have not yet identified a sole cause for necrotizing enterocolitis (NEC), a serious bowel disease that most often affects preterm babies (see Chapter 10). One study, however, showed that preterm babies who were fed formula developed the disease more often than babies fed human milk.[11] Studies are continuing regarding causitive factors of NEC and possible ways to prevent this disease.

Brain growth and development is rapid in the final three months of gestation and continues well into the second year of postnatal life. Several studies have suggested that breastfeeding improves mental development.[12]

Although breastfeeding requires skill and maturity on your baby's part, it can be less stressful than bottle feeding. Possible difficulties of bottle feeding (because of the fast flow of milk from a bottle) are so common that doctors and nurses have come to think of them as "normal" responses to feeding: irregular or absent breathing (apnea) with a resulting drop in oxygen, slowed beating of the heart (bradycardia), and blue skin color (cyanosis). Paula Meier, a nurse researcher who has studied the feeding behaviors of premature infants for many years, discovered that breastfeeding is less stressful than bottle feeding because the baby can "pace" the feeding, controlling the flow of milk and pausing when necessary.[13] Meier's research shows that, during breastfeeding, a baby stays warm, his heart rate remains regular, and oxygen levels stabilize (or even improve). She recommends that healthy preterm babies begin breastfeeding at 32 weeks gestational age but not begin bottle feeding until 34 weeks gestational age.

Advantages for Mothers

Breastfeeding has decided advantages for the mother, too. It causes your uterus to contract, decreasing the chance of postpartum hemorrhage (bleeding). Breastfeeding delays the return of your menstrual periods for several months after childbirth—which allows your body to rebuild its store of iron and is a nice convenience. It also has a contraceptive effect.[14] If you are exclusively breastfeeding (feeding or expressing your milk every couple of hours around the clock), have had no vaginal bleeding after the 56th postpartum day, and are less than six months postpartum, your risk of getting pregnant is only 2 percent in the first six months of breastfeeding. Pregnancy can occur, however, so don't depend on breastfeeding as a primary method of birth control if family planning is important to you.

Breastfeeding also burns calories—an estimated 600 to 900 calories to produce a liter of breast milk per day, or the equivalent of playing basketball for an hour and a half. Studies have shown that breastfeeding women have a smaller hip circumference at six months postpartum than bottle feeding women.[15]

Women who breastfeed may have a lower incidence of breast cancer and ovarian cancer. One study showed that women who breastfed for more than two years had a 43 percent lower risk of breast cancer than women who had never breastfed.[16]

But most NICU moms say that the best thing about breastfeeding is that it is something they (and they alone) can do for their baby. When your baby's survival depends to a great degree on the expertise of doctors and nurses, you may feel insignificant—as if your role doesn't matter. When you bring your breast milk to the NICU, you declare loudly and clearly that you are your baby's mother. You know you are making an important and tangible contribution to your baby's well-being. You feel confident that your baby needs you.

Breastfeeding also restores a sense of normalcy to your birth experience. One mother said, "I never got to wear pretty maternity dresses or go to childbirth classes. Then when the baby was born, I didn't get to hold her right away or room-in like the other mothers on the maternity unit. But at least I could breastfeed. It's the one thing I could do right."

So, although it may be challenging to provide breast milk for your special-care baby, consider the good feelings it can provide:

- Reassurance of your role as the baby's mother
- A sense of normalcy about the pregnancy and birth
- The satisfaction of providing something tangible for your baby
- The knowledge that you are important to your baby's health and survival
- The joy that comes from providing some physical comfort to your baby
- More confidence when it's time to take your baby home
- Pride in accomplishing something worthwhile

When Not to Breastfeed

In some situations, it may not be safe to provide breast milk for your newborn. Mothers with certain infections or those whose milk may contain specific prescription medications or nonprescription drugs should not provide breast milk. In rare instances, jaundice in your newborn can be a reason to temporarily stop breastfeeding.

Maternal Infections

A few infections can be transmitted to your baby through your breast milk. The main ones you should know about are these:[17]

- **Human immunodeficiency virus:** The Centers for Disease Control recommend that women who test positive for HIV use formula instead of giving their breast milk to their babies.
- **Cytomegalovirus:** Almost half of all adults test positive for cytomegalovirus (CMV). This virus is shed in the pharynx, urine, genital tract, and breast milk. In theory, infants who are born very early could become infected by breast milk from a CMV-positive mother because they did not receive the transplacental immunity the mother would have conferred to them in the final three months of the pregnancy. Most NICUs do not screen for CMV, however, nor do they restrict CMV-positive mothers from providing breast

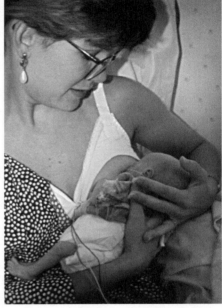

Breastfeeding.
This very small baby (actually born at 29 weeks gestation and 6 weeks old here) breastfeeds well for short periods of time. Her mother pumps breast milk for the baby's supplemental gavage feedings.

milk. If you know you are CMV-positive and your baby was born before 28 weeks gestation, ask your baby's doctor for advice.

- **Herpes:** Some women get recurrent herpes lesions on their breasts. Just like the virus that causes cold sores on the lips (herpes type 1) or genital herpes (herpes type 2), the virus that causes these sores can be life-threatening for newborns. If you have a herpes sore on your breast, discard the milk from that side and don't breastfeed on that side until the sore is completely healed. Also note that the herpes virus is shed before the appearance of a sore; you may wish to weigh the risk and benefits of breastfeeding in this situation. Ask your lactation specialist and physician for advice. Some women who experience recurrent herpes on one breast will choose to nurse their baby only from the unaffected breast. Although this takes more planning on the mother's part, the baby can usually breastfeed successfully from one breast.

- **Breast infection:** If you develop fever, chills, and flulike symptoms, along with a hot, red, tender area on your breast, you probably have a breast infection (called mastitis). You'll be given an antibiotic to treat the infection. Under ordinary circumstances, women with mastitis should continue to breastfeed; the baby probably has the germ in his mouth already. In fact, the baby probably brought the germ to the mother's breast. In the special-care nursery, if your baby has not yet suckled at your breast, it's probably a good idea to discard the milk from the infected breast(s) until the antibiotic starts to work and you feel better.[18] Although you should discard your milk, continue to pump your breasts so you can resume breastfeeding as soon as the infection clears up.

Drugs

Always tell your baby's nurse or doctor about any medications you are taking. Usually, the benefits of breast milk outweigh the risk of a trace of prescription drug in your breast milk, but a few medications are considered unsafe during lactation. Others, although safe, may cause symptoms in your baby; the staff needs to know to watch for these symptoms.

Don't forget to mention substances such as alcohol, tobacco, street drugs, and over-the-counter drugs. Alcohol and all street drugs pass through to your breast milk and can have tragic side effects. Seek professional help for your alcohol and/or drug-use problem, and protect your baby from affected breast milk.

Breast Milk Jaundice

You may also need to stop providing milk or breastfeeding temporarily because of jaundice. Some babies have such high blood levels of the substance bilirubin that the doctor may recommend discontinuing breastfeeding for a day or two. In very rare cases, the bilirubin level comes down with this treatment. This does not mean that anything is wrong with your milk; you can resume breastfeeding without fear as soon as the baby's bilirubin level drops to normal. Chapter 9 contains more information on physiologic jaundice, which is different than breast milk jaundice.

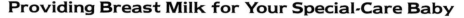

Providing Breast Milk for Your Special-Care Baby

Every family has a lot to think about after labor and birth are over. You'll receive an overwhelming amount of information. Amid all the excitement, if you have decided to breastfeed, be sure to tell your nurse and the NICU nurse.

Providing breast milk for your special-care baby means expressing milk from your breasts every two to three hours. Experts don't agree on the number of times per day a mother should express her milk.[18-21] Most NICUs recommend that you express your milk at least six times per day, and preferably more. Pumping both breasts simultaneously (which requires a double pump setup) with a hospital-quality electric pump usually takes only 10 to 20 minutes (15 minutes average). Short, frequent pumping sessions are necessary to keep up your milk supply.

How the Breasts Make Milk

To appreciate the importance of emptying your breasts frequently and completely, it helps to have an understanding of how the breasts work.

By week 16 of pregnancy, your breasts start producing a thick, clear or yellow-gold secretion called colostrum. Within two or three days after you give birth, the colostrum begins to change to a thinner, whiter milk called mature milk. The amount of milk your breasts produce also increases dramatically at this time, and you may notice that your breasts are swollen hard and painful. This happens as a result of the hormonal changes that accompany birth—whether your baby is born early or on time and whether you breastfeed or not.

When a baby sucks (or a pump exerts suction) on your nipple, it signals your brain to release two hormones: prolactin and oxytocin.

Prolactin causes the milk glands in your breasts to start secreting milk. You may notice a side effect of sleepiness or peacefulness when prolactin is released into your bloodstream.

The other hormone, oxytocin, may be familiar to you as the hormone of labor. Just as it causes the muscles of the uterus to contract, it also causes contractions of tiny muscles that surround the milk glands in your breasts. These contractions squeeze the milk down into small reservoirs just behind the nipples. This is called the milk-ejection reflex, or the let-down reflex. An early sign that this is occurring may be menstrual-like cramps in your uterus. You'll notice these cramps only in the first week or two after birth, and you may not notice them at all if this is your first baby. After a week or so, you may notice a feeling of thirst a few minutes after you begin to pump, a gripping sensation or a sensation of "pins and needles" in your breasts, or milk dripping from your nipples. After pumping, you may notice distinct softening of your breasts (like deflated balloons). These are all reassuring signs that the oxytocin-induced milk-ejection reflex has occurred.

Prolactin is released every time your nipples are stimulated and only when your nipples are stimulated. Nothing else signals your body to make and keep on making milk. Oxytocin is released in response to sucking, but it can be released in response to other stimuli, too—such as sitting in the same chair to

"My pregnancy was difficult. My baby's birth was complicated and frightening. Thank goodness my body made breast milk perfectly."

nurse or to pump your breasts, hearing the sound of the pump, or just relaxing. This is called a conditioned response.

What to Expect in the First Few Days

Soon after you give birth, your nurse will bring a breast pump to your room. (If your medical condition allows, ask for it by six hours after birth.) She'll show you how to hold the milk-collecting cups up to your breasts and turn on the pump. Many mothers laugh about feeling "like a dairy cow." You may feel awkward and embarrassed—and possibly discouraged when only a drop or two of milk appears on your nipple. But every drop is precious. Try to save whatever you can in a small container. The volume of your baby's first feeding is very small, perhaps only 1–2 milliliters (ml) (about ⅕–⅖ tsp).

Practice pumping every three hours, even if little milk comes out. Your milk supply will increase dramatically by the third to fifth day, and for a few days you may need to pump more often to keep up with the production. Don't worry about producing too much milk; it's much easier to reduce a plentiful milk supply than to build up one that's flagging.

In the first few hours after giving birth, especially with everything that is happening with your baby, trying to learn about expressing and storing your milk may feel overwhelming. Admittedly, this is not the best time to take in new information. Don't be ashamed to ask the same questions over and over again. Watch videos if they are available, and ask for written materials that you can take home with you. Arrange to have a family member or friend in the room when the nurse or lactation consultant is explaining everything; chances are that between you, you'll remember the important points.

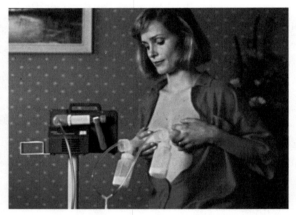

Using the breast pump.

A double breast pump expresses milk from both breasts at the same time. This not only saves time pumping, but produces more milk than if the mother pumps each breast separately. (Courtesy of Medela, Inc., McHenry, Illinois.)

Learning about the Breast Pump

If your baby were going home with you, he would be breastfeeding around the clock. Your baby would fuss every hour or two and stop crying when put to your breast. You'd feel proud of your ability to console him. If your baby slept longer than three or four hours, your breasts would begin to swell with milk—you'd literally ache to nurse and feel welcome relief when that happened. These events, repeated over and over again—more than a hundred times in the first two weeks after birth—soon condition not only a fast and easy milk-ejection response, but also a feeling of pleasure, joy, and great contentment in the process of feeding your baby.

Breast pumping is not like that. Your baby doesn't cry or fuss to tell you it's time to pump. The satisfaction of knowing that you can console your baby, the physical pleasure and pride as your baby nurses at your breast—all are missing. The pump may give you physical relief if your breasts are overly full, but soon even *that* feeling goes away as the early postpartum engorgement subsides.

When you first learn how often you'll need to pump, you may think that it will be too much trouble. Keep in mind that very young babies suckle frequently, on demand, 10 to 14 times a day. If you pump infrequently or skip a pumping here and there, your milk supply will dwindle. This usually results in feelings of discouragement and failure.

The cost of renting an electric breast pump—from $1.00 to $2.50 per day—may also be a concern. At a time when you are rightfully concerned about medical bills, eliminating the breast pump may seem like one way to cut costs. Keep in mind, though, that formula costs more and will be necessary through-out the first year. Also check to see if insurance or Medicaid will cover the cost of breast pump rental.

If pumping seems like too much trouble, try to focus on why you are expressing your milk. You are pumping not only to give your baby your milk now but also to preserve your ability to make milk until your baby is ready to breastfeed. Make this your goal. Remind yourself of the long-term benefits for you and your baby. Talk to other breastfeeding mothers in the special-care nursery. Ask your baby's nurse if there is a parent support group, or call one of the national support groups listed in Appendix D. If you are lucky enough to have a lactation consultant at your hospital, she can give you the support you need. Breast pumping requires commitment on your part and encouragement from the people around you. Remember: *It is worth it*.

Using the Electric Pump at Home

To establish and maintain a milk supply, you really can't depend on small, hand-operated or battery-powered pumps. Only hospital-quality, fully automatic electric breast pumps are adequate for the job (brands include Medela [800-TELL-YOU] and Ameda-Egnell [800-323-8750]). These pumps empty both breasts at the same time. This not only saves time but also increases your pro-lactin levels. To use a pump of this sort, you hold two plastic, funnel-shaped cups over your breasts, and the pump automatically collects your milk in bottles or bags attached to the cups. These collection kits are attached to the pump by tubing. The pump has an on/off switch and a dial for adjusting the suction.

How Long and How Often to Pump

The guidelines that follow are general ones. Your NICU may have slightly different or more detailed rules. Your nurse or the lactation specialist should be able to answer your questions.

In the beginning, before your milk supply is established, you'll need to pump for about five minutes. Once your milk supply is established, you can use the flow of milk as your guide: Pump until the flow slows down or stops. If you are trying to increase your milk supply, pump more often—not longer. It's much more effective to pump every three hours for 10 to 20 minutes than to pump for a longer time but at wider intervals. Whether to pump during the night depends on several things: Are you awake anyway? Are you trying to build your milk supply? Is your baby coming home soon? An answer of yes to any of these questions is a good reason to pump at night. If you decide that uninterrupted sleep is more important than pumping, don't let more than eight hours go by without emptying your breasts, and pump at least six times during your waking hours.

Keeping Milk and Equipment Clean

Breast milk is not sterile; the bacteria in the milk probably help the development of beneficial microorganisms in a healthy newborn. Before your NICU baby receives your milk, however, it will have been expressed, stored, exposed to light, handled by nurses, and sent through feeding tubes, so it makes sense to be extra careful about keeping it clean. The best way to keep your breast milk safe and clean is to wash your hands before you pump. Washing your nipples before pumping also decreases the bacterial count in breast milk and doesn't appear to cause skin irritation.[22] Most NICUs don't require it, however.

Only those parts of the pump that actually come in contact with your milk require cleaning after each use. Rinse them well in cold water, wash them with hot, soapy water, and rinse again—or wash them in the dishwasher. Many special-care nurseries ask you to sterilize your breast pump parts once each day. Sterilize by boiling them in water for at least five minutes. Allow clean pump parts to air dry, touch only the outside of the parts, and store them in a clean, covered container between uses.

Storing and Labeling Your Milk

Your hospital may provide a supply of sterilized containers for storing and transporting your milk. They may be glass or hard plastic containers or plastic bags. Each medium has its advantages and disadvantages, but all are safe for storing human milk.

Immediately after pumping, label the container with your baby's name and the date and time you pumped the milk. If there is another baby on the unit with a last name similar to yours, be extra careful with labeling. Ask the NICU staff for "name alert" stickers, and add your baby's hospital number to the label. If you are thawing frozen milk, also write on the label the date and time that you took the container out of the freezer.

Several studies have been done on the effects of various methods of storing human milk, but more research is needed. You may get conflicting advice about storage. A general rule is that the longer breast milk is stored, the more nutrients and immunologic properties it loses. Some NICUs are more conservative than others in trying to preserve and protect milk quality. Most allow breast milk to be stored in the refrigerator for at least 48 hours and in the freezer for at least three months.[23] For older babies, it's probably safe to hold milk for up to five days in the refrigerator and six months in the freezer.[24] Once frozen milk is thawed, most NICUs like to use it within 24 hours. Be sure to consider the quality of your refrigerator/freezer: How cold is it? Do frozen foods stay frozen hard? How often is the door opened?

Transporting Your Milk to the Hospital

To take your milk to the hospital, pack it in a small cooler or an insulated bag. If you must transport frozen milk a long distance (requiring several hours out of the freezer), pack it in dry ice in a sturdy, insulated container. You may wish to ask your nurse for advice on transporting milk safely.

Learning to Breastfeed

At about 32 weeks gestational age, preterm babies begin to develop the ability to take the nipple into their mouth, suck effectively, and swallow breast milk without interference with breathing.[1] As your NICU baby approaches this age, keep your expectations in line. Although your 32-weeker may nurse well once, he probably won't be able to do it again for at least another day. Also keep in mind that 32 weeks is the earliest age at which babies are capable of breastfeeding. If your baby has health problems or other complications, the first feeding at your breast may have to be delayed.

An excellent way to prepare for breastfeeding is to hold your baby skin-to-skin. This practice, called kangaroo care, is simple, safe, and beneficial for preterm babies (see Chapter 4). It is especially beneficial for breastfeeding mothers and babies. Its benefits are documented in the medical literature; however, it is still a new concept in most NICUs.[9] If your baby is stable enough to be held in your arms, he can (and should, if you're planning to breastfeed) be held skin-to-skin. Ask for this opportunity if the staff doesn't suggest it.

For as little as 20 minutes a day, or as much as several hours a day, you can snuggle your baby against your chest. You wear clothing that opens in the front, and your baby wears only a diaper. Warm blankets can be draped over the two of you. In experiments comparing mothers and babies who were given the opportunity to use kangaroo care with mothers and babies who were not offered this opportunity, the effects of kangaroo care on breastfeeding were dramatic:[9]

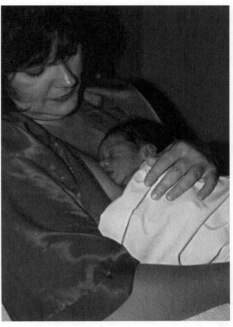

Kangaroo care for mothers and babies.

Snuggling your baby skin-to-skin increases your milk production and provides special moments of intimacy for you and your baby.

- Breastfeeding incidence is increased by at least 25 percent and up to 50 percent
- Mothers' average daily milk production is higher
- Mothers and babies breastfeed more often per day
- Mothers and babies breastfeed for more weeks' duration

Getting comfortable enough to breastfeed in an intensive care setting is not easy. Nursing amid bright lights and alarms sounding and with strangers milling about takes getting used to. Give yourself lots of time to learn to relax. You may find that one chair fits you better than the others and that it helps to rest your feet on a small footstool. Experiment with pillows: One on your lap usually helps. There are special U-shaped pillows designed for feeding twins simultaneously.

While you and your baby are learning to breastfeed, keep pumping your breasts on your regular routine. Many mothers think they should skip pumping on the days they feed their babies. They want to be sure to have plenty of milk for the baby. What happens instead is that they arrive in the NICU with engorged breasts and nipples that are hard to compress—and, later, their milk supply decreases. Instead, try pumping or massaging your breasts for a few minutes right before the feeding. This not only softens your nipples and makes it easier for the baby to latch on, but also stimulates your milk-ejection reflex.

Positioning Your Baby and Your Breast

A breastfeeding position that works especially well for preterm babies is the cross-cradle hold. Lay your baby on the pillow, on his side facing you, with his mouth right beside your nipple. Add pillows to bring the baby's mouth to the level of your nipple rather than trying to lift or lower your breast. Encircle your baby's body with the arm opposite the breast that your baby is about to nurse from, and grasp the back of the baby's head in your hand. With the same-side hand (left hand on left breast, for example), cup your breast and present the nipple to your baby. Place your four fingers underneath and your thumb on top of your breast.

Compressing Your Breast

With your fingers cupping your breast, you can shape your areola (the dark area around the nipple) to fit your baby's mouth. Although the mouth forms a circle when open wide, as soon as it clamps onto your nipple, the lips and gums form a flattened oval. If you compress your breast in that same oval shape, your baby is likely to be able to suck longer. Consider this technique especially if your baby latches onto your nipple just fine and sucks three or four times but then quits. If the concept seems hard to understand, think about how you squeeze a very thick sandwich just before you take a bite or how you turn an oval peg to fit it into an oval hole. Be sure that your thumb is parallel to your baby's upper lip and your index finger is parallel to your baby's lower lip. Some mothers find a U-shaped hold works better than a C-shaped hold. To do this, slide your fingers toward the center of your body and your thumb toward the outside of your breast. Your nurse or lactation consultant can help you with positioning.

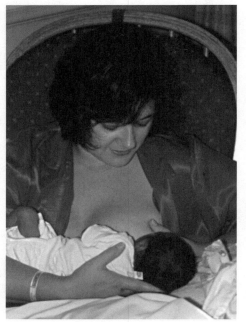

Positioning for breastfeeding.

This position works well for breastfeeding a preterm baby. Support his head with the hand opposite the breast that he is about to nurse from. With the hand on the same side as the breast he is to nurse from, cup your breast and present the nipple to the baby.

Tickling Your Baby's Lower Lip

It's important to learn this next step so that you can use it when your baby is mature enough to respond, but it rarely works before 34 to 36 weeks gestation.[1] The idea is to get your baby to open his mouth. To do this, stroke the center of your baby's lower lip with the tip of your nipple. Brush your nipple lightly, delicately, and repeatedly over the lower lip, as if giving a signal. When your baby is older and more experienced, this technique will be a powerful cue: Your baby will open his mouth wide. Then, with a quick movement of the arm encircling your baby, you'll pull him onto your breast. When you are both learning about feeding, though, your baby will probably just lie there. The lactation specialist can hold the infant's chin down with a finger or help to shape your nipple and aim it toward the roof of your baby's mouth.

Bringing Your Baby onto Your Breast

With one hand shaping your areola and the other hand holding your baby's head, you are in a perfect position to bring your baby onto your breast. As you do so, aim your nipple up toward the roof of the baby's mouth. This helps ensure that you get your nipple above your baby's tongue. Pull him in so close that the tip of his nose touches your breast. Continue to compress your breast throughout the *entire* feeding. You'll notice that your hand gets tired. That hints at why this technique works so well with premature babies: It probably keeps the tiny muscles around the mouth from getting fatigued.

Making Sure Your Baby Is Latched On

You can tell that your baby is well latched on by looking for these signs:

- A wide-open mouth with lips spread out around your breast
- Your baby's mouth covers all of your nipple and some of the areola
- A firm tug on your breast every time your baby sucks
- Your baby's ability to suckle for more than three or four sucks in a row
- Your baby's ability to hang on to your nipple during pauses between bursts of sucks

Determining Your Baby's Intake

Once your baby is latched on well, he will suck in small, quick bursts until your milk begins to flow. Then the sucking pattern will change to slower, deeper, more rhythmic sucks. If the NICU is quiet enough, you may be able to hear your baby swallow. This is a sure sign that he is getting milk.

When you first begin to breastfeed, your milk-ejection reflex may not occur until after your baby has tired of sucking and fallen asleep. But, just as your body became conditioned to respond to the breast pump, you will learn to respond to your baby's suck. One clever mother brought the breast pump to her baby's bedside for the first few feedings: She knew that her milk would let down as soon as she heard the sound of the pump.

You can assess how well the breastfeeding is going by counting the number of sucks and listening for the swallowing sounds. Every baby has a unique "suck signature." You will soon learn your baby's. Maybe your baby always sucks ten times in a row and then pauses. In general, the more sucks a baby takes before pausing, the more milk he is taking. Also, if your baby swallows with every suck, he is obviously getting lots of milk.

After a few minutes of sustained, rhythmic sucks, your baby will revert to bursts of little sucks with long pauses in between. The swallowing sounds will be further and further apart. It's time to take your baby off your breast (few mothers need to break the suction with a preterm baby), burp him, and switch to the other breast. On the second side, watch again for the sucking pattern to slow down and swallowing to become less frequent. You can take your baby off the breast and switch him back and forth as many times as necessary to arouse him to take more milk.

During early feedings, some babies may not be able to tolerate this "burp and switch" technique. They'll do better if you let them nurse on only one breast at a feeding. To encourage your baby to stay awake, you can gently massage your breast when the sucking pattern slows down. Breastfeeding on only one side at a feeding may also improve your baby's weight gain, because the milk that comes at the end of the feeding (called hindmilk) is higher in fat and calories than the first milk. This is good to remember if you're producing much more milk than your baby can take at one feeding. In fact, if your baby is having trouble gaining weight, you may want to pump before nursing and freeze the thinner "foremilk" for later feedings. One-sided nursing is also a good approach if it takes a long time (ten or more minutes) to get your baby latched on. If you interrupt the baby's suction to switch sides, you may be back to square one. It's better for your baby to nurse well on one breast than to nurse ineffectively on both.

"When my baby could finally try to breastfeed, a light came on between us. Pumping was easier after that because I knew we were going to make it."

The only accurate way to determine how much milk your baby is getting is to weigh the baby on an electronic scale before and after feeding.[25] When you feel confident that your baby is getting milk and you'd like these breastfeeding sessions to "count," you can ask the nurse to help you weigh the baby before your next feeding session. Then breastfeed until the baby's sucking and swallowing slows down, and put the baby back on the scale without changing his diaper or clothes. Each gram of weight gain is equal to approximately 1 milliliter of milk. If your baby took very little milk (less than half the amount needed), the nurse will need to supplement the breastfeeding with a gavage feeding. In time, the amount your baby takes will gradually increase until he is taking all he needs from your breast.

At first, you will be able to breastfeed only once or twice a day. Few babies under 36 to 37 weeks are able to suck more than this. They become tired and begin to lose weight if you push them to suckle more than they are developmentally capable of doing. Your baby's other feedings will be by gavage. Continue to pump immediately after each nursing until supplemental feedings are not necessary. Although it's tempting to say, "I breastfed the baby, so I don't need to pump," if you don't keep pumping after every breastfeeding, you'll risk losing your milk supply.

As your baby matures, he will start to wake up and show signs that it's time for a feeding. At that point, gavage feeding is no longer appropriate. If you have been breastfeeding for a few days, bottle feeding by the nursing staff when your baby is awake and hungry but you are not there does not usually cause a problem with breastfeeding success.

Sometimes NICU parents and staff worry about nipple confusion, in which a baby develops difficulty with breastfeeding after exposure to bottles. To avoid giving bottles to breastfeeding babies, some nurseries use techniques such as finger feeding or cup feeding. With finger feeding, the baby is encouraged to suck on a clean, gloved finger (nail bed down, pad up toward the roof of the baby's mouth), and a feeding tube is slipped into the baby's mouth along with the caregiver's finger.[26] With cup feeding, the baby is held upright, and small amounts of milk are placed on the baby's tongue with a small cup or spoon.[27] (Medela makes a soft cup-feeding device that fits on a standard infant feeding bottle, especially for this purpose.) Although finger feeding and cup feeding preterm infants are methods commonly used in developing countries, few NICUs in the United States consider them as options. These methods have not been carefully researched, and it has not been proven that they enhance breastfeeding success, but many mothers and breastfeeding specialists who have tried these methods believe that they do help prevent nipple confusion.

Because bottles are a routine part of a breastfed baby's care in most NICUs, observe for difficulties with breastfeeding after bottles are introduced. If you notice that breastfeedings aren't going as well now that your baby is being bottle fed, your best alternative is to spend more time at the hospital so that you can be there for most of his feedings. If this is impossible and you'd like to try finger feeding or cup feeding, discuss it with your baby's nurse or doctor.

Solving Breastfeeding Problems

Breastfeeding is not easy for everyone and can be especially challenging for NICU mothers and babies. Give yourself time to learn, and ask for help when you encounter problems.

Baby Cannot Latch On

If you can't get your baby latched on to your breast, ask for help. Your baby may be turning his head to reach your nipple, or the weight of your breast may be pulling the nipple out of your baby's mouth. Another position might work better (a football hold, for example, with the baby tucked under your arm at your side). An extra pair of helping hands, from a knowledgeable nurse or a lactation specialist, can help you through the awkwardness of learning what works for you and your baby.

Perhaps your baby is holding his tongue against the roof of his mouth. First check to be sure that your baby's head and neck are well supported. Then let your baby suck on your clean or gloved finger for a few minutes before feeding. Gently stroke the roof of his mouth several times to elicit the sucking reflex. Let your baby suck on your finger until the suck becomes rhythmical. The baby's tongue will drop down, and its sides will cup around your finger, forming a channel, or "trough," for your finger to lie in. This technique works like warming up a pitcher in a bullpen. It seems to help babies get organized, which improves their suck.

In some cases, your nipple can be difficult for your baby to latch on to. If your nipple is short or inverted, first try pulling it outward with your fingers, then rolling it between your thumb and forefinger to make it erect. If that doesn't work, try pumping for five or ten minutes before the feeding to soften the areola and elongate the nipple. Don't worry about removing milk that your baby might have taken at the feeding. The first step is to get your baby latched on; milk intake can come later. Wearing breast shells (a plastic dome with a center hole that allows the nipple to come forward) inside your bra before feedings can also encourage your nipples to stand out. When these techniques don't work, a nipple shield (an artificial nipple placed over your own nipple) sometimes helps. Ask the lactation specialist for assistance.

A few conditions make it difficult or impossible for a baby to latch on. Infants with cleft lip may eventually learn to breastfeed, but those with a cleft of the gum or palate (roof of the mouth) are unable to create suction. Babies with abnormalities of the skull and face may be unable to latch on effectively. A very small, recessed chin (a condition called micrognathia) may also interfere with breastfeeding. So can a very short frenulum (a baby with this condition is sometimes called tongue-tied because of the unusually short tissue attached to the base of the baby's tongue), but this problem can be alleviated by clipping the frenulum. Some babies with nervous system or heart problems don't have enough strength or coordination to suck effectively. Consult with the NICU's lactation specialist or physical therapist—many of these experts are trained to assess and treat infant feeding problems such as these.

Diminishing Milk Supply

You might notice that you are producing less milk after the second or third week of pumping. This is less likely to happen if you have a hospital-quality electric pump in good working order, are using the double pumping kit, are using breast massage before pumping, and are pumping eight times a day. But if you skip a pumping session and let your breasts become overly full, your milk supply will go down. Pumping frequency is important. If two women each spend 100 minutes a day pumping but one does ten 10-minute sessions and the other does five 20-minute sessions, the first mother will have a larger milk supply.

On the other hand, some mothers who pump religiously have trouble making enough milk. If you are one of them, you will find it frustrating to ask for advice and to be told only, "Pump more often." Feeling anxious about your baby's condition, feeling exhausted, taking birth control pills, not eating or drinking enough, coming down with the flu—these can all have an adverse effect on your milk supply. Consider low milk supply a signal to take extraordinarily good care of yourself. Read up on and practice stress management techniques. (Medela makes a relaxation audiotape especially for breastfeeding mothers; see Appendix D.) Ask your health care professional or pharmacist if any drugs you are taking might be affecting your milk supply. As a last resort, you might ask your physician to prescribe metoclopramide hydrochloride (Reglan), which some studies have shown may improve milk supply. As with any body system, recognize that individuals vary; some women can't make more than a limited amount of milk. If you've tried everything and still can't build your milk supply, consider the possibility that it's a system (not a personal) failure.

Failure of Milk-Ejection Reflex to Kick In

If you feel as if your breasts are bursting with milk but nothing comes out when you pump or feed your baby, you may need to enhance your milk-ejection reflex, also called the let-down reflex. You can condition your milk-ejection reflex to respond to familiar ritual. When you pump or feed, sit in the same comfortable chair, sip the same beverage, apply a warm washcloth to your breasts, and massage them beforehand. If you get no results within 24 hours, ask your lactation specialist for help.

Sore Nipples

If your nipples become sore from pumping, try turning the pump's suction down, temporarily limiting pumping time to no more than ten minutes, and applying modified lanolin around the areola before pumping. Also, Egnell makes a soft, flexible insert (called a Flexishield) for the electric pump that may take the pressure off your sore spot. Preterm babies exert much less pressure when they suckle than a pump or a full-term baby exerts and rarely cause sore nipples.

If your nipples suddenly become sore after being pain free, you may have a yeast infection. Babies often get yeast infections, also called thrush, which appear as a milky white coating on the tongue or as a persistent red diaper rash. Thrush is particularly common in babies who have been on antibiotics. In mothers, the symptoms of thrush are very sore nipples—which may look perfectly normal or be quite pink—and burning/shooting/stabbing pains in the breasts. To treat the yeast infection, you'll need prescriptions for antifungal medicine: an oral suspension for your baby and a topical cream for your nipples. During the treatment, you and your baby's caregivers must sterilize pacifiers, breast pump parts, bottle nipples, and anything else that might reinfect your baby's mouth or your breasts. You can continue to breastfeed during treatment.

Clogged Ducts

A clogged duct produces a red, hot, tender lump on one breast. Take it seriously, because it could progress to a breast infection (called mastitis, described earlier in this chapter). Treat yourself as if you were coming down with the flu: Take it easy for a couple days, rest in bed, drink extra fluids, soak your breast several times a day in a tub of warm water, massage it gently, and pump more frequently. The clogged duct may take two or three days to resolve. Sometimes, as the clog moves down the duct, you'll develop a painful white spot on the tip of your nipple. Clogged ducts are sometimes caused by a mechanical obstruction—an underwire bra that presses in on the breast, a shoulder strap, or your sleep position, for example. Talk to a lactation specialist if you get clogged ducts repeatedly.

Making the Change to Home Feeding

A few common concerns parents have about breastfeeding at home are addressed here. Chapter 16 provides more information on home feeding. Once you are breastfeeding independently, you may have many more questions. Call your hospital's lactation specialist with your questions, or find a support group in your community to help you stay inspired and confident in your abilities.

When your baby is finally ready to go home from the hospital, your biggest concern may be whether he is getting enough milk by breastfeeding. How are you going to manage breastfeeding at home, away from the scale, the staff, and the security of the NICU? In preparation for discharge, you need to know two things: (1) whether your baby's suck is effectively extracting milk from your breasts, and (2) whether your milk supply is adequate.

"I was so embarrassed to use the breast pump at first. But when I saw the containers filling up, and I saw the nurses giving my milk to Ryan, I got over it. The breast pump is a great tool for NICU mothers who want to breastfeed their babies."

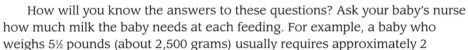

How will you know the answers to these questions? Ask your baby's nurse how much milk the baby needs at each feeding. For example, a baby who weighs 5½ pounds (about 2,500 grams) usually requires approximately 2 ounces (56 ml) every 3 hours. If you have not been weighing your baby on an electronic scale before and after each breastfeeding, ask for this to be done now, in the final days of hospitalization, so that you can know the effectiveness of your baby's suck. Is he capable of taking his minimum requirement directly from your breast by breastfeeding?

For several days before your baby comes home, keep track of the amount of milk you produce. Add up all the milk you remove by pumping, *plus* the before-and-after breastfeeding estimates measured on the electronic scale at each breastfeeding. Figure out your daily total. If it is high (about 24 ounces per day, or at least several ounces more than your baby requires), you may be able to go to exclusive breastfeeding at home.

A scale for test weighing.

Your health care professional may recommend an electronic scale to determine if your baby needs supplemental feedings. (Courtesy of Medela, Inc., McHenry, Illinois.)

Effective Suck/High Supply

If your baby is sucking well when he is discharged from the hospital and your milk supply is high, you'll quickly progress to complete breastfeeding. How glad you'll be to get rid of that pump! But usually your baby's suck is not consistently strong immediately after discharge, and you'll need to depend on the pump for a few more weeks.

To find out whether your baby is getting enough milk, you have a few options:

1. Stay in the hospital with your baby for 24 hours, feeding exclusively by breast around the clock. See if your baby gains weight (at least 15 to 30 grams each day) on breastfeeding alone.
2. Stop at your pediatric office on the way home from the hospital. Get a baseline weight on the office scale (scales are often slightly different). Make an appointment to go back in a day or two for another weight check, to confirm that your baby is gaining the required 15 to 30 grams per day.
3. Count the average number of wet and dirty diapers your baby produced each day in the week prior to discharge. Use this number as a guide at home. A baby who was gaining steadily in the hospital with an average of seven wet diapers and three bowel movements per day, for example, is likely to be gaining well if he keeps up this pattern at home. Get a weight check right away if his output drops.

Ineffective Suck/High Supply

Sometimes, despite a high supply of breast milk, test weights reveal that your baby doesn't take his required amount of milk by breastfeeding. Perhaps he bottle feeds well but hasn't mastered breastfeeding yet. So now you're taking him home, knowing that you have a good supply of milk but a baby who isn't able to breastfeed well. Try some of the following suggestions:

- Pump before nursing to stretch out your nipple, soften the areola, and get the milk flowing. If you notice that your baby chokes when your milk begins to flow, try pumping before nursing to help remove enough milk so that your initial "let down" is not too forceful.

- If your baby takes a bottle well but can't seem to latch on to your breast, contact a lactation specialist. This consultant might suggest trying a nipple shield. If you use a nipple shield, you will need close follow-up to make sure that your baby is getting enough milk through the shield, and also to help wean your baby from the shield. This usually takes several weeks.
- To determine whether supplements are needed, rent an electronic scale for home use. Medela's new BabyWeigh scale is as accurate as hospital scales and can be rented for under five dollars a day from most Medela rental stations (800-TELL-YOU).[25]

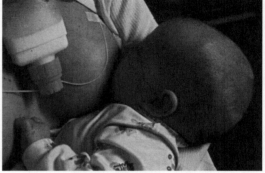

Nursing supplementer.
Your breast milk or formula is delivered to the baby from a tube taped alongside your nipple. This way, your baby receives supplemental feeding while nursing at your breast. (Courtesy of Medela, Inc., McHenry, Illinois.)

Effective Suck/Low Supply

If your milk supply is low even when your baby sucks effectively, your baby will need supplements at home. During breastfeeding, massage your breast whenever your baby's sucking slows down. Use a nursing supplementer at your breast to give the extra milk your baby needs. This device, a bottle or bag that delivers milk to your baby through a tube that can be taped alongside your nipple, has special benefits:

- It gives your baby the necessary supplement at your breast rather than from a bottle, teaching your baby the correct way to suck and avoiding nipple confusion.
- It makes for a one-step feeding process: breastfeeding only, rather than breastfeeding followed by bottle feeding.
- It gives your breasts more stimulation, which should help you produce more milk.

Pump after every breastfeeding. Test weights are the only accurate means of knowing how much milk your baby is taking from your breast. Without weight checks, you have no idea when to stop giving supplements. Either rent a scale for home use or arrange for frequent appointments (every two to three days) with a health care provider who is knowledgeable about both breastfeeding and preterm infants. The health care provider can advise you when you can safely stop giving supplements, refer you to other infant feeding specialists if needed, and counsel you about your chances of regaining a full milk supply if things don't improve within a week. You might also refer to the section "Diminishing Milk Supply" earlier in this chapter.

Ineffective Suck/Low Supply

If your baby is not effectively breastfeeding at discharge and your milk supply is low, pump religiously—8 to 12 times a day. Don't depend on breastfeeding to bring in a good milk supply. You will need to pump for at least two weeks after discharge. Use whatever milk you can express plus stored breast milk or formula to feed your baby the amount specified by the NICU. If you can get your baby latched on, a nursing supplementer at your breast is the best way to accomplish your two goals of teaching your baby how to nurse and building your milk supply. Massage your breasts whenever the baby's sucking slows

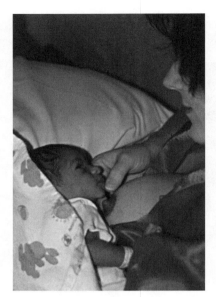

Awake and hungry.

An alert baby is ready to practice breastfeeding.

down. Adjust the supplementer so that the milk flows easily. If you cannot get your baby latched on, get help from a lactation specialist and ask about alternative methods of feeding your baby. Sometimes, cup or finger feeding may keep your baby from becoming completely bottle fed while you increase your milk supply. Breastfeeding takes a lot of hard work. Don't attempt to go it alone; arrange for frequent appointments with a lactation specialist.

Watching for Feeding Cues

If your baby doesn't demand to be fed at least eight times a day, you'll need to encourage more frequent nursing. During the day, if your baby sleeps for more than two or three hours at a time, look for subtle signs that he is ready to feed: rooting, bringing his hands to his mouth, making sucking motions, or simply moving about in sleep. When you see these cues, pick up your baby and encourage breastfeeding. A good way to bring your preterm baby to a quiet alert state is to allow him to suck on a pacifier for five to ten minutes before breastfeeding.[28]

Meeting Your Baby's Needs

Learning to breastfeed your special-care baby may be one of the most challenging things you'll ever do—but the rewards are worth it. You'll look back on this experience as something to be proud of. After weeks of pumping and days of awkwardness at breastfeeding, you'll finally take your baby home. This leap of faith—leaving behind the monitors, scales, and professional consultants—requires courage and a commitment to breastfeeding. Eventually all the pumps, tubes, and devices will be gone, and you will be feeding your baby on your own.

If You Must Stop Breastfeeding

Even under the best of circumstances, not all mothers and babies can breastfeed. It's normal to grieve the loss of something you looked forward to and valued. If you pumped for even a few days, you truly did "breastfeed." Your baby will experience some long-lasting health benefits if he received even a little of your milk. Give yourself credit for your hard work. Don't let anyone make you feel guilty that you didn't try hard enough or long enough. Recognize that you made the best decision for yourself, your baby, and your family under very difficult circumstances.

Emotional Responses

For a while, you may feel waves of guilt or sadness about not breastfeeding. Also, expect to feel angry if you believe you didn't get the help or support you needed to breastfeed successfully. On the other hand, you may take on the task of learning to bottle feed without much emotional response to the "loss" of breastfeeding. A mother's response usually depends on how much discrepancy there was between what happened and what she had hoped would happen. In other words, if breastfeeding meant a great deal to you, expect to feel a sense of loss.

Physical Responses

If you are able to stop breastfeeding over a period of days or a few weeks, your milk supply will gradually diminish and cause little discomfort. But if you have an abundant milk supply and stop breastfeeding suddenly, the physical pain may be unbearable. One mother whose baby died said that her continued milk supply was a sad and painful reminder that she had lost her baby: "It was like salt in a wound." If you too experience painfully full breasts when you stop breastfeeding, read ahead to the section entitled "Breast Engorgement."

When You Decide to Bottle Feed Your Baby

Families bottle feed their special-care babies for many different reasons. Sometimes a mother tries and is unable to produce enough milk, or the baby is not able to breastfeed. Sometimes medical complications in the mother or baby make breastfeeding inadvisable. For other women, bottle feeding is a personal choice, perhaps influenced by culture and background. Whatever the reasons, the NICU staff will support your decision and encourage your active participation in feeding your new baby.

Even though you have decided to bottle feed your baby, your body naturally begins to produce milk. This may cause an uncomfortable condition called breast engorgement. The following information will help you cope with your milk production.

Breast Engorgement

After you give birth, your body experiences a dramatic hormonal shift. Levels of estrogen and progesterone, the major hormones of pregnancy, fall. Prolactin, the hormone that tells your body to make milk, rises. The effect of this shift is seen approximately 48 to 60 hours after birth, when your breasts swell with milk. If you don't remove the milk by nursing your baby or by pumping, your breasts will become rock hard and painful. The swelling may extend up into your armpits, making even simple movements uncomfortable. You may develop a mild fever. This combination of symptoms is called postpartum engorgement.

You may have heard about medications to dry up your milk and may wonder why your doctor doesn't prescribe them for you. Most physicians no longer prescribe bromocriptine mesylate (Parlodel) and related drugs to suppress milk production, because these drugs can have dangerous side effects. Stroke, heart and urinary system changes, and seizures have been reported.[29] In addition, many women report that their breasts become engorged when the medicine wears off—a phenomenon called rebound engorgement. So most doctors recommend letting the breast milk dry up naturally.

When milk is not removed from the breasts, your body stops making breast milk. Pressure from the excess milk inside the mammary glands signals the pituitary gland to shut down the milk supply. (Many breastfeeding mothers learn this only after they've skipped a pumping session and let their breasts get overly full—their milk supply drops dramatically.) Also, the absence of nipple stimulation—no baby sucking, no pump pumping—means that you won't have regular surges of prolactin and oxytocin. These two hormones signal your milk glands to continue making and releasing milk.

Comfort Measures

While you wait for the engorgement to resolve naturally, try these comfort measures:

- Apply cold compresses. (Use gel-packs made for this purpose, a bag of frozen peas, wet washcloths chilled in the freezer, or the classic Australian remedy of cold raw cabbage leaves.)
- Wear a bra *if* it fits well and feels good. Don't wear one if it digs into you and leaves red marks. Some mothers wrap a stretchy Ace bandage around their chest to reduce pain and keep their breasts from bouncing uncomfortably. If you have a stretch bra designed for athletic exercise, try that. Wear it to bed if the pain is keeping you awake at night.
- Take a pain reliever containing acetaminophen (Tylenol) or ibuprofen (Advil or Motrin)—these not only relieve pain but also reduce swelling. (While you're still bleeding vaginally, avoid aspirin. It reduces blood-clotting ability.)
- Try heat to relieve the pain: Wrap your breasts in warm wet washcloths (covered with plastic wrap to keep the heat in), dip your breasts in a basin of warm water, or take a warm shower, allowing any milk produced to flow down the drain.
- If you are comfortable with the idea, use a breast pump or hand express to remove some of the milk. Don't worry that this will increase your milk supply. Express just enough to relieve the pain, and only as often as you need to. You can either discard the milk or ask the hospital staff for sterile containers in which to store it so that it can be given to your baby for these few days. As the swelling subsides, gradually pump or express less often. In a few days, you'll be able to stop altogether.

After two or three days of engorgement, you'll notice that your breasts are getting softer and more comfortable. They won't return to their pre-pregnancy size for several weeks. Until then, you may notice milk leaking from the nipples. Some women continue to notice leaking for several months after giving birth. This is normal, but leaking can be prolonged by anything that causes nipple stimulation—for example, jogging or other exercise that causes your breasts to bounce and sexual play that involves your breasts and nipples. If you still have milk 6 to 12 months after giving birth, or if you think the leaking is excessive (and you've tried reducing the amount of nipple stimulation), talk to your health care provider.

> "I had planned to breastfeed my baby. But after four months of bedrest, I needed my body back. Bottle feeding was the right decision for me."

Bottle Feeding Basics

Providing adequate nutrition for special-care babies is a complex process, one in which the NICU team carefully assesses the best approaches to helping your baby grow and get well.

Formulas for NICU Babies

At birth, the organ systems of all babies—particularly the stomach and intestines, the liver, and the kidneys—are immature. This is even more true of preterm infants. When medical illness is combined with organ immaturity, nutritional support becomes difficult. That is why most NICU babies receive special formulas designed to help preterm or ill infants grow and gain.

Ask your baby's nurse or physician about your baby's nutritional status and what types of formula enrichments are being provided. Your baby may receive a preterm infant formula containing extra protein, calories, sodium, calcium, phosphorus, copper, zinc, and selected micronutrients. Additives such as Polycose or MCT oil may be used to provide extra carbohydrates or fats to the formula. A vitamin and mineral supplement may be added as your baby grows.

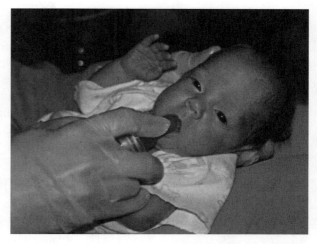

Positioning the nipple.

A preterm baby may try to bottle feed with his tongue on top of the nipple. You can help position the nipple correctly by guiding the nipple, with your finger on top of it, into his mouth.

Bottles and Nipples

Bottles designed for feeding babies in special-care nurseries usually hold 1½ or 2 ounces, and measurements are marked on the side of the bottle in tiny increments. The NICU staff measures formula using the more accurate metric system. You may hear the terms ml (pronounced M-L [which stands for milliliter]) and cc (pronounced C-C [for cubic centimeter]) used interchangeably. One ounce contains about 30 milliliters or cubic centimeters. A preterm infant's first feeding is usually 1–2 milliliters (about ⅕–⅖ tsp).

The nipples for bottles come in a variety of shapes and sizes. The smallest, softest, most pliable nipples—called premie nipples—were originally designed to make feeding easier for babies with a weak or immature suck. It now appears that these nipples may actually make feeding more difficult for some babies, however, because even a slight movement of the baby's mouth results in a flow of milk.[30] This may be more milk than the baby can cope with. Ordinary nipples (designed for full-term babies) often work just fine for preterm babies and for babies with breathing problems.

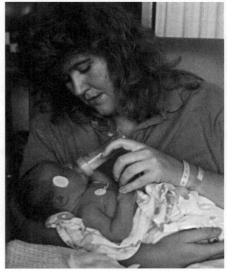

Positioning for bottle feeding.

Hold your baby close during bottle feeding. Flex the baby's hips, and hold his head higher than his bottom. This mother is helping the baby keep his hands in midline by supporting the baby's right hand with her little finger.

Preparing Your Baby for the Bottle

In the early weeks of life, before your baby is ready for bottle feedings, much of the oral stimulation he receives is unpleasant. Endotracheal intubation and suctioning, gavage tubes, and even a nasal cannula taped to the cheeks provide unpleasant sensory stimulation to your baby's face and mouth. You can make it your job to offer some pleasant forms of oral stimulation for your baby.

Gentle, loving stroking of your baby's lips and the area around his mouth can improve success at feeding.[31] The nurses will make sure that your baby gets opportunities for sucking during gavage feedings; this has been documented to prepare preterm babies for successful nipple feeding.[31] You can also offer opportunities for nonnutritive sucking when you notice signs that your baby would like to suck. These signs include bringing his hands close to his mouth, turning his head and opening his mouth, and making sucking motions. Even if you don't see these cues, next time you're holding your baby, try slipping your clean finger into his mouth (nail bed down) and gently stroking the roof of his mouth with the pad of your finger.

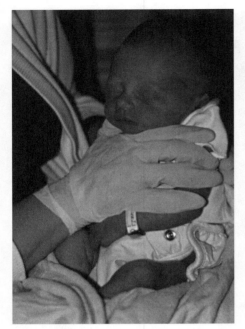

Burping position.

Your baby can rest and burp in the middle of the feeding by sitting upright on your lap. He is also more likely to stay awake when held upright. Support his head and neck, and pat his back gently. A lot of patting, jiggling, and position changing may cause your baby to spit up his feeding.

Learning to Bottle Feed

Feeding an NICU baby offers many challenges. Here are some tips for bottle feeding your newborn when the time comes. Chapter 16 offers suggestions for successful bottle feeding after your baby comes home.

Watch Your Baby's Signals

Do what you can to help your baby be alert and ready when you offer the bottle. If you notice that preparations for feeding (temperature taking, diapering, dressing) seem to tire your baby, for example, next time feed him first, straight from the bed. Save the diapering for later.

Position Your Baby Properly

Hold your baby comfortably in your arms and close to your body, with his head slightly raised. You may wish to ask about warming the formula; however, most babies accept room-temperature formula just fine. If your baby's arms and legs are limp, bend them into a flexed position to imitate the feeding posture of a healthy full-term baby. Hold your baby in your right arm at one feeding and in your left arm at the next to help him develop strong eye muscles and a symmetrical body. Notice your baby's response to light and sound. Don't sit where bright lights will shine in your baby's face, and take a break if the noise in the NICU becomes too loud. Never prop the bottle: Your baby could choke or could spit up the milk and breathe it back into his lungs.

Establish a Bond

Even if you are bottle feeding, you need to take primary responsibility for your baby's feedings. Resist the temptation to let others feed your baby too often—so that you can "get something done." Breastfeeding mothers know that feeding is a great excuse to take a break, relax, put their feet up, and focus on their baby. Babies who are bottle fed also need this one-on-one time with a consistent person. Bottle feeding mothers, too, need extra rest to recover from childbirth.

If you are interested, ask your baby's nurse about kangaroo care (see Chapter 4). This method of skin-to-skin holding is not just for breastfeeding mothers. Most NICU parents and babies enjoy the soft warmth of this experience and appreciate the family closeness it offers. After you take your baby home, find times to hold him right next to your skin during bottle feeding—for example, after a bath or first thing in the morning. Allow yourself and your baby the pleasure and the tactile stimulation of skin-to-skin contact during feedings.

Let Your Baby Set the Pace

Relax, and let your baby set the pace during feeding. Don't try to hurry the process by manipulating the nipple in your baby's mouth. If your baby stops sucking, let him rest. Prodding the baby to take more milk by jiggling the nipple, moving it back and forth, or twisting and turning it may result in what *seems* like a successful feeding. In the past, NICU staff took pride in their success at using these techniques to get the required amount of milk into very young premature babies. But they now know that forcing milk into a baby's mouth without the infant's active participation can make the feeding more stressful for the baby. In fact, pauses in breathing (apnea) and slowing of the heart rate (bradycardia) often result from this type of feeding.[32] If the baby can't control the fast flow of milk from the bottle, there is also an increased risk that he will breathe the milk into the lungs (aspirate it).

On the other hand, a feeding that lasts longer than 30 minutes may leave your baby exhausted. Try to learn to interpret your baby's cues; they'll tell you whether to stop feeding or to continue.[33] Developing this partnership with your baby—this mutual understanding—takes time, but it's basic to successful feeding.

Your Baby's Need for You

Feeding is a common area of concern for the families of both full-term and preterm infants, for parents of babies who are healthy at birth and of those who need special care. Not only is nourishment vital to your baby's well-being, but feeding is closely related to many other areas of your baby's care and progress. Whatever your concerns, questions, or struggles as you take on more of the responsibilities for nourishing your baby, specialists in the NICU will help you find the best approaches.

Chapter 6

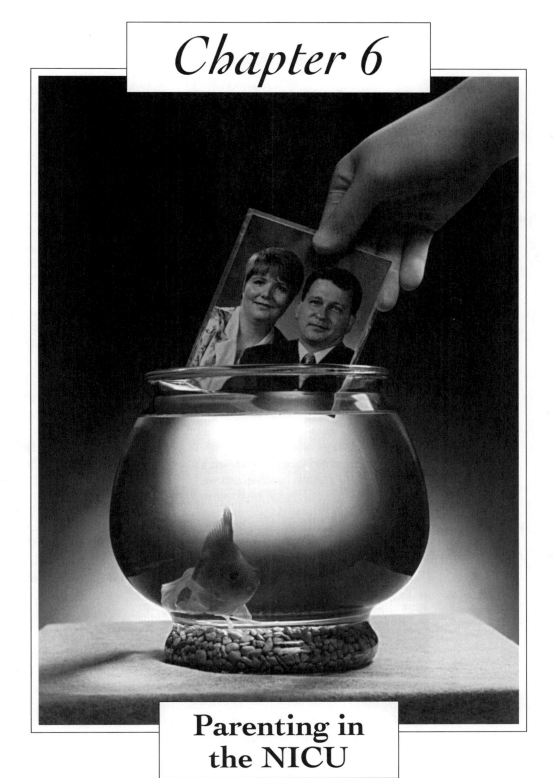

Parenting in
the NICU

Carole Kenner, RNC, DNS, FAAN
Ann Flandermeyer, RNC, PhD
Patricia Thornburg, RN, PhD

> **"**"And I know it *seems* easy," said Piglet to himself, "but it isn't *every one* who could do it."**"**

You are an important part of your baby's life in the NICU and a valuable member of your baby's health care team. You may feel intimidated by the technology and outnumbered by the NICU staff, but you have a bond with your baby that no other member of the NICU team can match. You will learn how to care for your baby in a context of love that will continue long after the NICU stay is behind you.

Parents of healthy newborns have time to gain confidence before they must give up some control to the daycare providers, teachers, and coaches who are an inevitable part of most children's lives. When your baby is admitted to the NICU, however, you are immediately forced to collaborate with others and trust them with your baby's welfare. Keep in mind that the NICU team members are only the first of many people you'll work with as your child grows to adulthood. These professionals present you with an early opportunity to learn how to work with those who will influence the course of your child's life.

The challenges of NICU parenting are great, but you can meet them. A positive NICU experience depends on forming a working partnership with the NICU health care team. Involvement helps you grow in your role as parent, learn about your baby, and prepare for a happy homecoming.

Overwhelming Beginnings

Even when you are prepared for the birth of a sick newborn, the actual event can be overwhelming. Some things may turn out better than expected; other complications may come as a surprise. The first hours or even days after your baby's birth may be chaotic and filled with unexpected events and emotions. You may feel off balance and out of control.

Family Imbalance

Separation is one contributor to this feeling of imbalance. It is not uncommon for the mother to be in the postpartum unit, the baby in the NICU, and the father, grandparent, or other support person running between units in the same hospital or even between hospitals. The support person's role becomes that of an information gatherer and messenger. This person is also expected to keep the rest of the family informed and, often at the same time, to care for other children.

As a result, the support person may be as stressed as the mother but feel there is no one to lean on. Furthermore, the partner may try to protect the mother by minimizing a bleak prognosis and maintaining a cool exterior or take the opposite approach by being totally honest about the prognosis. In some cases, the mother may think that her partner and others are holding back information. Other family members may feel, at times, that they are not hearing the whole story. Fathers and other support people, especially grandparents, also need nurturing and may have no one available to provide that support.[1]

Some couples offer each other remarkable support, growing closer and strengthening their bond through this experience. More typically, though, this is a highly stressful time for parents, marked by feelings of both physical and emotional separation. You and your partner may feel separated by anger, guilt, denial, blame, or feelings of failure and ambivalence. Mothers and fathers, as well as other family members, may be using all the resources they can muster to cope with the situation and not have any energy left over to support each other. In these cases, stress and misunderstandings can multiply, because all parties are too exhausted to sort things out.[2]

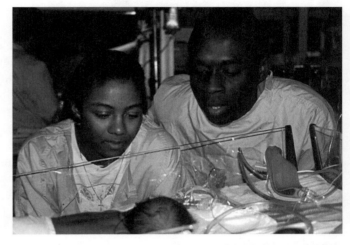

Differences in moms and dads.

Because men and women are different, mothers and fathers often react differently to the NICU experience. It is important to keep talking to each other during this stressful time.

Moms and Dads Cope Differently

Because men and women are different, fathers and mothers often use dissimilar coping strategies to deal with the situation. These variations in perspective can create difficulties between partners and cause problems that are difficult to resolve on your own. Many parents say that they don't tell each other what they are thinking or feeling. When issues are not discussed, marriages, partnerships, and family relationships can suffer.

As an NICU mother, you may be getting less sleep than you need and catching meals on the run. You may feel that you have more responsibilities than your partner—and no time for yourself or the rest of your family. You may be making daily visits to the NICU and wonder why your partner does not seem more involved.[3]

The father's tendency is often to back off, leaving the mother to assume the predominant parenting and visiting role. Many men busy themselves at work in an attempt to feel productive and to restore normalcy and control to their lives. Fathers, feeling uncomfortable in the NICU, may cope with their sense of powerlessness by avoiding the situation. Fathers often say, "Why should I go and sit by that glass house? I can't do anything, and I'm just in the way. When she's bigger, I'll come in."

On the other hand, the father who touches and cares for the baby early on usually continues to visit regularly and becomes an active participant in the baby's care. However, the daily responsibilities of work and home cannot be ignored for long. At first, even the strongest partnership can become tense as you reposition and balance the new responsibilities of NICU parenting.

If both partners are feeling stressed but coping in very different ways, it is no wonder that the relationship seems strained. When you are both in crisis, you may not have the energy to help each other. It can be difficult to talk to one another and understand the other's point of view.

Although open, expressive communication between you may be difficult, it is important to maintaining your relationship. Seek help from other parents who have experienced the NICU, from your pastoral counselor, or from caring professionals who have helped many couples through this crisis. You may need emotional support and professional assistance to work through difficulties and keep your relationship strong.

It may be hard to take time out for yourself, as well as ask for help; however, taking time is important to restore the energy you need to deal with the NICU. As soon as you feel you are able, take a day off from the NICU, make a date with your partner, and meet your own personal needs. This time-out is essential for your well-being. Don't think of it as taking time away from your baby.

Drugs and alcohol may temporarily help you forget your problems, but they only complicate things in the long run. If you have a substance abuse problem, you will not likely be able to face the realities of parenting without professional help. If your problems seem overwhelming, seek help from a trusted professional who has experience working with substance abuse problems.

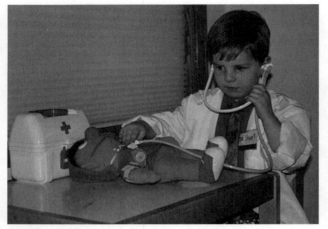

Figuring it out.

This big brother plays hospital with his doll in order to figure out the NICU experience. This is a good opportunity for parents to answer questions and give information at the child's level of understanding.

What to Tell Siblings

If you have other children, they will want to know when the baby is coming home or where the baby is. Tell them as simply as you can about "their baby." Be honest, and try to answer your children's questions at their level. Remember that for younger children, a baby they cannot see is difficult to imagine. Showing them pictures of the baby can help them see her as a real person.

It can be especially difficult for toddlers and preschoolers to understand what is happening. They need to be reassured that the baby's illness is not their fault. Young children may be jealous of the new baby and say things like, "I hate that baby." These feelings are normal.

Simple explanations and "exchanging" gifts with the baby help small children to feel important and involved. Parents can also tell a sibling, "When you're sick, Dad and I are worried and sad about it. Now your new baby sister is sick, and we're worried and sad about her." Sometimes attendance with you at sibling support classes offered by many NICUs can help even toddlers.

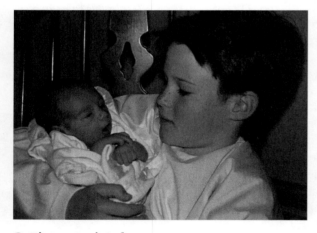

Getting acquainted.

Take advantage of sibling visitation in the NICU. This big brother will feel more involved and less anxious now that he has seen and held the new baby.

You will be understandably upset by the birth of a sick baby, and even young children will know something is wrong. If you leave your children out of this experience or neglect to discuss everyone's feelings, they are likely to respond with regressive, acting-out behavior. These behaviors can include temper tantrums, crying episodes, clinging behaviors, or acting on fears that had previously been resolved. Your children know no other way to compete for your attention. They are likely to manage better if you keep them informed without overwhelming them with complex information.

If the NICU permits sibling visitation, take advantage of this policy so that your children can see the baby. Older children, especially, benefit from visiting the NICU. Rarely are they overwhelmed by the sights and sounds that bother adults. They tend to focus on the little human being that they, too, have been planning for. A visit, along with updates about your baby's progress, will help make the baby real and make siblings feel involved.

Involving Grandparents

Grandparents often feel they should not voice their frustrations or fears. One grandmother said, "It is so hard to watch my daughter suffer and know there is nothing I can do to make it better. I don't know what to say. I am too far away to care for the other children, so all I can do is listen." A mother-in-law stated, "We have never had a close relationship. I know she thinks I blame her, but I don't at all. I just don't know how to tell her so she will believe me. I can't talk to my son about this because he has enough on his mind." Feelings such as these need to be addressed before the infant's discharge, or the relationship between parents and grandparents may never be the same. You may be reluctant to rely on grandparents for help after your baby's discharge unless you work things out before she comes home.

Grandparents benefit from talking with other grandparents who have gone through the NICU experience. Referral to a support group, even when the grandparents live in another city, may be beneficial.

Visiting the NICU when possible allows grandparents to understand the true situation. Their fears about the child are often worse than the reality. During their visit, you and your nurses may be able to find concrete tasks that will make grandparents feel helpful, without interfering. In some families, putting the grandparents in charge of family communication helps ease the pressure on parents and gives the grandparents an active role to play. Grandparents can also be helpful in caring for other children and keeping up with the daily household routine so you are able to visit the NICU.

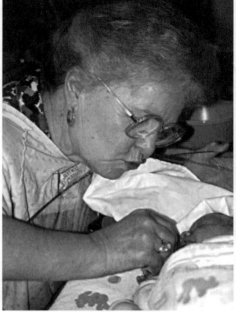

Special grandparents.

Grandparents worry about their new grandchild and about the baby's parents, too. By visiting the NICU, this grandmother gains an understanding of the challenges facing NICU parents and can provide better support for the family.

Where To Find Support

Your Partner

No matter how well-meaning, those closest to you cannot always provide the support you need. Your partner's support can be important in coping with the NICU experience. But because men and women often cope differently, communication with your partner may be difficult at times and may not meet all your needs.

Others Who Can Help

Other sources of support include extended family members, friends, nurses, social workers, the NICU staff, and other NICU parents. You may find that as your needs change over time, so do your support people.

Friends can be a source of stress as well as support. If they fear saying the wrong thing, they may cope by avoiding you and the NICU situation at a time when their support would be helpful. Pregnant friends or childbirth class buddies may feel guilty for being pregnant or having a healthy baby. Just when you need their support, they seem to pull away. Health care professionals can help you realize that this avoidance reflects your friends' feelings of inadequacy, rather than lack of caring. If you feel awkward or do not have the energy to do so, a steadfast friend, your partner, or your parents or partner's parents can tell your friends exactly what you need or how they can help. Friends usually have to be told only once, and then they'll make dinner, pick up your children at daycare, run errands, or help in other directed ways. Don't concern yourself with those who cannot seem to help. Accept help from those who can.

Support Groups

At some point in your NICU experience, you may need to talk to someone about questions that your baby's caregivers cannot answer. "Why do I hear different opinions about how to care for my baby?" is one example. These questions can often be addressed in support groups that are offered at the hospital or in your community. These support groups provide a "safe" place for you to express your feelings and frustrations and to find support from people who can relate to your situation. Support groups are sponsored by many different organizations and are led by people both with and without professional training.

Dynamics within the group can affect how much support you will find. Many groups work very well to provide you with the support you need. In some groups, however, one or two vocal parents may take over, giving the others little time to discuss or share their parenting experiences; or perhaps the group leader feels a need to "control" the group, limiting open communication. Some parents in hospital support groups fear that staff will see their negative feelings as poor attachment to their baby or bad parenting and that expressing such feelings will affect their baby's care.

Many parents and families feel that support groups organized by nonprofessionals but led by a professional not directly associated with the NICU provide the "safest" and most supportive setting for sharing feelings. In this safe

"We had perfect lives—nice jobs, a great marriage, and a long-awaited pregnancy. Now our baby weighs 2 pounds in the NICU. This must be our reality check."

setting, parents and grandparents can work through their fears and share their concerns about having a baby in an intensive care unit. Hearing other parents tell about their parenting successes and failures provides reassurance. And if a baby dies, the group can provide "family" support during the initial grief period.

Most groups encourage parents and grandparents or other relatives to get involved during the infant's hospital stay and then to continue attending, if possible, after the baby is discharged. After your baby's home-coming, the support group meeting may become just one more thing to do or one more time to hire a baby-sitter. The answer for some parents is for one partner or a relative to stay home while the other attends the meeting. Unfortunately, this limits the family sharing that can be so beneficial.

If you feel a support group might help you cope, then attend one or two meetings. If you don't find the meetings particularly helpful, you needn't continue. Seek the support that works best for you. Don't try to please the health care staff by attending a group that isn't meeting your needs just because they think it's important for you to do so.

Just as the NICU team shouldn't pressure you to attend a support group, you shouldn't pressure your partner to use only your method of support. Resentment can build at a time when you need each other the most. Some couples find that one of them does better in a group and the other does better with a one-on-one relationship. Seek the support that works for each of you; then share the benefits of that support with one another.

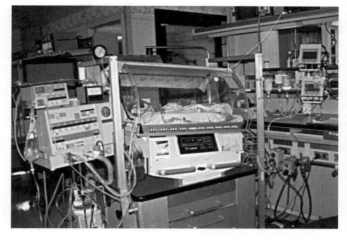

The NICU as parents see it.

The NICU setting presents many barriers to parenting. As you get acquainted with NICU staff and learn about NICU equipment, you will focus less on the technology and more on your baby.

Chapter 4 discusses many of the feelings NICU parents experience during their early visits with their baby. With time, you will feel more at home in this busy environment your new baby calls "home." Even so, the NICU presents challenges to parenting. Here are some tips for dealing with some of these barriers.

Challenges of NICU Parenting

Geographic Barriers

If your baby is in an NICU some distance from your home, family members may be separated from one another. It may be difficult to find an affordable place to stay near your baby. Low cost temporary housing such as the Ronald McDonald Houses are available for parents near some hospitals. Other hospitals may make rooms available in school or nursing dormitories or have accounts with nearby hotels for parents or visitors. Ask about these resources and use them when you are able.

Physical and Mechanical Barriers

Some parents find the overall atmosphere of the NICU overwhelming. Bright lights, excessive warmth, and noise make it difficult to manage an already stressful situation.

Rest is essential to maternal healing and milk production, as well as to the emotional well-being of both parents. New parents need to be able to lie down or put their feet up when they become tired or overwhelmed. Meeting those physical needs in the NICU is not always easy, however. Your orientation should provide you with information about the locations of telephones, restrooms, and parent lounges.

Many mechanical barriers come between you and your baby in the NICU. Your baby's incubator can be intimidating at first. You may hesitate to break through this barrier and touch your baby. Intravenous tubing and monitor wires can tangle like vines in the jungle, and you don't want to risk pulling something loose. The humidity inside an oxygen hood creates a fog and makes it difficult for you and your baby to see each other. A nasal cannula can sometimes be substituted for the oxygen hood, but you still have to deal with oxygen tubing that can't stretch too far from the wall. All of these barriers make caring for your baby a challenge.

Psychologic Barriers

When you visit the NICU, you may feel like a guest in the health care providers' home—one who must obey the rules of your host. You may feel that, to keep on the staff's good side, it's best to do as you're told and not rock the boat. You may fear that, if you ask too many questions or become demanding, you will be labeled bad parents, and your baby may not receive as high a quality of care as she otherwise would. These fears are normal. They will lessen as you become more familiar and involved with the staff and with NICU routine.

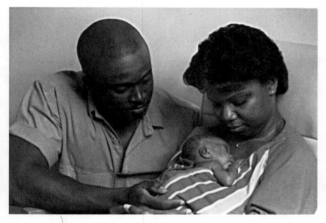

Feeling like a family.

Private moments are difficult to come by in the NICU, but your baby's nurse will help you find opportunities. These parents enjoy kangaroo care with their infant.

You may need to ask who may visit your baby with you to provide support. Some NICU policies limit visitors to parents and grandparents, but you may find better support from a neighbor or friend. A skilled NICU nurse or social worker can help you define your "family" and allow you to work out your own visiting policy. This cooperation helps you feel more in control and fosters a partnership between you and the NICU team.

Psychologic barriers may also include lack of privacy to spend quiet time together as a family. Some families report that they just can't be themselves in the NICU. Parenting within the NICU fishbowl creates stress; you may feel your caregiving skills are under constant scrutiny and are inferior to those of the nurses. You may feel shy and rigid as a family, with your usual warm, spontaneous family interactions inhibited. In part, these feelings resolve with time and experience.

Attachment Barriers

You want your baby's nurses to have both a professional and an affectionate bond with your baby, but it can be frustrating when the nurses seem to know your baby better than you do. You may hear the nurses refer to your baby as "my baby." Some parents admit feeling jealousy toward their baby's nurses, because the nurses do everything well and seem to meet their baby's needs better than they themselves can. Spending time with your baby and participating in her care will help you feel more like a parent and resolve many of those feelings.

Another barrier to attachment is the fear that your baby may die or get sick again after discharge. Some professionals refer to this as chronic sorrow (see Chapter 13), whereas others believe it is a symptom of grief. Grief for the loss of the hoped for, healthy infant you pictured during pregnancy may delay feelings of love for and attachment to your special-needs baby. Give yourself some time to sort out your feelings. You may find it helpful to discuss your concerns with your baby's nurse, the social worker, or another support person.

Forming A Partnership with the NICU Team

Time and familiarity with NICU routine eliminate much of the discomfort of NICU parenting. But your NICU experience will be much more positive when you and the NICU team work as partners to care for your baby. Because your baby requires intensive care, immediate decision making and interventions in the best interest of your baby are often necessary. Obviously, parents are not included in every medical or nursing care decision on a moment-to-moment basis. However, the NICU team should strive for a working partnership with parents, which means that parents are included in the baby's *overall* plan of care. For this to occur, you need to learn appropriate skills that allow you to participate in your baby's daily care, and you need to be involved in any decision making that affects your ability to care for your baby when her hospital stay is over. By working together, you and the NICU team achieve two important goals:
1. You help your baby reach her highest level of wellness.
2. You gain the confidence and skills you'll need to parent your special-care baby.

You are an important member of your baby's health care team. Your comments are important in working out strategies to involve the family in your baby's NICU care. In a successful partnership, planning for your baby's discharge begins early in the NICU stay.

The Nurse-Parent Partnership

Nurses in the NICU have chosen a career that enables them to make a difference in the lives of families. However, NICU nurses must budget their time carefully so that they can spend time with you. Nurses are assigned one or two "vents" (infants who require mechanical ventilation) or three or four "feeders" (babies who are growing and doing well). Unless discharge teaching is scheduled, time for family intervention is rarely allotted when daily assignments are made. Time constraints usually don't reflect the nurses' lack of commitment to you, but rather represent the reality of a hospital budget.

Even in the face of nurses' heavy workloads, many parents form close and significant relationships with members of the NICU team. Your baby's nurses usually become your main source of information and insights and gain your trust. Nurses also act as liaisons between you and your baby's physicians. They are individuals who explain your baby's condition in understandable terms and answer your questions as they arise.

The better acquainted you are with your baby's nurses, the more likely you are to form trusting bonds with them. Units that assign primary nurses (one nurse or a nurse team assigned to coordinate the family and infant's care throughout the entire NICU stay) or a neonatal nurse practitioner to direct your baby's care encourage this type of relationship. Whatever their approach, most NICUs will try to assign the same team of nurses to your baby. This is most satisfying for you and for the nurses because it gives you the chance to learn about each other and form a good working partnership.

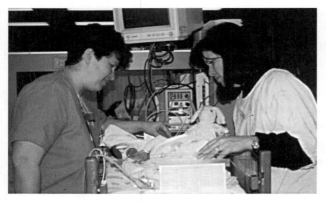

Nurse and parent.

Nurses and parents often form a bond through mutual caregiving to the baby. A team approach involves the parent at the bedside and increases your confidence as you make the transition to home.

Black Cloud Days

Just as nurses learn to tune in to parents' moods, parents soon become attuned to those of the nurses. You'll begin to notice that, on good days, everyone works as a team, and the unit functions smoothly. But when unit politics or family crises sour the day, strong nursing leadership and cohesive staff are required to keep things running smoothly.

On these "black cloud" days, you may feel in the way, both physically and psychologically. Although your baby's nurse will try to make you feel comfortable and included, you may notice that she has less time and patience for you on these days. Try to be flexible when the NICU is stormy. If possible, wait until the mood has lifted a bit to ask lengthy questions or to ask about trying new and complicated care techniques. Sometimes it helps to tell your nurse that you've noticed the unit is extra busy. This opens communication and allows both of you to discuss what you can realistically accomplish during your visit. These black cloud days should not be frequent, but they do occur. They demand extra patience from parents and NICU staff.

Communication as a Building Block

Open, honest, and clear communication between parents and NICU staff is the key to a caring partnership. This takes effort on everyone's part. Chapter 3 addresses many communication issues. Here are some other points to keep in mind.

Clarifying What You Overhear

You want to be valued as unique individuals. As consumers of health care services, you feel your needs deserve attention. It's common for NICU parents to believe that everything they see or overhear has something to do with them.

Innocent comments taken out of context can sound frightening. Ask for clarification about anything you overhear that worries you. Your nurses can correct misconceptions and allay unnecessary fears.

For example, a mother overheard one nurse reporting to another that housekeeping had not had time to clean the empty incubators. This mother did not realize that this was part of the change-of-shift report and that the nurse was passing on the information so that the next shift would clean the beds. Instead, the mother worried that her baby had been placed in a "dirty" bed and that perhaps that was why her baby had an infection. In addition to increasing her stress, misinterpreting these comments increased her fear of leaving her baby with strangers.

Don't feel shy about voicing your concerns. Tell the staff about any worries you have about your baby's quality of care—both for your peace of mind and to maintain good communication with the NICU team.

"The nurses became our anchors. We will never forget how they helped us get through this experience."

Getting Your Questions Answered

You need information. You want to know about your baby's medical condition, bowel movements, and feedings.[4] You may also want to know the unknown. For example, you may ask, "Will my baby be okay?" or "When will my baby be able to go home?" Lack of concrete answers is frustrating for parents and health care providers alike.

You may also encounter different viewpoints. Some nurses may reassure you that your baby is okay. Others may not commit. Then you become suspicious: Does the nurse who won't commit know something the optimistic nurse doesn't? Is someone hiding something from us?

No one withholds information on purpose, but members of the NICU team may choose not to offer their own opinions. Nurses don't always feel comfortable sharing their personal thoughts about how your baby is doing. They may "feel" your baby is doing well but have no solid evidence to back up their hunch. Rather than sharing those vague feelings with you, they may say nothing. If you are not getting all the information you want, you need to ask for it. (Chapter 3 offers some suggestions.)

Be wary of filling in the blanks yourself. Imagination is often more frightening than reality. Parents are commonly frightened when they see an IV line in their baby's scalp, for example. They may worry that the IV fluid is going directly to the baby's brain. In truth, many NICU nurses prefer a scalp site because it frees the baby's hands from IV tape and tubings and lets the baby bring her hands to her mouth. By asking about the IV placement, you learn that the IV fluid does not go directly to your baby's brain. You become more knowledgeable about her treatment and more confident of the nurse's abilities. You may also feel more comfortable about asking your next question.

"Our four-year-old daughter was there when the doctor first told us, in very big words, about respiratory problems, infections, and other problems our baby could face.
My daughter summed up the whole thing when she broke in and said,
'The baby's not done yet, Mom. Just put it back in.'"

The language health care professionals use when they talk to you can be a source of support or stress. If the language is simple and easy to understand, you're less likely to be intimidated and more likely to ask further questions. But if NICU staff use professional double-talk or answer a simple question with a long and complicated response, they create confusion and put up barriers to communication.

You should expect the NICU team to simplify complex information for you, to get to the point, and to reinforce what they tell you with written information whenever possible.[5] They should validate their explanations with you—that is, they should make sure you understand what they have told you. They may do this by asking you to repeat what they have told you in your own words. If an explanation you receive from a caregiver does not make sense to you, ask for clarification.

Making Your Needs Known

Developing open and honest communication requires that you tell your baby's nurses about your needs and feelings. Although NICU staff members should anticipate your needs, they are human and sometimes miss your signals. Help those helping you by asking for what you need and being honest about what you don't understand. Clear communication establishes the basis for an ongoing partnership.

Learning Care Skills

Parenting in the glass house of the NICU is intimidating. At first, you may believe that your caregiving skills can never measure up to those of the nurses. The first step to active parenting is to recognize that your role is different from that of the nurses but just as important to your baby's health.

Your involvement in your baby's care is essential from the very beginning. Otherwise, you become more an NICU visitor than an involved parent. This does not help anyone, because when it's time for your baby to go home, you'll feel unprepared and resentful.

Your involvement in your baby's care usually begins on a basic level. When you first visit your baby, the NICU team provides you with information and perhaps encourages you to touch your baby. This slow beginning gives you a chance to recover from the excitement surrounding the birth and learn about the NICU routine.

Later, when the reaction to having a baby in the NICU has passed and you are more comfortable in the NICU, your involvement moves to a different level. The information you are given becomes more detailed, and you begin to participate more in your baby's care. You may help by changing your baby's diaper or assist in changing the bed. This is a beginning. Because health professionals are individuals, the degree to which parents and family participate in care depends, to a certain extent, on each nurse's level of comfort with you and on her own style of working with families.

A skilled NICU nurse will involve you in your baby's care and help parenting feel "real." You'll be encouraged to call your baby by name and talk to her about your day or play audiotapes of your voice or soothing songs. Changing your baby's diaper or perhaps bringing baby clothes from home may bring some normalcy to your relationship. Ask if you can personalize your baby's bed with name and birth date cutouts, family pictures, and special toys from home.

As you spend more time at your baby's bedside, you start to recognize what your baby likes and dislikes. For instance, you may notice that your baby sleeps more soundly on the right side or spits up less when stroked and calmed after feeding. These "little" things are subtle but just as important to your baby's care as anything the nurse may note about the baby. Talk about the cues you see, and encourage the health care team to use these suggestions during caregiving. This little person is your child, and nurses are her guest caretakers for a short while. Health care professionals know that first you enter *their* "home," and then, with their help, you and your baby make your way back to *yours.*

You will learn new things about your baby every day that will help ease the transition from hospital to home. Some aspects of your baby's care will make perfect sense and come easily to you. Others may be more complicated and take longer to learn. Here are some things to keep in mind as you learn care skills in the NICU.

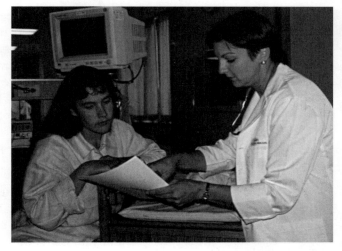

Vital communication.

Ask questions and be clear about what you want to know. The NICU team should keep you informed and involved in your baby's care.

Keep Focused for Learning

It's very hard to pay attention or to understand new information if you are distracted by pain, hunger, fear, or exhaustion. Take care of yourself so that you can give your baby your best. This means you must spend some time away from the NICU to rest. In the same vein, your baby won't respond well to care if she is in pain, tired, or uncomfortable. If you are learning something with your newborn and she begins to cry, the teaching session needs to stop until your baby is consoled. The same holds true for you. If you feel "weepy" or sad, stop and take a break. Share your feelings with a nurse who can help you sort out your feelings and provide support. When you feel better, you will have more confidence in your ability to learn about your baby.

Figure Out What You Know

Your teachers will spend lots of time asking you questions before they give you information or begin instruction. This process may seem time-consuming, but assessing what you already know is an important first step in the learning process.

Learn the Basics First

Because they know that parents may hesitate to ask for clarification or to admit they don't understand something, most NICU staff give plenty of basic information. They aren't talking down to you; they just want to be sure they are not talking over your head. Even if this is your second or third baby, most NICU nurses won't assume that you know everything there is to know about newborn care. Unless you tell them otherwise, your NICU team will teach you the basics first.

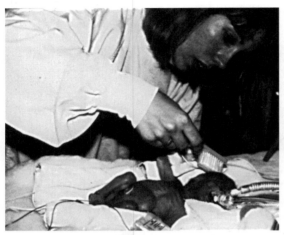

Parent time.

Parents can do much of the baby's daily care. This is an important part of feeling like a parent in the NICU.

Ask Questions

No question is silly or unnecessary. Take as much time as you need to discuss your concerns and questions. Don't be afraid to say that you just don't understand something or need the information presented in a different way. People learn in many different ways and at different paces. The NICU team expects you to have plenty of questions. Many times you can watch a video-tape to help you learn. Take notes if doing so helps you learn, or ask for a demonstration.

Learn Bit by Bit

Most NICU parents report thinking, "I know the nurse gave me that information, but I have no idea what she said." Not remembering everything you're told is normal when you're distracted by the NICU environment. Printed information, videotapes for review, and your own notes may help the information sink in. Don't be embarrassed or afraid to ask for the information again. The nurses are there to help you learn about your baby.

Get On-the-Job Training

At first, you may be hesitant to dive in and care for your new baby. Most parents begin to learn by watching the nurse provide care and then asking the nurse questions about what she is doing. Observing care is a comfortable way to begin to learn, because there's no pressure to "prove yourself" as a competent parent.

While you observe caregiving, ask questions. Encourage your baby's nurse to talk with you about how your baby is doing, how to know when to stop what you're doing and allow the baby to rest, why certain procedures are necessary, and how much care you can provide as a parent.

As you become more comfortable touching your baby, the nurse should give you opportunities to provide more care, such as taking your baby's temperature. When it's time for diapering or bathing, for example, the nurse may first demonstrate the procedure and then ask you to do the same task, either immediately or later. As you care for your baby, your nurse will probably coach you through the procedure and stand ready to help if you need it.

During your baby's NICU stay, you'll learn to do much of your baby's care. Some parents are immediately comfortable with activities such as diaper changing, bathing, and feeding; others require some practice. When you and your baby are ready, ask your baby's nurse to "reserve" feeding, bathing, and other care activities for you. This helps you learn to manage your baby's care before you take her home, helps define you as the parent, and allows you to maintain some control over certain areas of your baby's life.

Hospital routines can sometimes be changed to accommodate your schedule. For example, if your baby is being fed every three hours on a 3–6–9 schedule but you can visit only from 6:30 to 8:00, ask if your baby's schedule can be changed. A 4–7–10 schedule would allow you to feed your baby as well as spend some time getting to know her.

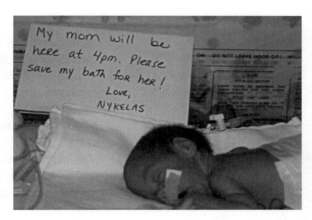

Give as much of your baby's care as possible. Caring for your baby builds your self-confidence for her homecoming. Even though you may continue to think of questions about each skill you learn, don't by shy about asking the nurse to teach you the next skill. For example, if you know how to take your baby's temperature, ask if you may learn how to give the bath. Continue learning new skills as your confidence builds. If your baby will need a special type of feeding at home, such as tube feeding, watch the feeding and ask questions. The next time, ask to do the feeding with the nurse as supervisor. When the nurse watches you care for your baby, she is better able to assess what else you need to know before discharge. As you cooperate together, you strengthen your partnership.

Learning by doing.
The NICU team encourages you to care for your baby as soon as you and the baby are ready. This baby's nurse put a sign in the baby's bed to alert other caregivers to save baby's bath time for his mother.

Be Flexible

Some nurses are better teachers than others. Ideally, your nurse will be diplomatic as she makes constructive comments or corrects you if your technique is not safe. You will also encounter nurses who have different opinions on how certain things should be done. Listen for the reasons each one gives for doing the task in a certain way; then do what makes sense to you based on those principles.

Your ability to be flexible is also appreciated when a "reserved" baby care activity, such as feeding, doesn't work out according to plan. Occasionally, your baby will awaken and fuss "off schedule," and if you are a distance away, the nurse will go ahead and feed her for you. If this happens, cuddle or stroke your baby when you arrive. Such a missed opportunity is disappointing, but this type of occurrence should not happen often. If it does happen often, discuss the problem with the primary nurse or the NICU charge nurse.

Be an Involved Long-Distance Parent

If you are parenting from a long distance, set up a phone call schedule and communicate frequently with your baby's nurses and physicians. Some nurseries have strategies to help you cope with long-distance parenting. These may include sending you postcards and photos to update you on your baby's progress and involve you in your baby's life. Don't feel guilty if you are not able to visit as much as you would like. Keep in touch with your baby's nurses—they know that you care. For parents at a distance, the opportunity to "room-in" with your baby before she is discharged is very valuable. Ask the team about the possibilities.

Continue to Learn After Your Baby Comes Home

The NICU staff will try to teach you what you will need to know to care for your baby after discharge. However, until you're home with your baby, anticipating what you don't know or will need to know can be difficult. Learning about some aspects of your baby's special care is like being asked if you have any questions about driving before you get behind the wheel of a car. You can expect to have questions long after your baby leaves the NICU.

If you are offered a home visit after discharge, take advantage of this important service. Home visits are most effective during the first week after discharge, when most questions and concerns arise. The visiting nurse can reinforce previous teaching, help you troubleshoot potential problems, and guide you in solving real ones. This visit can help you anticipate possible problems and therefore avoid crises. Families of newly discharged babies are under tremendous stress and may need to cope with new situations, sometimes daily. A home visit can reassure you that many things are going well, building your confidence. It can also help you cope with difficulties you may encounter.

The Parenting Process

It may take some time for you to feel that you are truly your baby's parent. Getting to know the NICU staff and routine and caring for your baby help break down some of the barriers to NICU parenting. Open and honest communication with family members and with the health care team creates trusting partnerships. Mutual respect and understanding of each person's contribution to your baby's care is a starting point. Everyone involved has a common goal: the health and well-being of your new baby. When parents and the NICU team work together toward this goal, each partner in care helps the others achieve success.

Chapter 7

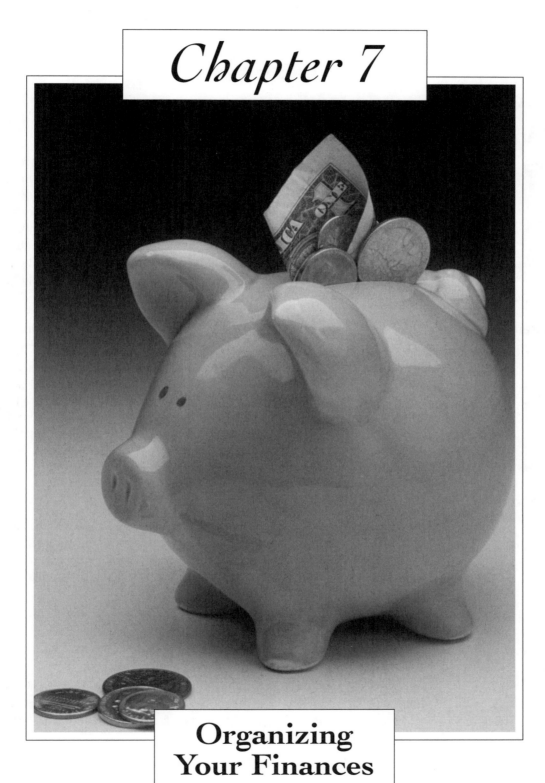

Organizing
Your Finances

Cathy Livingston, MSW, LCSW-C

❝"Nobody knows anything about this....This is a Surprise."❞

Eeyore–

Can you place a price tag on the life of your child? Of course not. Yet the care of your NICU baby does come at a very real cost. It may be overwhelming to think about the financial challenges facing you, but the sooner you get organized, the better you will be able to manage this part of the NICU experience. The first part of this chapter provides general information for NICU parents. The second section addresses health insurance issues, and the final section offers information and resources that will be helpful if your baby lacks health insurance coverage.

Survival Basics

Amid health care reform, it's risky to give absolutes for managing your health care dollars. A few survival basics apply no matter what, however.

Take Care of Business

Dealing with health care bureaucracies is difficult enough without the added weight of your baby's condition on your mind. Because of your stress level, you may find it difficult to make the many phone calls and appointments that are necessary to get organized. Try to set aside time at least once a week for financial housekeeping.

Manage Your Bills

Throwing all your bills into one big box to figure out later is not a good idea. The complications only multiply as time passes. Open each bill as it arrives and decide how to deal with it. If you are employed but have no health insurance, keep your bills organized and seek help from the hospital financial counselor as soon as possible.

Use Resource People

Do not hesitate to ask the hospital social worker and/or financial counselor to assist you in getting information. Nurses and doctors who are familiar with your baby can address your questions concerning the potential length of your baby's hospital stay. The personnel department at your place of work may be able to help you regarding the specifics of your health care benefits.

Work with the Hospital Financial Office

With the stress and responsibilities of NICU parenting, paying your bills may seem like a low priority. Calls from a collection agency will only increase your stress level, however. Make an appointment with the hospital financial office and establish a cooperative relationship as soon as possible after your baby's birth. Here are some tips for building a good working relationship:

- Communicate. You cannot avoid the bill by avoiding the billing office.
- Get the name and phone number of the person responsible for your child's account. This person is usually called an account manager. Try to direct your questions to this person every time.
- Make sure the billing office has your complete insurance information: insurance company name(s), account numbers, group numbers, and so on.
- Ask if your account manager has been in touch with your insurance company case manager. The insurance company case manager can sometimes authorize services that are not typically covered by your insurance policy but that would be cost-effective in the long run.
- If you cannot pay the full amount due, work with your account manager to arrange a payment plan under which you pay something every month, even if only a small amount. If you find you will not be able to make a payment, notify the office *before* your payment is due.
- If you do not have adequate insurance coverage, ask about local charity funds. Some hospitals have access to funds to help their patients cover their bills. Ask your social worker about United Way agencies, Easter Seals, March of Dimes, and other organizations that may offer financial help, as well as about possible government assistance programs.

Keep Accurate Records

Keep a file folder of receipts and canceled checks related to your baby's medical expenses. When tax time approaches, seek help from a qualified tax consultant or accountant to help you claim the tax deductions to which you are entitled.

Stand Your Ground

Most of the people you talk with will do their very best to be helpful. If you are not getting adequate service, however, ask to speak to a supervisor, who may be of more assistance.

I mmediately notify your insurance company of your baby's birth. If you delay or forget to call, you may find that you are not covered for those "lost" days. Ask if the provider requires written verification of the birth and, if so, within what time frame. Your NICU nurse or social worker will help you contact the person in the hospital's medical records department who can provide the required paperwork.

"I was uninsured, but soon discovered that I wasn't in this alone. The NICU social worker and the hospital financial people were very helpful."

When You Have Insurance Coverage

If you have given birth to twins or more, emphasize to the insurance carrier the fact that there is more than one baby. Otherwise, duplicate bills may be confusing.

Know What Your Coverage Is

The financial counselor at the hospital, a representative of your insurance company, or your employer's personnel or benefits office can help you understand your health care coverage. If you aren't completely familiar with the "fine print" of your coverage, it's time to find the answers to some important questions:

- What are the terms of your policy?
- What does your policy cover in this situation?
- What does your policy not cover in this situation?
- How much is the deductible (the amount you pay before your insurance "kicks in")?
- What percentage of the bill will your insurance cover?
- Is there a catastrophic illness clause (100 percent coverage above a certain dollar amount)?
- Is there a limit to the total amount of insurance coverage?
- Are you required to use certain physicians or designated hospitals?
- Who is the primary carrier for your baby's hospital bills?
- Who is the primary carrier for your baby's doctor bills?
- Will the insurance carrier assign you a case manager? What is that person's name and phone number?

Know Who Pays—and How Much

If you and your partner each have health care coverage, figure out which one of you carries the primary coverage. Each bill should first be submitted to the primary carrier. The balance not paid by the primary carrier may be paid by the partner's coverage.

You may receive two kinds of bills: those that have been submitted by the hospital or physician to your insurance carrier for you and those that you must submit to the carrier yourself. You should submit any bill that does not say on it that it has already been submitted to your insurance company for payment. You'll need to obtain the proper insurance claim forms and know where to mail them. You should not resubmit a bill that has already been submitted.

After a bill has been submitted to your insurance company, you'll receive a statement from them of amounts they have paid. Then you'll receive follow-up bills from the hospital, doctor, and others stating the original amount due, the amount the insurance company has paid, and the amount you now owe. If you do not have additional insurance, you need either to pay the amount due or to contact the source of the bill to arrange a payment plan.

Sometimes, if your insurance carrier is not aware that your baby's care involves specialized treatments and procedures, the carrier will pay only the going rate for routine nursery care. If you submit a bill from the neonatologist

> *"At first we called our box of hospital bills the Boo Box. But once we understood how to submit claims and who to call with our questions, it wasn't so frightening."*

for NICU care and your insurance covers only the standard rate for a pediatrician's routine hospital visit, ask the hospital financial office or the physician to call or write to your insurance company to justify the higher fee. The insurance company may make an adjustment in your favor.

If you notice errors in any of the statements, call immediately for clarification and corrections. Look for written instructions on the bill telling you how to report errors or ask questions.

Family and Medical Leave Act

If you are employed by a company that has at least 50 employees and have worked for that company for at least one year for at least 25 hours per week, you may be covered by the Family and Medical Leave Act of 1993. This federal legislation mandates that employers provide up to 12 weeks of unpaid leave for the birth of a child or the care of a seriously ill family member—with continuation of the employee's usual health insurance.

Health care programs offered at the federal level are likely to change. Stay informed about political and legal changes that may affect the status of any benefits you receive or may quality for.

To apply for any government program, you will need to have your child's birth certificate and social security number. You will be able to obtain a valid birth certificate shortly after the baby's birth. Call your local Social Security Administration office for information on obtaining a Social Security number for your infant. When you apply for government assistance, be prepared to provide information regarding your income and your assets. You will also be asked to provide names, addresses, and telephone numbers of doctors and hospitals your child has visited. Keep a record of this information and of dates of service and account numbers used by these facilities.

The following public agencies provide benefits to those who meet certain requirements. The hospital social worker may be able to help you identify possible sources of financial aid. If you think you may qualify for assistance, contact one or more of these agencies.

Social Security Administration

Your NICU baby might qualify for benefits from Social Security under one of two programs:

1. Social Security Dependents Benefits. A child under age 18 (age 19 if in school) is eligible for Social Security if he is a dependent of someone receiving either retirement or disability benefits or is a survivor of a parent with a Social Security record.
2. Supplemental Security Income (SSI) Benefits for Children. An affected child under age 18 who comes from a home with limited income and resources and who has disabilities or is of low birth weight qualifies for these benefits.

Many rules and regulations apply to dependents and SSI benefits. Check with your local Social Security office for a complete description, or call

U.S. Government Agencies and Programs

(800) 772-1213 any business day between 7:00 AM and 7:00 PM. You may wish to ask for this publication, also available in Spanish: *Social Security and SSI Benefits for Children with Disabilities* (SSA Publication No. 05-10026).

State Department of Health and Human Services

Medicaid

State social service agencies (the name varies from state to state) are responsible for Medicaid or medical assistance. Medicaid is a federal/state program available for families who qualify based on both medical and financial need.

Spend Down

If your income level exceeds eligibility requirements for Medicaid in your state but your medical costs are extraordinarily high, another program, called Spend Down, may help. Under this program, after you have been charged a specified amount in medical expenses, the state will contribute to the remainder of your debt.

Pregnant Women and Children

Another program that may be of help is PWC. Similar to Spend Down in that the income threshold for assistance is higher than for Medicaid, PWC covers costs related to pregnancy and children's health care needs.

Public Health Departments

Children with Special Health Care Needs (CSHCN) programs help provide specialized services to eligible children through arrangements with clinics, private physicians, hospital-based outpatient and inpatient treatment centers, or community agencies. The names by which CSHCN programs are known vary from state to state. A couple of examples are Children's Special Health Services, Children's Medical Services, and Handicapped Children's Program.

Staying Financially Healthy

Your hospital financial counselor and social worker can help you find local addresses and telephone numbers for the agencies that will be most helpful to you. Be prepared to spend time waiting in offices, filling out forms, and meeting with people who will repeatedly ask you the same questions. Once the application process is completed, though, the benefits can be very helpful. Your financial health can affect your future. It pays to stay informed and communicate closely with those people who are most in touch with your financial status.

Chapter 8

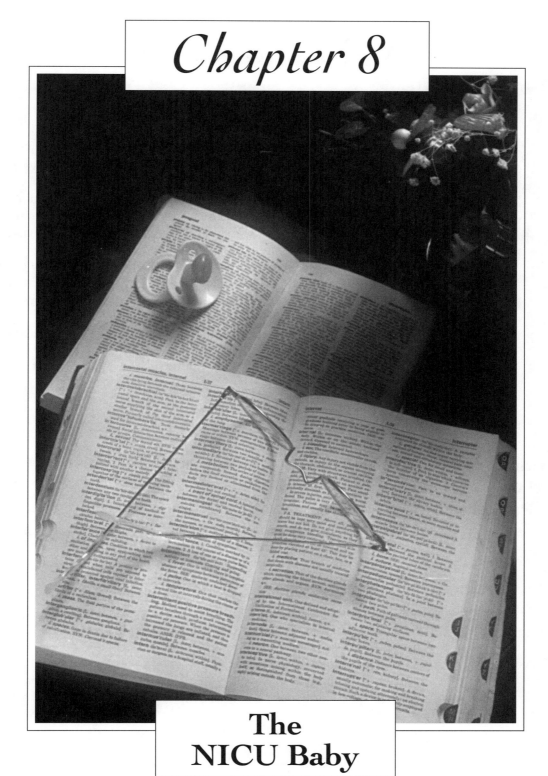

The
NICU Baby

Kathleen M. Pompa, RNC, MN, NNP

"It is hard to be brave," said Piglet, sniffing slightly, "when you're only a Very Small Animal." Rabbit, who had begun to write very busily, looked up and said: "It is because you are a very small animal that you will be Useful in the adventure before us."

After birth, babies may need the kind of special care provided by a neonatal intensive care unit for many different reasons. The most common reason newborns need intensive care is that they are born early (they are premature or preterm). The first section of this chapter explains the relationship between the length of your pregnancy and your infant's weight at birth. It also describes how premature infants differ from term infants in their level of maturity at birth and lets you know what to expect if your newborn arrives earlier than anticipated.

Other factors, explained later in this chapter, that can determine whether your newborn will need special care include the following:[1]

- The mother's health before and/or during pregnancy (called maternal factors)
- The health of your unborn baby as she grows and develops in the uterus (called fetal factors)
- Conditions your infant experiences during labor and delivery

Gestational Age and Growth Patterns

As a new parent, the first question you usually hear from relatives and friends is "How much does your baby weigh?" This information is important, but weight alone does not give a complete picture of your newborn's growth, development, and maturity status. A newborn's weight is important in relation to the length of the mother's pregnancy—the period called gestation. So to a care provider in the NICU, an equally important question is "How many weeks gestation is this newborn?" The answer tells the caregiver if the baby is full-term, preterm (premature), or postterm ("overdue").

Health care providers sometimes have difficulty identifying the length of a pregnancy from the information parents can provide. A direct examination of the newborn, however, is a reliable way to identify gestational age (the number of weeks from the mother's last menstrual period before conception to birth). As a pregnancy progresses, the baby's brain, nerves, and muscles develop, as do many physical characteristics, in a predictable fashion. These indicators of maturity can be used to pinpoint your baby's gestational age within two weeks. Combined with your baby's birth weight, length, and measurement of head circumference, this information makes it possible to categorize your newborn as appropriate for gestational age (AGA), small for gestational age (SGA), or large for gestational age (LGA).[2] The intrauterine growth chart on page 121 will help you find your baby's classification of size based on gestational age.

Small for Gestational Age

A newborn can be small for her gestational age whether born at term (after a full-length pregnancy) or prematurely (before the end of the 37th week of pregnancy). If a newborn is very underweight for gestational age, the condition is called intrauterine growth retardation (IUGR). Slow growth, development, and maturation in the uterus—either throughout the pregnancy or just during the last portion of it—cause low birth weight.[3] Slow growth can be the result of maternal problems during pregnancy (including infection or reduction in placental blood flow to the fetus) or of fetal development problems (genetic defects). It is also possible for a newborn's weight to be low at birth simply because both parents are small.[1]

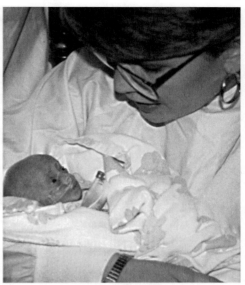

Small-for-gestational-age infant.

This baby's tiny size is deceptive. Although she is preterm, she is more mature than her size would indicate. About six weeks old in this photograph, she was born at 29 weeks gestation and weighed 1 pound, 9 ounces (about 710 grams).

Newborns who are small for gestational age and who have experienced slow growth and development throughout the pregnancy often appear "old looking" for their tiny birth size. They are generally short in length and have a small head. Infants whose growth and development slowed only during the final weeks of the pregnancy often appear scrawny, but their length and head size are normal. The skin of postterm SGA newborns is often loose, dry, and scaly. SGA babies have little fat and muscle tissue development. These infants are usually alert and active, however, and seem hungry.[4]

Newborns who are both SGA and preterm may experience complications related to their prematurity. Those who are SGA but who are born at term are at risk for the following:[1]

- Complications related to the stress of labor and delivery
- Difficulty making the change from fetal to newborn blood circulation
- High red blood cell count
- Low blood sugar level
- Infection
- Difficulty "catching up" in their growth to babies born at an average weight

Large for Gestational Age

Some babies grow larger than usual during gestation and so weigh more at birth than the average baby of the same gestational age. These babies are called large for gestational age. The infants may be born preterm, at term, or postterm. Fast growth often occurs in babies whose mothers have diabetes, babies whose parents are larger than average, and babies who have certain congenital (genetic) syndromes. Infants who are LGA show the physical characteristics appropriate for their gestational age—that is, they do not develop and mature faster than AGA babies—but they have above-average amounts of fat tissue at birth.[4,5]

The size of a preterm LGA baby can be deceptive because she may weigh as much as an "older" baby who is born closer to term. But the preterm LGA

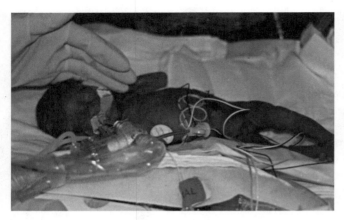

Baby at 25 weeks gestation.

This baby is very premature and requires a ventilator for breathing assistance. The umbilical catheter is also visible in this photograph.

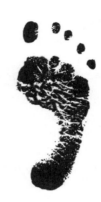

Baby at 28 weeks gestation.

This baby is premature and also requires ventilator assistance. Note the round leads for the cardiorespiratory monitor placed on her chest and the IV line in her left hand.

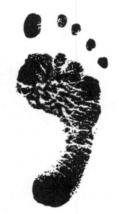

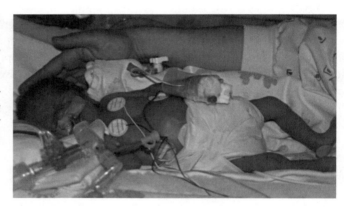

Baby at 32 weeks gestation.

This premature baby receives breathing assistance from nasal CPAP (see Chapter 10). She also has an IV line in her left hand and an umbilical catheter.

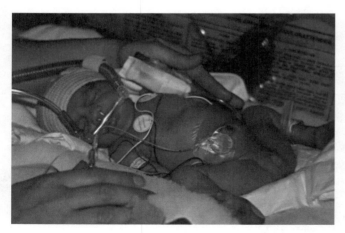

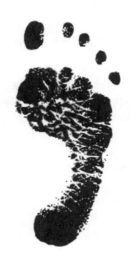

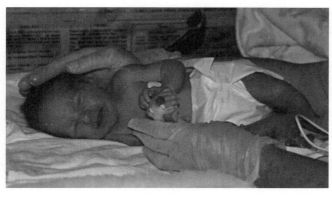

Baby at 35 weeks gestation.

Although still considered premature, this baby does not require breathing assistance or supplemental oxygen at this time. She has an IV line in her right hand.

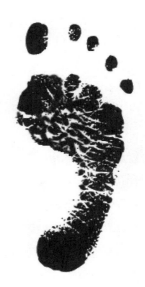

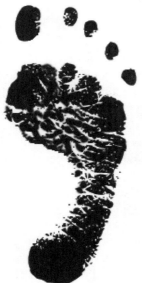

Baby at 38 weeks gestation.

This baby is considered full-term. Note the rounded appearance of this mature newborn, her flexed position, and her good muscle tone.

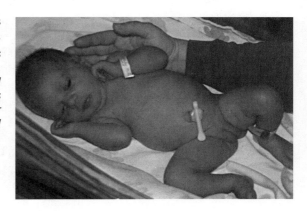

baby can experience many of the same problems that other preterm babies do. All LGA babies are also at risk for the following:[1]

* Complications related to the stress of labor and delivery
* Birth injuries
* Low blood sugar and calcium levels
* High red blood cell count
* Immature lung development

The Term Baby

A term (or full-term) baby is one who is born between weeks 38 and 42 of gestation. Term babies who are appropriate for gestational age average about 19½ inches (49 centimeters) long and weigh about 7 pounds (3,200 grams) (see Intrauterine Growth Chart on page 121), but term newborns may also be SGA or LGA.[2] The skin of term newborns is soft, and the blood vessels underneath do not show through. Vernix (a greasy white or yellow material made up of secretions and dead skin cells) is usually present at delivery only in skin creases. There may be a bit of soft, downy hair—called lanugo—on the newborn's shoulders and upper back.

The hair covering a term newborn's head is rich and silky. The nails may extend past the tips of the fingers, and the soles of the feet show creases. Term newborns have strong muscle tone, and healthy term newborns readily curl up into the familiar fetal position. A term newborn's cry is strong and sounds healthy.[4]

The Premature Newborn

A premature—or preterm—baby is one who is born before week 38 of gestation.[3] Premature infants can be SGA, AGA, or LGA, but most are either small or appropriate weight for their gestational age.[3]

The gestational age of a baby born prematurely determines the problems for which she is at risk. In general, the earlier in the gestational period your infant is born, the more risk there is of complications—and the higher the level of care she will likely need. Your baby's appearance at birth is directly related to length of gestation. The table on page 121 shows how to correlate the infant's physical characteristics with gestational age. Your infant's level of maturity at birth determines how she will interact with her new environment outside the uterus.

A baby born at 24 weeks gestation usually weighs about 1 pound, 12 ounces (800 grams) and is about 12½ inches (32 centimeters) long.[2] The skin is red and immature, with a shiny, transparent appearance that allows the blood vessels beneath to be seen easily. The skin is often described as gelatinous. There may be traces of lanugo, and some vernix is visible at delivery. There are no creases on the soles of the newborn's feet. The eyelids are fused, and the earlobes are flat and soft and can be folded easily. This newborn has little fat or muscle tissue beneath her skin. Because muscle tone has not yet developed, a 24 weeker has limited ability to bend her arms and legs and does not breathe regularly on her own.[4]

A baby born at 28 weeks gestation usually weighs about 2 pounds, 7 ounces (1,100 grams) and is about 15 inches (38 centimeters) long.[2] The skin is less red now and more pink* because it is becoming less transparent, although the veins can be seen through it. Thick vernix covers the skin at birth, and long, thick lanugo is present, especially on the back. The nails on the fingers and toes are developed. There are faint red marks (the beginnings of creases) on the soles of the feet near the toes. The eyelids are now open. The earlobes are soft and easily folded but are beginning to spring back on their own if folded. The baby has developed some fat and muscle tissue under the skin and can bend her arms and legs a bit.[4]

"I looked at my baby and wanted to say how beautiful she was. But she wasn't beautiful. She was long and skinny and furry. She was not very cute for quite a while."

---

* Pink refers to the color of the skin's undertones. Full-term newborns of dark complexion are pink over their palms, soles, and mucous membranes (especially inner lips and gums). Very preterm babies may lack the dark complexion of their parents until close to term gestation.

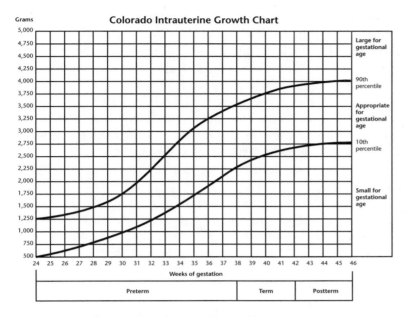

Colorado Intrauterine Growth Chart

Intrauterine growth chart.

Find your baby's gestational age in weeks on the bottom line of the chart. Then find her weight on the side of the chart. The intersection of the two lines determines whether your baby's weight is small for gestational age, appropriate for gestational age, or large for gestational age. For example, a baby born at 32 weeks gestation and weighing 1,100 grams would be classified as small for gestational age.

From: Battaglia FC, and Lubchenco LO. 1967. A practical classification of newborn infants by weight and gestational age. Journal of Pediatrics *71(2): 159–163.* Reprinted by permission of *Mosby-Year Book.*

Your Baby's Appearance

Physical Appearance		Weeks Gestation																				
		24	25	26	27	28	29	30	31	32	33	34	35	36	37	38	39	40	41	42	43	44
Typical Weight	lb-oz	1-12		2-1.5		2-7		2-14		3-10		4-10		5-12		6-10		7-1				
	gm	800		950		1,100		1,300		1,650		2,100		2,600		3,000		3,200				
Skin		thin, translucent; red, puffy, visible veins over abdomen								smooth, thicker; no puffiness						pink; few visible veins			pale, pink, some peeling	thick, pale, peeling		
Hair		eyebrows and lashes						fine, woolly hair bunching out from head								silky, single strands lying flat				receding hairline or loss of baby hair		
Ears	Form	flat, shapeless										beginning curve		upper 2/3 curved		well-defined curve to earlobe						
	Cartilage	soft, stays folded if pressed against head								more firm, springs back slowly from folding				thin, springs back readily from folding		firm, stays erect from head						
Nipples		flat and barely visible										slightly raised			increased in size and height							
Genitalia	Testes			felt above scrotal sac									in upper scrotum			in lower scrotum						
	Scrotum			few wrinkles									wrinkles in front			wrinkles overall		pendulous				
	Labia and Clitoris					prominent clitoris; labia majora small, widely separated						labia majora bigger, nearly covering clitoris			labia minora and clitoris covered						
Creases on Sole of Foot		smooth soles, no creases								1–2 creases on ball of foot		2–3 creases on ball of foot	creases on 2/3 of ball of foot		creases on heel			deeper creases over entire sole				
Resting Posture		⟨image⟩		⟨image⟩		⟨image⟩		⟨image⟩		⟨image⟩		⟨image⟩		⟨image⟩		⟨image⟩						

Adapted from: Lubchenco LO. 1976. *The High Risk Infant.* Philadelphia: WB Saunders, 59. Reprinted by permission.

A baby born at 32 weeks gestation usually weighs about 3 pounds 10 ounces (1,650 grams) and is about 16 inches (41 centimeters) long.[2] The skin is pale pink and thickening and may be peeling. Only a few of the larger blood vessels (in the abdominal area) can be seen through the skin. Vernix covers the skin at birth, but lanugo (especially over the lower back) is thinning. This newborn has definite sole creases near her toes, with red marks reaching the middle of her soles. The eyelids are open. The earlobes are soft but show some cartilage development; they will spring back if folded. At this age, the newborn has developed some muscle tone and can keep her arms and legs slightly bent at rest.[4]

A baby born at 36 weeks gestation usually weighs about 5 pounds, 12 ounces (2,600 grams) and is about 19 inches (48 centimeters) long.[2] Her skin is pale overall, appearing pink only over the ears, lips, palms, and soles. The skin has thickened and has begun to crack and peel on the hands and feet. Only a few large blood vessels can be seen faintly in the abdominal area. Lanugo has diminished, and areas without it are visible. Hair on the head is fuzzy or woolly and sticks together. The skin has a thick covering of vernix at birth. Creases extend to the middle of the soles of the feet. The earlobes are firm, with well-formed cartilage, and spring back immediately if folded. Muscle tone is quite developed; the newborn's legs are usually in a froglike position, and the arms are bent at the elbow.[4]

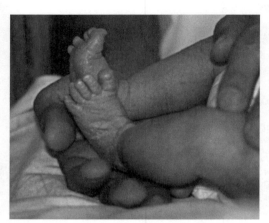

Postterm baby.

This baby has the typical peeling skin of an "overdue" newborn.

The Postterm Newborn

Babies born later than week 42 of gestation are called postterm newborns. Most are healthy, but as the pregnancy continues past 42 weeks, the placenta becomes less efficient at supplying the fetus's nutritional needs, which increase as the baby continues to grow. Many of the physical characteristics postterm newborns show are associated with this decline in nutritional sustenance. Sometimes called the syndrome of postmaturity, these characteristics include a somewhat malnourished appearance (despite large size) caused by loss of fat tissue. The postterm newborn's skin appears dry, cracked, peeling, loose, and wrinkled (especially at the ankles and wrists and on the palms of the hands and soles of the feet). The postterm baby may be meconium stained. Meconium, a sterile, dark green substance produced in the fetus's bowel that may be released into the amniotic fluid before birth, will color ("stain") the skin and umbilical cord.[5]

Posterm infants are at risk for the following:[1]
- Complications due to the stress of labor and delivery, including meconium in the amniotic fluid or meconium aspiration syndrome (see Chapter 10)
- Birth injuries

Maternal Conditions that Can Affect a Developing Baby

- Age over 40
- Age under 16
- Poverty
- Infertility
- Cigarette smoking
- Drug or alcohol abuse
- Diabetes
- Thyroid disease
- Kidney disease
- Urinary tract infection
- Heart disease
- Lung disease
- High blood pressure

- Anemia
- Low platelet count
- Blood-type incompatibility
- Increased amount of amniotic fluid
- Bleeding
- Premature rupture of membranes
- Infection
- History of past high-risk births
- High temperature

Adapted from: Pursley DM, and Cloherty JP. 1991. Prematurity, postmaturity, large-for-gestational-age, and small-for-gestational-age infants. In *Manual of Neonatal Care*, Cloherty JP, and Stark AR, eds. Boston: Little, Brown, 85–103. Reprinted by permission.

- Low blood sugar and calcium levels
- High red blood cell count
- Feeding difficulties (baby feeds slowly, tires easily)
- Difficulty making the transition from fetal to newborn blood circulation

Maternal Factors That May Affect Your Baby

An unborn baby (a fetus) grows and develops within the complex environment of the mother's uterus. This is called the baby's prenatal environment. The fetus depends on its mother for oxygen and nutrition. During development, babies do not easily adapt to stress or changes in their surroundings. This dependence means that a mother's health and well-being are very important to her growing baby.

A mother's medical condition both before and during her pregnancy affects the prenatal environment in which her baby grows and develops. Use of alcohol, nonprescription drugs, and cigarettes creates a hazardous environment for a growing baby. Certain medical conditions can cause specific problems for the developing baby or produce effects seen only after birth. Health care providers who have cared for the woman during her pregnancy, labor, and delivery generally inform the pediatrician or neonatologist about her health during her pregnancy so that the health care team can anticipate any immediate or long-term consequences her condition might produce in her newborn. Many maternal conditions can affect a developing baby. The most commonly monitored conditions include:[1,6]

- Diabetes
- Heart disease
- High blood pressure
- Bleeding
- Infection
- Blood-type incompatibilities

Diabetes and How It Might Affect Your Baby

Diabetes is a condition in which the body either does not make enough of, or does not use normally, the hormone insulin, which is necessary to keep healthy blood sugar levels. Pregnancy changes the way a woman's body uses sugar. Some women already have diabetes when they become pregnant. Others are unable to produce enough insulin during pregnancy, a condition called gestational diabetes. Whether the condition exists before pregnancy or develops during it, the increased sugar available to the fetus from the mother's blood alters the environment for fetal development. Chapter 9 has more information about maternal diabetes and the newborn.

If you are diabetic, the key factor to the well-being of your baby is keeping your blood sugar at a safe level throughout your pregnancy. Possible complications for the baby of a mother whose blood sugar levels are difficult to control include:[7]

- Low blood sugar
- Low calcium

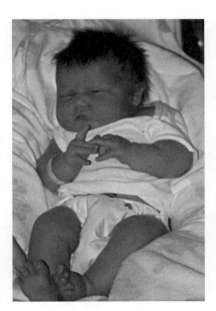

Infant of a diabetic mother.

This large baby is actually about 35 to 36 weeks gestation. Infants of diabetic mothers are often preterm and large for gestational age.

- Low magnesium
- Respiratory distress syndrome (see Chapter 10)
- Jaundice (see Chapter 9)
- Increased number of red blood cells
- Increased birth weight, which can increase the risk of birth injuries
- Premature birth
- Small size for gestational age (if maternal diabetes is chronic and advanced)
- Increased incidence of birth defects (affecting the heart, kidneys, stomach and intestines, brain and spinal cord, and/or bones)

If you have diabetes, caregivers will monitor your newborn closely. They will take frequent blood samples to evaluate her blood sugar level, as well as the levels of sodium (Na) and potassium (K)—called electrolytes—in your baby's blood. Caregivers will also closely watch your baby's breathing; babies of diabetic mothers sometimes need extra oxygen and even the assistance of a ventilator to help them breathe. Medical staff will assess your baby's heart (this may involve an electrocardiogram [EKG] or an echocardiogram) and closely monitor your baby's ability to keep down feedings, pass stool, and make urine to be sure that her stomach, intestines, and kidneys are healthy.

Maternal Heart Disease and How It Might Affect Your Baby

When you are pregnant, your heart and circulatory system must work harder than when you are not pregnant. The amount of blood in your system increases, raising the rate at which your heart beats and the amount of work it must do.[6] These changes provide adequate blood flow through the placenta supplying the developing fetus with the oxygen and nutrition necessary for healthy growth and development. If you have heart disease, pregnancy can have important medical consequences for you and for your baby.

Although your heart disease may not worsen during pregnancy, the increased work your heart must do may cause your symptoms to worsen. To cope with the increased work of pregnancy, your heart may reduce blood flow to your placenta and baby so that it can provide enough blood flow to your brain, liver, and heart. These disturbances in blood flow to the placenta can result in loss of the pregnancy (spontaneous abortion), premature birth, abnormal growth and development, and/or inadequate supply of oxygen to the baby at various times during development.

Babies of mothers with serious heart disease are also at risk because of the medications their mothers must take to manage their condition. A wide variety of drugs is used to manage cardiovascular disease in pregnant women. Although some can affect the developing infant, most can be used safely during pregnancy.[1,5,6]

If you have congenital heart disease, your doctor will probably recommend a procedure called fetal echocardiogram (heart ultrasound) during pregnancy to examine your infant's heart. Evaluations after birth may include a chest x-ray, an electrocardiogram, and an echocardiogram. The baby of a

"We had good prenatal care. We simply had really bad luck."

mother with heart disease is likely to be preterm and/or small for gestational age. The NICU team will perform a detailed physical examination and manage complications related to these problems.

High Blood Pressure and How It Might Affect Your Baby

Blood pressure does not usually increase during pregnancy, but for unknown reasons, high blood pressure does complicate about 6–8 percent of pregnancies in the United States.[8] A woman who has high blood pressure before she becomes pregnant, or develops high blood pressure before the 20th week of gestation, is said to have chronic hypertension. A woman who develops high blood pressure after 20 weeks gestation is said to have pregnancy-induced hypertension (PIH). PIH is a disease that involves more than just high blood pressure.[8] PIH can occur in a pregnant woman who has no history of high blood pressure. However, a woman with chronic hypertension is more at risk for developing PIH than a woman who does not have chronic hypertension.

When PIH affects the woman's kidney function, the disease may be called pre-eclampsia. If PIH leads to seizures in the pregnant woman, the disease may be called eclampsia. If PIH leads to serious problems with blood clotting abilities and liver function, it is called HELLP syndrome.

If you develop PIH, you will probably respond to medications to lower your blood pressure so that you can continue your pregnancy. If your blood pressure stays high, however, blood flow to your kidneys, liver, brain, and uterus can be reduced. This can limit your baby's supply of oxygen and nutrients. If your hypertension is serious and does not respond to medical treatment, the only solution is delivery of your baby.

Because they lower the mother's blood pressure, the drugs used to treat PIH—among them methyldopa (Aldomet), propranolol hydrochloride (Inderal), and magnesium sulfate—may reduce blood flow through the placenta. The risks of PIH to your developing baby are generally associated with this reduction in blood flow. An additional risk of PIH is that you may not be able to carry your baby to term; many mothers with PIH begin labor and deliver their babies prematurely. Because babies of mothers with PIH experience periods of decreased blood flow during their growth and development in the uterus, they frequently are small for gestational age at birth; this is evidence of slow fetal growth.[1,5,6]

Blood tests after delivery may also show your newborn to have a high red blood cell count, a lower than normal number of platelets and white blood cells, and a higher than normal level of electrolytes. Babies of mothers treated with magnesium sulfate for PIH may have high levels of magnesium in their blood. Symptoms include poor feeding, intolerance to feedings (vomiting, residuals, abdominal swelling), easy tiring, muscle weakness, and/or apnea (pauses in breathing). If apnea is severe (which is rare in this case), your baby may need breathing assistance. As long as your baby's kidneys are functioning normally, the magnesium level usually reduces on its own.

"This was our first baby who made it as far as the NICU. For us, this was a joyful birth."

Bleeding During Pregnancy and How It Might Affect Your Baby

Some women experience vaginal bleeding during pregnancy. This bleeding can be ongoing (chronic) or a one-time event (acute). Chronic bleeding can lead to anemia (a low red blood cell count) in the mother, decreasing the oxygen available to her developing baby. Acute bleeding decreases the mother's blood volume, which reduces blood flow (and thus oxygen and nutrients) to her developing fetus.

Bleeding during pregnancy occurs for two common reasons. The first, called placenta previa, occurs when the placenta lies abnormally low in the uterus, near to or covering the cervical opening. Placenta previa may cause occasional painless bleeding and often results in premature labor.

Placental abruption, separation of the placenta from the uterine wall before delivery, is life threatening for both mother and baby. This separation limits the flow of blood and oxygen the baby needs to survive and can cause severe maternal and fetal hemorrhage. A woman with placental abruption usually experiences abdominal pain and rigidity. Vaginal bleeding may occur, or it may be hidden if the blood from the placental site stays within the uterus. When placental abruption occurs, the baby must be delivered as rapidly as possible. A baby born following placental abruption can be severely ill, requiring a high degree of breathing and blood pressure support. The newborn's red blood cell count may be low, and she may need emergency blood transfusions. Lack of oxygen may cause damage to major organs. Caregivers will evaluate the infant's brain, kidneys, liver, and heart to determine whether they are functioning normally.[5]

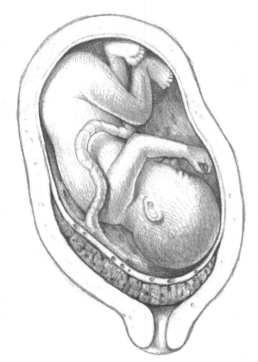

Placenta previa.

The placenta normally lies near the top of the uterus. With placenta previa, painless vaginal bleeding may occur when the placenta partially or completely covers the cervix. This bleeding is potentially dangerous for the mother or her baby.

From: Mayo Foundation for Medical Education and Research. 1994. The third trimester. In Mayo Clinic Complete Book of Pregnancy and Baby's First Year. New York: William Morrow & Co., 195. Reprinted by permission.

Infection During Pregnancy and How It Might Affect Your Baby

When a pregnant woman develops an infection, it is cause for concern. Infections can be caused by a virus or by a bacterium or fungus—and you can pass an infection to your developing baby. Among the risks of maternal infection are premature birth, stillbirth, abnormal fetal growth and development, abnormal blood cell count in the baby's blood, jaundice, seizures, pneumonia, and infection of the fluid that surrounds your baby's brain.

Certain infections are most threatening:

- TORCH—a group of viral infections that may affect a baby while in the uterus and/or during the birth process (The infections are **t**oxoplasmosis, **o**ther, **r**ubella virus, **c**ytomegalovirus, and **h**erpes simplex virus.)[9]
- The human immunodeficiency virus (HIV)—the virus that causes AIDS
- Any infection of the female reproductive or urinary tract, including sexually transmitted diseases (STDs) such as chlamydia or syphilis

Chapters 9 and 10 discuss these and other infections—including those a mother can pass to her baby before or during birth. Those chapters also explain why newborns are especially susceptible to infection when exposed and detail the consequences of infection for the baby.

Blood-Type Incompatibility and How It Might Affect Your Baby

To understand blood-type incompatibility, you need to know something about human blood cells. Blood cells have substances called antigens attached to their surface. Blood-type identification is based on these antigens. Our immune system (which protects our bodies from invasion by "foreign" cells) recognizes antigens as either "friendly" (compatible) or "foreign" (incompatible). Foreign bodies are usually bacteria or viruses that cause infection. If the immune system recognizes a blood cell carrying a foreign antigen, it takes the same action it would for an infection-causing agent—it produces antibodies to destroy or deactivate the antigen. When that happens, the antibody destroys the blood cell carrying the antigen along with the antigen itself. Antibodies can affect two types of blood cells: red blood cells and platelets.

Red Blood Cells

All human beings have a blood type, depending on the type of red blood cells they have. Blood types are identified by the ABO system: type O (the most common), type A, type B, and type AB. Blood types are either compatible or incompatible when mixed—that is why any blood used for transfusion must be tested carefully (typed and cross-matched) to be sure it is compatible with the blood of the person who is to receive the transfusion.

In addition to your blood type, human blood also has an Rh factor—a positive or negative designation (for example, blood type A positive or A negative). Both your blood type and your Rh factor are determined by genes that are passed from mother and father to child. It is possible for a mother and fetus to have incompatibilities due to the difference in their blood types and/or due to the difference in their Rh factors.

A blood type incompatibility between the mother and her baby is often referred to as ABO incompatibility, or an ABO "setup." This complication occurs most often when the mother's blood type is O and the baby's blood type is A or B. Incompatibilities of this type are rare for mothers whose blood type is A or B. Blood type incompatibility does not present as great a threat to the fetus and newborn as Rh incompatibility. The newborn with the ABO type incompatibility is at risk for jaundice and hyperbilirubinemia soon after birth. (See Chapter 9 for information about hyperbilirubinemia.)

Problems caused by Rh incompatibility are usually more serious for the fetus and newborn than ABO problems. Rh incompatibility is possible if the mother is Rh negative and the father is Rh positive. This is because the fetus could be Rh positive, having inherited this factor from the father. Problems are possible when the Rh negative mother carries an Rh positive fetus.

Pregnancy complications that are caused by Rh incompatibility are not a concern if the mother is Rh positive or if the mother and father are both Rh negative.

"The NICU staff kept calling my baby a '25 weeker.' I knew my baby was sick, but why did every baby get called 'weeker': 32 weeker, 34 weeker, like that?"

The problems of blood type/Rh incompatibility occur when the fetal red blood cells cross the placenta and enter the mother's circulation. This happens commonly during birth, but can occur during pregnancy or during a previous pregnancy, abortion, or birth. This introduction of Rh positive blood cells or an incompatible blood type sensitizes the mother to this type of cell. The mother's immune system then produces antibodies against the fetus's "foreign" blood antigens. When the antibodies travel back into the fetal circulation, the maternal antibodies destroy the fetus's red blood cells. If this incompatibility occurs in future pregnancies, the mother's body quickly produces this antibody and puts the fetus at risk for red blood cell destruction.

The medical term for destruction of red blood cells is hemolysis. In the case of ABO incompatibility, the fetus usually compensates for hemolysis by increasing its production of red blood cells. After birth, a newborn whose blood type is not compatible with her mother's may develop anemia (a low red blood cell count) because hemolysis continues after birth, but the newborn cannot produce red blood cells fast enough to keep up with their destruction. With red blood cell destruction, a waste product of destroyed red blood cells (bilirubin) may build up more quickly than it can be eliminated, causing jaundice (see Chapter 9). The baby's blood type will be checked, and red blood cell and bilirubin counts will be monitored frequently. The baby may require phototherapy (treatment with light) to reduce jaundice and intravenous fluids to prevent dehydration. In rare cases, the baby may require an exchange transfusion (see Chapter 9).

If the mother's antibody response against her fetus is particularly strong, as is often the case with Rh incompatibility, hemolysis may result in severe fetal anemia and jaundice. Sometimes the fetus can receive a blood transfusion while within the womb. This type of fetal therapy can be lifesaving for the unborn baby because a severely affected fetus can be born with heart failure, edema, shock, an enlarged liver, and bleeding problems. These babies usually require help breathing, IV fluids, blood transfusions, and medications to maintain an adequate blood pressure and antibiotics to fight infections.

To anticipate any potential incompatibility problems, pregnant women have their blood type and Rh factor determined during prenatal care. Because Rh incompatibility produces more serious complications for the fetus and newborn baby than does ABO (blood type) incompatibility, mothers who are Rh negative are followed very closely throughout their pregnancies. In most cases, the first pregnancy is not affected; however, sometimes the fetal red blood cells cross the placenta and enter the mother's circulation before delivery. Rh negative mothers usually receive a medication call RhoGAM (WinRho in Canada) at the beginning of the third trimester of pregnancy (at about 28 weeks gestation) and again right after they give birth. RhoGAM destroys fetal cells in the mother's circulation and therefore blocks the production of antibodies against Rh positive red blood cells. (RhoGAM is effective only for women who have not already formed antibodies against the Rh positive factor.) RhoGAM is given to protect not only this baby, but also future fetuses. Unless the antibody-producing response is blocked with medication, an Rh negative mother begins to make antibodies against the fetus's Rh positive cells. If a future fetus is Rh positive, the mother's immune system may begin to produce antibodies quickly, even before she knows she is pregnant, putting her growing fetus at high risk for complications of Rh incompatibility.

Platelets

Blood cells that control bleeding are called platelets. Platelets have antigens on their surfaces; these antigens determine the platelet "type." The antigen system that identifies platelet type is known as the PLA system. Platelet type is determined by genes that are inherited in the same way that red blood cell type is. You and your baby may have the same platelet type (platelet compatibility) or two different platelet types (platelet incompatibility).

Your growing baby's platelets can cross the placenta and circulate in your bloodstream if there is a capillary break in the placenta. If the fetus's platelet type and your own are not the same (incompatible), your body will produce antibodies against your fetus's platelets. When these antibodies return to your fetus through the placenta, they can destroy the fetus's platelets and cause low platelet counts.

A maternal disease called idiopathic thrombocytopenic purpura (ITP) can also cause destruction of fetal platelets. Some women who have this disease produce antibodies directed against all platelets. These women have frequent problems with low platelet counts because the antibodies their immune systems make destroy even their own platelets. During pregnancy, these antibodies cross the placenta and destroy the fetus's platelets. The babies of these women may be born with low platelet counts.

The medical term for low platelets is thrombocytopenia. Babies with a low platelet count may look healthy or may show bruising; a purplish, speckled "rash" (called petechiae and pronounced pe-TEE-kee-eye) that is actually due to tiny hemorrhages of the blood vessels just under the skin surface; and bleeding that is difficult to control because of the decreased number of platelets. Some of these babies require only protection from injury that could cause bleeding. Others may need transfusions of platelets or medications to reduce platelet destruction. Blood tests to check blood and platelet type, red blood cell count, and platelet count will be done. The baby's platelets will be low only until the antibodies from the mother are eliminated from her system. This can take a few days to a few weeks. When the antibodies have been eliminated, the baby's platelet count will be normal.

Although blood typing is a routine part of prenatal care, platelet typing is not. If your newborn baby has low platelets, the physician may want to test your blood and the baby's father's blood to see if you have platelet antibodies or to determine your platelet types. Knowing if you carry antibodies against platelets or if your platelet type is incompatible with your newborn's can give the NICU team certain clues about how to treat your newborn's low platelet count. This information will also be important to your obstetrician for future pregnancies.[10]

"We knew that pregnancy was a risk to my health. But we planned carefully, got excellent prenatal care, and everything turned out fine. We were lucky."

Fetal Factors That Affect Your Baby

As babies grow and develop throughout pregnancy, they interact with their environment. That environment is their mother's uterus and the amniotic fluid surrounding them in the uterus. The rate of growth of your uterus and the amount of amniotic fluid surrounding your baby are valuable clues to your baby's growth and development status.

Multiple Pregnancies

If you are pregnant with more than one fetus (called a multiple-gestation pregnancy), lack of uterine space can affect your fetuses' weight gain in the final third of your pregnancy. Through week 29 of a healthy pregnancy, the growth rate of more than one fetus is nearly the same as it is for one. But at 30 weeks and later, multiple fetuses do not gain weight as rapidly as a single fetus does. In fact, with more than one fetus, the babies may not gain weight or grow in length at all after week 37 or 38 of pregnancy. In contrast, a single fetus is able to gain weight and grow until term.

A second risk associated with more than one fetus is abnormal blood flow through the placenta. If your multiple gestation pregnancy resulted from a single egg, the fetuses are called identical and usually share one placenta. If more than one egg was fertilized, the fetuses are fraternal, and each has its own placenta. With more than one fetus, the connection of the umbilical cords to the placenta (in the case of identical fetuses) can develop abnormally, or the separate placentas (in the case of fraternal and some identical fetuses) can connect to one another abnormally. These abnormal connections can cause differences in blood flow between or among the fetuses. This is known as twin-to-twin transfusion syndrome. Newborns who have received reduced blood flow during pregnancy can show signs of low birth weight, low red blood cell count, reduced blood volume, and perhaps altered kidney function and congestive heart failure. Newborns who have received greater than normal blood flow during pregnancy are generally sicker than those who have received limited amounts. They often show a high red blood cell count, signs of jaundice, an overworked heart, a high blood volume, and abnormal liver function. Multiple-birth newborns who show symptoms of these two opposite situations are called discordant.

If you are pregnant with more than one fetus, you are at risk for developing gestational diabetes, pregnancy-induced hypertension, and anemia. These conditions were discussed previously in this chapter—and all can be problematic for your developing babies. An additional risk with multiple births is the presence of above normal amounts of amniotic fluid (see the next section). More than one infant also increases the risk of premature birth and/or injury during labor and delivery for both mother and babies.[1,5,6]

Amniotic Fluid and Its Effects on Your Baby

Your developing baby is surrounded by amniotic fluid in your uterus. This fluid cushions your fetus against jolts and bumps, helps control fetal temperature, protects the umbilical cord, and prevents infection.

Amniotic fluid is made up of fetal urine and lung fluids, as well as fluid made by the lining of the sac that holds your baby. The fetus regulates the amount of amniotic fluid present by swallowing, "breathing" (the amniotic fluid moves in and out of the fetus's lungs), and urinating. Presence of a normal amount of amniotic fluid indicates that the fetus's lungs, esophagus, nervous system, and kidneys are developing as they should be. If a fetus has problems swallowing, "breathing," or making urine, greater or less than normal amounts of amniotic fluid will likely be present.

Oligohydramnios is the medical name for a lower than normal amount of amniotic fluid surrounding the fetus. This condition is most commonly the result of a pregnancy that extends beyond 40 weeks gestation; in this case, a combination of fetal, placental, and maternal factors contributes to the reduced volume. Oligohydramnios may also occur if the fetus's kidneys are improperly formed or improperly functioning. Maternal causes of oligohydramnios include a small tear in the amniotic sac, permitting a slow leak of fluid over time, and inadequate maternal nutrition.

When the fetus is not surrounded by enough amniotic fluid during development, the environment is cramped and constricted, causing compression (pressure) and dehydration. The newborn may display physical features characteristic of this environment: a set of facial features that develop due to the compressive forces around the baby's head (short neck; tiny nose; wide-set eyes; small chin; large, low-set ears), small, undeveloped lungs, wrinkled skin, stiff joints, and bone problems. In addition, the umbilical cord can become compressed during labor and delivery because of the restricted space and lack of cushioning fluid. This can limit blood flow to and from the fetus, placing her at risk for complications during labor.

If oligohydramnios has been a problem during pregnancy, your newborn's caregivers will observe her closely to see whether her kidneys are working properly. They will monitor the relationship between fluid intake and urine output and will also check the level of electrolytes in her urine and blood. Ultrasound evaluation of the kidneys may be used to determine kidney structure. Newborns whose kidneys are not functioning normally often require bladder catheterization (insertion of a tube into the bladder) for accurate measurement and/or collection of urine. Newborns who have developed in less than normal amounts of amniotic fluid may also have underdeveloped lungs (called pulmonary hypoplasia). They will need help breathing. Chest x-rays and measurement of blood gases will likely play a part in the assessment of your newborn's lung development.

A greater than normal amount of amniotic fluid—a condition called polyhydramnios—may also occur during pregnancy. Causes of polyhydramnios include an improperly formed or improperly functioning gastrointestinal tract

"The ultrasound technician discovered our triplets. She was very quiet, staring at the screen, then she cleared her throat and asked, 'Are you and your husband planning a large family?'"

(stomach and intestines) or an improperly formed or malfunctioning brain and spinal cord. Fluid builds up when the fetus cannot swallow effectively because of a blockage in the gastrointestinal tract or a problem in the nervous system. It also increases if the fetus cannot absorb the amniotic fluid it swallows. Finally, fluid volume can grow if the fetus's nervous system is leaking cerebrospinal fluid. This occurs with conditions such as spina bifida.

When polyhydramnios is present, the baby is often in either the breech (buttocks or feet first) or oblique (shoulder first) position at delivery. These infants rarely show any physical features indicating their developmental condition. Caregivers will assess the newborn's breathing patterns, muscle tone, and response to stimuli (to determine nervous system status) and her ability to suck and swallow, tolerate feedings, and pass stool (to determine the condition of the gastrointestinal tract).[1,5,6]

Birth Defects

Some newborns show physical abnormalities at birth. The medical term for these abnormalities is congenital (meaning "existing at birth") anomalies, and they are more commonly called birth defects. For information on specific birth defects, see Chapter 10.

Structural malformations are seen when organs or organ systems develop in an unusual fashion. The changes may be genetic (inherited) or may be caused by some environmental or maternal factor. Structural malformations often occur early in the pregnancy (between the third and eighth weeks), before many women are even aware that they are pregnant. They include heart defects, cleft lip/cleft palate, a defect of the spine called spina bifida, and defects of the abdomen in which internal organs protrude outside the body (for example, omphalocele and gastroschisis). Structural malformations require medical, surgical, and/or cosmetic treatment.

Many babies are born with minor anomalies (small variations in appearance), which are caused by mechanical pressure on the fetus in the uterus. For example, bowed legs or a turned-in foot can be caused by positioning in the uterus and usually resolves without treatment. Other variations include skin tags (small outgrowths of the skin) on the earlobes or extra fingers or toes. These variations can occur in families as a hereditary trait.

Malformations may appear singly or in patterns (several defects together), a situation called multiple congenital anomaly (MCA) syndrome. Many congenital malformations are discovered only after birth, during the first physical examination, but more are now detected during pregnancy through ultrasonography.[11]

The process of labor and birth is greatly influenced by the health of the mother and her unborn baby. Many of these factors have been discussed previously in this chapter. The birth process involves an amazing chain of events that are all interrelated and dependent on the healthy functioning of the mother's body and on her baby's ability to tolerate the stresses of labor and the transition to extrauterine life. A healthy fetus will be able to withstand the normal stresses of labor and delivery with no ill effects. A fetus that has developed in a problematic environment (and thus is at risk even before the birth experience) or a baby who experiences a greater than normal degree of stress during labor and delivery may need special care immediately after birth.

Major risk factors for mother and baby are usually anticipated prior to labor and birth. Appropriate prenatal care and ongoing assessment during labor enable your health care team to make decisions that result in the best possible outcome for you and your new baby. Chapter 1 discusses what you may expect if you experience a complicated labor. This section discusses some of the occurrences of labor and birth that may result in a newborn who requires special care.

How Your Baby Is Affected by Factors Associated with Labor and Delivery

Problems with Oxygen Supply and Delivery

The unborn baby must have a sufficient supply of oxygen during labor and birth. If the mother's own oxygen supply is at risk (perhaps because of cardiac or respiratory problems or serious blood loss), the fetal supply is also in jeopardy.[12] Problems with placental function (perhaps because of infection, poor placental development, or decreased efficiency late in pregnancy) can influence oxygen supply to the unborn baby. The fetus can also have heart or circulation problems before labor that further stress abilities to use oxygen efficiently.

Maternal, placental, and fetal problems are usually discovered before the baby's birth. Adequate prenatal care is important for discovery and management of these conditions. In some cases, newborn intensive care may be inevitable, but good prenatal care and close monitoring before and/or during labor enable the health care team to deliver the baby in the best possible condition.

The oxygen supply to the fetus is decreased during labor contractions—this is a normal and expected part of the labor process. Even a healthy baby can experience distress, however, if the mother experiences unusually forceful contractions, contractions that are too close together, or that last an unusually long time.[12] These abnormalities in the labor process can cause an inadequate oxygen supply to the baby. The health care team takes steps as necessary to ensure an oxygen supply to the fetus by administering extra oxygen to the mother and by attempting to restore normal labor contractions.

The unborn baby can also have problems with oxygen supply if the umbilical cord becomes squeezed or compressed.[12] The cord can become trapped between the baby and the mother's uterine wall during contractions, or the baby's head or body may press on the cord, limiting oxygen supply to the baby. Compression can also occur if the cord slips past the baby and enters the mother's birth canal before the baby. This event is called umbilical cord prolapse and requires emergency delivery of the baby.

Newborns whose oxygen supply is inadequate during labor may require resuscitation at birth to breathe and to achieve or maintain an adequate heart rate (see Chapter 2). Infants have an amazing capacity to overcome serious problems at birth, but extended lack of oxygen during labor and birth can damage the infant's major organs. These complications are discussed in Chapter 10.

Lung Preparation During Labor and Birth

During labor, the fluid that has been in the fetus's lungs during growth and development begins to be absorbed. This process of fetal lung-fluid absorption during labor prepares the newborn's lungs to breathe air and absorb oxygen immediately after birth. Lung preparation is believed to be an important function of labor.

Vaginal birth also helps prepare the lungs for breathing. As the baby passes through the tight birth canal, her chest is squeezed, aiding in expulsion of any remaining fetal lung fluids. Infants who do not experience labor (those born by cesarean section, for example) or whose mothers have only a very brief labor can have problems breathing immediately after birth. If this respiratory distress is severe, it may require a brief stay in intensive care. The situation usually resolves rapidly, however.

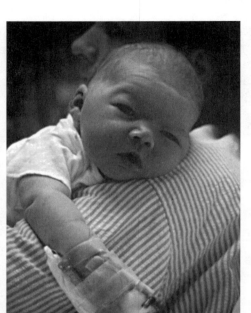

Relaxing with Mom.

The NICU cares for babies of all sizes with many different problems. But every baby needs a parent's special care.

Precipitous Labor and Delivery

A labor and delivery that lasts less than three hours is called a precipitous labor. In such labors, the mother's uterine contractions are very strong, and they push the fetus through the birth canal quickly. Problems associated with precipitous labor include reduced blood and oxygen flow to the baby (because of the strength of the contractions). They may also include injury to the infant's head (because the cervix has not dilated sufficiently to allow the baby to pass through easily).[13]

Birth Trauma and How It Might Affect Your Baby

Birth injuries—often called birth trauma—can occur during a difficult labor or birth. These injuries may be minor, with no long-term consequences for your baby, or they may be more serious. Birth injuries are more frequent among babies who are large in weight for their gestational age, babies who are born prematurely, those born following a precipitous labor (see previous section) or a lengthy labor, those not born headfirst, or, rarely, those delivered with mechanical assistance (forceps or vacuum extraction).[13]

There are three categories of birth injuries: (1) head and neck, (2) nerve, and (3) bone. The more common injuries are discussed here.

Head Injuries

A cephalhematoma occurs when blood from a broken blood vessel collects between the surface of the skull bone and the tough membrane that covers the skull bone. It is normally seen only on one side of the head. Most often, a cephalhematoma is small and resolves without causing the baby any problems, but in rare cases, it can become quite large. Bleeding from a large cephalhematoma in a newborn may cause a low red blood cell count, low blood pressure, and jaundice. Cephalhematomas usually resolve without treatment over the first months of life.

Rarely, fracture of the skull can occur during birth and may cause a serious birth injury.[14] In addition to the bone damage, the fracture can cause the brain to be bruised, or damage can occur to the blood vessels in the brain, causing bleeding. An x-ray and sometimes a CT scan are performed to aid diagnosis. Superficial fractures that do not involve the brain heal without treatment or complications in 8 to 12 weeks. If the newborn's brain has been bruised or if bleeding in the brain has occurred, the baby's brain or nervous system development can be affected.

Nerve Damage

Erb's palsy is the most common birth injury affecting the nerves. It involves the roots of the nerves at the base of the newborn's neck. These nerves may swell, become irritated, or be damaged due to stretching and twisting during delivery. Erb's palsy usually affects only one side of the body and causes paralysis of the arm, hand, and/or fingers only on the affected side. Healing generally occurs naturally, but range-of-motion exercises and maintenance of joint alignment can help. If the injury does not heal on its own, growth of the affected arm may be stunted.

Bell's palsy involves damage to the newborn's facial nerve. It causes paralysis (lack of movement) on one side of the face. The damage heals on its own without treatment or complications. During recovery, the infant may have difficulty sucking and may need eye drops to keep the eye on the affected side moist.

Damage to the phrenic nerve (another nerve root at the base of the baby's neck) during delivery can cause paralysis of the diaphragm. The diaphragm is the muscle under the lungs that assists in breathing. Because the phrenic nerve controls this muscle, damage to that nerve can cause paralysis of the diaphragm on one or both sides, affecting the infant's breathing. Some babies require assistance with breathing. An x-ray and an ultrasound examination are used to diagnose the problem. Recovery usually takes from one to three months. During recovery, caregivers focus on keeping the infant from developing pneumonia (an infection of the lungs).

Paralysis of the vocal cords can result from damage to the laryngeal nerve at the base of the baby's neck. Diagnosis of vocal cord paralysis is made by examining the newborn's vocal cords. One or both can be affected. During recovery, the newborn may receive help in breathing and feeding, to prevent choking. If only one vocal cord is involved, the infant will usually recover in four to six weeks. When both are involved, the infant will need mechanical help to breathe, and recovery will likely take longer.[15]

Bone Injuries

Term infants born in the breech position and term babies who weigh more than average for their age at birth are the most likely to sustain birth injuries to their bones. The causes of these injuries are stress to and twisting of the bones during birth. The most common location for bone breakage is the clavicle (collarbone). A newborn with a fracture of the clavicle may show limited movement of the arm on the side of the break and may also have muscle spasms. An x-ray may be taken to diagnose the injury. Caregivers will limit the infant's arm movements during the healing period, which takes seven to ten days.[5,14]

Your Baby's Special Needs

Most of the time, the circumstances that result in an NICU admission are beyond anyone's control. Even though your health care team is able to plan ahead for most factors that place the mother or fetus at risk, an NICU admission is sometimes inevitable. This is especially true for preterm birth. Other babies admitted to the NICU are those who have problems resulting from a complicated labor and birth, infection, birth defects, or maternal problems that affect the unborn baby's growth and development.

The delivery of a newborn is a time of emotional highs and lows. If your baby needs intensive care, the joys and fears of this emotional roller coaster will be even more extreme. You will need some time to begin to understand why your baby is in the NICU. Soon you will realize the challenges facing your baby. Remember that even if your baby requires special care for the same reason as another baby, your child's needs will be unique. As parents, you will discover how to work with the NICU team to best meet those special needs.

Chapter 9

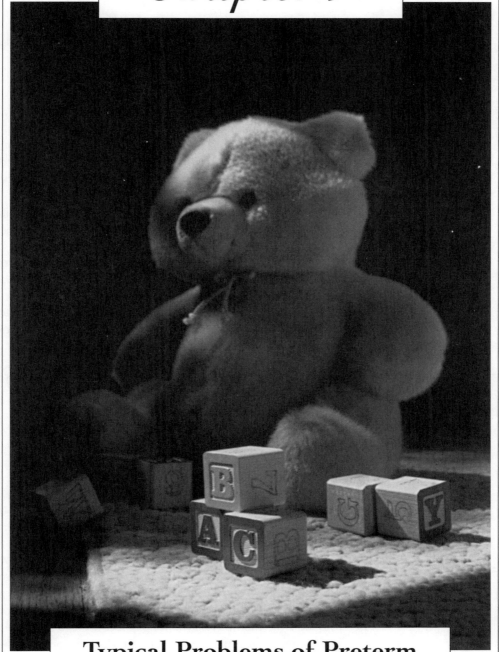

Typical Problems of Preterm Babies and Other Sick Newborns

Susan Tucker Blackburn, RN,C, PhD, FAAN

**❝"Listen to this, Piglet,"
said Eeyore, "and then you'll
know what we're trying to do."❞**

We often hear it said that babies are different. Babies are different from older infants, children, and adults in many ways, including how they behave and respond to things and how their bodies function. This doesn't mean that babies cannot cope with the world around them. It simply means that they may respond differently than older infants would and that some of their responses and body functions are still immature.

By the time your baby is born, even if he is born prematurely, all the major body systems have been formed. Even in term infants, however, these organs and systems continue to mature after birth. The more premature a baby is, the more maturing these systems need to do. Many of the problems premature and other sick newborns experience are because of the immaturity of their organs and body systems, not because of a disease.

Babies in intensive care, especially premature babies, share many common problems. Little can be done to prevent many of these problems; they are just part of being a small or sick baby. The good news is that your baby's health care providers know what these potential problems are. They can recognize babies who are at risk, identify signs of developing problems, and do something about them to minimize their effects and to keep minor problems from becoming major ones.

This chapter describes possible problems that NICU babies may experience because of the immaturity of one or more of their major body systems. Your baby may or may not be at risk for developing one of these problems. Also keep in mind that a baby at risk does not always develop the problem. Talk with your baby's nurses and doctors about any concerns you have for your special baby.

Problems Related to the Heart and Lungs

The cardiorespiratory system includes the heart, blood vessels, and lungs. This system is essential for movement of oxygen into the body and through the lungs and for getting rid of carbon dioxide. Humans cannot survive without adequate oxygen because cells need oxygen to function properly and to prevent damage. Carbon dioxide, a by-product of energy production, must be removed from the body by the lungs, because too much carbon dioxide in the body can be harmful. The heart pumps blood from the body to the lungs, where oxygen is added (the blood is oxygenated) and carbon dioxide is removed. The heart then pumps the oxygenated blood to the rest of the body.

Many aspects of an infant's heart and lung functions are immature at birth, even when the infant is born full-term. The more premature a baby is, the more immature the cardiorespiratory system. Immaturity of this system can increase the risk of problems such as apnea (absence or pause in breathing), bradycardia (slow heartbeat), and cyanosis (blue color).

Potential Breathing Problems

Premature babies often stop breathing for brief periods. What this condition is called depends on the length of the pause in breathing and whether the breathing pause is accompanied by changes in heart rate and skin color.

Periodic Breathing

Periodic breathing is a cyclic pattern in which the infant briefly pauses in breathing (usually for about 5 to 10 seconds) and then assumes regular breathing.[1] Infants who have periodic breathing always start to breathe again on their own and never show any changes in heart rate or skin color. Periodic breathing is a common pattern in premature infants and may last for many weeks after birth. Healthy term infants may also exhibit this pattern in the first few days after birth. Because this is a normal pattern, no special care is needed.

Apnea of Prematurity

In preterm infants, episodes of periodic breathing that involve pauses in breathing of 20 seconds or longer or pauses of any length accompanied by changes in heart rate and/or skin color are called apnea of prematurity, or primary apnea. This type of apnea is related to the immaturity of the infant's central nervous and respiratory systems.

One of the most common problems of premature infants, apnea is seen in 25 percent of all premature babies and in more than 80 percent of babies born weighing less than 2½ pounds (about 1,100 grams). Periods of apnea usually begin during the first week after birth and may continue for a few days or for many weeks.

Three main types of apnea are seen in premature infants: central apnea, obstructive apnea, and mixed apnea. Central apnea is a result of immaturity of the brain, especially the area known as the respiratory center, which controls breathing. Obstructive apnea occurs when the upper portion of the baby's breathing tube (called the upper airway) becomes blocked. This is also related to immaturity. It can be caused by flexion of the baby's neck or by the decreased muscle tone of the tongue and upper airway during sleep, which can cause blockage of the passage of air into the lungs. Mixed apnea is a combination of central and obstructive apnea. It is the most common type of apnea in premature infants.

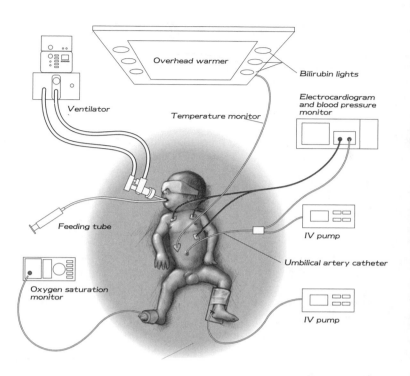

Typical NICU baby with support equipment.

While every baby's hospital course is different, many babies share typical problems. This drawing depicts the equipment commonly used to support the NICU baby.

From: *Mayo Foundation for Medical Education and Research. 1994.* Mayo Complete Book of Pregnancy and Baby's First Year. *New York: William Morrow & Co., 360. Reprinted by permission.*

Characteristics of the Cardiorespiratory System in Term and Preterm Newborns

Aspect	Characteristics	Significance	Examples of Care Provided
Heart rate/rhythm	Faster than in adult; may be irregular	Uses oxygen more rapidly than adults therefore needs to breathe faster	Infant watched carefully; stress reduced by gentle, minimal handling; decreasing noise in the environment; maintaining a normal temperature; and nesting the infant in blankets
Blood output of heart (cardiac output)	2–3 times higher than in adult	Heart rate higher (120–160 beats per minute) than in adult	Cardiorespiratory monitor used to observe heart rate and detect changes from normal range
Blood circulation	Transition must be made from fetal circulation to newborn circulation; if ductus arteriosus remains open (patent) some blood bypasses lungs, thereby reducing blood oxygenation	Risk of lower blood oxygen levels and cyanosis	Infant watched carefully; oxygen and medications given as needed Pulse oximeter and/or transcutaneous monitor used to assess respiratory status
Small blood vessels (capillaries)	Fragile	Risk of bruising and bleeding	Infant handled carefully
Rib cage and muscles	Less well developed and not as firm as in adult	Less effective breathing; abdominal muscles used to help with breathing	Infant positioned to enhance breathing
Lung and chest wall elasticity (compliance)	Stiffer (less elastic) lungs and floppier chest wall than in adult	Harder work required to expand lungs; leads to retractions of floppy chest wall during intake of breath	Infant positioned to enhance breathing; ventilator used if needed
Diaphragm	Less well developed than in adult; fewer muscles that can work hard for a long time	Uses abdominal muscles to breathe; tires more quickly and develops weaker breathing efforts	Infant positioned to enhance breathing; stress reduced by gentle, minimal handling; decreasing noise in the environment; maintaining a normal temperature; nesting in blankets; ventilator used if needed
Airway (nose and trachea, or breathing tube)	Narrower and more flexible than in adult	Mucus may block passage of air	Infant suctioned as needed
Air sacs (alveoli) in lungs	Fewer than in adult; immature	More work required to get oxygen into body	Reduce stress by gentle, minimal handling; decrease noise in the environment; maintain normal temperature; nest in blankets; give extra oxygen as needed
Surfactant (substance that prevents air sacs from collapsing at end of each breath)	Production immature; some air sacs collapsed	More work required to expand air sacs; more oxygen used	Ventilator or CPAP used (see Chapter 10); extra oxygen given as necessary Surfactant replacement therapy, if appropriate
Oxygen consumption (needs)	Higher than in adult	Faster breathing required to take in enough oxygen (30–60 breaths per minute)	Cardiorespiratory monitor used to observe breathing rate and detect changes from normal range
Breathing control	Immature development	Risk for apnea of prematurity; irregular breathing	Cardiorespiratory monitor used to detect apnea; Medication (theophylline or caffeine) given as ordered (see Appendix B)

As the infant's central nervous system and respiratory system mature, apnea of prematurity disappears. Most premature babies develop control of their breathing before they are discharged home. Rarely, premature infants develop long-term apnea. These infants may require home apnea monitoring after discharge (see Chapter 16).

Other kinds of apnea

Especially when it begins suddenly, apnea may be an early sign of other diseases in term or preterm infants. This is sometimes referred to as secondary apnea. Disorders sometimes associated with sudden-onset apnea in the first few days after birth include a low temperature (hypothermia), infection, low blood sugar (hypoglycemia), necrotizing enterocolitis (NEC), intraventricular hemorrhage (IVH), and shock. See Chapter 10 for more information on NEC and IVH.

Management of apnea

Periods of apnea can be frightening to parents. Many apneic spells end spontaneously, with the baby beginning to breathe again on his own. Infants at risk for apnea are attached to a cardiorespiratory monitor that tracks their heart and breathing rates. They may also be attached to a pulse oximeter that monitors the oxygenation of their blood. (Both monitors are described in Chapter 2.) Alarms on these machines are set to sound when the heart rate, breathing rate, or oxygen level falls below a specified level. The level at which the alarm will activate is set high, so it sounds before the baby is in serious trouble. When the alarm sounds, a caregiver helps the baby begin breathing again.

Although babies often start breathing again by themselves, the nurse may gently rub the baby's side or foot to stimulate respirations. This is known as tactile stimulation. Sometimes the nurse also needs to give the baby extra oxygen, especially if the baby's response to tactile stimulation is slow or if the baby develops a very low heart rate and a blue color along with the apnea. Extra oxygen to raise the pulse and make the baby pink can be given by blowing the oxygen near the baby's face if he has begun to breathe normally again or by "bagging" if the baby is not breathing well on his own. "Bagging" means that the caregiver gently pumps oxygen into the baby's lungs with an oxygen bag and a face mask. (Chapter 2 provides more information on both interventions.)

Two therapies used with infants who have frequent apneic spells are nasal CPAP—continuous positive airway pressure—and medications. Nasal CPAP involves providing air or air mixed with oxygen at low pressures through small, short tubes placed in the baby's nose. This air helps keep the airway and air sacs in the lungs (alveoli) from collapsing and open to the passage of air. Nasal CPAP works best for obstructive or mixed apnea.[2] To help reduce central apnea, medications that stimulate the central nervous system are used. The most common are theophylline and caffeine. Appendix B discusses both.

Apnea and sudden infant death syndrome

Parents of infants with apnea of prematurity are often concerned about a possible relationship between apnea and sudden infant death syndrome (SIDS). Apnea of prematurity is a developmental event that disappears as the infant matures. Apnea of prematurity is not the same as SIDS and is not considered to be a specific risk factor for SIDS.[3] The cause of SIDS is unknown (see Chapter 16).

Bradycardia

Changes in heart rate often accompany apnea but may occur independently. A temporary slowing of the heart rate—called bradycardia—is the most frequent heart-rate change seen with apnea. In most babies, the heart beats between 120 and 160 times every minute (twice as fast as an adult heart beats). With bradycardia, the heart may slow to 60 to100 beats per minute, but it does not stop or even come close to stopping. Like apnea, bradycardia usually resolves with tactile stimulation. Occasionally, additional oxygen may be required.

Cyanosis

Cyanosis is the term for a bluish color of the skin. An infant may have acrocyanosis (bluish color of the hands and feet), circumoral cyanosis (bluish color around the mouth), or generalized cyanosis (bluish color of the entire body). A bluish-pinkish skin color may be described as "dusky."

Acrocyanosis is a common and often normal response. Infants often have acrocyanosis for a few hours after birth and may develop it if their limbs are cold. Generalized cyanosis, duskiness, or circumoral cyanosis may occur with apnea and/or bradycardia. These forms of cyanosis indicate that the infant's cells are not receiving adequate oxygen. The infant may not be breathing, the infant may not be breathing effectively enough to take in adequate oxygen, or the infant's heart may be pumping too slowly to send enough oxygen to the skin cells. The cyanosis often disappears once the infant's breathing rate and heart rate return to normal. Sometimes the baby needs additional oxygen for a short period.

Problems Related to the Skin

The skin has many functions, including sensation and protection. Through touch receptors in the skin, your baby interacts with and learns about the world. Touch sensation is one of the earliest senses to develop. The fetus begins to respond to touch early in development. After birth, touch is an important way that parents and other caregivers can relate to a baby. Gentle touching—a hand placed on the infant's head or back—is soothing to many babies. Chapter 4 provides more information on the sensory capabilities of newborns.

The skin's protective functions are sometimes called its barrier properties. The skin acts as a barrier to keep out bacteria and viruses that can cause

"Our nurse told us that apnea was a typical problem for a baby like Jason. My imagination ran wild. If turning blue was typical, what other death-defying tricks could we expect from Jason?"

infection. Through fat, the skin also provides insulation, helping to keep in heat and fluid and preventing your baby from becoming cold or dehydrated.

Characteristics of the Newborn's Skin

The skin consists of three layers: an outer layer (the epidermis), a middle layer (dermis), and an inner layer (the subcutaneous tissue). In preterm infants, the skin is immature and unable to act as much of a barrier. One reason is that the epidermis is thinner and less firmly attached to the dermis than in term and older infants. Also, the preterm infant's subcutaneous layer is thin and initially contains little insulating fat.

Four problems can arise because of the immature barrier properties of the skin in preterm infants: (1) increased water and heat loss, (2) increased permeability of the skin to lotions and other substances, (3) increased risk of infection, and (4) increased risk of skin breakdown, especially with the removal of tape.

After birth, the skin matures quickly. Within two to three weeks, a preterm infant's epidermis and skin permeability are quite similar to those of a term infant. As the skin matures, the cells of the skin continue to develop, through a process called keratinization, and the skin dries out. You will notice your baby's skin becoming dry and flaky. This is a normal (and healthy) change. Even though your baby's skin may not look as nice as it once did, it's best not to apply lotions, powders, and other substances. These may increase your baby's risk for problems related to the skin's immature barrier function. In addition, absorption of some of these substances across the permeable skin can further alter the immature skin barrier and increase the risk of problems such as skin breakdown and infection.[4]

Newborn skin care is not an exact science, and new research is constantly influencing nursing practice. The fragile skin of a preterm infant poses incredible challenges for nursing care. Every NICU has its own protocol for skin care; ask your baby's nurse for information on your baby's care plan.

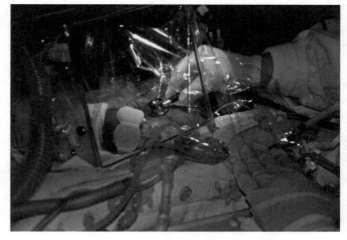

Skin care for a very premature infant.

This baby is intubated and using a ventilator to breathe. In this case, a plastic oxygen tent is used to decrease the amount of heat and fluid lost through his very thin skin. Eye patches are in place because he is under phototherapy lights.

Special Skin Care for Babies

To protect their skin and to prevent skin breakdown, all babies receive special skin care. Babies are generally bathed only with warm water as needed. Skin care also includes use of heat shields or a sheet of plastic stretched over the baby to reduce water and heat loss from the skin; gentle handling; avoidance of lotions, ointments, or other substances (unless medically indicated); use of special tape that is gentle to the skin; avoidance of adhesives; and use of special transparent dressings. These dressings can be used over skin irritations to promote healing or over places where intravenous (IV) lines or catheters have been inserted to protect these sites and reduce the risk of infection. A soft, easy-to-remove barrier can be placed between the tape and the infant's

Characteristics of the Skin in Preterm Infants

Aspect	Characteristics	Significance	Examples of Care Provided
Epidermis (top layer of skin)	Thinner	Provides less protection; is more permeable	Only essential substances applied; use water only, for routine bathing
Dermis (middle layer of skin)	Thinner; fewer elastic fibers and less adhesion to epidermis than in term infant	Increased risk of skin breakdown with removal of tape	Special tape used; barriers used between tape and skin
Permeability	More permeable than in term infant	Increased water and heat loss; caution required in application of skin ointments and other substances	Fluid balance and temperature monitored; humidity increased as needed; only essential substances applied
Touch sensation	Present (one of earliest senses to develop)	Gentle touching important	Gentle touching provided

Characteristics of the Renal (Kidney) System in Term and Preterm Babies

Aspect	Characteristics	Significance	Examples of Care Provided
Rate at which kidneys remove water and other substances from blood (glomerular filtration rate)	Slower than in an adult	More time needed to remove excess water, medications, and substances such as electrolytes (i.e. sodium, potassium, etc.)	Fluid and electrolyte balance carefully monitored; medication levels in the blood monitored and infant watched carefully for side effects
Ability of kidneys to remove substances from blood without also causing much water loss (ability to concentrate urine)	Less efficient than in adult; more water lost in urine	More frequent urination; risk of dehydration	Fluid intake and output monitored; additional fluids given by IV therapy
Ability to retain essential substances (such as glucose, sodium, and potassium) in blood	Less efficient than in adult; more of these substances lost in urine	Risk of imbalances	Blood levels of these substances monitored; additional amounts provided by IV therapy if needed

skin. Even with careful attention to skin care, however, some babies may develop some areas of skin irritation because of the immaturity of their skin.

Problems Related to the Kidneys

At birth, your baby's kidneys do not function as well as yours do. In term babies and in preterm babies born after about 35 weeks gestation, however, the kidneys mature rapidly in the two weeks following birth. Renal (kidney) function takes longer to mature in babies born earlier than 35 weeks. The more premature a baby is, the more immature the renal system.

Dehydration (inadequate body fluids) is a common problem for preterm infants. It has two main causes: (1) high water requirements because of immature functioning of the renal system and (2) increased water loss through immature skin. (See "Problems Related to Temperature Control," later in this chapter, for more information on this type of water loss.) At the same time, premature infants also have difficulty getting rid of excess water—again, because of the immaturity of their renal system. To guard against both these problems, caregivers calculate your baby's fluid needs carefully—to the drops needed per minute.

Problems Related to The Gastrointestinal System

Good nutrition is an essential component of your baby's care. Making sure special-care babies get enough food and fluid to support their growth can be a challenge to caregivers, because functioning of both the stomach and the intestines is limited in these tiny infants.

The more premature a baby is, the more immature the gastrointestinal (GI) function. These infants have limited protein and energy reserves. Cold, infection, or pain can increase an infant's energy needs. Energy balance in the infant can be thought of as the balance between intake (food taken in by mouth or IV feeding), energy lost (energy used to produce heat, be active, eat, breathe, fight infection, respond to pain, or cry), and energy stored (leftover energy that can be stored to produce weight gain). Preterm infants have very small stomachs, limiting the amount of food they can take in at one time. Because their GI system is immature, they also have more difficulty digesting and absorbing food, especially fats, sugars, vitamins, and minerals. These factors make provision of adequate nutrition more difficult.

Meeting Your Baby's Nutritional and Fluid Needs

Each infant's fluid and nutrient needs are unique. Working from established estimates of protein, carbohydrate, fat, vitamin, mineral, and water needs for infants of various gestational ages, caregivers individualize these guidelines to meet your baby's situation. For example, some babies may lose more fluid through their thin skin and therefore need more water. Others may need additional glucose to maintain a normal blood sugar level.

Intravenous Feeding

Your baby may not be fed by mouth immediately after birth. Instead, he may be fed through an IV line (see Chapter 2). At first, this type of feeding usually consists of glucose (sugar) water. After a day or two, electrolytes—substances or elements that are essential for the proper functioning of each cell of the body—are added. Electrolytes include sodium, chloride, calcium, potassium, and magnesium. All babies have sodium, potassium, and chloride added to their IV by a few days of age. Other electrolytes may be added depending on the baby's individual situation.

As your baby's physical condition improves, he will be given the opportunity to get started on nipple (breast or bottle) feedings. When this occurs depends on the maturity of your baby's feeding reflexes (sucking, gagging, swallowing)

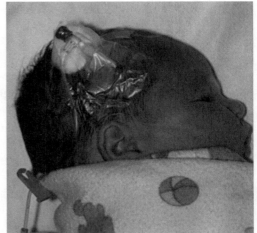

Scalp intravenous site.

The scalp is often used as an IV site. The IV catheter is placed in a vein just under the skin. Unlike an IV line placed in the baby's hand or foot, the scalp IV allows the baby full mobility of hands and feet.

and on his ability to coordinate those reflexes. While your baby's reflexes and coordination remain immature, feedings will be primarily by gavage.

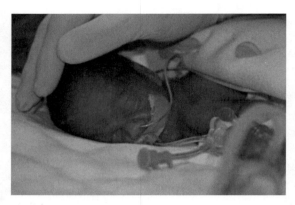

Nasogastric tube.

This narrow feeding tube is passed through the baby's nose and into his stomach to provide gavage (tube) feedings. The tube is taped into place, eliminating the need for insertion and removal at every feeding. Also visible is the baby's endotracheal tube, secured over his lip with tape.

Gavage Feeding

Gavage (tube) feeding is a common way to provide nutrition to preterm and ill term infants. A narrow tube is inserted through the infant's mouth or nose into either the stomach or the intestine. Because babies who need gavage feeding generally do not have a strong gag reflex, insertion of the tube is usually easy on the baby. The most common methods of gavage feeding are orogastric (tube through the mouth into the stomach) and nasogastric (tube through the nose into the stomach). The tube may be inserted for each feeding or left in place for a period of time. Giving your baby a pacifier to suck on during gavage feeding (an approach called nonnutritive sucking) may enhance digestion and absorption of food.

A gavage feeding consists of breast milk or formula. Your baby may receive small amounts of milk on a regular schedule, such as every two or three hours (intermittent gavage feeding), or may receive milk from a feeding pump that provides a steady infusion through the gavage tube (continuous gavage feeding). With continuous gavage feedings, the feeding tube is inserted and left in for a period of time. Milk is slowly dripped down the tube at a set rate (such as 1 to 2 milliliters, [or about ⅕–⅖ tsp] every hour). Sometimes the feeding tube is placed in the intestine (transpyloric feeding) rather than in the stomach.

The type of gavage feeding selected for each baby depends on many factors, including health status, size, and maturity. Infants who are gavage fed are carefully monitored to make sure that they are taking and absorbing (tolerating) the whole feeding. Tolerance of gavage feedings is assessed by observing for distention (enlargement) of the abdomen, spitting up, and for the amount of food remaining in the stomach (called residuals) just before the next gavage feeding. Increasing amounts of residuals over time may indicate an intestinal problem such as necrotizing enterocolitis (see Chapter 10).

Each type of gavage feeding has advantages and disadvantages. Intermittent gavage feeding produces normal cyclic variations in GI hormones and helps to stimulate the normal hunger cycle and stomach emptying. It is also easier to monitor for signs of feeding problems such as delayed emptying of the stomach (transfer of the feeding from the stomach to the intestines). Disadvantages of this type of feeding include risks of effects on breathing patterns and risk of feeding problems such as vomiting.

Continuous gavage feeding is often used for very small or ill infants. Advantages include reduced effects of the feeding on breathing patterns, reduced risk of stomach distention (enlargement), and less need to handle a baby who does not tolerate handling. Disadvantages include difficulty in monitoring feeding problems, lack of the normal cyclic changes in GI hormones, and risk of tube dislodgement.

Transpyloric feeding (continuous feeding into the upper intestine) is used less frequently than the other methods. This type of feeding may reduce problems such as markedly delayed stomach emptying or severe spitting up, help the infant tolerate larger amounts of feeding, and have less effect on breathing patterns. Disadvantages of transpyloric feeding include increased difficulty in placing and securing the tube, need for x-rays to check tube location, and risks of complications such as diarrhea, tube obstruction, abdominal distention, and intestinal perforation.

Parenteral Nutrition

If your baby cannot begin oral feedings for a long period (perhaps because of GI problems, surgery, extreme immaturity, or chronic respiratory problems) or if your baby does not grow on standard feedings, an approach called parenteral nutrition will be used. The term *parenteral* refers to food that enters the body through a blood vessel. In total parenteral nutrition (TPN), all of the essential nutrients (carbohydrates, protein, fat, vitamins, and minerals) and water are provided in a special solution delivered through an IV line directly into one of the baby's veins. Sometimes a baby will receive part of his feedings by gavage and part by IV or parenteral nutrition. This type of feeding is also called hyperalimentation.

Nipple Feeding

Caregivers base the decision to start nipple feeding (breast or bottle) on your infant's maturity and health status. Factors they consider are:
- Development of the gag, suck, and swallow reflexes and ability to coordinate those reflexes with breathing
- Breathing rate. It is difficult to coordinate sucking and swallowing with a very rapid breathing rate
- Growth (consistent pattern of weight gain)
- Tolerance of gavage feedings

Chapter 5 explains the challenges of both breast and bottle feeding and how to do each.

Breast Milk

Breast milk is the ideal food for a newborn.[5] It contains essential nutrients in forms that are easy for the baby to digest. The advantages of breast milk for preterm and sick babies include:
- Presence of components that help protect your baby against infection
- Presence of enzymes that help your baby digest and absorb fat
- Presence of essential amino acids (proteins) that meet your baby's unique needs
- Presence of components that enhance growth and metabolism
- The development, perhaps, of fewer intestinal problems than when fed formula
- Waste products that are easy for your infant's kidneys to handle after his body uses the nutrients in your milk

"We eventually figured out that Matthew would have good days and not-so-good days. On the good days, we would feel great. On the bad days, we knew we would just have to hold on until another good day came along."

Characteristics of the Gastrointestinal System in Preterm Babies

Aspect	Characteristics	Significance	Examples of Care Provided
Suck and swallow reflexes	Weak in preterm infants before 32 to 34 weeks gestational age; coordination of feeding reflexes poor	Possible inability to breastfeed or bottle feed	Infant fed by gavage (tube)
Stomach	Small capacity; more time required to empty; immature sphincter (valve) at top of stomach	Only small feedings may be accepted; spitting up likely	Small amounts of food given more frequently, or slow, continuous feedings given; amount of food left in stomach (residual) measured before next gavage feeding
Intestines	Reduced area; irregularity in movements that propel food through intestine (peristalsis)	Poor absorption	Weight gain and growth monitored; breast milk or special formulas used
Intestinal enzymes (substances that help to digest food)	Decrease in amount and/or effectiveness of some digestive enzymes*	Poor digestion and absorption of protein, carbohydrate, fat, vitamins, and minerals	Breast milk, special formulas, or parenteral feeding used if needed
Liver	Immature*	Reduced ability to break down medications and other substances	Medication levels in blood monitored; infant watched carefully for side effects of medications

*Also true in term infants

Average Weeks of Gestation for Development of Feeding Reflexes in Newborns

Reflex	Functional	Mature
Suck	13–15	32–33 (NNS*) 32–34 (NS**)
Gag	18–20	34
Swallow	28–32	34
Suck/swallow coordination	32–34 (earlier for breastfeeding)	36–38
Suck/swallow/ breathing coordination	32–34	38

* nonnutritive sucking (for example, on a pacifier)
** nutritive sucking

For very premature infants, however, breast milk may not contain enough protein, calcium, phosphorus, and sodium. For the first few weeks after giving birth, mothers of preterm babies produce milk that contains higher levels of these substances than does the milk of mothers of term babies. Even the increased levels of these substances may not be enough for some immature babies, however. If your gavage-fed baby needs more of these substances than your milk provides, special supplements such as Enfamil Human Milk Fortifier (Mead Johnson) and Similac Natural Care (Ross Laboratories) may be added to your breast milk until your infant is more mature.

Formula

Commercial formulas were first developed to meet the needs of term infants. Now there are special formulas that are soy based or that have low levels of certain proteins or other nutrients for infants with allergies or for those who cannot tolerate cow's-milk formulas. Formulas have also been developed to meet the unique nutritional needs of preterm infants. Many of these formulas are patterned on breast milk, with the addition of some components that may be low in breast milk. They do not mimic breast milk, however, because they are cow's milk based and do not contain components that provide protection against infection.

Rate of Weight Gain

Weighing your baby is important for monitoring his growth. In the nursery, your infant's weight is usually measured in grams. Because a gram is a smaller unit than an ounce, it gives a more precise measurement than pounds and ounces and makes it easier to recognize small changes in your infant's weight. One ounce equals 28 grams. Appendix A contains a chart to help you convert grams to pounds and ounces.

Your baby's birth weight reflects the amount of growth and development experienced in your uterus. The relationship between your baby's birth weight and gestational age indicates how well he grew before birth and whether he is small, appropriate, or large for gestational age (see Chapter 8).

Babies in the NICU are weighed daily or every few days depending on their health status. The nurses will usually try to weigh your baby on the same scale each time, because scales can differ from one nursery to another or even within the same nursery.

After birth, all infants lose weight. This is a normal process that reflects changes in water balance with birth. The fetus is composed of large amounts of water and sodium (salt). After birth, your baby must excrete extra water and salt that he no longer needs. Term infants may lose up to 10 percent of their birth weight after birth; preterm babies may lose up to 15 percent. If your son is preterm, weighs 1,200 grams at birth, and loses 15 percent of his birth weight, for example, his weight would fall to 1,020 grams (15 percent of 1,200 is 180 grams). Smaller or sicker babies tend to lose the most weight.

Term infants usually lose weight only for the first few days of life. Sick preterm infants may lose weight for a few days to several weeks before starting to gain it back. At first, your baby may not gain weight regularly. His weight may increase on some days, stay the same on others, and occasionally go down. Even when your baby does begin to gain weight regularly, there will be occasional days of no gain or even a slight loss. This is normal. Factors that can

"I measured Katie's progress by how much weight she gained every day. I was so proud when she topped 3 pounds and her favorite nurse nicknamed her Cannonball."

influence weight gain include health status; activity level; energy needs; discomfort or pain; fluid, nutrient, and calorie intake; and temperature regulation.

The average daily expected weight gain in a healthy growing preterm infant is about 10 to 15 grams per day for each kilogram of body weight. To convert grams to kilograms, divide the grams by 1,000. For example, a 900-gram baby weighs 0.9 kilogram. The daily expected weight gain for this baby would be about 9 to 13.5 grams. ($10 \times 0.9 = 9$; $15 \times 0.9 = 13.5$). An 1,800-gram baby weighs 1.8 kilograms, so this baby's daily expected weight gain would be 1.8×10, or about 18 grams. Remember, however, that each baby is unique and will establish an individual weight gain pattern. In addition, few babies gain exactly the expected daily amount each day. One day the baby may gain more, another less, and another none at all, or he may even lose a little weight. To assess your baby's progress against the expected weight gain, average his actual daily weight gain or loss over a few days to a week.

Rate of Growth

Weight is not the only measure of growth and development. Your infant's body length and head circumference are also important and will be measured periodically. Length and head circumference are usually measured in centimeters. Appendix A provides a chart for converting centimeters to inches. Your baby's caregivers may plot your baby's growth—weight, length, and head circumference changes—on standard charts. These charts assume that a preterm infant will grow at a rate similar to that of a fetus until he reaches the gestational age of a full-term infant. Note, though, that research has not confirmed that this assumption is correct.[6] The extrauterine world is much different from the world of the uterus, a fact that may affect the validity of this assumption.

Problems Related to Temperature Control

At birth, an infant moves from the warm environment of the uterus to the cooler delivery room. For the first time, the infant must control his own temperature.

Body Temperature Control

Because infants have less fat for insulation and a larger surface area in proportion to their size than older children or adults do, they lose body heat more easily. *Surface area* is a term to describe the expanse of the external surface of the body. The outer surface area of the body of an infant is about 15 percent of an adult's surface area. The body size of an infant (referred to as the volume [mass] of the body), however, is only about 5 percent of the body mass of an adult. The greater the difference in surface (heat-losing area) to volume (including available heat-producing areas of the body), the greater the heat loss. Older individuals produce heat primarily by shivering. Newborns usually do not shiver. Instead, they produce heat to warm themselves by increasing their energy and heat production (called metabolic activity) or by burning something called brown adipose tissue (BAT), also known as brown fat.

Brown fat, a special kind of fat found in newborns and in hibernating animals, is present around the shoulders, base of the neck, sternum (chest bone), and organs such as the liver, kidneys, and adrenal glands. Brown fat breaks down more easily and generates heat more quickly than does the more common white adipose tissue. The brownish red color of brown fat comes from the many blood vessels it contains. When the fat is broken down, this good blood supply works to carry the heat produced to the rest of the body.

Babies produce heat mainly by breaking down brown fat. But premature infants (especially those born at less than 30 weeks gestation) have only small stores of brown fat. Premature newborns can use up these stores quickly. Other infants may use up all of their brown fat keeping warm if exposed over a long period to a cool environment. Whatever the reason, infants who have exhausted their brown-fat stores must then use metabolic energy to produce heat when they are cold. But producing heat with metabolic energy uses up oxygen and glucose (sugar) that these infants need for other purposes. This puts them at risk for problems in those areas.

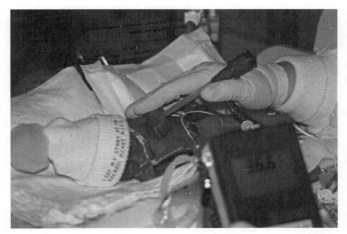

Temperature check.
Many body functions depend on temperature regulation. A digital thermometer is used here to assess the baby's axillary temperature.

Effects of Coldness

Hypothermia and cold stress are both terms related to low body temperature. Infants who become cold (hypothermic) can also become cold stressed and develop other complications, including breathing problems, low blood sugar, and weight loss. Respiratory problems occur because these infants try to take in the extra oxygen they need to produce heat energy by breathing faster. Immature infants or infants with breathing or heart problems may not be able to take in enough extra oxygen to meet both their heat needs and the needs of their cells. Insufficient oxygen can lead to increased acidity of the blood (low pH), hypoxia (inadequate oxygen for the cells), and respiratory distress. Metabolic heat production also uses up glucose (sugar) stores and can lead to inadequate blood sugar levels, a condition called hypoglycemia (explained later in this chapter). Infants who are cold stressed over a period of time often will not gain and may lose weight because they are using the energy (calories) that would normally produce growth to produce heat.

Management of Temperature

Because temperature changes can cause serious complications in newborns, maintaining a normal body temperature is a major focus of infant care from the moment of birth. Your baby's temperature and the temperature of the environment (for example, the incubator) are measured regularly, and adjustments are made to keep your baby's body temperature normal. Temperature may be measured in degrees centigrade (most common) or Fahrenheit.

Temperature Control in Term and Preterm Newborns

Aspect	Characteristics	Significance	Examples of Care Provided
Heat production	Produced by increasing metabolism rather than by shivering; much heat also generated by breakdown of brown fat	Oxygen and glucose (sugar) used; brown fat stores possibly used up	Temperature monitored regularly; incubators and radiant heaters used to maintain normal body temperature
Heat loss	Less fat for insulation; more surface area for heat loss relative to body size than in adult; heat lost through conduction, convection, evaporation, and radiation	Risk of low body temperature (hypothermia) and cold stress, which can lead to breathing and metabolic problems	Temperature monitored carefully; automatic temperature control devices and head coverings used to reduce all four types of heat loss
Sweating	Poor sweat production	Risk of overheating (hyperthermia)	Body and environmental temperatures monitored carefully

Types of Heat Loss in Infants and Preventive Techniques

Type	Definition	Examples of Care Provided*
Convection	Transfer of heat from baby's body to air	Baby protected from drafts Side guards used on radiant warmers; plastic wrap stretched across baby and attached to side guards
Conduction	Transfer of heat from baby's body to objects that touch baby	Blankets, clothing, and mattresses prewarmed Warm blankets placed on scales, x-ray plates, and other surfaces before baby placed on them Incubators and radiant warmers preheated
Evaporation	Loss of heat in water that evaporates from baby's skin or lungs	Baby dried after birth and baths Oxygen warmed and humidified before administration Humidity in incubator increased in some cases
Radiation	Transfer of heat (as heat waves) from baby's body to cooler objects in room	Baby kept away from cold windows or walls Double-wall incubators and heat shields used

*The interventions exemplify some ways to reduce each type of heat loss. Most babies will not require all of these interventions.

Possible Causes of Hyperbilirubinemia in Infants

Cause	Underlying Physiology or Pathophysiology
Higher-than-normal bilirubin production	Higher-than-normal red blood cell destruction because of Rh or other blood-type incompatibilities, bruising, and/or hemorrhage Higher-than-normal number of red blood cells in circulation (polycythemia)
Greater-than-normal enterohepatic circulation (return of bilirubin from intestine to bloodstream)	Delay in first bowel movement Sluggish intestinal movement Delay in first feeding Intestinal blockage
Altered liver functions involved in bilirubin conversion	Decreased blood flow to the liver (possibly because of breathing or heart problems or infection)

Note: No cause is ever found for hyperbilirubinemia in some infants.

Appendix A provides a chart for converting centigrade temperatures to Fahrenheit.

Two common temperature-monitoring approaches are axillary (armpit) and skin. To monitor skin temperature, a temperature probe is placed on the infant's skin, usually on the belly. The skin temperature probe may just record the temperature, or it may control the thermostat and help maintain the baby's temperature within specified limits. Combination monitoring and control involves a device called a servomechanism, or servocontrol. Servo-mechanisms are used with all radiant (open) warmers and can also be used with incubators.

Because premature and sick babies have difficulty maintaining their temperature by themselves, they are placed in special environments. The incubator and the radiant warmer, both described in Chapter 2, are two such environments. Babies lose heat through convection, conduction, evaporation, and radiation. These terms are explained in the table on page 152.

Problems Related to Bilirubin

When the body breaks down used red blood cells, a substance called bilirubin is released. Before the body can dispose of the bilirubin, the liver must change (convert) the form released—called indirect bilirubin—into the form called direct bilirubin.

A specific enzyme is required for this bilirubin conversion. In most newborns—and especially in preterm babies—this enzyme is not very active for the first few days after birth. In other words, it takes a few days for this liver conversion function to "turn on." Until the liver begins to convert large amounts of indirect to direct bilirubin, the indirect form may build up in a newborn's blood. Some of the indirect bilirubin may leave the blood, deposit in the skin tissue, and cause jaundice (yellow skin color).

When indirect bilirubin is changed to the direct form, the liver releases the direct bilirubin into the upper part of the intestine, where it is broken down further and eliminated in stool (feces). While the direct bilirubin is waiting in the newborn's intestine to be eliminated, another enzyme acts upon it, converting some of it back into indirect bilirubin and undoing the work of the liver. The newly formed indirect bilirubin returns to the infant's bloodstream and must go back through the liver for reprocessing before it can be eliminated. This "undoing" process is called the enterohepatic ("entero" = intestine; "hepatic" = liver) shunt.

The high activity level of this "undoing" enzyme in newborns is held over from fetal development. Because the fetus does not normally have bowel movements, its bilirubin is removed through the placenta. For the placenta to remove bilirubin, it must be present in the fetal bloodstream. The high activity level of this intestinal enzyme in the fetus ensures that much of the bilirubin that reaches the fetus's intestines is returned to the blood. Activity of this enzyme gradually decreases after birth. In the first few days after birth, the longer the direct bilirubin stays in the intestine, the more time this intestinal enzyme has to work on it, resulting in more direct bilirubin being changed

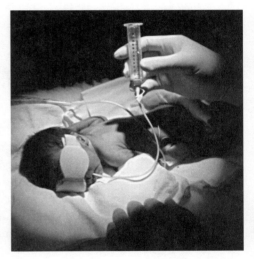

Phototherapy.
The white spotlight of phototherapy is a common sight in the NICU. This baby is being tube fed while under phototherapy lights. Usually the eye patches are removed for the feeding; this baby spits up his feeding if moved afterward, however. He was cared for and held first, therefore, and then prepared for a nap prior to feeding. When the gavage feeding is over, the nurse will offer him a pacifier.

back into the indirect form. The initial bowel movements help to move direct bilirubin out of the intestines and reduce enterohepatic shunting.

Physiologic Jaundice

Because indirect bilirubin is attracted to fatty tissue, such as the fat layer in the skin, some of it may leave your baby's bloodstream and collect in fatty tissue during the first week after birth. This gives your baby's skin a yellow color. In infants, this yellowing is called physiologic (or normal) jaundice. This is not the same type of jaundice that occurs in older individuals, and it does not mean that something is wrong with your baby's liver. It is simply a result of your infant's immature liver function.

Physiologic jaundice is a normal condition in newborns, with 45 to 60 percent of full-term infants and up to 80 percent of preterm infants developing it. Visible jaundice (yellowish skin color) appears as the infant's bilirubin levels rise above about 5 to 7 milligrams per deciliter. Physiologic jaundice occurs in two phases. During phase 1, bilirubin levels reach their highest point: by about three to four days in term, bottle-fed infants; by about four to five days in term breastfed infants; and by about five days or later in preterm infants. The levels then gradually fall over the next few days. In phase 2, bilirubin values are stable for several days, then fall to minimal levels over one to two weeks. The pattern of bilirubin blood levels for preterm and for full-term infants is similar. Peak levels are higher in preterm babies, however, and fall gradually over several weeks. Although physiologic jaundice usually needs no treatment, some infants may require a few days of phototherapy treatment (described later in this chapter).

Hyperbilirubinemia

Infants whose blood bilirubin level is higher than normal or rises faster than normal have a condition called hyperbilirubinemia (an increased level of bilirubin in the blood, usually of the indirect form). Hyperbilirubinemia may be caused by an exaggeration of the normal bilirubin process in the newborn, such as above-normal enterohepatic shunting; by excessive production of bilirubin (for example with more red blood cell breakdown such as occurs with bruising during birth); or by other problems, such as infection, that alter liver function.

Hyperbilirubinemia is a concern for two reasons. First, it may be a symptom of another problem. If another problem is suspected, tests will probably be done to eliminate possible causes. In most cases, however, no cause other than the high bilirubin levels is found, and there are no aftereffects. Second, very high levels of bilirubin can cause a disorder called kernicterus if bilirubin passes into the brain. Kernicterus can result in permanent brain damage.

If your infant is at risk for or has hyperbilirubinemia, his blood bilirubin levels will be monitored very carefully. Infrequently, a baby's bilirubin quickly reaches levels that are of concern. In this case, an exchange transfusion may be necessary. During this procedure, a calculated amount of the baby's blood is withdrawn through an umbilical catheter and replaced by fresh blood from a blood donor.

Fortunately, few babies with hyperbilirubinemia require exchange transfusions; most are successfully treated with phototherapy (treatment involving lights). In very immature babies, phototherapy may be started within a few days after birth to prevent bilirubin concentrations from reaching excessively high levels.

Phototherapy

Phototherapy was developed in England after nurses there noticed that babies near the window (in the sunlight) did not become as jaundiced as other babies in the nursery. Bilirubin is very sensitive to light waves. Phototherapy is a form of treatment that uses light waves (from "bililights" or "lights") to break down indirect bilirubin into products that the infant's body can eliminate in urine.

There are three major methods of providing phototherapy: bank bilirubin lights (a row of fluorescent lights), spotlights (a single spotlight focused on the baby), and fiberoptic blankets (which can be wrapped around the baby's body). Sometimes a baby will lie on a fiberoptic blanket to expose the underside of his body to phototherapy and at the same time have a bank light or spotlight shining on the upper side of his body. Babies under bank lights, under a spotlight, or lying on flat fiberoptic blankets wear protective shields over their eyes while the lights are on. The lights can be turned off for short periods while the infant is being fed or receiving other care or so that you can hold your child. Babies under phototherapy often have more frequent and looser bowel movements than do infants not receiving the therapy and may therefore need more fluid. Caregivers take this into account in calculating the baby's daily fluid needs. Phototherapy lights have been used since the 1960s with no serious or permanent side effects.

Problems Related to the Metabolic System

The word *metabolism* comes from a Greek word meaning "to change." Metabolic processes refer to chemical reactions in which the body converts the nutrients in foods (such as carbohydrates, protein, fat, vitamins, and minerals) into substances that the body uses to function (for example, to contract muscles, to transmit nerve impulses, and to produce energy) or to build new cells and tissues. The levels of some of these substances can become too high or too low in infants, leading to problems that are commonly seen in babies who are preterm or sick. Glucose, calcium, and electrolytes (such as sodium, and potassium) are examples of these substances.

Glucose

Your baby uses glucose (sugar) to produce energy for cells, to drive chemical reactions within the body, and to build new tissue for growth. Before birth, the fetus gets a constant supply of glucose from the mother across the placenta. The fetus uses this glucose for energy and growth. The fetus also stores some of the glucose as a reserve for use during birth, when energy needs are high. Immediately after birth, the infant depends on two sources of glucose: the stored glucose (called glycogen), and the glucose in breast milk or formula or in the IV fluid if the infant is not being fed orally. In all infants, the blood glucose level falls during the first few hours after birth, then stabilizes. In some infants, the blood glucose level may become too low (a condition called hypoglycemia) or too high (hyperglycemia).

Hypoglycemia

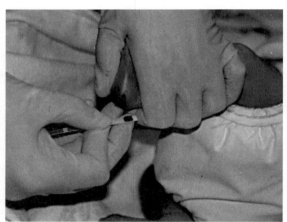

Heelstick blood test.

The baby's heel is pricked, and a drop or two of blood is used to screen his blood sugar.

Hypoglycemia refers to a blood sugar that falls below a critical level, generally considered to be 30 to 40 milligrams per deciliter depending on the infant's age. Hypoglycemia is a common problem among NICU infants. Babies most likely to develop hypoglycemia are preterm babies, small-for-gestational-age babies, infants whose mothers are diabetic, and infants who required resuscitation because of breathing problems at birth. Hypoglycemia is a temporary problem and may or may not develop in these groups of at-risk babies. If hypoglycemia does occur, it is quite treatable.

Preterm babies develop hypoglycemia for two major reasons: (1) they have smaller stores of glycogen (stored glucose) than do term babies, and (2) their immature livers cannot produce glucose from substances such as fat and protein as easily as can the livers of term infants. Preterm infants with respiratory distress have higher energy needs than other infants—and therefore, higher glucose needs. Babies of mothers who have taken medications to stop preterm labor occasionally develop hypoglycemia as a response to those drugs.

Small-for-gestational-age infants develop hypoglycemia because they have higher energy needs, higher glucose use, and lower glucose stores than larger infants. They may have decreased stores because an SGA baby has a smaller placenta that was unable to transfer enough glucose to the fetus or because the infant used up existing stores during labor and birth. The increased energy use of babies who require resuscitation at birth can also deplete glycogen stores and increase the risk of hypoglycemia.

Infants of insulin-dependent diabetic mothers develop hypoglycemia because these infants produce too much insulin (a condition called hyperinsulinemia). Insulin, a hormone produced by the pancreas, helps to move glucose from the blood into the cells. If a baby has too much insulin, too much glucose may be removed from the blood. The result is hypoglycemia.

Why do babies of diabetic mothers produce too much insulin? These babies had higher-than-normal glucose levels (hyperglycemia) during fetal development. Glucose rapidly crosses the placenta from mother to fetus. If a mother has above-normal glucose levels (as is the case for many diabetic women), her fetus will also develop hyperglycemia, because the fetus's blood glucose level is always related to (but slightly lower than) the mother's level. Maternal insulin itself does not cross the placenta to the fetus. The fetus's pancreas is stimulated by the higher-than-normal glucose levels in the blood.

At birth, the newborn stops receiving glucose from the mother through the placenta. His blood glucose falls, but his pancreas continues to produce extra insulin. The extra insulin causes too much glucose to move out of the baby's blood, which can cause hypoglycemia. After a few days, the baby's insulin level begins to return to normal, and hypoglycemia is no longer a problem.

Babies who are hypoglycemic may or may not have obvious signs. Even when signs are present, however, it can be difficult to know whether hypoglycemia is causing them. This is because the signs of hypoglycemia are often nonspecific: Many of them are also indicative of other disorders. Signs of hypoglycemia may include tremors or jitteriness, irregular breathing, decreased muscle tone, decreased temperature, and cyanosis (a bluish skin color). Hypoglycemia can be dangerous because it can lead to convulsions.

Because the signs of hypoglycemia are nonspecific or may be absent, any baby who is at risk for hypoglycemia is carefully monitored. One monitoring method is to test a few drops of blood from the baby's finger, heel, or toe. The drops of blood are placed on a special test strip that changes color. Each of the colors signifies a different range of blood glucose values. Another device used to screen blood glucose is a digital glucose meter, which analyzes a drop of blood and gives a number value instead of a color value. If the test indicates that an infant's blood glucose level is low, a blood sample will be sent to the laboratory to determine the exact level so that therapy can be started if necessary. Therapy consists of additional glucose provided to the baby through an intravenous line.

"I am a diabetic, and our baby weighed over 12 pounds. I felt so guilty for having a huge baby in a unit full of 2-pounders. I wanted to scream at those other moms, 'Hey, my baby is sick! Just because he's huge, don't think he isn't sick!'"

Hyperglycemia

Occasionally an infant develops hyperglycemia: a blood glucose (sugar) greater than 125 milligrams per deciliter. Hyperglycemia is seen most often in very premature infants who have difficulty regulating their metabolic processes because of their immaturity. Infants may also develop hyperglycemia after surgery or if they have an infection. Hyperglycemia can be treated with infusions of insulin.

Calcium

Calcium is a mineral that is critical for bone growth and development, heart function, blood clotting, muscle contraction, and other body processes. The fetus receives a steady supply of calcium from the mother. After birth, infant calcium levels fall over the first few days, then become stable. Your baby must now get calcium and other minerals from feedings.

Hypocalcemia

Hypocalcemia—a too-low calcium level in the blood, below 7 to 8 milligrams per deciliter—is a common metabolic problem in sick infants. Calcium levels are determined by a blood test. Infants who are at highest risk of developing hypocalcemia are preterm infants and babies of insulin-dependent diabetic mothers. Altered levels of the hormones that control calcium levels, decreased intake of calcium after birth, and impaired calcium absorption by the immature intestinal tract are among the reasons for hypocalcemia in premature infants. In infants of diabetic mothers, increased levels of maternal hormones that control calcium may build up in the fetus's blood, temporarily suppressing the infant's production of these hormones after birth.

Signs of hypocalcemia may or may not be present and, as with hypoglycemia, are often nonspecific. Signs of hypocalcemia may include tremors, twitching, irritability, a high-pitched cry, and an altered heart rate. Hypocalcemia is of concern because it can affect the function of the cardiovascular and nervous systems. Hypocalcemia is a temporary problem that responds readily to treatment, which involves giving the infant calcium.

Electrolytes

Electrolytes ("lytes") are elements found in the blood, in cells, and in body fluids. They are critical to the functioning of all body cells. If the levels of electrolytes in the body are too high or too low, the cells will not function properly, and the infant can become ill. Electrolytes are often referred to by their abbreviations: Na for sodium, K for potassium, Cl for chloride, Ca for calcium, and Mg for magnesium.

Electrolytes are found in breast milk and in formula. Levels of electrolytes in your infant's blood will be monitored regularly. Babies whose electrolyte needs are not being met by feeding will need additional amounts of some of these elements. For these infants, sodium, potassium, chloride, and possibly others will be added to the IV fluid.

Problems Related to the Blood

The blood and its components (including the plasma, or liquid, portion of the blood and the cellular components) are called the hematologic system. Plasma contains plasma proteins, electrolytes, and other substances. Cellular components of the blood include red blood cells (RBCs), white blood cells (WBCs), and platelets. Red blood cells are important for carrying oxygen from the lungs to the cells. White blood cells (which include neutrophils, basophils, monocytes, and lymphocytes) are part of the body's defenses against infection. Platelets play a role in blood clotting and thus in preventing bleeding. The cellular components of the blood can be measured by a test called a complete blood count (CBC).

At birth, your baby's blood has all of the components yours does. The components may function in an immature fashion, however, and their levels may differ from those of older children and adults. Levels of many of the blood components change during the first week after birth.

A newborn's red blood cells are more fragile and have a shorter life span than do those of an adult. Newborns are therefore at increased risk for RBC breakdown, which can contribute to physiologic jaundice and hyperbilirubinemia (explained earlier in this chapter). In newborns, RBCs use more glucose to produce energy, which increases the risk of hypoglycemia (low blood glucose level).

Anemia

Hemoglobin (Hgb) and hematocrit ("crit") levels are used to monitor RBCs. Hemoglobin is the component of RBCs that carries oxygen molecules to the cells. The hematocrit is the percentage of red blood cells in the blood. Infants with lower-than-normal hemoglobin and hematocrit levels are said to be anemic.

Anemia is a common problem in NICU infants. These babies are more likely to develop anemia because of the amount of blood drawn for tests such as blood gases, blood glucose, and electrolytes. In addition, all infants experience a "physiologic anemia" after birth. This physiologic anemia is more marked in immature infants and increases their risk of lower-than-normal hemoglobin and hematocrit levels.

Physiologic anemia develops because RBC production temporarily stops after birth. A hormone called erythropoietin controls production of RBCs. After birth, an infant's blood oxygen level increases from the low fetal level to the higher newborn level, and erythropoietin secretion—and therefore RBC production—stops. The hemoglobin level falls gradually over several weeks to a few months. Eventually the hemoglobin reaches a level where erythropoietin is again secreted, and RBC production resumes.

Your baby's hemoglobin and hematocrit are monitored to ensure that the RBC level does not fall too low. If an infant becomes anemic, a blood transfusion may be necessary.

Likelihood of Infection

Defense mechanisms are factors within our bodies that protect us from infection. Because the defense mechanisms of babies are still immature, infants are at greater risk for developing an infection than are older children or adults. Also, because of their immature defense mechanisms, babies tend to develop a general infection (sepsis) rather than a local (limited) infection. In addition, some microorganisms (germs)—such as the herpes simplex virus—may cause much more serious infections in babies than they do in adults.

Babies' Defense Against Infection

The baby's immune system fights infections. Defense mechanisms can be general or specific. One of the first lines of general defense against microorganisms that enter the body is the inflammatory response. In newborns, the inflammatory response does not function very well. This means that newborns usually do not "localize" infection—that is, they cannot keep microorganisms at the point where they first enter the body. As a result, newborns tend not to have specific, localized infections, such as ear infections or infected fingers. Instead, they experience general infections of the blood. This type of infection is called sepsis. Sometimes a general infection also involves the fluid surrounding the brain and spinal cord (the cerebrospinal fluid); this type of infection is known as meningitis.

Babies also have other immature defense mechanisms, limiting their ability to respond rapidly and effectively to specific organisms. One reason for this is that babies have fewer antibodies (disease-fighting substances) in their blood than do older individuals. Babies receive antibodies from their mothers before birth. These antibodies provide initial protection against some, but not all, organisms. This transfer of antibodies across the placenta occurs late in pregnancy, however. This means that preterm infants (especially those born before 30 weeks gestation) have lower levels of protective maternal antibodies than do term babies. Preterm babies are therefore at greater risk for developing sepsis.

In newborns, the body cells (called B and T lymphocytes) that fight off bacteria, viruses, and fungi do not function in a mature fashion. This reduces the infant's infection-fighting abilities.

Finally, babies have fewer memory cells—cells that develop only after contact with a specific virus or bacterium. Memory cells remember specific microorganisms. If the same microorganism invades the body again, memory cells tell the body to quickly produce antibodies to destroy that microorganism.

Common Infectious Organisms

Common organisms that cause infection in newborns include bacteria such as Streptococcus (especially Group B), *Escherichia coli* (commonly called *E. coli*), Pneumococcus, Staphylococcus, and Listeria, as well as fungi such as *Candida albicans*. Microorganisms such as herpes simplex virus, hepatitis B virus, human immunodeficiency virus (HIV), cytomegalovirus, and *Toxoplasma gondii* can invade the fetus before or during birth, later causing infection in the newborn. Chapter 10 gives more information about some of these infectious agents.

Signs of Infection in Newborns

One of the most common notations on the charts of NICU babies is "Rule out sepsis." This notation means that the baby has some factors that increase the risk of an infection or has some signs that may indicate sepsis or meningitis. Factors that increase the risk for sepsis are prematurity, prolonged rupture of the membranes prior to birth, maternal infection, infection of the amniotic fluid, and any newborn complications.

Signs of infection in babies often are not specific. Because the temperature-regulating center in the brain is immature, babies do not usually develop a fever when they have an infection. If an infected infant shows a change in temperature (and many do not), it will usually be a decrease (hypothermia) rather than an increase (fever). Other signs sometimes associated with infection in babies are poor feeding, irritability, lethargy, respiratory distress, a drop in the heart rate (bradycardia), abdominal distention, and diarrhea. None of these signs is specific to an infection; all can be signs of other problems. Trying to figure out whether a baby has an infection is a challenge.

Treatment of Infections in Newborns

Any baby who is suspected of having an infection will have a blood culture. Cultures may also be done of other fluids, such as the spinal fluid if

Characteristics of Infection-Fighting Defense Mechanisms in Babies			
Aspect	**Characteristics**	**Significance**	**Examples of Care Provided**
Initial defenses and inflammatory response	Newborn unable to localize infection	General infection more likely than a specific infection	Careful infection control practiced, especially hand washing; infant continuously monitored for signs of infection
Specific defenses (B and T blood cells, antibody formation)	Infant has fewer antibodies than adult, immature B and T cell function, lack of memory cells	Risk for bacterial, viral, and fungal infections; more rapid development of infections	Careful infection control practiced, especially hand washing; infant continuously monitored for signs of infection
Intestinal defense mechanisms	The barrier to microorganisms and protein molecules is immature	Risk of intestinal infection and allergy	Careful infection control practiced, especially hand washing; extra protection given through breastfeeding; foods containing potential allergens (such as wheat or eggs) not given in early infancy

meningitis is suspected. For a blood culture, a sample of your baby's blood is taken using sterile procedures. The sample is sent to the laboratory, where the blood is placed on special dishes to see if any microorganisms grow. It can take days for some organisms to grow and be identified. Because it is difficult to determine whether a baby is infected and because babies who are infected often quickly become critically ill, treatment is often started before the culture results are known.

Antibiotic therapy is used to treat infection. Babies are usually started on two different antibiotics. These antibiotics are known to kill the most common organisms that cause sepsis in newborns. If infection is confirmed and the organism causing the infection is identified, the two initial antibiotics may be replaced by antibiotics to which that specific organism is most sensitive. Most babies turn out not to be infected. See Chapter 10 for more information about treatment of infections.

This chapter described many of the common problems seen in infants in a neonatal intensive care unit or special-care nursery. Most babies who require care in these units experience at least one of these problems. Many experience several, and unfortunately, some experience many. Being at risk for a problem does not mean that a newborn will develop the problem, however. Knowledge of your baby's risk status for specific problems enables the NICU team to monitor your baby carefully to identify early signs of any problems and to start treatment immediately.

The Key: Knowledge

Chapter 10

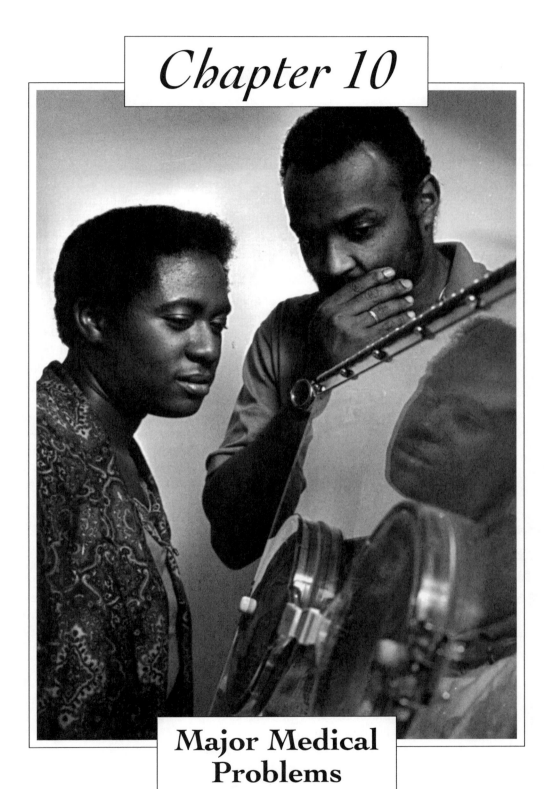

Major Medical Problems

Debbie Fraser Askin, RNC, MN

❝"This is Serious," said Pooh. "I must have an Escape."❞

Some babies complete their NICU experience without many problems. Others face serious difficulty. This chapter explains many of the major medical problems faced by infants needing intensive care. These problems can affect both preterm and term infants. Remember that no baby will experience more than a few of these problems. You may want to refer only to those sections that talk about your baby's current problems. Use these explanations as you prepare questions for your baby's health care team and interpret the information you're given.

The information in this chapter is meant to serve as a base on which to build your knowledge about your baby's special needs. Each child is unique (and none has read this book!), so your baby's situation may differ a bit from the descriptions you read here. Above all, ask as many questions of your baby's caregivers as you need, to feel comfortable. There is no such thing as a bad question or a question asked too often.

This chapter begins by looking at problems that affect specific body systems: the brain and nervous system, eyes, heart, lungs, stomach and bowels, and immune system. The explanations are designed to answer common questions parents ask about these problems. Then the focus turns to birth defects, with explanations of some common conditions that may require special care after birth.

Problems Affecting the Brain and Nervous System

Brain and nervous system development begins in the third week of pregnancy and continues well beyond the second year of life. When development is complete, the brain consists of many interconnected areas capable of performing all of the tasks that make human beings unique.

The outer layer and largest part of the brain is the cerebral cortex. Made up of billions of nerve cells (neurons), the cerebral cortex is the nerve center of the brain. Underneath, white matter links the nerve cells of the brain and spinal cord.

The lower part of the brain is the cerebellum, or brain stem. It is responsible for many of our reflexes and for vital body functions such as breathing. The spinal cord sends information the body feels or senses to the brain and carries action messages from the brain back to the body. Some reflexes are also controlled by the spinal cord.

Because of its complex nature, the developing brain is vulnerable to injury and to influences from environmental agents. Many factors play a part in brain development both before and after birth. These include nutrition, oxygen and blood circulation, genetic makeup (cell structure), and cell function.

If these factors are limited or do not perform properly, the result can be brain injury. If brain injury occurs during fetal development, the tissue in the brain may not develop normally, producing a congenital malformation—commonly called a birth defect (explained later in this chapter). Brain injury that occurs at or near the time of birth is usually the result of insufficient oxygen delivery to brain tissue.

Asphyxia

Asphyxia occurs when the cells of the body do not receive enough oxygen because a life-threatening situation severely impairs oxygen delivery. The cells, said to be hypoxic in this situation, cannot work properly without oxygen and begin to produce waste products in the form of acids. These acids build up, causing a condition called acidosis, which can temporarily damage many of the body's cells. Severe or prolonged lack of oxygen may result in permanent cell damage. The brain is especially sensitive to damage from asphyxia because its cells need a lot of oxygen.

Causes of Asphyxia

When the baby is still in the uterus, asphyxia may occur at any time the blood flow through the placenta is critically inadequate. A table on page 167 of this chapter lists factors that can cause a critical lack of oxygen. Following delivery, a baby who does not start to breathe and circulate oxygen-rich blood through her body for a prolonged period of time will experience asphyxia.

Signs and Treatment of Asphyxia

One of the goals of the health care team is to identify any pregnancy that may be at risk for asphyxia and to intervene before the baby is in critical condition. When the potential for birth asphyxia is identified during pregnancy (if you have high blood pressure or diabetes, for example, or if the fetus is not growing or gaining weight appropriately), prenatal testing—such as frequent ultrasounds—may be done to measure fetal well-being. Induction of labor may be done or cesarean birth may be necessary if the health care team determines that the baby's chances for continued growth and survival are better outside the uterus or if the team determines that spontaneous labor could jeopardize fetal well-being.

During labor and delivery, fetal heart rate monitoring can help detect trouble. Additionally, the pH and acid content of the baby's blood may be measured from a sample taken from the baby's scalp. (Fetal scalp sampling is possible when the amniotic sac has broken and the baby's head is far enough down in the mother's pelvis for the nurse or doctor to reach up and obtain the sample.) With careful monitoring of the baby, birth is accomplished before a severe chemical imbalance (acidosis) is present.

Severe birth asphyxia is an unusual pregnancy complication, with most factors being outside anyone's control. Asphyxia is often undetected until a pregnant woman presents with a problem or complaint, such as decreased fetal movement or severe abdominal pain. During the mother's examination,

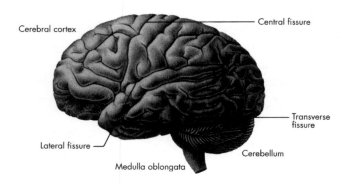

Cerebral cortex

Central fissure

Transverse fissure

Lateral fissure

Cerebellum

Medulla oblongata

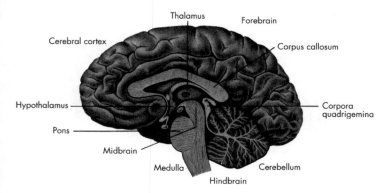

Thalamus

Forebrain

Cerebral cortex

Corpus callosum

Hypothalamus

Corpora quadrigemina

Pons

Midbrain

Medulla

Cerebellum

Hindbrain

Structure of the brain.

Upper diagram shows the external surface of the brain. The folds and grooves of the surface are called convolutions. The lower diagram is a cross-section of the brain, and shows important internal structures.

From: Burke S. 1992. In Human Anatomy & Physiology in Health and Disease, *3rd ed. Albany, New York: Delmar, 180. Reprinted by permission.*

the nurse or physician may detect a fetal heart rate that is tachycardic (unusually fast), or bradycardic (unusually slow), or unusually steady and does not change in response to fetal movement or stimulation. On examination, the nurse or physician may find vaginal bleeding, unusual uterine tenderness, a prolapsed umbilical cord (part of the umbilical cord slips into the birth canal ahead of the baby), or the presence of meconium in the amniotic fluid (discussed later in this chapter).

If an emergency delivery is done, additional people may attend to assess your baby and provide care as needed. (See Chapter 2 regarding newborn resuscitation.) If your baby is mildly asphyxiated, the resuscitation team may be able to quickly revive her by providing breathing support, using bag-mask ventilation with 100 percent oxygen. After the baby is stabilized, she will be closely monitored.

Babies who are severely asphyxiated require a more complex and prolonged resuscitation. If the baby's blood oxygen level is very low, the blood carbon dioxide level very high, and the resulting chemical imbalance (acidosis) severe, the baby may need more than breathing support. Lifesaving techniques such as intubation, cardiac compressions, and emergency fluids and medications may be necessary. Your baby will require close monitoring in the NICU and may develop serious complications as a result of the asphyxia.

Complications of Asphyxia

When the oxygen supply begins to fall early in asphyxia, the body automatically restricts the blood supply in the bowels, kidneys, muscles, and skin. This helps to redistribute available oxygen to the heart and brain, where it is needed most. If oxygen supply continues to be inadequate, and as the body continues to respond, the heart loses power and efficiency, also affecting the blood supply to the heart and brain. After delivery, the infant recovering from asphyxia may show signs of tissue injury. The severity of the symptoms and the length of time they last depend on the severity of the asphyxia. A table on page 167 lists complications of asphyxia.

Mild asphyxia usually resolves without long-term problems. In the short term, though, hypoglycemia (low blood sugar level) may mean your baby will need an intravenous (IV) line. Because the intestines are sensitive to lack of oxygen, feeding may be delayed for 24 to 72 hours to allow the bowel to rest and recover. Severe asphyxia affects all body systems.

Factors that Can Cause Critical Lack of Oxygen to the Fetus

- Separation of the placenta from the uterine wall (abruption)
- Compression of the umbilical cord during labor and delivery; a cord tightened around the baby's neck (nuchal cord); a cord dropped below the baby in the birth canal (prolapsed cord)
- Prolonged or difficult delivery
- Unusual presentation during vaginal birth, such as buttocks-first (breech presentation)
- Life-threatening maternal or fetal infection
- Certain medical conditions of the mother, such as severe hypertension (high blood pressure), severe hypotension (low blood pressure, as in shock), or maternal hypoxia (lack of oxygen to the tissues related to acute asthma, severe pneumonia, or apnea during maternal seizures)
- Umbilical cord accident (a cord that knots *in utero* or tangles with a twin and cuts off circulation to the fetus, for example)
- Traumatic injury to the mother (from a motor vehicle accident or domestic violence, for example) causing maternal hypotension, maternal hypoxia, or placental abruption

Complications of Asphyxia

- Seizures
- Swelling of the brain
- Temperature instability
- Low heart rate
- Changes in circulation
- Persistent pulmonary hypertension
- Congestive heart failure
- Respiratory distress
- Kidney damage
- Damage to the bowel
- Necrotizing enterocolitis
- Low blood sugar
- Hormone and chemical imbalances in the blood
- Blood-clotting problems

Seizures

Seizures occur when the electrical signals in the brain short-circuit. Seizures are a sign of brain injury or irritation. In term infants, in fact, seizures are the most common sign of brain injury.

In term babies, seizures may appear as jerking movements of the arms or legs; stiffening or arching of the back; or rhythmic movements of the eyes, lips, or tongue. Apnea and bradycardia (periods with no breathing and a low heart rate) may also occur. In preterm babies, the signs of seizures may be quite difficult to detect, because premature babies are normally quite jerky or jittery. Normal jittery movement stops when a hand is placed on the baby's arms or legs, however, but seizure activity does not.

Causes of Seizures

Many seizures are idiopathic—that is, no cause can be found. Others may result from infection, chemical imbalances in the blood (i.e., low blood sugar or low calcium), bleeding in the brain or surrounding tissues, swelling of the brain, or malformation of the brain.

Diagnosis of Seizures

If physicians suspect seizures, they will study your baby's brain waves using a painless test called an electroencephalogram (EEG) to help diagnose the problem. This test involves placing electrodes on the skin of the baby's scalp and recording the electrical activity in the baby's brain. Seizures appear as abnormal patterns of electrical activity on the brain-wave tracing.

Tests that may be done to determine the cause of seizures include:

- An ultrasound of the brain: to look for bleeding, swelling, or abnormalities in the brain's structure
- Computed tomography (CT) scan or magnetic resonance imaging (MRI): to look for bleeding, swelling, or abnormalities in the brain's structure
- Blood tests: to look for chemical imbalances (sugar, sodium, calcium, etc.) or abnormalities in function of some of the body's cells
- Blood and spinal fluid tests: to look for infection

A neurologist (doctor specializing in disorders of the brain and nervous system) may also examine your baby.

Treatment for Seizures

Seizures cause the brain to use large amounts of sugar, oxygen, and other nutrients. Continued seizures may harm the cells of the brain and interfere with normal breathing patterns. Seizures are treated with medications such as phenobarbital (phenobarb for short) or phenytoin (Dilantin) (see Appendix B).

Potential Outcome for a Baby with Seizures

The long-term prognosis for a baby who has seizures depends on what is causing them, how severe they are, and the number of days over which they occur. Many babies recover completely, with no long-term signs of brain damage. Seizures occurring because of severe asphyxia or disease of the brain may persist for a longer period. Follow-up visits with the neurologist will be needed to evaluate your baby's progress.

Intraventricular Hemorrhage

An intraventricular hemorrhage (IVH) is bleeding in the area near the ventricles (small central chambers) in the brain. It is sometimes referred to as a *bleed*.

As the fetus's brain develops, an area rich in blood vessels is responsible for producing cerebrospinal fluid, a substance that cushions the brain and spinal cord. In the fetus and premature baby, these blood vessels are immature and quite fragile. After birth, the premature baby's brain is exposed to changes in blood flow and oxygen levels. Those changes may cause these blood vessels to break and bleeding to occur. A hemorrhage is most likely to occur during the first four days after birth, but IVHs can also occur before birth or later, in the first two weeks of life. When bleeding occurs, the blood collects in an area of tissue known as the subependymal region (the area beneath the lining of the ventricle). If the bleeding progresses, blood spills into the ventricle. As blood fills the ventricle, it may enlarge. In severe cases, the blood may be forced out of the ventricle into the surrounding brain tissue. If the hemorrhage is small, the body gradually reabsorbs the blood over two to three weeks, similar to the way in which a bruise gradually fades. Larger bleeds may leave damaged tissue as they are absorbed. Sometimes the damaged tissue causes fluid-filled cysts in the brain. This can result in a condition called periventricular leukomalacia (PVL).

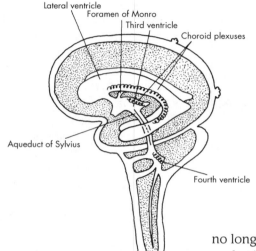

Lateral ventricle
Foramen of Monro
Third ventricle
Choroid plexuses
Aqueduct of Sylvius
Fourth ventricle

Structure of the ventricles.

Chambers of the brain are called ventricles. Cerebral spinal fluid is produced in the ventricles and circulates around the brain and spinal cord. Intraventricular hemorrhage occurs in an area near the ventricles. A severe hemorrhage can cause blood to spill into a ventricle.

From: Minarick CJ Jr, and Beachy P. 1993. Neurologic disorders. In Handbook of Neonatal Intensive Care, 3rd ed., Merenstein GB, and Gardner SL, eds. St. Louis: Mosby-Year Book, 451. Reprinted by permission.

Symptoms of an Intraventricular Hemorrhage

Most often, a baby with an IVH shows no symptoms of bleeding. If the bleed is large, the baby may show signs such as apnea (pauses in breathing) and bradycardia (low heart rate), anemia, seizures, poor muscle tone and decreased activity, and a bulging fontanel (the soft spot on the top of the baby's head).

Diagnosis of an Intraventricular Hemorrhage

Ultrasonography is used to diagnose an IVH. Many NICUs, in fact, routinely do an ultrasound of the head during the baby's first or second week of life, even in babies with no symptoms. The ultrasound scanner (transducer) is placed over the baby's fontanel, and sound waves provide images of the baby's ventricles. These images show the presence and extent of bleeding. The bleeding is assigned a grade from I to IV based on its amount and location and on the extent of dilation (swelling or enlargement) of the ventricles. The progress of the bleed and reabsorption of blood will be followed with additional ultrasounds. (Both of these diagnostic imaging techniques are explained further in Chapter 12.)

Potential Outcome for a Baby with an Intraventricular Hemorrhage

As many as 60 percent of babies born weighing less than 1,000 grams (about 2 pounds, 4 ounces) have intraventricular hemmorhages. Most of these bleeds are mild (Grades I or II), and about 90 percent resolve with few or no long-term problems. More severe bleeds, especially Grade IV, result in more significant short- and long-term problems. Short-term problems include dilation (enlargement) of the ventricles and hydrocephalus (see next section). Long-term problems include cerebral palsy (spasticity), hearing loss, vision problems, and learning disabilities.

Hydrocephalus

Your baby's brain and spinal cord are surrounded by cerebrospinal fluid (CSF). This clear fluid is produced constantly in the ventricles (small chambers in the brain) and circulated around the brain and cord. It is then reabsorbed by the membrane covering the outside of the brain. Cerebrospinal fluid acts as a shock absorber to cushion the nervous system.

Hydrocephalus (literally, "water on the brain") occurs when the circulation of CSF is blocked or when the reabsorption of the fluid is delayed. The CSF then backs up in the ventricles, causing them to expand and push on the surrounding brain tissue. As the ventricles expand, they push on your baby's skull bones, causing the baby's head to enlarge. Continued accumulation of fluid and pressure result in damage to the tissue of your baby's brain.

Causes of Hydrocephalus

Some infants develop hydrocephalus while in the womb when the flow of CSF is blocked by a malformation. The blockage may occur in the spinal cord

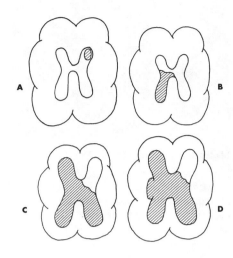

Classification of intraventricular hemorrhage.

Diagrams show views of intraventricular hemorrhages, looking down into the brain structure.

A: *Grade I: shows a small amount of bleeding near the ventricle (in the subependymal area).*
B: *Grade II: shows an extension of blood into the ventricle, but no enlargement of the ventricle.*
C: *Grade III: shows enlargement of the ventricle as it fills with blood.*
D: *Grade IV: shows enlargement of the ventricle and bleeding into the surrounding brain tissue.*

From: Minarick CJ Jr, and Beachy P. 1993. Neurologic disorders. In Handbook of Neonatal Intensive Care, 3rd ed., Merenstein GB, and Gardner SL, eds. St. Louis: Mosby-Year Book, 452. Reprinted by permission.

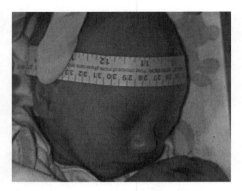

Measuring head circumference

This measurement allows the health care professional to monitor normal growth, and also to assess abnormal enlargement of the head caused by pressure within the brain from dilated ventricles or hydrocephalus.

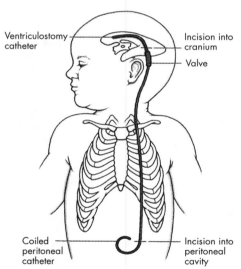

Ventricular shunt.

A ventriculoperitoneal shunt may be needed to relieve the pressure in the ventricles of the brain of a baby with hydrocephalus.

From: Hill CJ. 1987. Nursing Management of Children, Servonsky J, and Opas SR, eds. Boston: Jones & Bartlett, 1297. Reprinted by permission.

when there is a myelomeningocele, (see page 196) or within the brain. In preterm babies with intraventricular hemorrhage, blood in the CSF may cause a blocking or scarring of the membranes responsible for reabsorption of the fluid, leading to hydrocephalus.

Diagnosis of Hydrocephalus

A brain ultrasound or a CT scan is used to diagnose dilated ventricles or hydrocephalus. (See Chapter 12 for an explanation of these diagnostic imaging techniques.) The effects of pressure within the brain are also monitored by measuring your baby's head circumference.

Treatment for Hydrocephalus

In some cases, dilation of the ventricles may stop on its own. Treatment becomes necessary when the ventricles continue to expand. A medication that slows down the production of CSF—such as acetazolamide (Diamox)—may be given. (See Appendix B for more information on this medication.) A lumbar puncture (spinal tap) can also be done to remove CSF and relieve the pressure on the brain. Surgery, to place a shunt for the fluid, will be needed if these measures fail to relieve the pressure in the ventricles.

During surgery, a thin tube known as a shunt is inserted into your baby's ventricle. The other end of the tube is passed underneath the skin and drains into the abdominal cavity, where the body reabsorbs the CSF. Some shunts have a pump or reservoir, which can be felt as a circular bump under the skin on your baby's scalp. Once inserted, the shunt usually remains in place and must be lengthened every two to four years as your child grows. Complications occurring with shunts include infection and blockages.

Cerebral Palsy

Cerebral palsy (CP) is defined as an abnormality of posture or movement resulting from damage to the brain. Up to 70 percent of infants weighing less than 1,500 grams (about 3 pounds, 5 ounces) at birth have increased or decreased muscle tone and reflexes. Most of these abnormalities gradually resolve over 12 to 18 months, leaving the incidence of true cerebral palsy in premature babies at 3 to 6 percent.

It is difficult to predict a baby's long-term outcome in the first year of life. The diagnosis of cerebral palsy is not usually made until 12 to 18 months of age. Criteria for diagnosis are based on the baby's age. In the 12- to 18-month-old infant, cerebral palsy is diagnosed if there are differences in strength and movement between the two sides of the body (asymmetry) and/or delayed or abnormal motor skills. (Chapter 17 discusses developmental milestones.) In infants less than 12 months old, cerebral palsy is diagnosed only if there is obvious asymmetry (paralysis) with a known risk factor such as periventricular leukomalacia or Grade IV intraventricular hemorrhage.

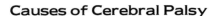

Causes of Cerebral Palsy

The cause of most cases of cerebral palsy is unclear. Risk factors in the development of CP in some babies include asphyxia during the perinatal period (from week 20 of gestation until 7 days after birth), prematurity, severe intraventricular hemorrhage, or periventricular leukomalacia (presence of brain cysts).

The body area affected by CP and the type of disability that results depend on the gestational age at which the brain injury occurs. In premature babies, the area involved is most likely to be the motor fibers supplying the legs. These babies usually have spastic diplegia (tight muscles) of the legs. In term babies, the injury is more likely to affect the arms, face, tongue, and speech areas.

Diagnosis of Cerebral Palsy

In the follow-up clinic, developmental clinic, or doctor's office, your baby will be tested for such things as muscle tone and strength, reflexes, posture and balance, quality or type of movement displayed, ability to achieve normal motor milestones (such as sitting, crawling, and walking), and gross and fine motor development. Abnormalities present at 6 to18 months will be monitored. Abnormalities that do not resolve lead to the diagnosis of cerebral palsy.

Potential Problems Caused by Cerebral Palsy

Children with cerebral palsy often have poor balance and difficulty walking. They may also drool excessively and have trouble with speech and eating. They may develop joint contractures (stiffness), scoliosis, hip dislocation, and out-turned ankles. Intelligence is often normal, but the child may experience learning disabilities. Mental retardation may occur with severe CP.

Treatments for Cerebral Palsy

If your baby is diagnosed with abnormal muscle tone, a team of health care professionals will follow her closely. Occupational or physical therapists may provide you with special exercises for your child and activities to aid with

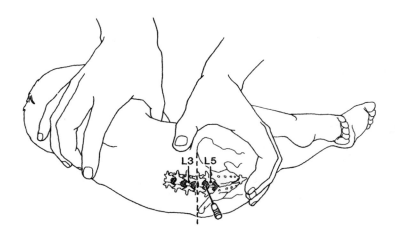

Lumbar puncture.

A lumbar puncture allows the practitioner to remove spinal fluid. A lumbar puncture may be part of a sepsis work-up to rule out infection or to remove spinal fluid and relieve the pressure on the brain of a baby with hydrocephalus. This diagram shows the anatomical location of the lumbar puncture. In order to access the spinal fluid, the baby is flexed to increase the space between the bony prominences of the backbone.

From: Gomella TL. 1994. Neonatology: Management, Procedures, On-call Problems, Diseases and Drugs, 3rd ed. Norwalk, Connecticut: Appleton & Lange, 157. Reprinted by permission.

muscle development and lessen complications. In some cases, surgery may be needed to correct muscle tightness.

Problems Affecting the Eyes

Your baby's eyes begin to develop in the first month after conception, but development is not complete until after birth. The eyelids in very preterm babies (less than 26 weeks) may be fused shut at birth but usually open within a few days to a week after delivery. Once open, your baby's eyes can see an object 8 to 10 inches away from her face but will be quite sensitive to bright light. All babies prefer the human face and black-and-white patterns, but premature babies may find visual stimulation overwhelming.

Retinopathy of Prematurity

Retinopathy of prematurity (ROP) is a disease of the developing eye. The retina (the lining or screen at the back of the eye) begins to develop a supply of blood vessels at about four months gestational age. This process begins in the center of the retina and progresses outward. Blood vessel development is complete shortly after birth in term infants.

With ROP, the normal growth of these blood vessels stops because of higher-than-normal concentrations of oxygen in the blood, combined with other factors. Rapid irregular growth of new vessels follows this pause. Continuation of this rapid growth can lead to bleeding and to the formation of scar tissue, which pulls on the retina. In the most severe cases, the retina may become detached, causing blindness.

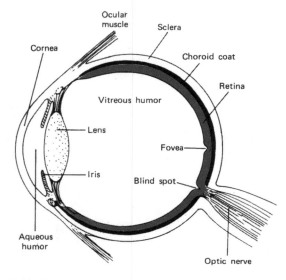

Normal eye anatomy.

The lens is at the front of the eye, on the left of the diagram. The retina lines the back of the eye, on the right of the diagram.

From: Burke S. 1992. In Human Anatomy and Physiology in Health and Disease, *3rd ed. Albany, New York: Delmar Publishers, 231. Reprinted by permission.*

Risk Factors for Retinopathy of Prematurity

- Complications of pregnancy
- Multiple gestation pregnancy (twins, triplets, or more)
- Apnea (pauses in breathing)
- Sepsis (bacterial infection in the bloodstream)
- Nutritional deficiencies
- Unstable blood pressure
- Blood transfusions
- Intraventricular hemorrhage
- Patent ductus arteriosus

Stages of Retinopathy of Prematurity

Stage 1	A thin line separating parts of the retina, with or without blood vessel development
Stage 2	The thin line developed into a ridge, with growth of new vessels
Stage 3	Extension of blood vessels beyond the retina
Stage 4	Retinal detachment

Babies Susceptible to Retinopathy of Prematurity

Retinopathy is usually seen only in babies less than 32 weeks gestational age, because most of the retinal vessels have developed by that age. The highest rate of ROP occurs in babies less than 28 weeks gestation at birth—with 10 to 30 percent of these babies developing some degree of retinopathy. The exact cause of retinopathy is not well understood, but the condition occurs most commonly in babies receiving supplemental oxygen and is believed to be closely associated with increased oxygen levels in the blood. (The amount of oxygen in a baby's blood may be quite different from the amount the baby is breathing, depending on the degree of lung disease the baby may have.) Risk factors for ROP are listed in a table on page 172.

Because the cause of ROP is not fully understood, it is not yet possible to keep babies from developing this disorder. Nor is it possible to predict which babies will develop ROP: Some babies with low blood oxygen levels show eye changes; some with high oxygen levels do not. There have even been cases of ROP in babies who did not receive supplemental oxygen at all. It's important that NICU nurses and doctors closely watch blood oxygen levels of all premature babies receiving oxygen.

Diagnosis of Retinopathy of Prematurity

Babies born at less than 32 weeks gestation usually have their eyes examined by an ophthalmologist (eye specialist) when they are approximately four to six weeks old. These examinations are usually repeated every two weeks until the blood vessel growth in the eye is complete. During these eye examinations, the ophthalmologist will place drops in your baby's eyes to enlarge (dilate) the pupils so that the retina can be viewed. The ophthalmologist will determine whether there is abnormal growth of the blood vessels in the eye and will look for evidence of scars. The ophthalmologist will stage (classify) the ROP according to the severity of the condition. A table on page 172 lists the stages of ROP. If ROP is present, your baby may be scheduled for more frequent eye exams to monitor the problem and its progress.

Long-Term Outlook for Babies with Retinopathy of Prematurity

Most often, retinopathy resolves on its own, and the vessels resume their normal growth pattern. In almost 75 percent of infants with mild ROP, the abnormal blood vessels do not cause scarring or damage to the eye. Some mild cases of ROP result in vision problems requiring glasses (such as near-sightedness) or problems requiring surgery or patching—for example, strabismus (crossed eyes) and amblyopia (lazy eye). Babies with moderate to severe ROP are more likely to need glasses than are those with mild cases.

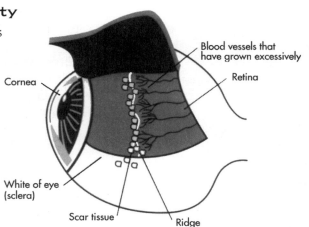

ROP scar tissue.

Retinopathy of prematurity (ROP) causes blood vessels to grow excessively at the back of the eye. If unchecked, the blood vessels can eventually bleed and form scar tissue, which pulls on the retina. In severe cases of ROP, the retina can detach from the eye and cause blindness.

From: IRIS Medical Instruments. 1991. In Understanding Retinopathy of Prematurity, 5. Reprinted by permission.

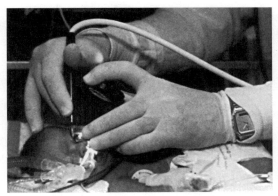

Cryotherapy.

A procedure called cryotherapy is used for some babies with ROP. An ophthalmologist uses a probe to freeze the abnormal blood vessels in the eye, which stops their growth and decreases the pulling on the retina.

From: IRIS Medical Instruments. 1991. In Understanding Retinopathy of Prematurity, 10. Reprinted by permission.

If ROP reaches Stage 3, with extension of blood vessels beyond the retina, the ophthalmologist may recommend that your baby undergo a treatment known as cryotherapy. Cryotherapy involves using a small probe with liquid nitrogen to freeze the abnormal blood vessels to stop their growth. This will help to decrease the pulling on the retina. This procedure may be done under local or general anesthetic. Your baby's eyes will be quite swollen for several days after cryotherapy. Eyedrops or ointment, as well as cold compresses, may be used to reduce the swelling.

A new laser treatment for ROP is being used in some areas. In this approach, a beam of light is directed into the eye to destroy the abnormal blood vessel growth. Advantages of laser treatment include less need for anesthesia and less pain and swelling. Trials are currently under way to test the effectiveness of laser treatment for ROP.

Problems Affecting the Heart

Development of the heart is complete quite early in pregnancy. The most common heart problem seen in preterm babies is a patent ductus arteriosus (described in the next section). Although the newborn's heart is usually strong and healthy, some babies experience congestive heart failure as a complication of other medical problems. This problem is also explained in this chapter. Congenital heart defects are explained in the second half of this chapter.

Patent Ductus Arteriosus

When your baby was in the womb, the blood circulating through her heart and lungs followed a path known as fetal circulation. This path allows some blood to bypass (not go through) the baby's lungs because the mother's lungs do the work of "breathing" for the baby.

Soon after birth, the two structures of the heart that allowed blood to bypass the lung—called the foramen ovale and the ductus arteriosus—normally begin to close. But in some newborns, especially those born preterm, the ductus arteriosus remains open after birth or reopens in the weeks following birth. This is referred to as a patent (open) ductus arteriosus. In the first few hours to days after birth, a patent ductus arteriosus directs blood away from the lung blood vessels, which are narrowed by the effects of respiratory problems such as respiratory distress syndrome, explained later in this chapter. This is called a right-to-left shunt and is similar to the circulation pattern the baby had in the womb. A right-to-left shunt allows blood without enough oxygen to travel to the body.

As the baby's lungs recover from RDS, the blood vessels in the lung relax, and blood can enter more easily. When that happens, a PDA will allow blood to flow back from the aorta into the lungs (a left-to-right shunt). Too much blood entering the lungs leads to many of the signs and symptoms of a PDA.

A patent ductus affects about 20 percent of babies weighing less than 1,500 grams (about 3 pounds, 5 ounces) at birth and 40 percent of babies weighing less than 1,000 grams (about 2 pounds, 4 ounces).

Signs of a Patent Ductus Arteriosus

The signs of a PDA depend on the size of the ductus and the amount of blood moving through it. (The ductus carries only a portion of the blood leaving a baby's heart.) A small ductus may cause few if any problems and requires no treatment. Signs of a large opening include a murmur (swishing sound heard with a stethoscope), an enlarged heart, and worsening respiratory problems. Other signs are visible movement of the baby's heart on the chest wall and throbbing pulses felt in the groin, over the wrist, or on top of the foot.

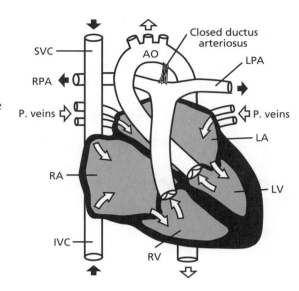

Chambers of the heart and heart valves.

The chambers of the heart are the left and right atria and left and right ventricles. The valves of the heart are the aortic valve, mitral valve, pulmonary valve, and tricuspid valve.

Normal cardiac anatomy and circulation. AO, aorta; AV, aortic valve; IVC, inferior vena cava; LA, left atrium; LDA, ligamentum ductus arteriosus; LPA, left pulmonary artery; LV, left ventricle; MPA, main pulmonary artery; MV, mitral valve; PV, pulmonary valve; P. veins, pulmonary veins; RA, right atrium; RPA, right pulmonary artery; RV, right ventricle; SVC, superior vena cava; TV, tricuspid valve.

From: Ross Laboratories. 1992. Clinical Education Aid. Columbus, Ohio: Ross Products Division, Abbott Laboratories. Reprinted by permission.

Diagnosis of a Patent Ductus Arteriosus

An echocardiogram (ultrasound of the heart) will show the open ductus. It can be used to estimate the size of the ductus and the amount of blood moving through it. (This diagnostic imaging technique is explained in Chapter 12.)

Complications Associated with a Patent Ductus Arteriosus

If untreated, a large ductus places a strain on your baby's heart, because the heart must work harder to circulate blood. This may lead to congestive

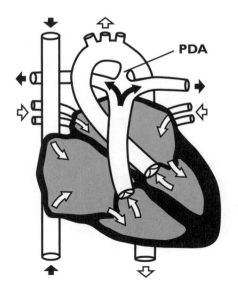

Patent ductus arteriosus.

The ductus arteriosus is a short vessel that connects the pulmonary artery with the aorta in the fetus, directing blood away from the fetal lungs. A patent ductus arteriosus refers to this connection that stays open (patent) after birth. A PDA directs blood away from the blood vessels of the lungs, especially if the lung blood vessels are narrowed by the effects of respiratory distress syndrome. This allows blood without enough oxygen to circulate in the body. As the baby's respiratory distress resolves, the vessels in the lung relax and allow blood to enter more easily. Now the PDA will allow some blood to flow back from the aorta in to lungs. Depending on the size of the PDA, the extra blood volume can cause heart and breathing problems.

From: Ross Laboratories. 1992. Clinical Education Aid. Columbus, Ohio: Ross Products Division, Abbott Laboratories. Reprinted by permission.

heart failure, a condition in which the heart has difficulty meeting the energy needs of the body.

Extra blood flow to the lungs may cause fluid to leak into the lung tissue. This condition is called pulmonary edema. It may increase your baby's work of breathing, making it more difficult to wean her from the ventilator or off supplemental oxygen. Your baby may have difficulty gaining weight because of the extra energy she is using to breathe.

Treatment for a Patent Ductus Arteriosus

Treatment of a ductus usually depends on its size and the degree of difficulty it is causing your baby. In very tiny or premature infants, the ductus may be treated before it begins to cause symptoms.

Medical treatment includes decreasing the amount of fluid given to your baby and use of the medication indomethacin (Indocin) (Appendix B). If medical treatment is unsuccessful in closing the ductus or can't be used because of other medical problems (such as hyperbilirubinemia, explained in Chapter 9), surgical closure will be needed.

Surgery for a PDA is done under general anesthetic. The surgeon makes an incision on the left side of your baby's chest wall under the arm. The ribs are gently spread apart and the lung moved aside. The surgeon then places a suture (clip) around the ductus and ties it off. Surgery takes approximately an hour, and babies generally do well. In addition to a dressing over the incision, your baby may require a chest tube for one to two days after surgery. The chest tube drains air from the chest cavity until it begins to heal. A chest tube is pictured on page 185.

Congestive Heart Failure

Congestive heart failure (CHF) is any condition in which the heart is under strain and is unable to meet the energy needs of the body.

Causes of Congestive Heart Failure

Any condition that makes the heart work harder, such as a patent ductus arteriosus, severe anemia, fluid overload, or a congenital heart defect, may cause CHF. Conditions that decrease the heart's ability to pump can also cause CHF. These include asphyxia, sepsis (an infection in the bloodstream), and arrhythmias.

Signs of Congestive Heart Failure

Babies with CHF show signs that their heart is working hard. These include tachycardia (rapid heart rate) and tachypnea (rapid breathing). Fluid may back up from the heart into the liver, causing it to enlarge, or into the lungs, causing pulmonary edema (fluid in the lungs). Babies with CHF may also produce less urine, and their skin may look pale or mottled (have a bluish, blotchy appearance) because of poor circulation. Babies with chronic CHF may experience feeding problems and difficulty gaining weight.

Treatment for Congestive Heart Failure

The ideal treatment for CHF is identification and elimination of the cause. When that is not possible, your baby's fluid intake is restricted. Drugs called diuretics (furosemide and aldactazide) are given to help your baby eliminate excess fluid and to reduce the load on the heart. Other drugs, such as dopamine or digoxin, may be used to strengthen the heart. (See Appendix B for more information on these medications.)

Other treatment includes supportive care—oxygen to maintain adequate levels in the blood and tissues, maintenance of normal temperature, and sedation (medication to help calm your baby) to conserve energy for growth. High-calorie formula or breast milk supplements and special feeding plans may be used for babies with chronic CHF.

Problems Affecting the Lungs

Many of the babies in an NICU have problems associated with their lungs. Some of these problems are because of the immaturity of the lungs at the time of preterm birth. Others are complications brought on by problems with other body systems. This section explains the lung and breathing problems NICU staff manage most often.

Transient Tachypnea of the Newborn

While your baby was in your uterus, her lungs were filled with fluid. During vaginal birth, much of this fluid was squeezed out of her chest as she passed through the birth canal. A baby's circulatory system absorbs the remaining fluid in the first few hours after birth. Transient tachypnea of the newborn (TTN, or "wet lung") develops when there is a delay in reabsorption of this lung fluid after birth.

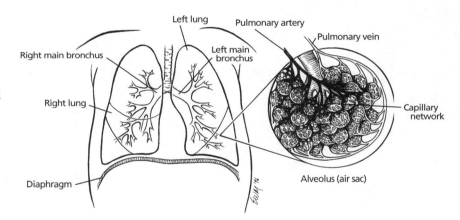

Breathing sacs in lungs.

An alveolus is an air sac in the lungs. Oxygen passes through the alveoli, into the tiny blood vessels called capillaries, and through the circulatory system to the body tissues. Alveoli are coated with surfactant, a soapy substance that keeps these tiny sacs open as the baby breathes in and out after birth. Surfactant production begins at about 24 weeks gestation, but is incomplete until about 34–36 weeks gestation; therefore a baby born prior to this time faces the possibility of respiratory distress syndrome.

Babies Susceptible to Transient Tachypnea of the Newborn

Term or near-term newborns are most likely to get TTN. Babies born by cesarean section or rapid vaginal delivery are at increased risk for developing TTN.

Potential Problems Caused by Transient Tachypnea of the Newborn

Fluid in the lung causes air to become trapped in the alveoli (small breathing sacs). This increases your baby's work of breathing and causes symptoms such as tachypnea (rapid breathing), cyanosis (bluish color of the lips or around the mouth and eyes), and moaning or grunting sounds heard with breathing. This increased work of breathing tires your baby and makes it difficult for her to take in enough oxygen and to get rid of carbon dioxide. Rapid breathing also makes sucking and swallowing difficult and may keep your baby from feeding.

Diagnosis and Treatment of Transient Tachypnea of the Newborn

An x-ray of your baby's chest will show increased fluid in the lungs. Transient tachypnea of the newborn can be difficult to distinguish from other lung problems, such as infection. Treatment includes giving your baby oxygen, fluids, and a warm environment. Some babies with TTN may require additional help with breathing. Prongs (short tubes) may be placed in your baby's nose so that nasal CPAP (explained on page 179) can be used to provide extra oxygen and apply a small amount of pressure to your baby's lungs. Usually TTN resolves in 24 to 72 hours. It should cause no further problems for your baby.

Respiratory Distress Syndrome

Respiratory distress syndrome (RDS) is the most common disease of the lungs that affects premature babies. You may hear RDS referred to as hyaline membrane disease (HMD). The earlier a baby is born, the more likely she is to have RDS, and the more severe the disease is likely to be. Physical immaturity of the lungs coupled with a decreased amount of a substance known as surfactant are the causes of RDS.

The lungs mature at different rates from one baby to the next. Some factors that may increase the likelihood that a baby will develop RDS include maternal diabetes, a difficult delivery, being the second-born of twins, and being male. Babies less likely to get RDS include those who experienced mild prolonged stress before delivery, such as ruptured membranes without infection, intrauterine growth retardation, and moderate maternal hypertension. These stresses seem to cause the baby to produce more surfactant. Health care providers can also speed up surfactant production in some babies by giving steroids to the mother 48 hours or more before delivery.

Surfactant is a soaplike substance that is produced by specialized cells in the lungs (see Chapter 12). Production begins at about 24 weeks gestation, but the surfactant production system is not fully developed until about 34 to 36 weeks gestational age. Surfactant coats the breathing sacs (alveoli) in the lungs, helping to keep them open as the baby breathes in and out. Without enough surfactant, the baby must use a great deal of energy to re-expand the alveoli with each breath. This leads to fatigue, which results in ineffective breathing. Collapse of the alveoli decreases the amount of oxygen available to the baby's body. Lack of oxygen causes some of the lung cells to die. Fluid then leaks into the breathing sacs, causing further damage to the lungs.

Signs of Respiratory Distress Syndrome

Premature babies may show signs of RDS moments after delivery, or they may develop breathing problems in the first few hours after birth. Initially your

One method of instilling artificial surfactant (plastic model).

For treatment of respiratory distress syndrome (RDS), "replacement" surfactant can be instilled into the lungs through a tube in the baby's trachea (windpipe). The surfactant coats the surfaces of the alveoli, and takes the place of the baby's own surfactant.

baby's breathing may be rapid or labored. You may notice retractions (pulling in of the skin and muscles between the ribs or just below the rib cage). You may also hear grunting or moaning sounds as your baby breathes out. Your baby may be dusky or cyanotic (having a bluish color of the skin and mucous membranes). As your baby tires, breathing becomes less regular, and there may be periods of apnea. The skin looks pale and mottled. Decreased oxygen levels in the blood cause the kidneys to produce less urine than normal. This means that more fluid is kept in the body for a 24- to 48-hour period, resulting in swelling of the tissues, especially around the eyes and in the hands and feet.

Respiratory distress syndrome may worsen over the first 48 hours as some of the breathing sacs (alveoli) collapse or close and lung-tissue damage continues. After 48 hours, as your baby starts to produce surfactant, the lungs stabilize and begin to recover.

Treatment for Respiratory Distress Syndrome

Treatment for RDS has changed greatly since the early 1990s with the introduction of a form of surfactant that can be given to babies after birth. This "replacement" surfactant is produced either from the lungs of cows or pigs, or from chemical compounds in a laboratory. The doctor introduces the drug into the baby's lungs through a tube placed in the baby's windpipe (endotracheal tube). The surfactant drains into the baby's alveoli, coating the surfaces and taking the place of the baby's own surfactant. Babies with RDS can receive an initial

Continuous Positive Airway Pressure

Explanation

Continuous positive airway pressure, or CPAP (pronounced See-pap), helps babies breathe without breathing for them. In CPAP, pressure helps the baby keep the small breathing sacs in the lungs from collapsing at the end of each breath but still lets the baby breathe on her own.

Methods

CPAP is usually delivered in one of two ways:

1. Through an endotracheal tube placed in the infant's windpipe. This type of CPAP is sometimes a final step in weaning the baby from mechanical ventilation.
2. Through short tubes (called prongs) inserted in the baby's nose. This approach is called nasal CPAP.

In both methods, a mechanical ventilator delivers a mixture of warmed and humidified air and oxygen to the baby at a set level of pressure. The pressure level can be adjusted to meet the baby's needs.

Complications

Possible complications of CPAP include:

- Air leaks, which can occur when any type of pressure is applied to the lung but which are less likely to happen with CPAP than with mechanical ventilation
- Irritation to the baby's nose, caused by nasal prongs and airflow
- Abdominal swelling, which occurs in many babies on CPAP because they swallow air, which can cause feeding problems.

surfactant dose soon after birth and may receive another dose 12 to 18 hours later. (Chapter 12 provides more details on surfactant replacement therapy.)

Instilled surfactant does not prevent the development of RDS, but it does significantly decrease the severity of the disease. Babies who receive surfactant have a higher incidence of patent ductus arteriosus (PDA) and of pulmonary hemorrhage (bleeding in the lungs) than do babies who are not treated with surfactant, however. The complications associated with those two problems can be treated and are less severe than are those of RDS.

In addition to surfactant, infants with RDS usually require help with breathing in the form of either nasal CPAP or mechanical ventilation. A table on page 179 gives more information about nasal CPAP, as do Chapter 2 and Chapter 9.

Potential Complications of Respiratory Distress Syndrome

The complications of RDS depend on the severity of the disease. They include air leaks, bronchopulmonary dysplasia (BPD), and infection. Hypoxia (reduced oxygen supply to the tissues), results from RDS and contributes to problems in other body systems, including intraventricular hemorrhage, retinopathy of prematurity, patent ductus arteriosus, and necrotizing enterocolitis. All are explained in this chapter.

Bronchopulmonary Dysplasia

Bronchopulmonary dysplasia (BPD) is a chronic lung disease occurring primarily in premature babies who have been ventilated for respiratory distress syndrome (RDS), just discussed. Bronchopulmonary dysplasia develops when air sacs in the lungs are damaged by RDS and hypoxia (too little oxygen reaching the tissues), as well as by waste products that develop when oxygen is broken down in the lungs. This damage leads to areas of bleeding in the lungs, followed by growth of new cells, which forms scar tissue. The presence of scar tissue causes small areas of the lungs to collapse (atelectasis) and other areas to trap air and overexpand. The new cell growth also increases mucus production and causes the walls of the breathing tubes to develop spasms or constrictions similar to those seen in asthma.

Babies Susceptible to Bronchopulmonary Dysplasia

It is not clear why some babies develop BPD while others do not. Premature babies with RDS who are mechanically ventilated are at greatest risk for BPD. Researchers believe that BPD develops because of damage to immature lung tissue resulting from the oxygen given and the pressure of the mechanical ventilation necessary to treat RDS. Prolonged exposure to high pressure and added oxygen increases the risk of BPD. Other factors associated with the development of BPD include the presence of a patent ductus arteriosus, increased fluid in the lungs, and a family history of asthma.

Some term babies—usually those who have significant respiratory problems requiring a great deal of ventilatory support—may develop BPD. Babies with severe meconium aspiration, persistent pulmonary hypertension of the newborn (PPHN), or diaphragmatic hernia are also at risk.

Diagnosis of Bronchopulmonary Dysplasia

Babies with RDS usually begin to wean from the ventilator after several days to a week of treatment. Infants who develop BPD often have more severe RDS initially, are slow to begin weaning, or may begin to wean and then stop making progress. Chest x-rays may show a bubbly or cystlike appearance in the lungs, reflecting areas of atelectasis and overexpansion. As BPD progresses, chest x-rays will be used to classify its severity.

Treatment for Bronchopulmonary Dysplasia

The lung area of a preterm baby is very small compared with that of a two-year-old child. The lung continues to grow and develop for up to two years after birth. The goal of BPD treatment is to allow the infant's lung to heal and new, undamaged lung tissue to develop.

Treatments for BPD include:
- Providing good nutrition, with extra calories for growth
- Avoiding fluid overload
- Reducing the use of mechanical ventilation and high oxygen concentrations as the baby's condition allows
- Providing chest physiotherapy, if indicated, to help eliminate extra mucus and prevent infection

A number of medications are used in the treatment of BPD. Steroids (dexamethasone) help by reducing lung inflammation. Theophylline (Aminophylline) and albuterol (Ventolin) help expand (dilate) the breathing tubes. Diuretics such as furosemide (Lasix) or Aldactazide help to reduce fluid in the lungs. Appendix B gives information on these medications.

A chronic disease, BPD can take months or occasionally years to heal. Because your baby could miss the exploratory stages of a healthy infancy, it is important to provide her with opportunities to develop and grow. Your baby's nurse or therapist will work with you and your baby on a variety of exercises and activities designed to promote optimal growth and development.

Potential Complications of Bronchopulmonary Dysplasia

Bronchopulmonary dysplasia represents a spectrum of illness. Mild BPD can mean your baby is on oxygen for a month or longer but able to go home without extra oxygen or medications. Most concerning for an infant with mild BPD are the consequences of viral illness; she can become more ill than expected after leaving the NICU, and may require rehospitalization because her lungs are not functioning at full capacity. At the other end of the spectrum are infants who are unable to breathe effectively without a ventilator or who eventually die from the disease. Most infants fall somewhere in between. If

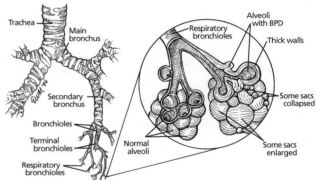

Lungs with bronchopulmonary dysplasia (BPD).

The enlarged portion of the diagram shows normal alveoli and alveoli with bronchopulmonary dysplasia (BPD). Alveoli with BPD have thick walls, making it more difficult to transfer oxygen through the alveoli into the circulatory system. Some of the alveolar sacs trap air and enlarge, and some collapse, forming areas of atelectasis.

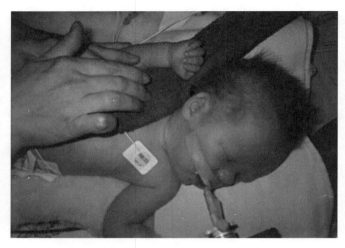

Chest Physiotherapy.

Chest physiotherapy, also called physio or chest PT, is sometimes used as part of the treatment for many types of lung problems in infants. Its purpose is to help the baby loosen and remove secretions in the lungs.

Chest physiotherapy can be given in a number of ways, depending on the preference of your baby's physician and/or nurse. Some babies also have a definite preference! With tiny preterm infants, physio may be given by gently tapping the chest with a finger or a small cup as in the upper photo. An electric toothbrush or mechanical vibrator may also be used.

Chest physio doesn't cause pain; however, some babies don't like to be touched or handled and therefore may show signs of distress during physio. Your baby's caregiver will watch to see how your baby is tolerating physio and adjust the treatment accordingly.

your baby has BPD, discuss her case with the members of her health care team.

Because BPD increases the production of mucus and requires continued ventilation, it increases your baby's risk of pneumonia. Also, air trapped in the lungs causes your baby's diaphragm to push down on the contents of the bowel. This slows emptying of the stomach, causing reflux (backward flow of stomach contents into the esophagus) and feeding problems. Feeding problems can also result from oral aversion—your baby's negative association with *anything* placed in her mouth because of her experience with such treatment aids as suction catheters.

Some infants with BPD develop "blue spells," or "snits." These spells can occur when the infant becomes upset or distressed and can cause cyanosis and more agitation leading to further hypoxia. Lack of oxygen is the most likely cause of these spells.

Bronchopulmonary dysplasia places a strain on the lungs and heart. This strain can lead to an increased heart size and, in severe BPD, to heart failure.

A few babies die of BPD. Infection or respiratory failure is the usual cause of death in infants with severe BPD. Babies who survive show gradual improvement over the first two years of life but may have some degree of abnormal lung function for a number of years. Asthma also occurs more frequently in this group of infants.

Meconium Aspiration Syndrome

Meconium is a sterile, dark green substance produced in the fetus's bowel and passed in the baby's first few stools (bowel movements). Sometimes meconium can be passed while the baby is still in the uterus, however, and can be inhaled (aspirated) into the lungs.

At or after term, a decrease in the amount of oxygen reaching the baby in the uterus may cause the release of meconium from the baby's bowel into the amniotic fluid (fluid surrounding the baby). As the fetus "breathes" (makes breathing movements), the meconium can enter the mouth and airway. Babies who have inhaled a large amount of meconium into their lungs can have severe breathing problems after birth. This condition is called meconium aspiration syndrome (MAS). About 10 percent of all deliveries are complicated by meconium in the amniotic fluid, but only a small number of these babies experience breathing problems.

Symptoms of Meconium Aspiration Syndrome

The presence of meconium in the amniotic fluid is the first sign that your baby may be at risk for MAS. Meconium may stain the baby's skin, fingernails, or umbilical cord. Babies who have inhaled meconium into their lungs may be quite slow to breathe after birth, or they may show tachypnea (rapid breathing) or labored breathing and cyanosis (blue color of the body and around the mouth).

Treatment for Meconium Aspiration Syndrome

The first goal in treating MAS is to remove the meconium from your baby's upper airway. The health care professional first suctions out your baby's mouth and nose as soon as the head is delivered. An endotracheal tube (breathing tube) may be inserted into your baby's airway so that any meconium in the airways can be suctioned out. Babies with mild meconium aspiration may require extra oxygen and intravenous (IV) fluids for several hours to days following delivery. Your baby may receive chest physiotherapy to help her cough up any remaining meconium from the lungs. Babies who have inhaled meconium into their lungs before delivery may be quite ill at birth, needing mechanical ventilation and drug and fluid support.

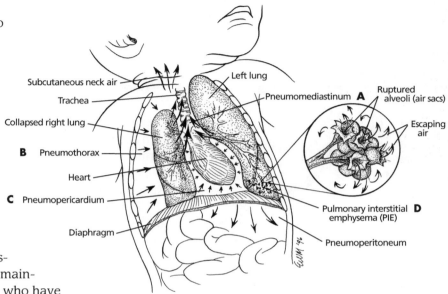

Potential Complications of Meconium Aspiration Syndrome

Mild meconium aspiration usually resolves with few complications. If your baby is breathing rapidly, feedings may be delayed. Whether your baby experiences long-term problems will depend on the degree of distress that occurred and on the severity of the MAS and pulmonary hypertension.

Some particles of meconium can be quite large and may block smaller airways. In some cases, a blockage traps air in the airway; in others, it keeps air from entering. This uneven inflation of the lung may lead to rupture of some air sacs and trapping of the air outside the lung (called a pneumothorax), discussed later in this chapter.

Meconium acts as a chemical irritant to the lungs, and although it is sterile, its presence may encourage the development of infection. In combination with hypoxia (reduced oxygen to the tissues), severe meconium aspiration can cause your baby to develop the serious complication of persistent pulmonary hypertension of the newborn (PPHN), explained later in this chapter.

Air Leaks

When a baby has trouble breathing, one possible complication is an air leak. This occurs when air ruptures one or several of the alveoli (breathing

Air leaks.
Arrows show the path of air out of the major airways that cause respiratory complications in babies.
*A: **Pneumomediastinum** occurs when air leaks into the space in the center of the chest containing the heart and major blood vessels.*
*B: **Pneumothorax** occurs when air collects in the space between the lung and the chest wall.*
*C: **Pneumopericardium** occurs when air collects in the sac around the heart.*
*D: **Pulmonary interstitial emphysema** occurs when air ruptures one or several of the alveoli (air sacs) and leaks into the spaces around the lung tissue.*

sacs) and leaks into the spaces around the lung tissue. Pulmonary interstitial emphysema (PIE) is the term for this type of air leak. Air may collect in the space between the lung and the chest wall (producing a pneumothorax), or it may leak into the space in the center of the chest containing the heart and major blood vessels (producing a pneumomediastinum). A pneumopericardium is a collection of air in the sac around the heart and is a life-threatening emergency.

Babies Susceptible to Air Leaks

Among healthy term babies, 0.5 to 1 percent may develop a pneumothorax shortly after birth. These air leaks are associated with aspiration of fluid or meconium and are usually quite small. Term babies with severe meconium aspiration or persistent pulmonary hypertension of the newborn may develop an air leak as a complication of ventilator treatment or bag-and-mask ventilation.

Preterm babies may develop air leaks because of the mechanical pressure needed to inflate lungs affected by respiratory distress syndrome (RDS). The incidence of air leaks in babies with RDS is about 4 percent but is decreasing as surfactant treatment increases.

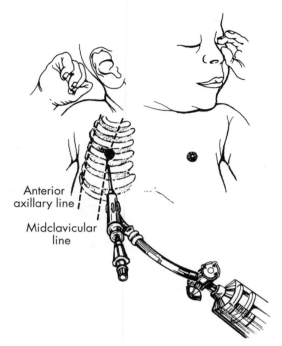

Needle aspiration of the chest.

To help treat a pneumothorax, a needle is inserted into the space between the lungs and the chest wall. The air is drawn out through the needle.

From: MDI, Inc., 537 Apple Street, West Conshohocken, Pennsylvania 19428. Reprinted by permission.

Signs of an Air Leak

Some term babies with a pneumothorax show no symptoms. Other babies have mild signs of respiratory distress, such as tachypnea (rapid breathing). Premature or unstable infants with a pneumothorax show more signs of distress, such as cyanosis (blue coloring), hypotension (low blood pressure), uneven chest movement, and decreased oxygen saturation. If you were to listen to the lungs of these babies with a stethoscope, you'd hear softer breath sounds over the area of the leak.

Babies with PIE usually show general signs of worsening respiratory status, such as an increased need for oxygen and poor blood gases. A pneumomediastinum produces no specific symptoms. A pneumopericardium produces severe distress, including low blood pressure and heart rate, severe cyanosis, and shock.

Diagnosis of Air Leaks

A chest x-ray is used to diagnose most air leaks. When a baby deteriorates suddenly, a bright light placed on the baby's chest (called transillumination) may show the collection of air outside the lung.

Treatment for Air Leaks

A high concentration of oxygen for several hours helps term babies with a small pneumothorax to reabsorb the trapped air. For term infants in greater distress or for preterm infants, the air may be removed by inserting a needle into the space between the lungs and the chest wall. The needle is then removed. If there is concern about the air reaccumulating, a chest tube is left in the lung space to drain the leaking air.

Pulmonary interstitial emphysema is more difficult to treat because the air is trapped in many small spaces and cannot be removed. Babies with PIE are given ventilator support until their lungs heal. In severe cases, special mechanical devices (such as high-frequency oscillatory or jet ventilators) help the baby breathe without further damaging the lung. (Chapter 12 explains how high-frequency ventilation works.)

A pneumomediastinum is not usually treated. The air is gradually reabsorbed on its own.

A pneumopericardium must be treated quickly. A needle is inserted into the space around the heart, the air is drawn into the needle, and the needle is removed.

Persistent Pulmonary Hypertension of the Newborn

Persistent pulmonary hypertension of the newborn (PPHN) occurs when a complex interaction of factors produces high blood pressure (hypertension) in the arteries supplying blood to the lungs. This forces blood away from the lungs and decreases the supply of oxygen to the body. Persistent pulmonary hypertension is a life-threatening problem for a newborn.

As the baby develops in the uterus, blood follows a path known as fetal circulation. This path allows oxygen-rich blood supplied by the placenta to circulate quickly to the baby's body. Much of this blood bypasses the baby's lungs, which do not function during fetal life. Two fetal shunts, the foramen ovale and the ductus arteriosus, produce the bypass. Because the lungs receive little blood flow, and little oxygen, the vessels are narrow (constricted). After birth, all blood must pass through the lungs to pick up oxygen for the body. The pressures in the heart change, and oxygen enters the lungs. The presence of oxygen relaxes the pulmonary blood vessels. These two factors cause the closure of the fetal shunts and the change to normal newborn circulation.

In term or close-to-term infants, several factors can interfere with this changeover from fetal to normal newborn circulation. These include asphyxia, meconium aspiration, infection, hypothermia (low body temperature), and occasionally respiratory distress syndrome. These problems trigger hypoxia (lack of oxygen in the tissues), which keeps the pulmonary vessels constricted, forcing blood away from the lungs. That, in turn, changes the pressures within the heart, keeping the fetal shunts open. Poor circulation to the lungs results in less oxygen in the blood for the body tissues, causing further hypoxia and a buildup of waste acid in the baby's body. This sets up a cycle of hypoxia and blood vessel constriction that is difficult to break.

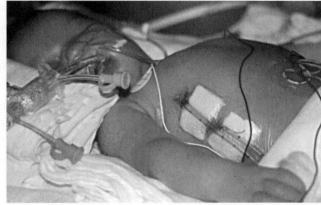

Chest tube.

A chest tube may be placed into the space between the lungs and the chest wall to draw out and prevent reaccumulation of air. The chest tube is a clear plastic tube that is sutured to the chest and secured well with tape and sterile dressings. This baby's chest tube enters the skin between his right nipple and armpit area. A baby can have multiple chest tubes if needed.

Signs of Persistent Pulmonary Hypertension of the Newborn

The signs of PPHN are difficult to distinguish from those of other major illnesses. Your baby may be either slow to breathe at birth or tachypneic (breathing quickly), be cyanotic with a low arterial blood oxygen concentration, be pale or mottled with low blood pressure, and have hands and feet that are cool to the touch or blue. As PPHN continues, your baby may become quite swollen because of low urine output.

Diagnosis of Persistent Pulmonary Hypertension of the Newborn

If your baby remains hypoxic despite good mechanical ventilation, PPHN is suspected. Additional tests can be done to show the presence of blood moving across the foramen ovale and ductus arteriosus. A cardiac ultrasound (echocardiogram) is done to examine the functioning of the heart and rule out other cardiac problems.

Treatment for Persistent Pulmonary Hypertension of the Newborn

The goals of treatment for PPHN are to improve oxygen levels in the blood, relax the blood vessels in the lungs, and maintain a normal blood pressure. Good ventilation helps to increase the oxygen in your baby's system and to relax the pulmonary vessels. In infants with diseased lungs, good ventilation may be difficult to achieve, requiring high concentrations of oxygen and increased amounts of pressure. Ventilation may be improved with high-frequency ventilation (Chapter 12). Another possible treatment for severe, life-threatening PPHN is extracorporeal membrane oxygenation (ECMO), explained in Chapter 12.

Normal blood sugar and blood pressure are maintained with intravenous (IV) fluid. Hypoxia may cause your baby's capillaries (tiny blood vessels) to leak fluid into the tissues. If that occurs, large amounts of a fluid such as albumin, the protein part of the blood, may help to stabilize the blood pressure.

Medications such as dopamine or epinephrine may be given to help to raise your infant's blood pressure. Other drugs, such as sodium bicarbonate, restore the chemical balance in the blood. Antibiotics prevent or treat infection. Medication will be given to sedate your baby, to decrease oxygen use. In some cases, medication will be necessary to paralyze your baby's muscles temporarily, to keep her from breathing against (fighting) the ventilator. Although unable to move her muscles, your baby can still hear your voice and feel your touch.

It's important that your baby be kept warm and away from drafts during this time. In addition, many babies with PPHN are very sensitive to noise, light, and handling. Your baby's nurse may use blankets and eye patches to protect her from light. Those around your baby will be asked to be especially quiet. You should discuss your baby's care with the nurse so that she can help you find the best way to communicate with your baby at this difficult time.

Necrotizing enterocolitis (NEC) occurs when the blood supply to the baby's bowel is decreased or interrupted. Hypoxia (lack of oxygen in the tissues) causes damage or death to cells of the bowel wall. Bacteria that are normally present in the bowel may invade the wall of the bowel, causing further damage. Bowel damage may be minimal or quite extensive, depending on the severity of the disease. In severe cases, the wall of the bowel may perforate (rupture), leading to peritonitis (infection of the abdominal cavity).

Necrotizing Enterocolitis: A Problem Affecting The Bowel

Babies Susceptible to Necrotizing Enterocolitis

Necrotizing enterocolitis is a disease that most often affects premature infants; however, some term or close-to-term infants may also get NEC. The reason babies develop NEC is not completely understood. Necrotizing enterocolitis most often occurs as the infant with risk factors begins oral feedings.

Signs of Necrotizing Enterocolitis

Infants with NEC may show a variety of signs, some of them quite subtle. Early signs show themselves as feeding problems and include abdominal distention (swelling), an increase in feeding residuals (milk left in the stomach when time comes for the next feeding), presence of bile (green-colored liquid) in the residuals, vomiting, blood in the stools, and decreased bowel sounds. More general signs include lethargy (less energy), apnea, bradycardia, and temperature instability.

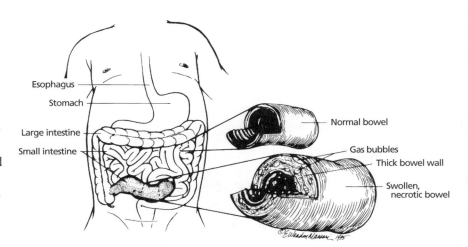

Necrotizing enterocolitis.

Enlargements of the gastrointestinal system show appearance of a section of normal bowel, and a section of bowel with necrotizing enterocolitis (NEC). The bowel with NEC shows bubbles in the bowel wall, along with swelling and thickening of the bowel wall. Necrotizing enterocolitis can affect the small or large intestine.

Possible Risk Factors for Necrotizing Enterocolitis

- Asphyxia (too little oxygen reaching the tissues) and/or hypoxia (lack of oxygen in the blood or body tissues)
- Low blood pressure or low blood volume
- Cold stress
- Receiving an exchange transfusion (discussed in Chapter 9)
- Patent ductus arteriosus
- Polycythemia

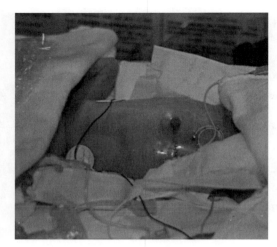

Ostomy site.

The dark circular opening on this baby's abdomen is the stoma (artificial opening) of his ostomy site. In this case, the ostomy (surgical opening into an organ) is into the intestine. The diseased portion of bowel has been removed, and a portion of the intestine has been brought to the surface and attached to the wall of the abdomen. An ostomy bag will fit over the opening to collect stool. An ostomy into the small intestine is called an ileostomy; into the large intestine, it is a colostomy.

Diagnosis of Necrotizing Enterocolitis

At the first sign of feeding problems, caregivers will watch your baby very closely. They'll check the amount of residuals in your baby's stomach and test the baby's stool for the presence of blood. If feeding problems continue or worsen, caregivers will begin diagnostic tests for NEC.

Abdominal x-rays will be done to look for bowel swelling and signs of gas in the wall of the bowel. Bacteria invading the injured bowel wall produce this gas, which appears as little bubbles on the x-ray. This sign confirms the diagnosis of NEC.

Treatment for Necrotizing Enterocolitis

Treatment for NEC depends on the severity of your baby's signs and symptoms. Babies with only one or two of the signs are given no feedings by mouth (kept NPO) for 24 to 48 hours. If caregivers consider NEC to be likely, your baby will be NPO longer, possibly for weeks while the bowel heals. In addition, a tube will be passed through your baby's nose or mouth and into her stomach to drain any mucus or swallowed air and allow the bowel to rest. Your baby will receive intravenous (IV) nutrition (total parenteral nutrition, or TPN) and may also be given antibiotics in case of infection.

Babies with NEC are quite ill and require close monitoring. X-rays may be done every 8 to 12 hours to check for rupture of the bowel wall. Your baby may require supplemental oxygen or ventilation because of apnea and shock. Additional fluids and medication may be needed to maintain your baby's blood pressure.

Potential Complications of Necrotizing Enterocolitis

Rupture of the bowel wall is a serious complication of NEC; it often requires emergency surgery. Scarring or narrowing of the bowel wall (strictures and adhesions) may also occur as the bowel begins to heal. These complications may require surgery later on. Surgical treatment of NEC involves removing the diseased or scarred portion of the bowel wall. Your baby may come back from surgery with a temporary ostomy in place to allow the bowel more time to heal. An ostomy is an opening on the surface of the baby's abdomen to allow stool to drain from the bowel into a collecting bag. If the intestinal diversion is in the large intestine, it is called a colostomy. If it is in the small intestine, it is called an ileostomy. More information on ileostomies and colostomies is found in Chapter 16. The opening onto the abdominal skin surface is called a stoma. A second operation may be possible at a later time to reattach the healed portion of the bowel and to close the ostomy.

Infants with NEC may also develop signs of shock or problems with blood clotting. If the disease is extensive, the amount of healthy bowel remaining may be quite short and therefore unable to absorb enough nutrients and water from the stool. This is called short bowel syndrome, or "short gut." Babies with short gut require intravenous nutrition (TPN) for a prolonged period. They also need special formula and nutrient supplements.

Advances in treatment have reduced the incidence of NEC in recent years, but very premature infants remain at significant risk.

Infection is a common problem in the NICU, especially among premature babies. They are especially vulnerable to infection for several reasons:

- During the final few weeks of a term pregnancy, protective substances called immunoglobulins cross the placenta from mother to baby. Babies born early may not receive these substances.
- Other infection-fighting mechanisms are not fully developed in the premature baby's body.
- Many of the diseases affecting preterm babies require invasive treatment procedures involving intravenous (IV) lines, catheters, and endotracheal tubes. These devices may introduce infection to the body.

Chapter 9 explains how a baby's immune system functions and why infections are especially problematic for newborns.

Problems Related to the Immune System

Infection

An *infection* occurs when a bacterium, virus, or fungus enters a part of the body where it is not normally found and causes a reaction. You may also hear the term *sepsis,* which means that infection is present in the blood. The two terms, *sepsis* and *infection,* have slightly different meanings but may often be used to refer to the same thing.

Causes of Infection

Three types of organisms are responsible for most neonatal infections: bacteria, viruses, and fungi. Some of these organisms are normally found in or on the body with no ill effects. They cause an infection only if they move to an area of the body where they are not normally found. Other organisms can be passed to the baby from the hands of parents, siblings, and caregivers. Still others live in the environment—in the water reservoirs of ventilators or incubators, for example. A table on page 190 gives information about various microorganisms.

Routes of Infection

Infections in the newborn fall into one of three categories, depending on how and when they occur: intrauterine (congenital), perinatal, and acquired.

Some organisms can cross the placenta and infect the baby while it is in the uterus. Called intrauterine or congenital infections, they are represented by the letters TORCH, which stand for their names: **t**oxoplasmosis, **o**ther, **r**ubella virus, **c**ytomegalovirus, and **h**erpes simplex virus. Human immunodeficiency virus (HIV) may also be transmitted in this way. Babies born following an intrauterine infection may show a variety of symptoms, including growth retardation (small for gestational age, or SGA), an unusually large or small head, a rash, an enlarged liver, and abnormal muscle tone and behavior.

Types of Microorganisms that Cause Infections

Bacteria are living, single-cell organisms. In healthy humans, bacteria cover much of the outside of the body. They also live in the bowel, vagina, and mouth. Bacteria are found in the environment—on plants, in soil, and in water. Most are harmless; some may actually help protect us from other, harmful bacteria. Problems occur when bacteria enter an area of the body where they are not normally found; then they may cause an infection. Bacterial infections are treated with medications called antibiotics.

Viruses are tiny structures that can survive only by living inside other cells. Those cells (such as the cells in our body) protect the virus and make it difficult to detect and treat. We associate viruses with the common cold and with the flu. Viruses are also responsible for illnesses such as measles, chickenpox, and herpes.

Fungi are another type of living organism can also cause infection. In infants, the most common fungal infection is yeast, caused by a group of fungi called Candida.

Some Microorganisms Responsible for Infections

Intrauterine or Congenital (Before Birth)

Toxoplasmosis

Other (such as syphilis)

Rubella virus

Cytomegalovirus

Herpes simplex virus

Human immunodeficiency virus (HIV)

Perinatal (Shortly Before or During Birth/Early Onset)

Group B β-hemolytic Streptococcus (β-strep)

Escherichia coli (E. coli)

Haemophilus influenzae (H. flu)

Chlamydia

Hepatitis B

Ureaplasma

Acquired (Late Onset)

Staphylococcus epidermidis (Staph epi)

Staphylococcus aureus

Group B β-hemolytic Streptococcus (β-strep)

Klebsiella

Pseudomonas

Enterobacter

Intrauterine infections are relatively rare but can be quite serious. If infection occurs early in the pregnancy, it can result in brain, nervous system, or tissue abnormalities or even in miscarriage.

The second route by which infants acquire infection is through the birth canal. These are called perinatal infections. Organisms may move up the birth canal and infect the baby in the womb, especially if the membranes rupture. A baby may also acquire an infection as she passes through the birth canal during delivery. Some organisms responsible for these perinatal infections may also cause illness in the mother. Others may live normally in the mother's vagina, causing no symptoms in the mother but producing significant illness in her baby. These types of infections are usually evident shortly after birth.

The third type of infection in the newborn is an acquired infection, meaning that the infecting organism was passed to the baby after delivery. Organisms that cause acquired infections may be passed to babies from their parents or siblings, health care workers, or the hospital environment. Symptoms usually develop several days to weeks after delivery. Acquired infections are commonly spread through poor hand washing. Before you visit your baby, always wash your hands. A table on page 190 summarizes more information on these types of infections.

Babies Susceptible to Infection

Premature or ill babies are especially susceptible to acquired infection because of an immature or weakened immune system. Other factors predisposing infants to infection are:
- Prematurity
- Low birth weight
- Prolonged rupture of membranes
- Maternal fever or infection at delivery
- Fetal distress
- Multiple fetuses (twins, triplets, or more)
- Invasive procedures (IVs, intravascular lines, catheters, and so on)
- Birth defects

Signs of Infection

Babies who are developing an infection often show general signs of illness or signs that mimic other problems. Newborns with perinatal or acquired infections most frequently show signs associated with breathing, such as tachypnea (rapid respirations), retractions (pulling in of the chest muscles while inhaling), cyanosis (blue color of the body or mucous membranes), and grunting while exhaling. Other signs of infection are:
- Lethargy or irritability
- Temperature instability
- Abnormal muscle tone
- Seizures
- Apnea (pauses in breathing) and/or bradycardia (low heart rate)
- Jitteriness

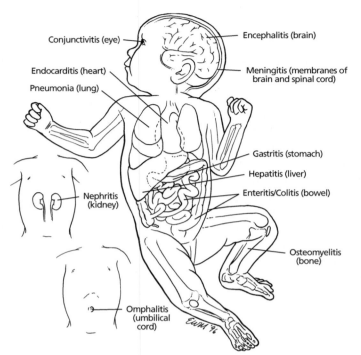

Conjunctivitis (eye)

Endocarditis (heart)

Pneumonia (lung)

Encephalitis (brain)

Meningitis (membranes of brain and spinal cord)

Gastritis (stomach)

Hepatitis (liver)

Enteritis/Colitis (bowel)

Nephritis (kidney)

Osteomyelitis (bone)

Omphalitis (umbilical cord)

Sites of infection.

Babies may develop infections in many areas of the body. The most common location for a neonatal infection is the lungs. Other sites include the skin, bowel, bladder, kidneys, heart, or bone. Infection may also occur in the lining of the brain or spinal cord, or as a generalized infection in the blood.

- Feeding problems (vomiting, diarrhea, increased amounts of the feeding remaining in the stomach)
- Unstable blood glucose levels
- Jaundice (different from physiologic jaundice)
- Poor perfusion (pale, mottled skin; cool hands and feet)

These signs may be subtle or quite dramatic, depending on the severity of the infection and the type of organism causing it.

Common Sites for Infection in Babies

Newborns may develop infections in many areas of the body. The most common location is the lungs—and the infection is pneumonia. Other sites include the lining of the brain or spinal cord (meningitis); the blood (septicemia or sepsis); the skin, especially around the umbilical cord; the bowel (gastroenteritis); and the bladder or kidneys (urinary tract infections).

Diagnosis of Infection

To see if your baby has an infection, caregivers do a sepsis workup. They take samples of your baby's blood, urine, and spinal fluid. These samples go to the laboratory where they grow in broth (cultures). If microorganisms (bacteria, viruses, or fungi) are present, the culture is positive, indicating an infection. Cultures usually take 24 to 48 hours to develop before a result can be read.

Samples will be taken from other areas of your baby's body—such as chest secretions or wound swabs—to check for specific types of infections. X-rays of the chest or abdomen may also be done. Less common infections require additional tests.

Treatment for Infection

The first treatment for infants suspected of having an infection is antibiotics—medications that are effective against bacteria. Initially, your baby receives antibiotics that are effective against a number of organisms. As caregivers learn more about the type of organism causing your baby's infection, they may give a more specific antibiotic.

Supportive care is also provided to increase your baby's ability to fight the infection. A warm environment, IV fluids, adequate nutrition (oral or intravenous), and oxygen or ventilation as needed are examples of supportive care.

Specific infections may require additional treatment. Pneumonia frequently requires intubation and ventilation until your baby's lung function begins to improve. Chest physiotherapy may help clear secretions from your baby's lungs. Sedatives or anticonvulsant drugs such as phenobarbital may be used in the treatment of meningitis.

Short- and Long-Term Complications of Infection

The problems resulting from infection depend on the severity of the infection, the type of organism causing it, and your baby's condition. Some organisms are aggressive, causing significant problems; others have only minor effects. Very low birth weight babies are more likely to be seriously ill with an infection than are larger, healthier babies.

In the short term: Significant infections cause several short-term problems. Some organisms release substances (toxins) into the bloodstream that can interfere with the blood's ability to clot. As a result, your baby may bleed at several locations in the body—a condition called disseminated intravascular coagulation (DIC).

Shock may accompany infection if the organism interferes with your baby's blood pressure, fluid balance, or heart function. Shock occurs when the blood circulation doesn't deliver enough oxygen to the body for its needs. This can occur for a variety of reasons:

- Hypovolemia (decreased blood volume)—caused by bleeding, vomiting, or diarrhea or because fluid has left the blood vessels and leaked into the body tissues
- Septicemia (sepsis)
- Heart failure—caused by congenital heart defects or damage from hypoxia

Any critically ill baby may show signs of shock. These signs may be seen immediately after birth or because of other medical problems:

- Increased heart rate
- Low blood pressure
- Pale, mottled skin
- Decreased oxygen in the blood
- Low urine output
- Chemical imbalance in the blood

Shock is treated by:

- Supporting the baby's blood pressure with fluids and medications
- Keeping the baby warm and well nourished
- Ventilating the baby to improve oxygenation
- Treating the cause of the shock where possible (for example, giving antibiotics to fight an infection)
- Correcting chemical imbalances
- Sedating the baby to decrease her oxygen use

Over the long term: Long-term complications of infection depend on the infecting organism and the site of infection. Treatment with antibiotics usually clears the infection from the body. Some types of infection may cause damage that takes longer to heal. Severe pneumonia requiring ventilator support may contribute to lung problems such as bronchopulmonary dysplasia (BPD).

Meningitis results in brain and nervous system complications, such as motor or mental disabilities, in 20 to 50 percent of cases. Infections of the kidney or bladder require follow-up investigations to rule out structural abnormalities that may have led to the infection. Blood, skin, and bowel infections usually do not cause long-term complications unless they are accompanied by severe illness.

Beta-Strep Pneumonia

Beta-strep—pronounced "BAY-tah STREP" and standing for Group B β-(beta) hemolytic Streptococcus (GBS)—is a type of bacteria found in the birth canal in up to one-third of healthy women. This organism does not usually cause any symptoms in the mother but in some cases may be responsible for chorioamnionitis (infection of the amniotic membranes). Colonization with Group B Streptococcus can be detected before the onset of labor if the birth canal is swabbed (cultured). If you have this organism in your birth canal, you may receive antibiotics during labor to prevent transmission of the organism to your baby after rupture of the membranes or during delivery through the birth canal. Beta-strep can cause pneumonia in newborns. Risk factors for the development of pneumonia include ruptured membranes for more than 12 hours, maternal fever, low birth weight, and a low one-minute Apgar score. Approximately 60 percent of babies born to mothers with GBS have the organism on their skin, but only a small number (1 to 2 percent) of those babies develop GBS pneumonia. Those who do become infected can become seriously ill. Often, infants with β-strep pneumonia show respiratory symptoms that mimic those of other respiratory problems, such as respiratory distress syndrome. The infection can progress rapidly, with development of shock, apnea, and persistent pulmonary hypertension of the newborn.

Treatment of pneumonia consists of antibiotics and supportive care (temperature control, ventilation, nutrition). In severe cases, your baby may receive immunoglobulins—substances found in the blood that fight infection. It is now possible to produce immunoglobulins that are specific to GBS. Given intravenously, these immunoglobulins help your baby's body fight the GBS organism.

Birth Defects

At birth, some babies show distinctive physical abnormalities. Others may have hidden abnormalities of the internal organs or organ systems. The medical term for these abnormalities is congenital (existing at birth) anomalies. The common name for them is birth defects.

Causes of Birth Defects

Abnormalities are generally identified as having one of four basic causes: genetic, environmental, a mixture of the two, or unknown. The remainder of this chapter looks at birth defects in each of these categories. It also includes an explanation of congenital heart defects provided by the American Heart Association.

Genetic Defects

As humans, we each have a genetic code that determines who we are: whether we are tall or short, blond or brunette. No two people share the same genetic makeup except identical twins.

The information that makes each of us unique is carried on genes found in the 46 chromosomes that make up the center of each cell in our body. All cells in the body contain identical genes. When a new life is formed, 23 of the 46 chromosomes come from the mother and 23 from the father. One pair of these chromosomes determines the sex of the unborn baby.

Problems at the time of fertilization can prevent the chromosome pairs from developing properly. This results in a chromosome, or genetic, defect. How severe the defect is depends on the type of problem it causes. In most cases, chromosome damage is so serious that the fetus cannot survive, and a miscarriage occurs. Sometimes the damage is so minor that it goes undetected. Occasionally, babies with chromosome defects are carried to term and are born with deformities or illnesses.

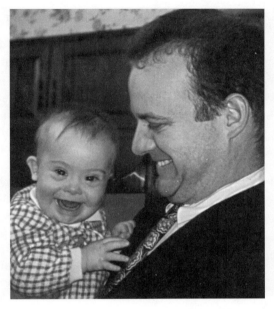

Down syndrome.
A baby with Down syndrome, showing some facial features typical of the syndrome: slanted eyes, and broad, flat nose.

Down Syndrome

The most common chromosome abnormality is Down syndrome—also called Trisomy 21. (The word *trisomy* means three, and babies with Down syndrome have an extra 21st chromosome.) A child with Down syndrome has 47 chromosomes. The extra chromosome affects the development of the body, causing the features of Down syndrome which may include: short wide hands; a crease across the palm of the hand; a fat pad at the back of the neck; slanted eyes, a broad, flat nose; low-placed ears; and decreased muscle tone. In addition to producing these visible features, the extra chromosome found in Down syndrome interferes with mental development and may affect structures such as the heart or bowel.

Down syndrome occurs more frequently, but not exclusively, when a woman becomes pregnant after age 35. Extra chromosomes also occur from time to time in other chromosome pairs. Trisomy 13 and 18 are two examples. These syndromes are less common than Down syndrome.

The Role of Environmental Agents in Birth Defects

Much has been written about the influence of the environment on the developing fetus. Although there is a great deal that we don't know, we have identified some specific drugs, chemicals, and toxins that can cause birth defects. These agents—called teratogens—can cause problems for the fetus if exposure occurs during a critical period of development, usually the first trimester. Remember that these agents do not always cause problems and that the benefits of some drugs must be weighed against the harm of untreated illness in the mother. Women attempting pregnancy and pregnant women should discuss both prescription and nonprescription drugs with their doctor before using them.

Birth Defects Having Mixed or Unknown Causes

Unfortunately, for the majority of birth defects, the cause is either not known or thought to be a combination of genes and the environment. Some of these problems may be detected before delivery, but many will not be diagnosed until after the baby is born. Some of the more common birth defects of unknown or mixed origin are described here.

Myelomeningocele

A type of spina bifida, myelomeningocele occurs during the third or fourth week of pregnancy. In this defect, the spinal column does not close completely, leaving a gap between the vertebrae. The covering of the spinal cord then pushes out through this gap, forming a sac. The sac can also contain spinal nerve fibers.

The incidence of myelomeningocele is one in 500 live births. Most defects occur in the lower back (lumbar region). Spina bifida often occurs with hydrocephalus, discussed earlier in this chapter. The location of the sac determines the types of problem that are likely to occur. Nerves supplying the areas below the defect are often damaged or nonfunctional, resulting in some loss of feeling and paralysis in the lower limbs. In addition, there may be a loss of bladder and bowel control.

Babies born with spina bifida require surgery to close the sac to prevent infection. If hydrocephalus is present, a shunt will be inserted. Extensive follow-up and ongoing treatments are required to optimize mobility and prevent bladder infections.

Cleft Lip and Cleft Palate

Problems in the development of the lip and palate may occur alone or as part of a pattern of defects, called a syndrome. A cleft lip is a defect that involves an opening from the upper lip to one or both nostrils. A cleft lip may be accompanied by a cleft palate, an opening on the roof of the mouth that connects the oral and nasal cavities. A small hole in the palate may cause minor feeding problems. The size and location of the defect, however, as well as any accompanying defects,will determine the scope of the baby's problems. Often, a baby with a cleft lip and/or palate faces serious feeding problems and requires extensive interventions for dental and speech problems.

If your baby's cleft lip is discovered by ultrasound before birth, you may have referrals to specialists even before she is born. By the time your baby arrives, you will already have received some education and guidance, and specialists will

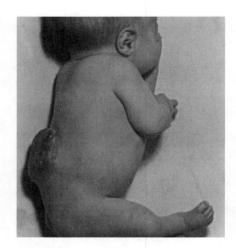

Spina bifida.

A baby with spina bifida. During early development, the spinal column does not completely close and the covering of the spinal cord pushes out through this gap, forming a sac. The sac can contain spinal nerve fibers.

From: O'Doherty N. 1986. Neonatology: Micro Atlas of the Newborn. *Basel, Switzerland: Reinhardt Communications. Reprinted by permission.*

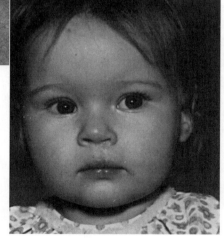

Cleft lip.

A cleft lip is a defect that involves an opening from the upper lip to one or both nostrils. This baby's defect involves both nostrils.

Cleft lip and palate after repair.

Improved surgical techniques promise good outcomes for children with cleft lip and palate.

From: O'Doherty N. 1986. Neonatology: Micro Atlas of the Newborn. *Basel, Switzerland: Reinhardt Communications. Reprinted by permission.*

be ready to help with your baby's care. In any case, early treatment involves the use of special feeding devices or a plate fitted over the palate defect to reduce feeding problems. Surgery to correct cleft lip and palate will be done either in the weeks shortly after birth or at three months of age, depending on the preference of the plastic surgeon. Prognosis is good following repair.

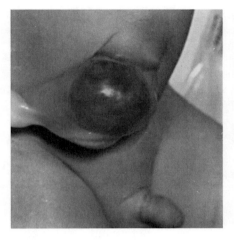

Omphalocele.

An omphalocele occurs when abdominal contents push out into the base of the umbilical cord. The abdominal contents are contained in a membranous sac; however, the sac may rupture at or before delivery.

From: O'Doherty N. 1986. Neonatology: Micro Atlas of the Newborn. Basel, Switzerland: Reinhardt Communications. Reprinted by permission.

Omphalocele

An omphalocele occurs when some of the contents of the abdomen (usually bowel) push out into the base of the umbilical cord. The bowel is covered by a membranous sac; however, the sac may rupture at or before delivery.

The presence of an omphalocele is often associated with other problems, such as heart defects and kidney and brain problems. Of infants with an omphalocele, 10 percent will also have blockages in the bowel.

After delivery, a baby with an omphalocele will be taken to surgery, where the surgeon will try to place the bowel back into the abdomen and close the defect. If the defect is large, the surgeon may place a pouch over the bowel and gradually ease it back into the abdomen in stages. Blocked or damaged areas of the bowel will also be removed.

Gastroschisis

Similar in appearance to an omphalocele, a gastroschisis occurs in a different way. In this defect, the contents of the abdomen (bowel, stomach, and liver) are pushed outside the abdomen through an opening in the abdominal wall. Because no membrane covers the exposed bowel or other abdominal contents, they are exposed to the amniotic fluid in the uterus and become swollen and matted.

Gastroschisis is rarely associated with other anomalies. It requires immediate surgery to prevent infection and large fluid losses. Putting the bowel back into the abdomen in one step is usually diffiicult, because of the amount of swelling present. Instead, a pouch or silo is placed over the bowel, and everything is wrapped in a sterile dressing. Over the next 10 to 14 days, the surgeon gradually pushes the bowel back into the abdomen by reducing the size of the pouch.

Infection is one complication of gastroschisis. Another is poor circulation to parts of the bowel because of the swelling. These parts may have to be removed.

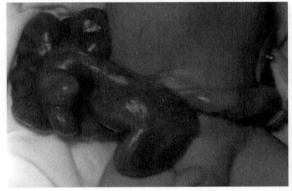

Gastroschisis.

A gastroschisis occurs when the contents of the abdomen (bowel, stomach, liver) are pushed outside the abdomen through an opening in the abdominal wall. Because there is no membranous sac to protect the organs from amniotic fluid, they can become swollen and matted.

Courtesy of J. Hernandez, MD, The Children's Hospital, Denver, Colorado.

Tracheoesophageal Fistula

A fistula is an abnormal passage. A tracheoesophageal fistula, or T-E fistula, is an abnormal connection between the trachea (windpipe) and the

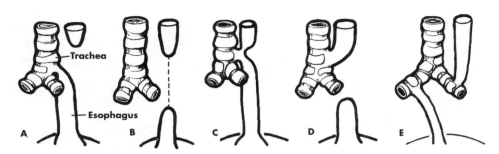

Tracheoesophageal fistula.

Possible variations of a tracheoesophageal fistula include:
A: *Atresia (blockage) of the esophagus with fistula from the lower esophageal segment. This is a J-type fistula, the most common type of fistula.*
B: *Absence of the middle third of the esophagus.*
C: *Atresia of the esophagus with fistulae from both upper and lower segments.*
D: *Fistula from the upper esophageal segment.*
E: *Fistula from both upper and lower segments.*

From: Gray SW, and Skandalakis JE. 1972. Embryology for Surgeons: The Embryological Basis for One Treatment of Congenital Defects. Philadelphia: WB Saunders. Reprinted by permission of the author.

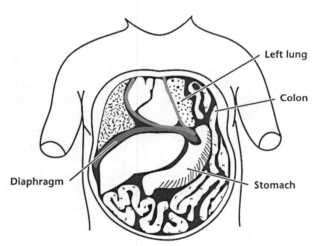

Diaphragmatic hernia.

A diaphragmatic hernia occurs when an opening in the diaphragm allows the bowel to push up into the chest cavity. As a result of the defect, the heart is pushed to the side by the bowel, while the lung on the affected side is compressed and may fail to grow properly.

From: Sadler TW. 1990. Langman's Medical Embryology, 6th ed. Baltimore: Williams & Wilkins, 170. Reprinted by permission.

esophagus (food pipe); it occurs during fetal development. Of babies with fistulas, 30 to 40 percent also have other types of anomalies. The J-type fistula, the most common type T-E defect, has a pouch where the upper part of the esophagus ends. This pouch collects saliva that cannot be swallowed.

Before birth, polyhydramnios (a greater-than-normal amount of amniotic fluid) is often the first sign of a fistula. Signs in the newborn include increased saliva, respiratory distress, and choking or blue spells during feeding. A fistula can be diagnosed with x-rays.

If your baby has a T-E fistula, she will be kept NPO (not fed by mouth), and a special suction catheter will be used to drain the saliva and prevent choking. Surgery will be scheduled to repair the defect. If the parts of the esophagus are close together, the surgeon will reattach them in one step. If they are too far apart, a two-step repair will be done. In the first step, a tube will be inserted into your baby's stomach to allow feeding. See Chapter 16 for more information about gastrostomy tubes. Four to six weeks later, a second operation will be done to reattach the esophagus and remove the feeding tube.

Strictures (narrowing) of the esophagus at the site of reattachment may develop. Reflux (food moving up the esophagus from the stomach) is another possible complication.

Duodenal Atresia

A duodenal atresia is a blockage of the duodenum (upper portion) of the small bowel. The reason blockages occur is unknown. Up to 70 percent of infants with duodenal atresia have associated defects.

Duodenal atresia causes abdominal distention (bloating) and vomiting. The blockage can be diagnosed on x-ray and is treated with surgery. Complications usually occur only if there are associated defects.

Diaphragmatic Hernia

For a baby with a diaphragmatic hernia, a hole in the diaphragm (the muscle separating the chest from the abdomen) allows the bowel to push up into the chest cavity. As the bowel enters the chest, it compresses the lung on that side and keeps it from growing. Diaphragmatic hernias that develop in the fetus early in the pregnancy result in a very small lung on the affected side. In severe cases, the opposite lung may also be smaller than normal. Hernias occurring later in fetal development do not cause such severe problems but still compromise the baby's health.

A diaphragmatic hernia seriously interferes with your baby's breathing and blood circulation. At delivery, your baby will have difficulty breathing and may be quite dusky or cyanotic (bluish in color). She will require intubation (insertion of a breathing tube into the windpipe) and transfer to an NICU. Once in the NICU, your baby will receive IV fluids, medications to stabilize blood pressure and circulation, and breathing assistance. A high-frequency ventilator may be used to help with ventilation. Some units also use a special technique called extracorporeal membrane oxygenation (ECMO) to help stabilize the baby's breathing and circulation. Both these techniques are explained in Chapter 12.

When your baby is stable, doctors will perform surgery to close the defect and return the bowel to the abdomen. Large defects may require a permanent synthetic fabric patch to the diaphragm to help with closure.

The complications of a diaphragmatic hernia are related to the impaired lung growth it caused and to the effects on your baby's circulation. Severe persistent pulmonary hypertension frequently occurs in babies with a diaphragmatic hernia and is difficult to treat.

Congenital Heart Defects

When the heart or blood vessels near the heart don't develop normally during pregnancy, the baby is born with a congenital heart defect. Some defects may be small and may cause your baby few problems; others are life-threatening. A great deal of progress has been made in recent years in the treatment of congenital heart defects.

At least 1 percent of all live-born infants have a heart defect. In the United States, that amounts to 25,000 to 30,000 infants born with defects each year. The percentage in Canada is similar. The cause of a heart defect is most often unknown. Sometimes, a viral infection such as rubella (German measles) contracted by the mother during pregnancy interferes with the heart's development. Other times, genetic problems such as Down syndrome result in a heart defect.

How the Heart Works

In adults, the heart is the size of a fist and consists of four muscular chambers that work together as a pump. The chambers are separated by valves,

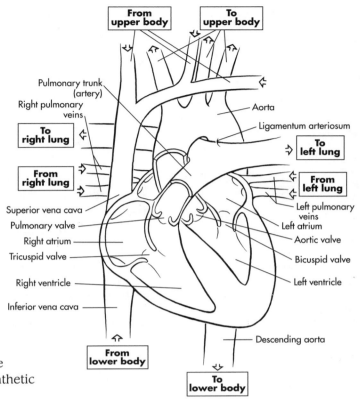

Chambers of the heart and heart valves.

The chambers of the heart are the left and right atria and left and right ventricles. The valves of the heart are the aortic valve, mitral valve, pulmonary valve, and tricuspid valve.

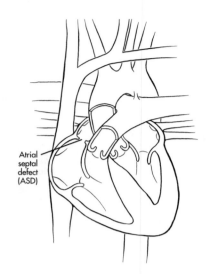

Atrial septal defect.

An atrial septal defect occurs when there is a large defect between the atria (upper chambers of the heart), that allows oxygen-rich blood from the heart's left side to leak back to the right side.

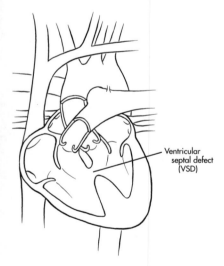

Ventricular septal defect.

A VSD is an opening between the ventricles. This allows oxygen-rich blood from the heart's left side to flow back to the right side. The blood is then pumped back to the lungs, instead of going out to the body tissues.

which control the flow of blood. Blood returns to the heart from the veins in the body. It first enters the right atrium and then flows into the right ventricle. From there it is sent to the lungs, where it picks up oxygen. Then the blood returns to the heart, first to the left atrium and then to the left ventricle, the strongest of the four chambers of the heart. The left ventricle must pump blood, rich in oxygen, out to the rest of the body through the aorta.

Diagnosis of Heart Defects

If your baby is suspected of having a heart defect, a number of tests will be done to help your baby's doctor and the heart specialists (cardiologists) gather information about the problem. The first test to be done is usually an echocardiogram, which is an ultrasound of the heart. (See Chapter 12.) This test gives a picture of the structure of the heart, as well as its function. An electrocardiogram (EKG) might also be done. This test measures the electrical impulses generated by the heart. A number of patches (called electrodes) are placed on your baby's skin and record the electrical patterns on paper. Chest x-rays and blood tests may also be needed. The information from all these tests helps the health care team develop a plan for caring for your baby.

Common Heart Defects

The American Heart Association (AHA) has provided these explanations of common types of congenital heart defects: septal, obstructive, and cyanotic. We acknowledge and appreciate the AHA's permission to use this information here.

Septal defects. In a heart that's working normally, low-oxygen blood from the body goes to the heart's right side. Then it's pumped to the lungs. In the lungs, it releases its carbon dioxide and is refreshed (supplied) with oxygen. After that, the oxygen-rich blood is pumped back to the heart's left side. From there, it's pumped from the left ventricle to the aorta and on to the rest of the body.

Sometimes a baby is born with a hole in the septum. (The septum is the wall that separates the left and right sides of the heart.) This defect may be between the two upper chambers or aortae (atrial septal defect) or between the two lower chambers or ventricles (ventricular septal defect). Sometimes, both upper and lower chamber are involved. This type of defect is sometimes called "a hole in the heart."

Atrial septal defect (ASD). When there's a large defect between the atria, a large amount of oxygen-rich (red) blood from the heart's left side leaks back to the right side. Then it's pumped back to the lungs, even though it's already been refreshed with oxygen. This is inefficient; blood that's already been to the lungs is returning there, and blood that needs to go to the lungs is being displaced.

Many children with this defect have few, if any, symptoms. Closing the atrial defect by open-heart surgery in childhood can prevent serious problems later in life. The long-term outlook is excellent.

Ventricular septal defect (VSD). When there's a large opening between the ventricles, a large amount of oxygen-rich (red) blood from the heart's left side is forced through the defect to the right side. Then it's pumped back to the lungs, even though it's already been refreshed with oxygen. The heart, which has to pump an extra amount of blood, is overworked and may enlarge.

Symptoms may not occur until several weeks after birth. Some babies with a large ventricular septal defect don't grow normally and may fail to thrive. High pressure may occur in blood vessels in the lungs, because more blood is there. Over time, this pressure may cause permanent damage to the walls of the vessels.

If the opening is small, it doesn't strain the heart. In that case, the only abnormal finding is a loud murmur. Closing these small defects with surgery may not be needed. In fact, they often close on their own.

Babies with a ventricular septal defect may develop severe symptoms or high blood pressure in the lungs, however. Early repair is often necessary. (The repair may be delayed in other babies.) If the opening is large, open-heart surgery is recommended to close it and prevent serious problems. This is usually done in infancy or childhood, even in patients with few symptoms; closing the septal defect will prevent complications later. Usually the defect is so large that a cloth patch is sewn over it to close it completely. Later this patch is covered by the normal heart-lining tissue and becomes a permanent part of the heart. Some defects can be sewn closed without a patch.

Defects causing obstruction in the heart or blood vessels. An obstruction to blood flow is a narrowing that may partly or completely block the flow of blood. Any one of the heart's four valves may be narrowed (stenotic) or completely blocked (atretic). The blockage may be above or below the valve. A blockage can also occur in vessels that return blood to the heart (veins) or that carry blood from the heart (arteries). The three defects that are the most common forms of obstruction to blood flow are pulmonary stenosis, aortic stenosis, and coarctation of the aorta.

Pulmonary stenosis. The pulmonary valve opens to let blood flow from the right ventricle to the lungs. Narrowing of the pulmonary valve (valvar pulmonary stenosis) causes the right ventricle to pump harder to get blood past the blockage. If the stenosis is severe, especially in babies, some cyanosis (blueness) may occur. Older children rarely have symptoms.

Treatment is needed when the pressure in the right ventricle is high (even though there may be no symptoms). In most children, the obstruction can be relieved during cardiac catheterization by balloon valvoplasty. In this procedure, a special catheter containing a balloon is placed across the pulmonary valve. The balloon is inflated, and the valve is stretched open. Other patients require surgery. During surgery, the valve can usually be opened so that it works well again.

Aortic stenosis. When the aortic valve opens, oxygen-rich (red) blood flows from the left ventricle to the aorta (the large artery that sends oxygen-rich blood through the body). Stenosis (narrowing) of the aortic valve makes it hard for the heart to pump blood to the body.

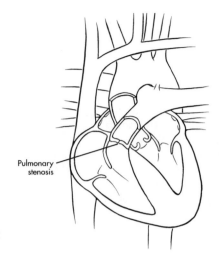

Pulmonary stenosis.

Pulmonary stenosis occurs when the pulmonary valve is narrowed (stenotic) and causes the right ventricle to pump harder to get blood past the blockage.

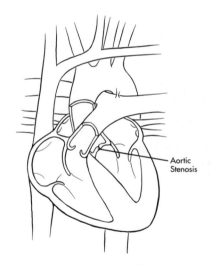

Aortic stenosis.

Aortic stenosis occurs when the aortic valve is narrowed, making it difficult for the heart to pump blood to the body.

Sometimes stenosis is severe, and symptoms occur in infancy. Otherwise, most children with aortic stenosis have no symptoms. In some children, chest pain, unusual tiring, dizziness, or fainting may occur. The need for surgery depends on how severe the stenosis is. In children, the surgeon may be able to enlarge the valve opening. Although surgery may improve the stenosis, the valve remains deformed. Eventually, the valve may need to be replaced by an artificial one.

Coarctation of the aorta. In this condition, the aorta (the main artery that carries blood from the heart to the body) is pinched or constricted. This obstructs blood flow from the heart to the rest of the body. Blood pressure also increases above the constriction. Symptoms rarely exist at birth, but they can develop as early as the first week after birth.

A baby may develop congestive heart failure or high blood pressure that requires early surgery. Otherwise, surgery can usually be delayed. A child with a severe coarctation should have surgery in early childhood to prevent problems such as high blood pressure as an adult.

Cyanotic defects. In these defects, blood pumped to the body has less than the normal amount of oxygen. This causes cyanosis, a blue discoloration of the skin. If cyanosis is mild, the complexion may look "ruddy." If it's severe, discoloration may be dark blue. The degree of cyanosis may vary with age, activity, or both.

Tetralogy of Fallot. The tetralogy of Fallot has four components: (1) a ventricular septal defect, described earlier in this section; (2) a stenosis (narrowing) at or just beneath the pulmonary valve, blocking the flow of venous blood into the lungs (this varies in severity from child to child); (3) the right ventricle is more muscular than normal; and (4) the aorta lies directly over the ventricular septal defect.

This combination of components results in blueness (cyanosis), which may appear soon after birth, in infancy, or later in childhood. "Blue babies" may have sudden episodes of severe cyanosis with rapid breathing and may even become unconscious.

Some infants with severe tetralogy of Fallot may need an operation, which will give temporary relief by increasing blood flow to the lungs with a shunt. During this procedure, the aorta and the pulmonary artery are connected so that some blood from the aorta flows into the lungs to get more oxygen. This reduces the cyanosis and allows the child to grow and develop until the repair can be done when she is older. Most children with tetralogy of Fallot have open-heart surgery before they reach school age.

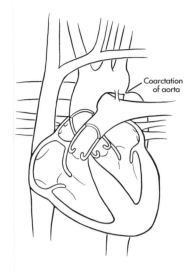

Coarctation of the aorta.

The aorta is pinched or constricted. Therefore the blood flow from the heart to the rest of the body is obstructed.

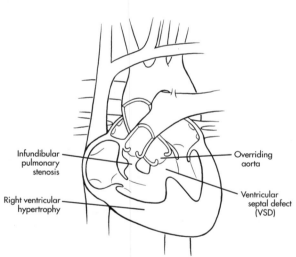

Tetralogy of Fallot.

Tetralogy of Fallot has four components: (1) ventricular septal defect; (2) narrowing at, or just below the pulmonary valve (blocks the flow of unoxygenated blood to the lungs); (3) the right ventricle is more muscular than usual; and (4) the aorta lies over the ventricular septal defect.

Transposition of the great arteries. Normally, the pulmonary artery carries venous (bluish) blood from the right ventricle to the lungs to get oxygen. Then the aorta carries the oxygen-rich (red) blood from the left ventricle to the body. In transposition of the great arteries, the vessels are reversed. The aorta is connected to the right ventricle so that venous (bluish) blood is carried to the body. The pulmonary artery is attached to the left ventricle so that oxygen-rich (red) blood is carried back to the lungs.

Infants born with transposition survive only if they have one or more connections that let oxygen-rich (red) blood reach the body. These connections may be in the form of a hole between the two atria (atrial septal defect), a hole between the two ventricles (ventricular septal defect), or a vessel connecting the pulmonary artery with the aorta (patent ductus arteriosus). Most babies with transposition of the great arteries are extremely blue soon after birth because these connections are not adequate.

To improve the body's oxygen supply, a special procedure called balloon atrial septostomy is used during heart catheterization. It enlarges the atrial opening and helps the baby by reducing cyanosis.

Tricuspid atresia. In this condition, no tricuspid valve exists, so no blood can flow from the right atrium to the right ventricle. As a result, the right ventricle is small and not fully developed. The child's survival depends on there being an abnormal opening in the wall between the two ventricles (ventricular septal defect). Venous (bluish) blood returns to the right atrium, where it is mixed with oxygen-rich (red) blood from the lungs. Most of this poorly oxygenated mixture goes from the left ventricle into the aorta and on to the body. The rest flows through the ventricular septal defect into the small right ventricle, through the pulmonary artery, and back to the lungs. Because of this abnormal circulation, the child looks blue.

Often these children require a surgical shunting procedure to increase blood flow to the lungs and reduce cyanosis. Some children with tricuspid atresia have too much blood flowing to the lungs and need a procedure (pulmonary artery banding) to decrease blood flow to the lungs.

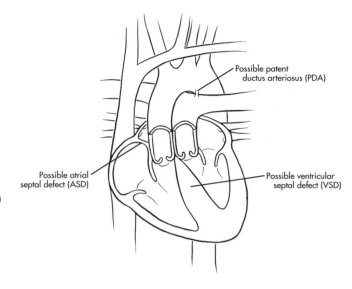

Possible patent ductus arteriosus (PDA)

Possible atrial septal defect (ASD)

Possible ventricular septal defect (VSD)

Transposition of the great arteries.

Transposition occurs when the two major arteries are switched.

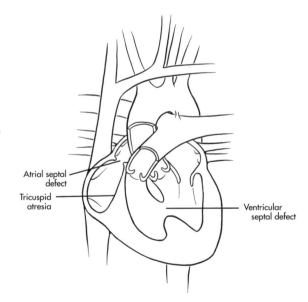

Atrial septal defect

Tricuspid atresia

Ventricular septal defect

Tricuspid atresia.

Tricuspid atresia occurs when there is no tricuspid valve. The baby's survival depends on there being an accompanying ventricular septal defect.

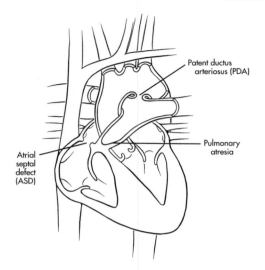

Pulmonary atresia.

There is no pulmonary valve, so blood cannot flow from the right ventricle into the pulmonary artery and on into the lungs. The right ventricle is small and undeveloped. An opening in the atrial septum lets blood exit the right atrium, so unoxygenated blood mixes with the oxygen-rich blood in the left atria. This mixture is pumped out to the body. The only source of lung blood flow is the open ductus arteriosus (PDA).

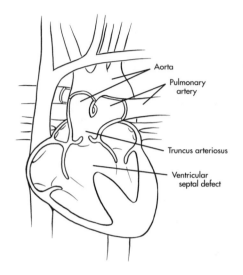

Truncus arteriosus.

There is only one artery from the heart that forms both the aorta and pulmonary artery. This defect is accompanied by a ventricular septal defect.

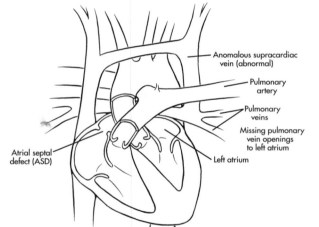

Total anomalous pulmonary venous connection.

In this defect, the pulmonary veins that bring oxygen-rich blood from the lungs back to the heart are not connected to the left atrium. Instead, they drain through abnormal connections to the right atrium. There, the oxygen-rich blood from the pulmonary veins mixes with the unoxygenated blood from the body. Part of this passes through the atrial septal defect into the left atrium, and out to the body. The rest of this mixture flows through the right ventricle, into the pulmonary artery, and on to the lungs.

Pulmonary atresia. In pulmonary atresia, no pulmonary valve exists. Consequently, blood can't flow from the right ventricle into the pulmonary artery and on to the lungs. The right ventricle functions as a fluid pouch that may stay small and not well developed. In addition, the tricuspid valve is often poorly developed.

An opening in the atrial septum lets blood exit the right atrium, so venous (bluish) blood mixes with the oxygen-rich (red) blood in the left atrium. The left ventricle pumps this mixture of oxygen-poor blood into the aorta and out to the body. The infant appears blue (cyanotic) because there's less oxygen in the blood circulating through the arteries. The only source of lung blood flow is the patent ductus arteriosus, an open passageway between the pulmonary artery and the aorta. If the PDA narrows or closes, the lung blood flow is reduced to critically low levels. This can cause severe cyanosis.

Early treatment often includes using a drug to keep the PDA from closing (prostaglandin E_1). A surgeon can create a shunt between the aorta and the pulmonary artery that may help increase blood flow to the lungs. A more complete repair depends on the size of the pulmonary artery and right ventricle. If the pulmonary artery and right ventricle are very small, surgery may not be able to correct the defect. In some cases, where the pulmonary artery and right ventricle are more normal in size, open-heart surgery may significantly improve how the heart works.

Truncus arteriosus. This is a complex malformation where only one artery arises from the heart and forms the aorta and pulmonary artery. Surgery for this condition is usually required early in life. It includes closing a large ventricular septal defect within the heart, detaching the pulmonary arteries from the large common artery, and connecting the pulmonary arteries to the right ventricle with a tube graft.

Total anomalous pulmonary venous connection. In total anomalous pulmonary venous connection (also called total anomalous venous drainage or total anomalous venous return), the pulmonary veins that bring oxygen-rich (red) blood from the lungs back to the heart aren't connected to the left atrium. Instead, the pulmonary veins drain through abnormal connections to the right atrium.

In the right atrium, oxygen-rich (red) blood from the pulmonary veins mixes with venous (bluish) blood from the body. Part of this mixture passes through the atrial septum (atrial septal defect) into the left atrium. From there it goes into the left ventricle, to the aorta, and out to the body. The rest of the poorly oxygenated mixture flows through the right ventricle, into the pulmonary artery, and on to the lungs. The blood passing through the aorta to the body doesn't have enough oxygen, which causes the infant to look blue.

Symptoms may develop soon after birth. This defect must be surgically repaired in early infancy. In surgery, the pulmonary veins are reconnected to the left atrium, and the atrial septal defect is closed. When surgical repair is done in early infancy, the long-term outlook is very good.

Staying Informed

This chapter has explained many of the serious medical problems that bring an infant to the NICU. No more than a few will apply to your baby. This information is intended to give parents a basic understanding of each problem, but it is not intended to replace detailed discussions with your baby's caregivers. Write down your questions, and discuss them with your baby's doctors and nurses. Keep in mind that just as each baby is unique, so is each NICU. There are different approaches to treating many of these problems. New discoveries are helping to improve the care of tiny and sick infants every day. Some of those discoveries may have an impact on the information in this chapter even before you read it. In medicine, as in many other areas of life today, things change quickly. The best approach is to keep asking questions.

Chapter 11

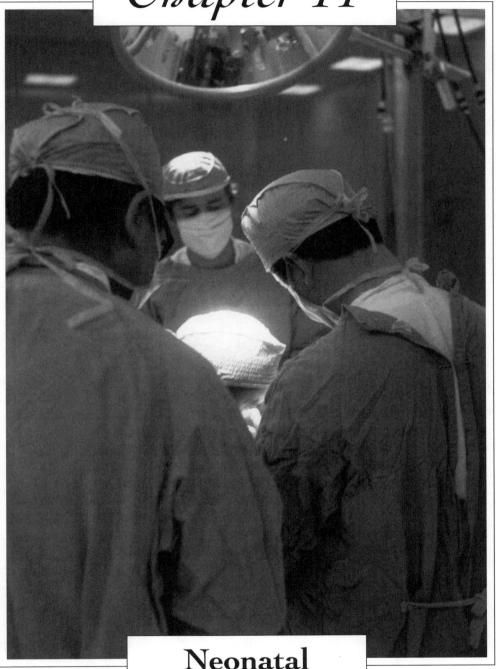

Neonatal Surgery

Kathleen A. Green, RNC, MSN, NNP

"Everybody was doing something to help. Piglet, wide awake suddenly, was jumping up and down and making "Oo, I say" noises; Owl was explaining that in a case of Sudden and Temporary Immersion the Important Thing was to keep the Head Above Water....**"**

Surgery on newborns—called neonatal surgery—is not an unusual event. Seriously ill infants may undergo surgery soon after birth to ensure their survival. Still other infants may need surgery during their hospital stay because of complications of prematurity, serious illness, or other factors. Still others may be in the newborn nursery or even discharged home when they develop life-threatening emergencies. And some parents have the dubious advantage of knowing far ahead of time that their baby will need to return to the hospital at some later time for a planned surgical treatment.

This chapter looks at common aspects of surgery and surgical care, including informed consent for the procedure, preparations for the surgery, anesthesia and pain relief, and what happens during recovery. This information is intended as a general guide for parents of infants undergoing surgery. Specific questions about your baby's procedure and care should be addressed to your NICU team.

Getting the Information You Need

When you first hear the words, "Your baby needs surgery," you may be overwhelmed by questions. For most parents, these questions fall into three basic categories: Who will be involved? What will the surgery itself involve? What is surgical consent?

The Surgeon

Pediatric surgeons are trained specifically for surgery of children. They perform a variety of surgeries involving the gastrointestinal tract and the chest region, as well as other procedures. They have experience with many of the surgically correctable congenital anomalies mentioned in Chapter 10. Surgery to treat disorders affecting other body systems—such as the brain, heart, kidneys, and bones—is performed by surgeons who specialize in the affected system and who may operate on adults as well as children and infants.

Not all hospitals treat enough critical congenital problems to be expert. If your baby needs a special type of surgery, such as cardiac surgery, he may be transferred to a larger university medical center or a children's hospital. The neonatology staff at your hospital will help transfer your baby to a center that specializes in the care required.

If your baby has a complex problem that requires surgery, you may want to research treatment options. Some neonatal problems are treated in basically the same way by most medical teams. Surgeons develop their own styles, however. Some perform single-stage corrective procedures—that is, they correct the problem in one operation—whereas others perform multiple-stage corrective procedures. Depending on where your infant is treated, who the surgeon is, and the extent of the problem, he may undergo several surgeries, while another infant with a similar problem may have the correction made in one surgery. Keep in mind, though, that your baby's condition may not be identical to another infant's. The specific physical characteristics of the problem may dictate the surgical option chosen for your newborn. If the surgery is not an emergency, it's often advisable to request a second opinion, as you would for any surgical procedure for yourself. This may entail meeting with different surgeons in different hospitals, bringing your baby's x-rays and lab information with you. This process may give you peace of mind about your baby's treatment. Your baby's neonatologist and surgeon can help you decide how much investigation of treatment options makes sense.

What You Should Know about the Surgery

Before you agree to a surgical procedure for your baby, you'll want the answers to questions like the following about the procedure itself, the anesthesia, and the recovery period.

About the Procedure

1. Why does my baby need surgery? What will happen if he doesn't have this surgery?
2. What type of procedure will be done?
3. Will my baby need more than one surgery?
4. How long will the operation take?
5. Who will perform the surgery?
6. How many times has the surgeon done this procedure?
7. When will I meet the surgeon?

About the Anesthesia

1. What type of anesthesia will my baby receive?
2. Will my baby be intubated (on a ventilator) during and/or after the surgery?
3. How long will the anesthesia last?
4. When will my baby wake up?
5. Who is the anesthesiologist?
6. When will I meet the anesthesiologist?

About the Postoperative Course

1. How soon will I see my baby after surgery? Where will my baby recuperate: in the NICU or in a different unit?
2. How will my baby look after surgery (for example, will he have an incision, tubes, bandages, or swelling)?
3. Will my baby be given pain medication? If so, what type?
4. Will my baby be given any other medications, such as antibiotics?

5. How long will the stitches (drains, tubes, and other medical equipment) stay in place?
6. How long will my baby need to stay in the hospital following the surgery?
7. When will we see the surgeon again for follow-up care?

Surgical Consent

Before any surgical procedure, the medical team must get the patient's agreement to the surgery—called consent. Because your baby can't speak for himself, you will be asked to sign the consent form. Consent forms vary from hospital to hospital, but all of them should include certain basic points:

1. The name(s) of the attending physician(s) (the surgeon[s] who will perform or oversee the procedure)
2. The name of the procedure that is to be performed
3. The fact that potential risks and complications have been explained to you

When you sign the consent, you are agreeing that the named physician(s) will perform the named procedure and that you understand the procedure, as well as the possible risks and complications. Some consents are all-inclusive —that is, they include consent for other actions that might be needed along with the surgery, such as a blood transfusion. Other hospitals obtain separate consents for blood transfusions. When you sign a surgery consent, consent for anesthesia is implied; a separate consent for anesthesia is not necessary.

In a teaching hospital, surgical residents may perform all or part of your baby's surgery, although the attending surgeon will be present in the operating room. The physician performing the surgery is usually the one who obtains the consent, so the attending surgeon or a surgical resident will present the consent form to you, rather than the neonatologist. For simple, straightforward procedures, such as central venous line placement or circumcision, a physician from the NICU may obtain the consent. The hospital's policies dictate who obtains consent and what the form includes.

Be sure to read the entire consent form before you sign it. There may be a lot of fine print, but you need to read that, too, so that you understand exactly what you are signing. The phrase "informed consent" means that you understand what you are agreeing to and that all your questions have been answered. If you have any questions about anything to do with the surgery, be sure you get answers to them before you sign.

The consent forms some hospitals use are relatively simple; others are very complex and difficult to read. Take as much time as you need to read and understand the form. Don't be intimidated by someone who may be in a rush. If your baby is having a procedure done to one side of the body (for example, eye surgery), make sure that the consent states the correct side of the body (for example, left eye). If the form contains abbreviations you don't understand, have them spelled out clearly. Before you sign the consent, be sure that you understand every word, especially the words that have been written in by the person obtaining your consent.

Common Neonatal Surgical Procedures

Central line placement: Insertion of an intravenous line for long-term use. The line is placed either by a needle stick (usually performed by a neonatologist or nurse practitioner) or by "cutdown" (an incision made into the vessel). The catheter is passed into the body or the right atrium of the heart to provide fluids, nutrition, or medications.

Circumcision: Removal of the foreskin from the tip of the penis. (See Chapter 15.)

Colostomy: A surgically placed opening on the baby's abdomen that allows stool (feces) to drain from the bowel into a collecting bag. A colostomy is most commonly placed after surgical removal of a portion of the large (lower) intestine. (See Chapters 10 and 16.)

Cryotherapy: A treatment for retinopathy of prematurity (ROP). Performed at the bedside or in the operating room, cryotherapy involves the "freezing" of blood vessels in the retina that are growing too rapidly. The frozen vessels die and become scar tissue. (See Chapter 10.)

Exploratory laparotomy: Surgery used to examine the abdominal organs and to aid diagnosis. Depending on what is discovered during exploratory surgery, major surgery may become necessary.

Fundoplication: A procedure used to treat severe gastroesophageal reflux. A procedure that tightens the valve between the esophagus (food pipe) and the stomach; prevents food from moving back up into the baby's esophagus.

Gastrostomy tube: A tube inserted through the abdomen into the stomach for feeding. (See Chapter 16.)

Hernia repair: A procedure performed in the inguinal area (pelvic region) to repair a weakness or gap in the muscle wall after contents of hernia (usually intestines) are pushed into an adjacent body cavity.

Ileostomy: A surgically placed opening on the baby's abdomen that allows stool (feces) to drain from the bowel into a collecting bag. An ileostomy is most commonly placed after surgical removal of a portion of the small (upper) intestine. (See Chapter 16.)

Orchiopexy: Correction for undescended testes in which the testis is sutured to the bottom of the scrotum.

Patent ductus arteriosus ligation: Cutting or tying off a PDA, a blood vessel used in fetal life that connects the aorta and the pulmonary artery. (See Chapter 10.)

Thoracotomy: A surgical incision of the chest, necessary for placement of a chest tube.

Tracheostomy: A surgical opening made in the neck and into the trachea (windpipe). The baby breathes through a tube placed in this opening instead of through his nose or mouth.

Ventriculoperitoneal shunt: A device used to drain excess fluid from the brain; used in treatment of hydrocephalus. (See Chapter 10.) A thin tube, called a shunt, is inserted into the ventricle of the brain, passes underneath the skin, and drains the excess cerebrospinal fluid into the abdominal cavity, where it is reabsorbed by the body.

Preparations for Surgery

Most of the time, neonatal surgery is not an emergency. You may know weeks ahead of time that your baby will need surgery (in the case of a hernia repair, for example) and may have just been waiting for your baby to grow large enough for the procedure.

In most cases, some preparation is required before surgery. The extent of the prep depends somewhat on the complexity of the surgery. Here are some basic preparatory steps most units take before surgery.

Anesthesia Support

If your baby requires anesthesia, you and your baby will meet the anesthesiologist. In addition, an anesthesiology resident may be working with the attending anesthesiologist. Some institutions utilize certified registered nurse anesthetists (CRNAs), who are specially trained to administer anesthesia in collaboration with the attending anesthesiologist. The visit from the anesthesia team is your chance to ask questions regarding your baby's anesthesia.

Laboratory Support

Depending on the type of anesthesia your baby will require, tests may be needed before surgery. Complete blood counts, measurement of blood electrolytes (such as sodium and potassium), and a chest x-ray are frequently performed on infants who will have general anesthesia.[1]

Respiratory Support

Even if your baby is breathing on his own, a tube may be placed in your baby's throat (intubation) and he may be attached to a ventilator before surgery. This enables the anesthesiologist to control your baby's breathing in case anesthesia or pain medications affect the baby's ability to breathe by himself.

Intravenous Support

Because the medications for anesthesia and pain relief can cause nausea and vomiting, your baby will be kept NPO (nothing given by mouth) for a specified period of time before surgery. Then if your baby vomits during or after surgery, the empty stomach helps prevent the possibility of choking and aspiration (fluid entering the lungs). Your baby will have an intravenous (IV) line to provide fluids and glucose until the surgeon determines that he can begin to eat again. The timetable for feeding depends on many factors, including the type of procedure and the medications used for anesthesia and pain control.

Temperature Support

Your baby must be kept warm during the ride to and from the operating room (OR) and in the OR itself, which is usually cooler than the NICU. Your baby may wear a hat, and his arms and legs may be wrapped in a soft material to retain warmth. Your baby may go to the OR covered in warm blankets in

"The day of our baby's surgery was almost as stressful as our first day in the NICU. We asked many questions, sometimes more than once. Information helped us to calm down and feel a little more in control."

the NICU incubator, on a radiant warmer, or in a warm battery-powered transport incubator. Whatever the transport method, most surgeons use a radiant warmer during surgery to keep the baby warm.

Parent Support

The NICU staff is aware that the prospect of surgery is very stressful for parents and will support you by providing information about your baby's condition. An NICU nurse, the NICU clinical nurse specialist, or a clinical nurse specialist who works for the surgical team will usually educate and inform parents before the surgery. Some parents also find it helpful to speak to other parents whose infants have had a similar procedure.

Another source of support may be your own clergy or the chaplaincy service at the hospital. If you have not yet done so, you may wish to have your baby baptized or blessed before surgery. Your NICU nurse or social worker can help you make arrangements.

O n the day of the surgery, you may wish to stay with your baby until he goes to the OR. Some hospitals even allow parents to accompany their baby to the OR. Others allow you only as far as the elevator or doors to the OR. Ask the nurse who provides your preoperative information about specific policies.

Your baby is probably on the OR "schedule" for a certain time. Remember that the schedule may change, depending on other surgeries and activities in the OR. The NICU or OR staff should let you know about major changes in the day's events so that you can adjust your expectations for receiving information and seeing your baby after the operation.

On the day of the surgery, make sure that you know where you can wait to be kept informed of the surgical progress and when you will be able to speak to the surgeon afterward. Some physicians have nurses (usually the clinical nurse specialists) who will keep you informed during the course of the operation. If not, remember that emergencies and delays in other areas of the OR may delay your child's surgery. Also, procedures sometimes take longer than expected.

Try to find a comfortable place to wait during surgery (some hospitals have special waiting areas for families), and bring a book or magazine to read, or something else to do. Make sure you eat something the day of surgery, especially if the procedure is a lengthy one. You don't want to feel faint when you're finally invited into the unit to see your baby.

I n the not-too-distant past, many in the medical community believed that babies did not need anesthesia during surgery because they did not "feel" pain.[1,2] This belief began to change in the 1970s, as research in this field intensified. As a result, pediatricians, surgeons, and anesthesiologists started to explore methods of safe anesthesia for infants. Even through the 1980s, giving term and preterm babies anesthesia, even for complex surgeries, remained controversial.

Waiting for the Outcome

Surgical Anesthesia

Research in two major areas has made neonatal surgery without anesthesia rare today. First, researchers have studied how newborns perceive pain and how their bodies metabolize (deal with) medications. Second, safer medications have been developed for anesthesia and pain relief in children and adults. The American Academy of Pediatrics now endorses the use of local or general anesthesia in all newborns undergoing surgical procedures.[3]

The type of surgery your baby needs dictates the type of anesthesia that will be used. The anesthesiologist, in conjunction with the neonatologist and the surgeon, will decide what is best for your baby. All anesthesia has risks, and the anesthesiologist will explain them to you. In addition, all types of anesthesia have the potential for side effects. Your baby may or may not develop these effects. You will be told about possible major side effects before the surgery.

Anesthesia types used in neonatal surgery include topical, local and regional (nerve blocks), and general. Each has its own special uses.

"When the doctor said Tyler would have an epidural, I felt better about the surgery. I had an epidural in labor, and knew it had worked well for me."

Topical Anesthesia

Topical anesthetics are those that are applied to the skin. Studies are currently under way in the United States and Canada to test the effectiveness of a topical anesthetic cream for circumcisions and central line placement. When applied two hours before a procedure, anesthesia develops within the underlying skin.[4] While not appropriate for major surgery, topical anesthesia holds promise for use in minor procedures.

A Nerve Block

When used in an awake or sedated patient, a nerve block eliminates the patient's ability to feel pain.[1] There are two types of nerve blocks: local anesthesia (in which a small, specific body area is "numbed") and regional anesthesia (in which a larger area of the body is "numbed"). Anesthetics used for dental procedures are classified as nerve blocks.

Local

Circumcision is the most common infant procedure utilizing local anesthesia.[1,2] Before the procedure, the baby receives an injection of lidocaine in the area above the penis. An effective block numbs the area, and the baby does not feel the pain of the circumcision. A number of studies have been done with various anesthetizing solutions used for nerve blocking prior to circumcision.[5–7] Few complications have been reported.[2]

Some physicians do not use any anesthesia during newborn circumcision. Ask your baby's doctor about his philosophy of pain control during this procedure.

Regional

The second type of nerve block, regional anesthesia, is familiar to many women who have received an epidural block or spinal anesthesia during childbirth. For preterm or formerly preterm infants undergoing surgical proce-dures, regional anesthesia has become more popular than general anesthesia because it does not have the undesirable side effects of general anesthesia. Regional anesthesia can be used when the operation is elective (planned), when the site of the surgery is below the level of the umbilicus (navel), and when the procedure is expected to take less than two hours.[1] Most of the stud-ies on regional anesthesia have been associated with its use in inguinal hernia repair, a surgical procedure that fits the three criteria.

Regional anesthetics can be administered by a single injection or through a catheter, a tiny tube placed in the spinal column. Catheter access allows the anesthesiologist to administer multiple doses of the medication rather than give multiple injections through the skin.[1,2] At the end of the operation, the catheter can also be used to deliver medication for postoperative pain. The catheter is removed before the infant leaves the operating room. The infant may be awake during regional anesthesia but is usually given a sedative. The benefit of regional anesthesia is that your infant does not need to be put to sleep and placed on a ventilator. After surgery, your baby may be groggy, but this effect subsides as the sedative wears off.

General Anesthesia

General anesthesia is used for neurosurgery, cardiovascular surgery, and abdominal surgery. This type of anesthesia is sometimes said to "make the baby sleep," but in reality the baby is unconscious and therefore unable to feel pain. Medications that produce general anesthesia are given through an IV line, or inhaled.

Administration through Intravenous Line

The IV approach to inducing general anesthesia uses a drug called fen-tanyl, a narcotic often used for pain relief in the NICU. Given at higher doses than those used for pain relief, fentanyl is an effective anesthetic for infants undergoing surgery for patent ductus arteriosus (PDA).[8] Fentanyl has also been used successfully for babies undergoing major cardiac surgery.[9,10] Other narcotics used as neonatal anesthetics include sufentanil and morphine sul-fate. A major side effect of all narcotics is respiratory depression (slowing of breathing). Infants who receive narcotics for anesthesia, therefore, require intubation in case of breathing difficulties, even when they are anesthetized intravenously.

Administration by Inhalation

General anesthesia may also be induced by using inhaled anesthetics. In this approach, the baby breathes in a gas form of an anesthetizing medication. This type of anesthesia works well, is easy to administer to a patient of any size, and is rapidly metabolized by the body.[2] Inhaled anesthetics have been widely studied in preterm and term infants, and recommendations for their use in babies have been developed and described in many medical texts.[2,11] Dosages can be titrated (adjusted) throughout the surgical procedure so that the baby can be extubated (taken off the ventilator) after the procedure and will wake up shortly afterward. If the baby will not be extubated for a day or two, extra anesthetic may be given toward the end of the operation to provide sedation and pain relief. Before the procedure, ask what the anesthesiologist and surgeon plan to do in the operating room and afterward. You will then be prepared if your baby is still asleep when you see him after surgery.

Side Effects

Although useful, effective, and easy to administer, general anesthesia has the most side effects of all anesthetics used for newborns. The most common side effect is apnea, or cessation of breathing for 15 to 20 seconds.[1,12] Apnea in a term infant is always considered abnormal unless it occurs within eight hours after the administration of general anesthesia.[1] Up to 80 percent of preterm infants develop apnea after surgery.[13] It is unclear exactly why postoperative apnea occurs, although it may have the same causes as apnea of prematurity (see Chapter 9). If your baby is or was premature but never had apnea before, he may develop it after surgery.[1] Apnea that occurs after surgery usually resolves within 24 hours.

To reduce the chances of postoperative apnea, elective surgery is usually postponed until the infant is at least 44 weeks postconceptional age. Some physicians prescribe caffeine before surgery, because it can regulate the respiratory center and reduce the occurrence of apnea.[12] If an infant is scheduled for a "same-day" procedure (one in which the baby goes home the same day as the surgery), the current recommendation is that the infant be 60 weeks postconceptional age.[1] Frequently, if a formerly preterm infant requires surgery, the procedure is performed a few days before discharge. In this way, the infant can be monitored for a day or two after the procedure without prolonging the hospital stay.

One study showed that those infants most likely to develop apnea had lower (less than 30 percent) hematocrits (a percentage measure of red blood cells to plasma, the liquid part of blood). Some physicians place infants on iron supplements before surgery and delay surgery if the baby's hematocrit is low. Rarely are infants transfused right before surgery unless the hematocrit is very low or the procedure is an emergency. It is impossible to predict exactly which infants will develop postoperative apnea, but adhering to guidelines about age and hematocrit appears to reduce risks.

When the Surgery is Over

Most babies return immediately to the NICU after surgery, bypassing the recovery room or postanesthesia care unit. In some hospitals, your baby may go to a specialized postoperative ICU, such as a neurologic or cardiothoracic unit. If that is the case, your baby may be transferred back to the NICU after a few days or may remain in the specialized unit until discharge.

What to Expect Right After Surgery

Immediately after surgery, the recovery nurse will be very busy assessing your baby's overall condition, recording frequent vital signs, and obtaining lab

specimens and x-rays. A baby who has undergone a simple surgical procedure, such as central venous line placement or hernia repair, usually requires
less intervention postoperatively than does a baby who has undergone a complex surgery. Again, these are general guidelines. Your baby's situation will be
unique, and policies vary from unit to unit. Once the immediate postoperative
tasks are completed, and as long as your baby is stable, you'll be encouraged
to visit. Your initial postoperative visit may be brief, but you'll be able to
resume normal visiting as your baby's condition improves.

You'll no doubt feel relieved when your baby comes through surgery,
things settle down a bit, and you can concentrate on his recovery. You'll want
assurances that your baby's pain is being controlled and that your role as a
parent is valued. Ask questions about your baby's condition, and participate in
your baby's care as he stabilizes.

Pain Relief After Surgery

The nurses and medical team caring for your baby will assess your baby's
pain by monitoring his vital signs and activity level and will then decide which
medications or techniques will provide the best relief. As it does in adults and
older children, pain perception appears to vary from infant to infant, and a
combination of medication and comfort measures may be necessary.

Most infants experience discomfort after surgery, but not all infants
require a lot of pain medication. For simple procedures, a couple of doses of
acetaminophen (Tylenol or Tempra) may be all that is required.
Acetaminophen is given by mouth or as a rectal suppository and will relieve
mild to moderate pain. It may be combined with a narcotic if your baby
requires more pain relief.

If your baby has undergone major surgery (cardiovascular, neurologic, or
gastrointestinal), narcotic pain relief may be used. Currently, most NICUs give
morphine sulfate and/or fentanyl.

Morphine sulfate is the most commonly used natural opiate in the NICU
and is the standard to which all other opiates are compared.[14] Morphine can
be administered through an IV, eliminating the need for yet another needle
stick. It can be given as a single dose, or if your baby requires pain relief for a
few days, it may be given continuously as an IV infusion. Morphine can cause
undesirable changes in a baby's heart rate or blood pressure, however, so it
isn't appropriate for every baby.[15]

Fentanyl is a synthetic opioid that has become a popular choice for pain
relief in the NICU. Unlike morphine sulfate, fentanyl does not cause blood
pressure or heart rate changes.[15]

Two side effects of both morphine and fentanyl are tolerance and dependence. Tolerance to a drug means that progressively higher doses are required
to achieve the same therapeutic effect. Babies seem to develop tolerance more
quickly to fentanyl than to morphine.[15] Dependence means that the recipient
becomes used to the effects of the drug, and stopping it abruptly can cause
withdrawal symptoms. If these drugs are administered at high doses or for

*"After surgery, the nurse
showed me how to cup my
warms hands around Brian's
feet. He seemed to like that,
and it made me feel better to
be doing something for him."*

more than a few days, your baby may be weaned from the drug (the dosage slowly decreased over time) rather than having the administration abruptly discontinued.

Touching, stroking, speaking softly to the baby, and other basic comfort techniques have been studied as nonpharmacologic methods of pain relief.[16] These methods have shown mixed results, with some infants experiencing pain relief while others become more agitated. If you have used a particular type of touch that has relieved your baby's discomfort in other circumstances, it may be beneficial after surgery. This may not be the time to introduce new techniques, which may heighten your baby's agitation rather than soothe him.

Be sure to ask what medications and techniques will be or are being used to control your baby's pain. Not all units manage postoperative pain relief in the same way, but understanding what is being done to relieve your baby's pain will help reduce your anxiety as well.

The Postoperative Period

As your baby heals, usual care patterns will resume. Vital signs will be needed less frequently, and your baby's sleep will be interrupted less often. Depending on the type of surgery, your baby's surgeon or neonatologist will decide when your baby can start eating.

As your baby stabilizes and makes progress, you'll be able to participate more in his care and visit for longer periods. The amount of equipment attached to your baby may determine when you can hold him. Until then, remember that your voice and touch are an important part of your baby's care and recovery. Babies generally recover more quickly than older children do, and your baby may rapidly shed the extra tubes and equipment. Ask your baby's nurse what she looks for as signs of recovery.

Depending upon the type of surgery your baby has had, sutures or staples may have been used to hold the skin together while it heals. Staples are generally removed one week after surgery, so if your baby is discharged before then, you'll need to return to the surgeon's office for staple removal. Some sutures are dissolvable. Bathing will remove them. The staff will tell you when you can bathe your baby. Other sutures are made from natural materials that the body will "absorb."

It's not always possible to determine immediately if a surgical procedure is successful. You may need to wait while your baby undergoes some tests (x-rays, scans, and so on) to evaluate the adequacy of the surgery. Often, gastrointestinal surgery requires a waiting period. Then your baby may have a test called a barium swallow. For this test, your baby is fed a small amount of barium and is then x-rayed. The barium shows up on x-ray and clearly defines the gastrointestinal tract for evaluation.

If your baby was cared for in a specialty unit postoperatively, he may be transferred back to the NICU after the evaluation. For some babies, surgery is the last hurdle before discharge. For others, it may be a step along the course of continued hospitalization.

The usual discharge criteria (adequate age, adequate weight, and ability to feed) apply postoperatively. If your baby has special needs or requires technologic assistance to be discharged home, you will be involved in the development of your baby's discharge plan and follow-up care.

Your baby's postoperative condition and whether or not your baby requires more surgery will determine how much follow-up the surgeon will do. If your baby has had a hernia repair, he will probably need to be seen only once after discharge to assess proper healing. If your infant has undergone complex surgery, however, you and your child may develop a long-term relationship with the surgeon.

Surgery, even on very small babies, is commonplace in most NICUs. Understanding your baby's condition and the procedures involved helps reduce anxiety. Be sure you understand what the surgery is supposed to accomplish, and ask as many questions as you can think of before and after the procedure. Seek support from your baby's nurses, your social worker, and friends and family who can be there for you during this stressful time.

Surgery may be the last major barrier to discharge—and for some, it can be the most difficult and frustrating. Your baby may have been almost ready to go home: taking all feedings from the nipple and off most medications. Immediately after the surgery, it may appear that your baby is back almost to where he started: not eating and on all the monitors again. Your baby may appear to be very sick after surgery; however, most babies heal quickly. This period will be short-lived. Remember: You are very important to your baby's recovery. Your voice and touch can do much to comfort your sick baby and make this difficult time pass quickly for both of you.

The Parent's Role in a Baby's Recovery

Chapter 12

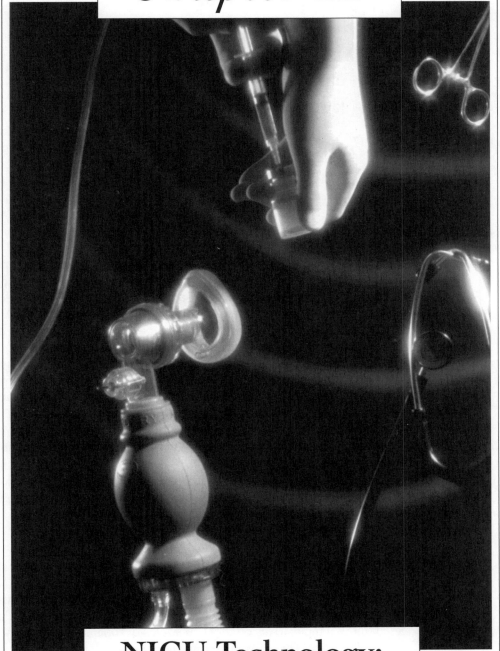

NICU Technology:
Promise and Progress

Ellen P. Tappero, RNC, MN, NNP

"Pooh!" cried Piglet, and now it was *his* turn to be the admiring one. "You've saved us!" "Have I?" said Pooh, not feeling quite sure.

The complexity of your baby's care in the NICU presents challenges to nurses and physicians. It also presents opportunities to use state-of-the-art technology. Since the 1960s, rapid advances in the computer industry have brought about an explosion of new NICU technology. These technologic breakthroughs have changed not only the way the health care team works with high-risk babies, but also the appearance of the NICU. Although the NICU may seem cluttered with lots of high-tech equipment, that "clutter" allows older, time-tested treatments to be monitored more closely and applied more effectively, with less risk of complications.

Like other specialty areas, neonatology has its own language and alphabet-soup shorthand. RDS, SGA, and premie—shorthand for respiratory distress syndrome, small for gestational age, and premature infant—may become part of your everyday conversation after only a day or two in the NICU. ECMO, HiFi, and MRI—shorthand for three of the state-of-the-art treatment and diagnostic approaches explained in this chapter—may seem more intimidating because you'll hear them less often. This chapter highlights and explains some of the new technical advances and procedures that are being used in many NICUs across the United States and Canada. If your baby's care involves any of these new technologies, you'll be better prepared to understand the health care team's explanations after you've learned a bit about them.

This chapter focuses on four treatment approaches and three diagnostic imaging advances:
- Surfactant replacement therapy
- High-frequency ventilation (HFV)
- Extracorporeal membrane oxygenation (ECMO)
- Nitric oxide therapy
- Computed tomography (CT) scan
- Ultrasonography
- Magnetic resonance imaging (MRI)

Not all of these complex therapies and diagnostic tools will be used for your infant. In fact, not every NICU will use or have all of them available. To keep things simple, focus on those therapies or tools that are playing a part in your baby's care. These explanations are of necessity somewhat general. You may need to ask your baby's health care team for more information.

Some of the most common problems NICU infants experience are associated with breathing and with getting enough oxygen to the body systems and tissues. Four relatively new treatments are having dramatic effects on seriously ill infants in many NICUs.

Therapeutic Treatments

Surfactant Replacement Therapy

A common serious problem facing premature infants is the limited ability of their lung cells to produce a substance known as surfactant. This substance, a mixture of compounds, is 80 to 90 percent fat and 10 to 20 percent proteins.[1] Surfactant appears in the fetal lung at about 24 weeks gestation and increases in amount as the fetus matures. It is rarely present in sufficient quantities before 36 weeks gestation.[2]

Surfactant lines the inner surfaces of the bronchioles (small airways) and the alveoli (small air sacs in the lung) and prevents their walls from collapsing at the end of each breath. Necessary gas exchange takes place in the alveoli. There the oxygen inhaled with each breath moves into the blood, and the carbon dioxide moves from the blood into the alveoli so that it can be exhaled.

How lung surfactant helps a baby breathe

At 22 weeks gestation, fluid fills the fetal airways. Air sacs (alveoli) are not formed. Lungs are not used for breathing.

At 24 to 34 weeks gestation, the fluid-filled air sacs begin to develop surfactant cells.

At 34 to 40 weeks gestation, nearly all the surfactant cells are formed. Most babies have sufficient surfactant by 36 weeks gestation.

a. A baby with surfactant can breathe easily. Surfactant mixes with the remaining lung fluid. Surfactant and lung fluid become a fine film, allowing air to slip in and out. Air sacs fully expand.

b. Without surfactant, air hydroplanes over the surface and prevents oxygen exchange. Alveoli are too sticky to fully expand. This makes it hard for the baby to breathe.

Airway

Alveoli bud

Alveoli

Surfactant cells

Birth through the vaginal canal helps squeeze out lung fluid. The first breath draws air into the lungs.

AIR

AIR

b.

Alveoli without surfactant

a.

Alveoli with surfactant

A lack of surfactant production leads, in part, to a condition known as respiratory distress syndrome, also sometimes called surfactant deficiency syndrome or hyaline membrane disease (HMD). Infants with RDS have a difficult time breathing, because the walls of their alveoli tend to collapse after each breath. The surfactant deficiency found in preterm infants is also said to cause a "stiff" lung—one with low compliance (flexibility). Low compliance means that the lung is hard to fill up with air, requiring the infant's respiratory muscles to work harder to bring in air.[3]

When a newborn takes her first breath, the air sacs in the lungs open for the first time. Just like blowing up a balloon for the first time, this breath takes a lot of effort. Each time that balloon is blown up again, though, inflating it takes less effort. The same is true of the breathing process in healthy term infants. But in babies without surfactant, alveoli that are inflated during a breath collapse at the end of that breath. Each breath an infant with limited or no surfactant takes, therefore, is like blowing up a balloon for the first time. If this condition is left untreated, the infant will eventually tire and go into respiratory failure, because when the alveoli collapse, oxygen and carbon dioxide exchange is limited. Once the infant slips into respiratory failure, she will need a mechanical ventilator to help her breathe.[4]

It has generally been accepted for more than 30 years that respiratory distress syndrome is associated with a lack of surfactant. A treatment for this deficiency has been elusive, however. Exogenous surfactant (surfactant that is not produced by the infant's body) was first given to premature infants as a treatment for RDS in the mid-1960s.[5] But not until the 1980s was the product perfected to the point that its benefits could be demonstrated in a convincing human study.[1,5]

There are two types of exogenous surfactants: (1) natural surfactants, made from animal lungs or human amniotic fluid, and (2) artificial (synthetic) surfactants, composed of a mixture of various chemicals. Currently, only two surfactant preparations, Exosurf and Survanta, have been approved by the Food and Drug Administration (FDA) for use in infants. A third, Infrasurf, although it has been shown to be safe and effective, is available only under research protocol in the United States.[1]

Exogenous surfactants are given through a tube placed in your baby's trachea (windpipe). A dose may be given within the first few minutes after birth (called preventive or prophylactic treatment) or only after signs and symptoms of RDS appear (called rescue treatment). Most NICUs give exogenous surfactant multiple times.

Surfactant replacement therapy doesn't prevent RDS. It only decreases the severity of the disease by stabilizing the alveoli.[5] The goal of this therapy is to reduce the amount of extra oxygen and to lower the ventilator pressures that must be used to maintain normal levels of oxygen and carbon dioxide in your baby's blood. An associated goal is to be able to wean your baby from the ventilator sooner, which decreases the chances that she will develop complications associated with ventilator therapy. See Chapter 10 for information on

Exogenous Surfactants		
Type	**Name**	**Source**
Artificial	Exosurf	Artificial
Natural	Curosurf	Pig
	Survanta	Cow
	Infrasurf	Cow

bronchopulmonary dysplasia (BPD) and retinopathy of prematurity (ROP), two possible complications of ventilator therapy.

Recently, there have been reports that surfactant therapy may also be useful in infants with respiratory failure whose condition is caused or complicated by surfactant inactivation (as seen with pulmonary hemorrhage) rather than just surfactant deficiency (seen with RDS). These reports provide encouraging information to support the use of exogenous surfactant in an expanded role. Further research will be conducted to evaluate the long-term effects of its efficiency when used for conditions that involve surfactant inactivation.[6,7]

High-Frequency Ventilation

Another relatively new technology for providing breathing support to infants in severe lung failure is high-frequency ventilation (HFV). Conventional ventilators require high pressures to deliver the volume of gas necessary to inflate a "stiff" (noncompliant) lung.[3] But medical professionals believe that the high pressures and high concentrations of oxygen required for conventional ventilators may cause air leaks in the lungs (called pulmonary air leaks) and bronchopulmonary dysplasia (BPD). High-frequency ventilation is a form of mechanical ventilation that delivers small tidal volumes (amount of air inhaled and exhaled with each normal breath) at rapid rates in an attempt to avoid those complications.[8]

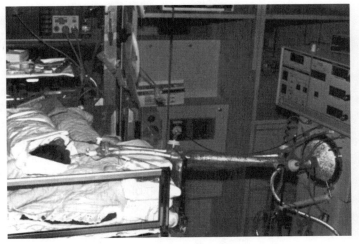

High frequency ventilation.

The baby on HFV rests on a radiant warmer surrounded by equipment.

From: Avila K, Mazza L, and Trujillo L. 1994. High-frequency oscillatory ventilation: A nursing approach to bedside care. Neonatal Network 13(5):23–30. Reprinted by permission.

In general, HFV has been used as a "rescue" therapy for infants with severe lung disease who appear to be "flunking" or who are not improving with conventional ventilation. Many studies have demonstrated that HFV is an effective method of providing both oxygenation (supplying oxygen) and ventilation (removing carbon dioxide from the blood). It has been used most successfully on infants with pulmonary air leaks, such as pulmonary interstitial emphysema (PIE), pneumothorax, and pneumopericardium. (See Chapter 10 for a discussion of pulmonary air leaks.) High-frequency ventilation may be used when all else fails and before an infant is placed on ECMO. It has also been used with limited success on infants diagnosed with diaphragmatic hernia, persistent pulmonary hypertension, and meconium aspiration.[9] (See Chapter 10 for information on these conditions.)

With conventional ventilators, the machine rate is measured in breaths per minute. When an infant is on HFV , the machine rate is so fast that counting the number of breaths per minute is virtually impossible. Instead, the health care team may use the term Hertz to state the HFV rate. One Hertz is equal to one cycle (breath) per second (1 Hz = 1 cycle per second or 60 breaths per minute). For example, a high-frequency ventilator set to run at 15 Hertz delivers 900 breaths per minute. The calculations are as follows: 15 Hz = 15 cycles/second.

Multiply by 60 to determine the number of cycles, or breaths, per minute—in this case, 900 breaths per minute. Between 10 and 15 Hertz is a typical setting for a high-frequency oscillatory ventilator. A ventilator set to operate at 7 Hertz would deliver 420 breaths per minute. This is a typical operational setting for a high-frequency jet ventilator. Both types are explained here.

Several techniques exist for producing high-frequency ventilation:

- **High-frequency positive pressure ventilation (HFPPV)** is produced using a conventional mechanical ventilator (CMV) at rapid rates of 60 to 150 breaths per minute.[3,9] One study has shown, however, that the rates at which these ventilators function most effectively range only from 75 to 100 breaths per minute, well below the 150-breaths-per-minute maximum. Main problems with this type of ventilation are inadequate oxygen delivery during inhalation and inadequate lung emptying during exhalation. For these reasons, HFPPV is usually used only as a short-term therapy.[10]

- **High-frequency jet ventilation (HFJV)** is produced by delivering short bursts (high-speed pulses) of gas directly into the trachea (windpipe) and down the airways to the alveoli at a rate of 150 to 900 breaths per minute.[9,10] The nursing staff and other members of the health care team refer to this type of ventilator as the "jet," or "HiFi." This type of high frequency ventilation was the first to be approved by the FDA for use in infants with RDS complicated by pulmonary air leaks. It is a popular form of HFV being used in NICUs today.[3] To allow for sighs (deep breaths) and continued expansion of the alveoli at the end of expiration, HFJV is used in conjunction with a conventional ventilator. It is similar to conventional mechanical ventilation in that the expiration phase is passive; air is exhaled by the "automatic" recoil (bounce-back) of the chest wall and lung. (During normal breathing, you actively bring air into your lungs by expanding your chest wall and thus inflating your lungs. In exhalation, you relax the respiratory muscles of your chest wall and diaphragm, passively deflating your lungs.)

- **High-frequency oscillatory ventilation (HFOV)** is quite different from the two methods discussed previously. HFOV actually vibrates the air; it uses a vibrating diaphragm or piston that alternates between pushing and pulling small volumes of gas within the airway. It operates at rates ranging from 300 to 3,000 breaths per minute.[3,11] In HFPPV and HFJV, passive recoil of the lungs and chest wall expels gas from the lung. In HFOV, the gas is actively pulled out of the lung during exhalation. This method of HFV is therefore classified as active expiration. Studies have shown that when conventional ventilation fails, HFOV can improve the condition of infants with RDS.[12,13] High-frequency oscillatory ventilators have been available only since 1990, however, and were not FDA approved until March 1991. The health care team may also refer to this type of ventilator as the "HiFi," or "oscillator." Research continues to be conducted to evaluate the long-term effects of this technique.

- **High-frequency flow interruption (HFFI)** ventilation delivers small tidal volumes of gas at rates of 300 to 900 breaths per minute.[3] In HFFI, a valve is used to intermittently interrupt a constant flow of gas that is forced into the tube in the infant's trachea. With this type of ventilation, expiration is once

"The NICU equipment is amazing. It's absolutely magic."

226

again "passive." There is little clinical experience or research using this type of ventilation. Consequently, you'll find this equipment only in NICUs in research or teaching hospitals.

Once high-frequency ventilation is started (it doesn't matter which technique is used), you'll notice that your baby begins to shake. Shaking of the chest and abdomen is the most obvious, but in very small infants, the whole body may appear to tremble. Don't be alarmed. This is a normal result of HFV therapy. The amount of vibration produced during HFV depends on the rate and pressure being used as well as on the size of the infant. When HFV is used in adults, patients describe the vibration as being "soothing."[14] The continuous motion appears to relax infants as well; as a result, fewer sedatives are needed to keep infants on HFV from fighting the ventilator. Infants can breathe on their own during HFV, but this usually does not happen unless they are upset or have increased levels of carbon dioxide in their blood. Infants are eventually weaned from HFV and placed on a conventional ventilator, nasal CPAP, or a nasal cannula, where they remain until they no longer require any breathing or oxygen assistance. (See Chapter 2 for information about the nasal CPAP and nasal cannula.)

Extracorporeal Membrane Oxygenation

The machine used for ECMO (pronounced "EK-mo") is a modification of a heart-lung bypass machine that allows for a longer period of therapy than the one used in the operating room for open-heart surgery.[15] Extracorporeal membrane oxygenation provides cardiac (heart) and respiratory (lung) support to the 2 to 5 percent of critically ill infants with severe lung failure who do not respond to the usual therapy of maximum conventional ventilation or medications and who are term or near term. These infants usually have one of the following problems: infection/pneumonia, meconium aspiration, respiratory distress syndrome, persistent pulmonary hypertension of the newborn, or a congenital diaphragmatic hernia.

There are two types of ECMO: venoarterial (VA) bypass and venovenous (VV) bypass. The method selected depends on whether the infant needs both heart and lung support or mainly lung support.

Commonly, ECMO is started by placing the infant on VA bypass. The surgical procedure required to put the ECMO catheters in place—called a cannulation—is usually performed by a surgeon with the operating room staff in attendance. Cannulation is commonly done at the infant's bedside to avoid the risks involved in moving a critically ill infant to and from an operating room. Before the catheters are placed, the infant is given medications for pain, for sedation, and to briefly paralyze her (stop all muscle movement) to prevent the formation of an air embolus (bubble) in the bloodstream. A tube (catheter) is placed in a large neck vein on the baby's right side and is then gently threaded (pushed or advanced) into the right atrium of the heart. A second catheter is placed next to the first one, but it is inserted into the carotid artery (a large artery in the neck that carries blood from the heart to the brain) and advanced to the infant's aortic arch (vessel through which the body is supplied with oxygenated blood).[3] After the catheters are inserted, an x-ray is taken to confirm that they are in the correct positions. The catheters are then connected to the ECMO circuit, which has been primed (filled) with heparinized adult donor blood. The heparin keeps the blood from clotting when it is exposed to the surfaces of the catheters and ECMO circuit tubing.

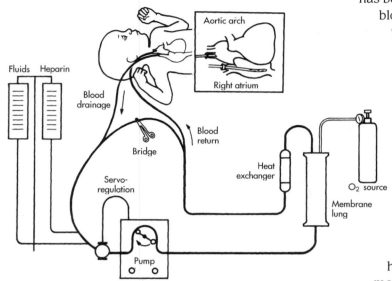

Venoarterial ECMO therapy—in which a catheter is placed in both a vein (veno) and an artery (arterial), as just described—is used for infants with heart or blood pressure problems. The advantage of VA bypass is that it supports not only the lungs but the heart. Therefore, if heart function is a concern, VA ECMO will be used.

The second method for initiating ECMO is a VV bypass. A single catheter is placed in a vein in the neck. This approach is used in infants who do not have blood pressure or heart function problems. The advantage to this method is that the carotid artery does not need to be tied off, as it must be in a VA bypass. Infants who are started on VV ECMO and later develop blood pressure problems or continue to have low oxygen levels can be changed over to VA ECMO if necessary.

How extracorporeal membrane oxygenation works.

Components of the ECMO circuit include cannulas, PVC tubing, a roller head pump, a membrane oxygenator (lung), gas source, a heat exchanger, and infusion pumps.

From: Nugent J. 1993. Extracorporeal membrane oxygenation (ECMO) in the neonate. In Core Curriculum for Neonatal Intensive Care Nursing, Beachy P, and Deacon J, eds. Philadelphia: WB Saunders, 180. Reprinted by permission.

In VA ECMO, dark blood (blood containing little oxygen—deoxygenated blood) is drained by gravity from the infant through the catheter that was advanced into the right atrium of the heart. The ECMO pump (which acts as an artificial heart) pushes this blood through the rest of the ECMO circuit. As the drained blood passes through the membrane oxygenator (which acts as an artificial lung), carbon dioxide is removed, and oxygen is picked up. The blood enters the oxygenator dark (deoxygenated) and comes out bright red in color (oxygenated). When the blood leaves the oxygenator, it is warmed in the heat exchanger and returned to the infant through the arterial catheter.

In VV ECMO, the procedure is the same as in VA bypass except that the blood is drained and returned through the same catheter, the one in the right atrium. This catheter has two lumens (openings). One-half of the catheter drains the dark blood, and then oxygenated (red) blood is returned to the infant through the other half.

Even if your infant is supported by ECMO, she will remain on the ventilator. Very low settings (low pressures and low oxygen concentrations) are used to "rest" your baby's lungs. The tube in the infant's trachea (windpipe) allows secretions to be suctioned out, and the light breaths from the ventilator help keep the baby's lungs inflated.

When ECMO is started, the pump is at first set at a low flow rate to check for leaks in the system and to ensure that the gravity flow of blood from the venous catheter is adequate. The flow rate of the pump is gradually increased until about 80 percent of the blood your infant's heart pumps out (cardiac output) is diverted through the ECMO circuit.[16] This usually requires flow rates of 120 to 150 milliliters per kilogram (of infant weight) per minute (ml/kg/minute). At maximum flow rates, your infant's arterial blood gases should be normal. This high flow rate means that ECMO is doing most of the work of providing oxygen to your baby's blood. While on high flow rates, infants usually remain quiet and may receive pain medications as well as a sedative to ensure comfort. Babies on ECMO may open their eyes, breathe on their own, and occasionally move their arms and legs in response to stimulation, such as your voice or a soft touch.

As your infant improves, the ECMO flow rate is decreased, and more blood then goes to her lungs for the exchange of oxygen and carbon dioxide. A decrease in the amount of ECMO support (or a decrease in the percentage of bypass) over a period of several days is an important sign that your baby is improving. Eventually, she will no longer need ECMO support to maintain adequate gas exchange at low ventilator settings.

When the ECMO flow rate is decreased to 50 ml/kg/minute, this is called "idling." If your baby's improved lung function remains stable at low ventilator settings during idling, the catheters are clamped, and a trial period off ECMO is attempted. If your baby's arterial blood gases deteriorate, the catheters are unclamped, and ECMO support is resumed. If blood gas values remain good while your infant is off ECMO, the catheters are removed from your baby's neck (decannulation). After decannulation, your infant will be weaned from the ventilator as tolerated, and routine NICU care will be resumed.

How long an infant remains on ECMO varies, depending on her condition and on the recovery of both heart and lung function. Most newborns average five to seven days on ECMO. Length of treatment depends on the age of the infant, the original illness, the amount of damage to the lungs before ECMO was started, and any complications that may have occurred during ECMO.

Although ECMO therapy has improved the outcome of infants with severe lung failure, there are risks associated with this procedure.

• **Bleeding:** Heparin is added to the blood in the ECMO circuit to prevent it from clotting when it comes in contact with the surfaces of the catheters and circuit tubing. The amount of heparin needed is monitored closely, and the infant's bleeding times (amount of time it takes for a small quantity of blood to clot) are tested frequently to minimize risks. The risk of bleeding depends on how closely the heparin is monitored and whether the infant is predisposed to bleeding—for example, due to necrotizing enterocolitis (NEC) or a previous Grade I or II intraventricular hemorrhage. Bleeding may occur anywhere in the body. If bleeding does occur and cannot be stopped, ECMO therapy may be discontinued.

• **Infection:** Any time a catheter is introduced into the body, there is always a risk of infection. Infants on ECMO may be given antibiotics (drugs to prevent or fight infections) throughout the ECMO run and are watched closely for signs of infection.

- **Transfusion reactions/complications/infections:** Infants on ECMO usually require several transfusions of some blood product. As with all blood transfusions, there is a risk of hepatitis, AIDS, and/or a blood transfusion reaction. All blood from the hospital's blood bank is screened for these and other viruses, but a small risk of acquiring a disease is always present.

- **Mechanical failure:** A mechanical failure can occur at any time. Although safety precautions are used, the circuit tubing could break, the neck catheter could accidently be pulled out, or there could be a power failure, to name only a few of the possibilities. The ECMO specialist watching the circuit is trained to handle just such emergencies. Should one occur, the infant will be placed on increased ventilator settings until the problem is resolved and ECMO can be resumed.

- **Emboli:** Air emboli and tiny clots can move from the ECMO circuit into the infant's bloodstream, leading to complications and possibly death. Safety precautions are taken, and the ECMO specialist monitors the circuit continuously for both air and blood clots.

Of babies on ECMO, 81 percent survive. This is impressive, because 80 percent of babies in respiratory failure are likely to die. For these sick babies, ECMO is indeed a lifesaver. Survival rates for infants on ECMO to treat each of these cases of lung failure are as follows: meconium aspiration—94 percent, persistent pulmonary hypertension of the newborn (PPHN)—84 percent; RDS—84 percent; infection/pneumonia—76 percent; congenital diaphragmatic hernia—58 percent; and pulmonary air leak syndrome—73 percent.[17]

Because infants who are treated with ECMO are critically ill at birth, it is difficult to determine whether the neurodevelopmental outcome is because of the original illness (there was a low oxygen concentration in the blood) or strictly related to ECMO therapy. Several follow-up studies have been conducted to assess both medical and developmental outcomes of infants treated with ECMO. One study reported that 90 percent of the infants treated with ECMO were normal at one year of age.[18] Other studies show that the neurodevelopmental outcome among infants treated with ECMO is consistent with the developmental outcome of infants who had severe respiratory failure and were treated with conventional therapy.[19,20] There is evidence of adequate blood flow to both sides of the brain in spite of the fact that the right carotid artery is tied off when VA bypass is used.[21] Further studies are needed, but it appears that ECMO can be given and that normal development is possible in infants who receive it.

Both the costs of the equipment and the personnel needed to provide it make ECMO expensive. Each baby on ECMO is staffed by an ECMO specialist (usually a nurse or a respiratory therapist) who has received hours of special training on both the equipment and the physiologic process. The staff is required to monitor and maintain a trouble-free ECMO circuit 24 hours a day, providing both routine maintenance of the circuit and taking emergency actions when unexpected, potentially catastrophic events occur. The baby's regular care is often the responsibility of another nurse while the baby is on ECMO. A physician familiar with ECMO and the infant's care must be available

"My own mother had a premature baby thirty years ago. When she visited Janis, I know she was thinking 'if only we had known about this back then.' But at the same time, she was glad that her grandchild was going to live."

24 hours a day; this may or may not be the infant's primary physician. The costs of the equipment and the staffing needed to run the circuit add up to a high daily ECMO charge. These charges are usually reimbursed by insurance companies, however, and should not play a part in your decision to use ECMO as a treatment for your infant.

Because ECMO is an invasive procedure, physicians will explain the process, the possible complications, and how they expect your baby to respond to the treatment. You will need to sign a consent form (see Chapter 11) giving them permission to insert the catheters and begin the therapy.

Nitric Oxide Therapy

One of the newest therapeutic advances to reach neonatal medicine is nitric oxide (NO). As recently as the mid-1980s, nitric oxide had a bad reputation as a common air pollutant found in cigarette smoke and smog. It was blamed for acid rain and the depletion of the ozone layer and was suspected of causing cancer. Nitric oxide is a small, light molecule that investigators have only recently discovered is a crucial part of the body's neurochemical system. It is essential for activities ranging from digestion to blood pressure regulation. It is not to be confused with laughing gas, or nitrous oxide (N_2O), which you may have received at the dentist's office or in the operating room.

In 1992, much attention was focused on nitric oxide's role as a blood pressure regulator. Cells that line the inner walls of both veins and arteries release NO; from there, it migrates to nearby muscle cells and relaxes them. This dilates (enlarges) the blood vessels and lowers blood pressure. Keeping this discovery in mind, neonatal physicians looked more closely at infants who had persistent pulmonary hypertension.

In the uterus, the fetus's lungs serve no respiratory purpose; the placenta supplies the fetus with oxygen. The alveoli of the lungs are filled with fluid rather than air. Therefore, the blood that flows through the lungs is unable to pick up oxygen and carry it to other parts of the body. The blood flow through the fetus's lungs is much less than what is needed after birth. This diminished blood flow is because of the partial closure of the arterioles (vessels in the lung) located next to the alveoli (see diagram above). The constriction (closure) of the arterioles results in a large amount of blood being diverted through the ductus arteriosus (a small blood vessel that connects the pulmonary artery to the aorta) (diagram at right).

At birth, infants take their first few breaths and expand their lungs. While the lungs are expanding, the arterioles also open up and let more blood flow through the lungs. Blood that was previously diverted through the ductus arteriosus while the baby was in the uterus now flows to the lungs, where it picks

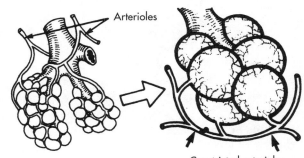

The fetal lung.

The fetal lung has diminished blood flow because of constricted blood vessels.

From: Bloom R, and Cropley C. 1994. Textbook of Neonatal Resuscitation. Dallas, Texas: American Heart Association, 1-7. Reprinted by permission.

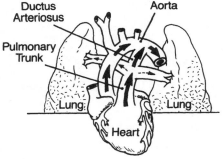

Patent ductus arteriosus.

The open ductus arteriosus allows blood to flow past the lungs of the fetus.

From: Bloom R, and Cropley C. 1994. Textbook of Neonatal Resuscitation. Dallas, Texas: American Heart Association, 1-7. Reprinted by permission.

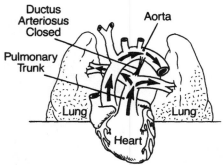

The ductus arteriosus beginning to close.

At birth, the ductus arteriosus closes off and allows more blood to flow to the lungs. The increased blood flow through the lungs supplies body tissues with oxygen as the baby breathes.

From: Bloom R, and Cropley C. 1994. Textbook of Neonatal Resuscitation. Dallas, Texas: American Heart Association, 1-8. Reprinted by permission.

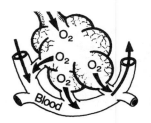

Healthy newborn at birth.

In a newborn with adequate oxygen, the blood vessels open, and blood flow through the lungs increases. With each breath, the baby supplies oxygen-rich blood to her body.

From: Bloom R, and Cropley C. 1994. Textbook of Neonatal Resuscitation. Dallas, Texas: American Heart Association, 1-9. Reprinted by permission.

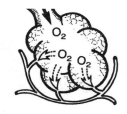

Newborn with asphyxia.

If the newborn does not have an adequate oxygen supply, the blood flow through the lungs decreases. The blood vessels constrict. This causes a cycle of inadequate oxygen causing inadequate blood supply to the lungs and decreased circulation through the lungs.

From: Bloom R, and Cropley C. 1994. Textbook of Neonatal Resuscitation. Dallas, Texas: American Heart Association, 1-9. Reprinted by permission.

up oxygen and carries it to the body. The ductus no longer serves a purpose, and it eventually closes (diagram at left).

In preterm infants with RDS or term infants with conditions such as meconium aspiration, infection/pneumonia, or congenital diaphragmatic hernia, the respiratory compromise may be complicated by persistent pulmonary hypertension (see Chapter 10) caused by low blood oxygen levels. In these infants, the nonoxygenated blood that would normally go to the lungs (diagram at left, below) is forced away from the closed arterioles and is channeled through the ductus (which never closed or which reopened after birth) to the aorta, leaving the blood unoxygenated. This creates a vicious cycle of unoxygenated blood in the body leading to further pulmonary arteriole constriction (diagram at right, below).

Currently, vasodilators (drugs used to open or widen the blood vessels) and ECMO are used to treat persistent pulmonary hypertension. In the past, vasodilators have had limited success because they performed inadequately. They either produced too little vasodilation or they produced too much, widening the blood vessels to the point where the blood pressure became too low. Extracorporeal membrane oxygenation has been effective in supporting these infants, but there are complications associated with that therapy also.

Nitric oxide was first described as an endothelial-derived relaxing factor (EDRF).[22,23] This relaxing factor has been shown to contribute to the normal opening of the pulmonary vessels after birth. Any alteration in the body's production of this molecule may result in failure of the pulmonary vessels to relax. Investigators believe that inhalation of NO (delivery of NO to the infant through a tube in the windpipe) allows the gas to diffuse directly into the smooth muscle of the pulmonary vessels, producing vasodilation. Giving NO by inhalation is thought to be most effective in dilating pulmonary vessels but not the systemic blood vessels, therefore avoiding the problem of a low blood pressure.

Two studies using inhaled NO for short periods on newborn infants showed that the gas improved oxygen and carbon dioxide exchange in the alveoli, and no signs of lung disease were found.[24,25] Nitric oxide therapy has also been used as a rescue treatment during the transport of critically ill infants from one hospital to another, more specialized hospital. It is used to stabilize severe swings in oxygen requirements so that the infant can be transported with fewer problems encountered during the trip.[26] Despite these findings, the risks and benefits of inhaled NO need careful consideration. This gas is presently approved for use only for babies involved in research protocols.

Low levels of inhaled NO for brief periods warrant further study as a selective pulmonary vasodilator in newborns. This new mode of direct delivery to the lung may allow for more new therapeutic applications that will increase understanding and treatment of persistent pulmonary hypertension in the newborn. Because this is such a new technique, the effects of breathing nitric oxide long term are not known. If long-term inhalation studies prove NO to be both safe and effective at decreasing pulmonary hypertension, a new era of treating infants with selective therapy will begin.

This gas is still under investigation and has not been approved by the FDA (except in approved FDA research studies). Therefore, it cannot be used in most NICUs. If your infant is in one of the approved research NICUs for trials of NO, the gas will not be used to treat your infant unless you sign a consent form granting the physicians permission to do so.

Diagnostic Imaging Techniques

Imaging techniques are simply methods for "seeing" inside something without opening it up. These techniques play a vital role in helping to identify (diagnose) the cause of medical problems. Important diagnostic imaging techniques developed since the early 1980s have revolutionized the field of diagnostic radiology by giving health care providers a better look at the internal structure and function of a baby's organs. Diagnostic imaging methods have gone from invasive examinations (tests in which catheters needed to be inserted or dyes had to be injected) to noninvasive and painless examinations, such as real-time ultrasonography and computed tomography (CT) scan. These techniques offer the health care team a tremendous amount of insight into such neonatal problems as congenital malformations, hydrocephalus, and intracranial hemorrhages (sometimes referred to as bleeds). (See Chapter 10 for an explanation of these problems.)

More recently, magnetic resonance imaging (MRI) has extended the health care team's ability to detect physical abnormalities in specific areas of the body. The potential diagnostic value of MRI for the newborn is just beginning to be appreciated. Each of these diagnostic imaging methods has its advantages and inconveniences, as the explanations that follow indicate.

Computed Tomography

The procedure called computed tomography—CT scan for short—became recognized as a diagnostic imaging tool in 1973. It involves aiming a very narrow beam of radiation at a specific layer of tissue and getting a computer-assisted reconstruction of the x-ray slices to provide a two-dimensional picture of internal structures.[27] Just as in a conventional x-ray, on a CT scan, bone absorbs the largest amount of x-rays and appears white; air absorbs the least and appears black. Because soft tissue is neither as dense as bone nor as thin as air, it appears as shades of gray. Computed tomography scanning is much more sensitive to tissue densities (thicknesses) than is a conventional x-ray. It can also detect changes in much smaller areas of tissue than a conventional x-ray can.

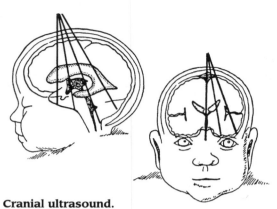

Cranial ultrasound.

The ultrasound Doppler is directed to scan different planes of the baby's head.

From: Hayden CK, and Swischuck LE, eds. 1987. *In* Pediatric Ultrasonography. Baltimore: Williams & Wilkins, 3. Reprinted by permission.

Computed tomography scanning is used to help determine the extent of a malformation or disease. It provides precise detail of the anatomy despite bone covering the area or overlapping of nearby body structures. In newborns, it is used most frequently to detect brain injury (cerebral lesions). It is not very useful in detecting chest (thoracic) defects because heart and lung movements distort the image. Injecting the infant with a contrast material through an IV site (known as contrast enhancement) can help measure blood flow to an area or define an abnormality. For most lesions in newborns, however, contrast enhancement for a detailed view of the blood vessels is not necessary.

Computed tomography scans are more reliable than ultrasonography or MRI in diagnosing or excluding certain kinds of brain and spinal cord hemorrhages, such as subarachnoid (below the innermost membrane covering the brain), subdural (below the outermost membrane covering the brain), and intraparenchymal (within the tissue of the brain). These small lesions may not be seen on ultrasound, and they may not be as easy to distinguish on MRI.[28] (See Chapter 10 for information on intraventricular hemorrhage and the "grading" of these lesions.)

Because motion distorts the CT scan image, newborns usually need to be restrained and often sedated for the study, a disadvantage in some cases. CT scanning is also unsuitable for repeated use because of the cumulative radiation dosages and the hazards of moving the infant from the NICU to the hospital's radiology department. For these reasons, real-time ultrasound has become the preferred method for diagnosing brain hemorrhages in newborns.

Ultrasonography

Ultrasonography uses high-frequency sound waves to evaluate internal anatomic structures, tissue movement, and blood flow. This diagnostic technique was first introduced into obstetrical practice in 1966 but wasn't used routinely with newborns until 1979.[27,29]

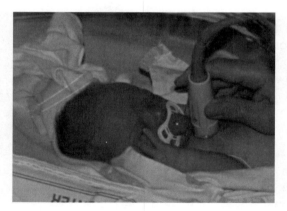

Echocardiogram.

The ultrasound machine can be used to scan the baby's heart.

Ultrasound imaging is based on mapping variations in reflected sound waves (echoes) within a specific region of the body. Using electronic mechanisms, a transducer in contact with the infant's skin sends brief ultrasound pulses through the tissue. These pulses are reflected by tissue interfaces (boundaries between two surfaces) and returned to the transducer as an echo. The transducer both sends (emits) the initial impulse and receives the reflected impulse.[30] A computer constructs a two-dimensional image from the reflected sound energy. Only tissues that are reflective enough to send back echoes are recorded and displayed on the scanner. Whether tissue is reflective depends on its density. The differences in the strength of the returning signals (echoes) are displayed on the scanner as various shades of gray. The stronger the reflection (the denser the tissue), the brighter (more echogenic) the image will appear on the scanner. Ultrasound cannot be used to scan bone, the lungs, or the bowel because the interfaces between soft tissues and bone and between soft tissues and air do not produce echoes. This method is used frequently in the NICU to scan the infant's brain to rule out intraventricular hemorrhages. If bleeding has occurred, its progression and the reabsorption of the blood will be followed with repeated ultrasounds.

The following are advantages of ultrasonography as a neonatal diagnostic tool:

- No ionizing radiation is necessary. Therefore, ultrasonography can be used frequently to evaluate the brain or to monitor the progression of bleeding inside the brain.
- No sedation is required. Injection of contrast material is not necessary.
- Ultrasound can be performed at the infant's bedside with portable equipment.
- Ultrasonography is less costly than CT scanning or MRI.
- The procedure is noninvasive and therefore considered mandatory in evaluating infants suspected of having heart disease.

Ultrasonography also has disadvantages:

- Bone, excessive fat, and gas act as barriers, totally blocking or distorting images. Certain parts of the body must be scanned through a "window"—in the case of the brain, through the anterior fontanel (soft spot). The useful-ness of echocardiography (ultrasound scan of the heart) is limited when overinflated lungs or chest wall deformities prevent adequate imaging.
- The usefulness of the scan depends on the operator's ability and the type of equipment used.
- Ultrasound scans cannot differentiate tissues with similar structure compo-sition: The interface (boundary) between the two tissue types is not well displayed on ultrasound. Computed tomography scanning is a superior method for imaging of tissues with similar structural compositions because it detects different densities. For example, a CT scan can differentiate the white and gray matter in the neonatal brain, because the two have different densities (white matter regions have more water). Ultrasonography cannot.

A technique called doppler ultrasound can be used along with regular ultra-sonography by simply "flicking" a switch on the machine. Doppler complements two-dimensional ultrasound because it detects disturbances in blood flow resulting from abnormal anatomic structure. Doppler-derived calculations are useful in estimating blood flow and the severity of stenotic (narrowing) lesions. From doppler ultrasound, estimates can be made about blood velocity (speed) and the direction of blood flow. These estimates are based on changes in sound wave frequencies reflected from moving structures, such as circulating red blood cells. Doppler ultrasound is most often used in echocardiography of the heart and in determining blood flow in the brain. Despite the availability of new imaging techniques, ultrasonography and doppler ultrasound remain the first choice in NICUs because they make a quick bedside diagnosis possible and lack side effects.

"I'm a computer engineer. For me, it was easier to understand what the nurses told me about the equipment than what they told me about our baby."

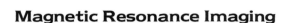

Magnetic Resonance Imaging

The theoretic basis of MRI is complex. The technique is based on interactions between the field of a large magnet in the imaging equipment and the atoms in the body. The magnetic field aligns the nucleus of a cell in the general direction of the magnetic field. Once aligned, these nuclei can be shifted out of alignment by using short bursts of radio waves. The atoms send out a signal that a specifically designed computer converts into thousands of mathematical calculations and then displays in the form of images. These images provide the health care team with a wealth of information for use in diagnosis and treatment planning.[30]

Particularly appealing for use in newborns, MRI is noninvasive, does not use ionizing radiation, and has no known adverse effects. It differs from CT scanning in that dense bone or fatty tissue does not affect the images produced. Magnetic resonance imaging produces better images of soft tissue than either CT scanning or ultrasound. It can show the degree of brain maturity in a premature infant, as well as allow earlier and more precise assessment of bleeding in both the gray and the white matter of the brain.

The disadvantages of MRI are its nonportability, its substantial equipment and operational costs, the length of time required to collect the necessary data, and the fact that access to the critically ill infant is limited during the procedure. The quality of the images produced by MRI is excellent, however. Magnetic resonance imaging holds great promise for future applications in the care of newborns.

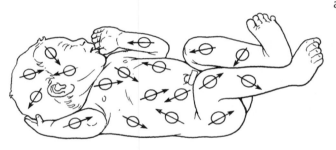

Magnetic resonance imaging—unmagnetized.

The body has randomly arranged spinning atoms.

From: Theorell C. 1993. Diagnostic imaging. In Comprehensive Neonatal Nursing, *Kenner C, Brueggemeyer A, and Gunderson L, eds. Philadelphia: WB Saunders, 869. Reprinted by permission.*

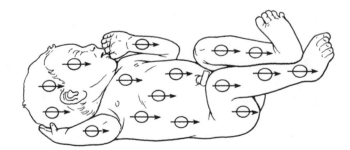

Magnetic resonance imaging—magnetized.

Once magnetized, the spinning atoms of the body are aligned in one direction. Short bursts of radio waves then shift the nuclei out of alignment. The resulting signal creates images that provide the health care team with information for use in diagnosis.

From: Theorell C. 1993. Diagnostic imaging. In Comprehensive Neonatal Nursing, *Kenner C, Brueggemeyer A, and Gunderson L, eds. Philadelphia: WB Saunders, 869. Reprinted by permission.*

The NICU you enter today is very different from the NICU of even a few years ago. Advances in respiratory care as well as in noninvasive monitoring and diagnostic techniques have been incredible. Both nursing and medical research are constantly changing the way sick babies are treated.

Understanding the basics of NICU technology prepares you to ask questions about your baby's treatment. The NICU team understands that this technology can be overwhelming for parents and that it may contribute to your feelings of powerlessness and frustration. Keep asking questions, and stay involved in your baby's care. The technology in the NICU is important to your baby's survival and holds promise for better neonatal outcomes but it cannot replace the importance of your voice, your touch, and your long-term commitment as an involved parent.

The Importance of Parenting

Chapter 13

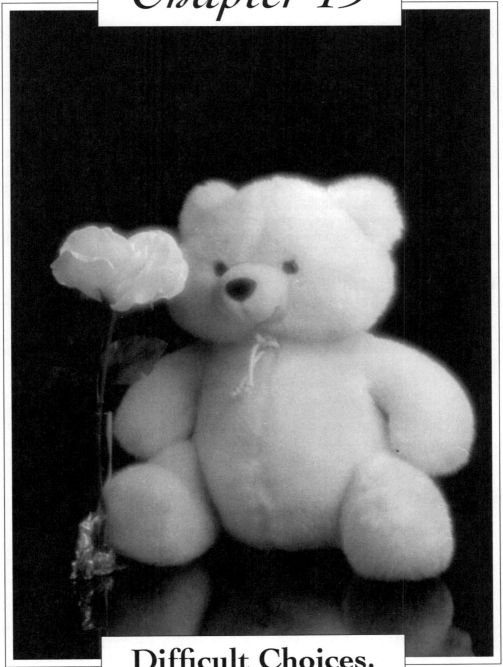

Difficult Choices,
Gentle Good-Byes

Kathleen A. Green, RNC, MSN, NNP

❝"Pooh, *promise* you won't forget about me, ever. Not even when I'm a hundred."❞

Christopher Robin—

Y ou'll face few struggles in life as difficult as the heartbreaking loss of your baby through severe disability or death. Not only must you face your own shattered dreams, you must manage the practical details of the situation and support those around you who are also trying to cope with this tragic loss.

This experience will change who you are and how you live. It may be difficult to find anything positive in these events. But as this experience unfolds, you will have opportunities to truly "parent" your baby, to share in important decisions, and to maintain some control over events that will affect you and your family for life.

Difficult Choices

A severely impaired child will change your family considerably. Recognition of this reality is important. There is no one right answer to the difficult questions facing you; each child and each family is different. Consultation with social workers, clergy, physicians, nurses, family members, and friends can provide you with information, but ultimately you must make the decision regarding your child's future.

Alternatives to NICU Care

The purpose of an NICU is usually to provide acute care—that is, highly skilled medical and nursing care for critically ill newborns. From the day a baby is admitted to the NICU, the final goal is discharge. The decision to discharge occurs when the infant is healthy (or has minor short-term or long-term problems) or when the infant has developed major long-term (chronic) problems better handled elsewhere. The time may come when decisions need to be made regarding continuing care of your infant in the NICU.

You shouldn't see transference of care as "eviction" or as failure of the NICU to complete the healing process. Rather, the NICU cannot be all things to all babies. Infants born with acute problems (congenital heart defects, kidney disorders, and seizure disorders, for example) may be stabilized but not cured in the NICU. Other infants develop severe complications and have physical or mental disabilities because of their prematurity or illness. Infants born with chronic syndromes may require long-term care after initial diagnosis and stabilization in the NICU.

If a decision for long-term care needs to be made, the medical team should provide you with a clear explanation of your infant's condition and their best guess at the prognosis (long-term outcome). Unfortunately, the prognosis for many problems is unknown, and the information you may want the most may be unavailable. As frustrating as it may seem, only time may clearly reveal your child's physical and mental abilities. At this point, your baby may benefit from a change in health care delivery to ensure individualized physical and developmental therapies and a health care team who may view problems in a different light.

Your baby's options for long-term care clearly depend upon his medical condition. As NICU care and technology have proliferated, so too have options for post-NICU care. Your options may include:

- Home care
- Transitional care facilities
- Long-term care facilities
- Foster care or adoption
- Abandonment (though not an acceptable option, it is discussed here)

As you sort through the various care options, your baby's social worker can be a valuable source of information and support. Generally, the social worker in your unit will know about suitable care facilities in the region. If you live far from the NICU, the social worker should be able to coordinate discharge activities with a social worker nearer your home. Financial assistance and regulations vary from state to state, and a social worker can describe the options available to you, based on your baby's condition and your family's situation.

Your baby's nurse or social worker may also suggest that you speak to a parent whose child has similar care requirements. Many parents find conversations of this sort helpful in some aspects of decision making. Appendix D lists parent organizations that may be able to provide support and answer your questions.

Home Care

Home care for babies who are very ill or seriously disabled (a small percentage of NICU survivors), can place tremendous hardships on the family. When the care decision is made, all members of the family need to be considered. This includes recognizing the impact that home care may have on the baby's siblings. Some children who have grown to adulthood with disabled siblings view it as the best experience of their life. Other children raised with disabled siblings grow up resenting the loss of parental attention and lack of financial resources. If you are considering caring for an ill or disabled infant at home, read Chapters 15 and 16, which explain what is involved on a day-to-day basis.

Transitional Care Facilities

A transitional care facility is usually a stopping place between an acute-care facility (such as the NICU) and home. This type of facility may also be called a rehabilitation hospital; its patients often include older children and adults. The goal at admission to a transitional care facility is discharge, and the possibility for discharge is the primary criterion for admission. Infants may be admitted to transitional or rehabilitative facilities to be weaned off a ventilator, for administration or weaning of total parenteral nutrition, or to address specific developmental issues. Usually, a team comes from the transitional care facility to the NICU to meet you and your baby, evaluate your infant's medical condition, and determine if the rehabilitation facility could meet your needs.

Shortly after your baby's admission to a rehabilitation facility, that facility's health care team develops a care plan, which it shares with you and everyone involved in your baby's care. This ensures that everyone caring for your baby knows the outcome goals. Parents are encouraged to assume more of their infant's care at transitional care facilities, and visiting policies are usually quite liberal. Most facilities allow the entire family to visit and really get to know the baby. The atmosphere in such facilities is more relaxed than in an NICU, and the care given and the decisions made are not emergent. Change proceeds at a slower pace than in the NICU. This enables rehabilitation facilities to be more "user friendly" for the parents and family than NICUs. The goal of the rehabilitation facility is to discharge your baby home. Rehabilitation facilities that encourage active parent participation can greatly ease the transition between hospital and home.

Long-Term Care Facilities

If your baby has a poor prognosis—for example, severe physical or mental disabilities or a condition that is ultimately fatal—a long-term care facility (also called a chronic-care facility) may be the proper placement. Infants who lack potential for rehabilitation are usually candidates for admission to a long-term care facility rather than for discharge home or to a transitional facility. Other factors that determine whether placement of your child in a long-term care facility is appropriate include your financial resources and the feasibility of home care.

Remember that few decisions are irrevocable. Eventually, you may be able to bring your child home from a long-term care facility. Home care does not work for every family, however, and a long-term care facility may offer options that best meet the needs of your child and family.

Foster Care or Adoption

Foster care or adoption are acceptable options when the NICU is no longer the place for your baby and you are unable to parent your baby. Relinquishment is a heart-wrenching choice, but it may be the best one for your family. Knowing that there are families who adopt or provide foster care for children with special needs and disabilities may make your decision easier.

This is a conscious choice you should make only after obtaining all the facts about your child's illness and prognosis from the medical team. You should also receive counseling from an adoption social worker, who can help you with decision making, facilitate the process, and provide resources for follow-up care for you and your family.

All parents who place a child in foster care or for adoption should see the child before doing so. If you have been told that your baby has some severe

"The decision to use a chronic care facility for our baby was the right decision for us. She gets loving care and we are still very much her parents."

deformities or abnormalities, this is especially important. Descriptions often make these defects sound worse than they actually are.

An important part of the adoption or foster care process is saying good-bye to your baby. Even though your baby has not died, you'll grieve the loss of your child and your role as parent and primary caretaker. You will never forget your baby and this chapter in your life. Saying good-bye is a concrete act that begins your healing process.

Abandonment

Some parents believe that abandonment relieves them of very difficult decisions regarding their baby's outcome. In actuality, abandonment is a very definite decision to relinquish your infant's care to others. Abandonment may not relieve you of financial responsibility, however, and may cause needless delays if consent is needed for a procedure that might improve your baby's condition. Also, abandonment may delay placement of your infant in a stable home environment.

There is no shame in realizing your limitations as a parent. Pursuing relinquishment through adoption or foster care is a more responsible and healthy way to manage your baby's future than is abandonment. Health care providers and counselors will support your decision and respect your ability to maintain control in a devastating situation. Abandonment is costly for you and your baby and will only complicate your lives psychologically, financially, and legally.

I n the delivery room, nurses and physicians cannot always identify babies for whom treatment will prove futile. Erring on the side of preserving life, they may vigorously try to stabilize the newborn. Not all attempts are successful, and some babies die despite vigorous treatment. Other babies may be stabilized, admitted to the NICU, and then on further evaluation found to have conditions incompatible with life. In addition, an infant may develop conditions that no longer respond to treatment. When this occurs, you may be asked to participate in making the most difficult decision of all—that of allowing your baby to die.

The Hardest Choice of All— Letting Go

Ethical and Legal Considerations

Until the 1980s, physicians and staff in labor and delivery units and NICUs made most of the choices about who lived and who died. Working mostly from a well-intentioned ethical perspective, health care professionals tried to protect parents from tragic situations by allowing extremely premature and disabled infants to die soon after birth. This was before widespread education about medical treatments and interventions empowered health care consumers to participate more actively in critical decision making. Although most health care professionals recognize that parents should participate in these decisions, it has taken time to change professional practices and beliefs.

Two important factors led to this change. First, some health care professionals follow the ethical principle that "all human life is equal" and do not believe that physicians and nurses should decide that one life is more valuable than another. Health care professionals with this belief chose to resuscitate and stabilize every live-born baby, regardless of how precarious that life might be. With a change to more conservative politics, stabilization of every newborn became the "correct" thing to do. After a complete assessment of the baby, however, it was not always clear who would make the critical decision to continue or discontinue treatment in the case of extremely premature or disabled infants.

The second factor was the enactment in the 1980s of federal guidelines known as the Baby Doe Regulations. These government rulings resulted from a case in which an infant known simply as Baby Doe was born with Down syndrome and esophageal atresia. The esophageal birth defect was surgically correctable, but the infant's parents refused to sign a consent, stating that because their infant would be severely disabled anyway, aggressive treatment was not in the baby's best interest. From birth, the baby was denied food, water, and medical aid. The hospital went to court to obtain permission for the surgery, the circuit court judge upheld the parents' decision, and the Indiana Supreme Court also agreed.[1,2] The infant died, and the case prompted widespread change in hospital treatment of disabled infants.

By March 1983, all delivery rooms and NICUs were required to post notices stating that all disabled infants would receive life-sustaining treatment. For a while, decisions were being made to support all infants regardless of the parents' wishes and the infant's best interests because hospitals feared legal reprisal and loss of federal funding. The controversy continued in and out of court, and legal opinions were repeatedly revised. Finally, in 1986, the courts decided that parents should be the primary decision makers for their child, so long as the decisions made were in the child's best interests.[2] In addition, the U.S. Supreme Court reiterated that child protection is a responsibility of the individual states and that each state, through its own child abuse and neglect laws, can intervene if it believes that parents are not acting in the best interests of their child.[2] Thus, four years of federal intervention ended with a clearer outline for decision making. Most important, the rulings included provision for parental input and supported the concept of multidisciplinary hospital committees to examine both medical and ethical aspects when critical decisions concerning disabled and gravely ill infants are being made.

The Role of the Ethics Committee

The concept of the Infant Care Review Committee was a beneficial result of the federal processes of the 1980s. In some hospitals, this committee may be part of a larger Bioethics Committee. The members of the Bioethics Committee may include physicians (neonatologists, pediatricians, or subspecialists), nurses, social workers, chaplains, and ethicists. The Bioethics Committee is asked to give an opinion to help resolve issues when there are no clear-cut answers. Cases involving complicated, difficult treatment decisions are presented to the committee for its opinion. The committee's decision is not binding but is carefully considered because it is based on the thinking of individuals with differing perspectives and ethical points of view. The table on page 246 explains these perspectives.

Not all decisions regarding whether to continue or stop treatment are difficult to make. Some may be straightforward; after a thorough assessment, it may be clear that the infant has a condition clearly incompatible with life, and futile medical therapies can be discontinued. Bioethics Committees arose because of the need to make decisions that are not straightforward. They allow a forum for those involved with the baby to offer facts, information, and opinions about the patient and his prognosis.

This does not mean that decision making has been standardized. Physicians in one hospital may treat an infant who physicians in another hospital would not treat. This is simply because caregivers cannot always predict who will benefit from care. With aggressive treatment and prolonged care, critically ill babies sometimes do well and survive with few complications; other babies are left severely impaired or even die.

In some hospitals, parents attend the Bioethics Committee's meeting or parts of it. In other hospitals, someone (usually a primary nurse or a social worker) acts as the parents' advocate.[2] You may be excluded from meetings to allow the committee to discuss the case freely and form a unified opinion. If you and the committee can then reach a mutually agreeable decision, you will work with the health care team directly involved in your baby's care to formulate a plan to implement the decision.

If the members of the Bioethics Committee are unable to reach a consensus, or if you disagree with their opinion, a court of law may be the forum for resolution. A child welfare agency may seek guardianship of your child if the hospital does not believe you are acting in his best interests. This is usually a last resort, after all avenues of conflict resolution have been utilized (second opinions brought in by you or the medical team, referral to the hospital Bioethics Committee, and so on). If your situation is presented in a court of law and one side presents the case for life, the judge(s) will usually rule for the life of the infant to be continued.[2]

The Rights and Responsibilities of a Parent

As a parent, you have the option of allowing your baby's care to continue, of adding no further treatment, or of stopping treatment and allowing your infant to die. The decision to stop treatment for your baby is very complicated. Unlike the members of the Bioethics Committee and the NICU staff, you will have to live with your loss every day.

Make this decision only when you are ready. When the medical team approaches you about making a decision, you may not be ready. As your baby's hospital course progresses, however, you may reassess the situation and conclude that it's time to make a decision. That is your prerogative as a parent. The medical team should respect your timetable. An action plan for treatment decision making is found on page 247.

Ethical Perspectives of the Bioethics Committee

1. *Your right as parents to decide.* Your right to decide in privacy is protected under the U.S. Constitution, as long as this right does not conflict with child abuse and neglect laws.

2. *The infant's best interests.* The infant's best interests are the primary issue in the decision-making process. It is usually not in the best interests of the infant to prolong futile treatments or suffering and dying.

3. *The parents' best interests.* The parents' best interests may be considered if the infant's best interests conflict with them. If the infant's care will place an undue burden on the family, this ethical precept may be used for decision making.

4. *The doctor's duties.* The doctor's duties can conflict with the infant's best interests. Some physicians feel strongly that they have to use all available medical technology, and this may conflict with their duty to relieve suffering. The line between helpful therapies and futile therapies may not always be clear-cut.

5. *Heroic measures.* Heroic measures or extraordinary means of support may be overutilized. The term extraordinary refers to therapy that is futile and a burden to the patient. A ventilator can be ordinary for a premature infant who is recovering from respiratory distress syndrome, but extraordinary for an infant who will never recover from multiple problems.

6. *Right to life versus a life worth living.* The concept of a "right to life" versus a "life worth living" is a particularly difficult one. Quality of life means different things to different people. In the 1990s, many view mental impairment as a tragedy, and the quality-of-life precept would therefore be important in their decision. Others believe all life is sacred, regardless of qualifiers. For those individuals, this precept would have no place in decision making.

7. *Fair share of resources.** Although financial considerations should perhaps not enter into the decision, more often now we are forced to think realistically about how to pay for such care.

Adapted from: Scully T, and Scully C. 1987. The Baby Doe dilemma: To treat or not to treat. In *Playing God: The New World of Medical Choices.* New York: Simon & Schuster, 202–208. Reprinted by permission of the authors.

Editor's Note: *In a perfect world, cost would not be a factor, and there would be enough medication and treatment for everyone who is ill. The current fiscal climate, however, requires that society as a whole think realistically about how to pay for expensive therapies. If one infant requires many days of intensive care treatment, does this mean that another infant will not receive therapy he may need? Some states have begun to evaluate costs versus benefits for adult patients who require expensive or scarce therapies and depend upon government health insurance. Decisions regarding provision of care are being made based on the likelihood of the patient benefiting from the therapy.*

Action Plan for Treatment Decision Making

1. Get all the medical facts about your baby's condition, his treatment options, and the likely outcome of each option.

2. Don't be rushed into making a decision. If a true emergency exists, the decision should usually be to treat the infant until there is time to consider the alternatives.

3. Be clear about whose needs will be met by any proposed decision—your needs, your infant's, the doctors', the nurses', the hospital's, or those of medical science.

4. Discuss your feelings, your anxieties, and all questions you have with your own physician, the baby's doctor, nurses, and specialists caring for your infant. Ask for a second or third opinion if you feel it might help in resolving your dilemma.

5. Talk to others who can assist you in making your decision, such as a minister, rabbi, or priest or the hospital pastoral counselor or social worker. Other parents who have made the difficult choice to withhold treatment and allow their baby to die may provide you with support in making your decision. Similarly, parents who are raising disabled children can often dispel myths and relieve anxiety about what the future may hold for your infant.

6. Consider the financial, physical, and emotional impact your decision will have on you and your family.

7. Ask to see your baby if you want to do so. When an infant is severely deformed, some physicians and nurses try to spare parents further emotional pain by advising them not to see the baby. It's all right to agree, but you should be the one to make that decision. Many parents who have imagined the worst have been glad to see their infant and even to hold him before he died.

8. If the hospital's infant Bioethics Committee reviews your baby's care, be sure you express your views, concerns, and preferences as fully as possible. Ask a friend, counselor, family member, or other supportive person to attend the meeting with you.

9. Read all informed consent documents carefully. Ask questions if you don't understand what you are being asked to agree to. You have a right to get information in words you can understand.

From: Scully T, and Scully C. 1987. The Baby Doe dilemma: To treat or not to treat. In *Playing God: The New World of Medical Choices.* New York: Simon & Schuster, 220–221. Reprinted by permission of the authors.

Physicians, nurses, and other health care team members will provide you with as much information as possible about your child's condition and prognosis. Ask as many questions as you need to, and then ask again, to make sure you understand the answers. Obtain a second opinion if you have access to resources and the time to do so. Generally, the neonatologists who work in any unit have reached their decision together. The decision to allow a baby to die is not made by one individual or by the parents alone.

Once a decision is made, parents often feel a great sense of relief. You may second-guess yourself and have some doubts, but these are normal feelings that will take time and sometimes professional help to resolve.[2] This may be the hardest decision you will ever have to make, but your participation in it ultimately gives you some control over the NICU experience. When treatment becomes futile and your baby is not going to get better, making the decision for a meaningful death is a parental right you can assert and will never regret.

Preparing to Say Farewell

You may feel very alone during this time, but you are probably surrounded by others who are also experiencing this loss. Grandparents, your older children, and close friends and relatives will grieve with you. Shielding them from the reality of the situation does not make the loss less acute.

Family Participation

Most NICU staff encourage family members, including older siblings, to share the death of the baby. Meeting the infant gives family members the opportunity to "know" him. Events may occur quickly: Birth, death, funeral, and burial may occupy only a few days. Sharing this time with others can make it more "real." In addition, when the family talks about the baby's death in the future, others will have known the baby and will be able to share precious memories and support.

Reuniting of Mother and Baby

If your baby was transported to another hospital, you may not be with him when difficult decisions are made or when your infant is near death. Find out what can be done to get you and your baby together. Laws, rules, and regulations vary widely, so ask the social worker and nurses for help when considering your options.

If you are the mother and you are medically stable, an early hospital discharge may be arranged to allow you to go to your baby. If hospital discharge is not an option, ask for a "pass" that allows you to leave the hospital but to return at a pre-arranged time for continued hospital care. In some cases, the hospital caring for your baby may authorize a back transport of the baby to the original hospital. Before agreeing to back transport, find out if your insurance carrier will cover the cost of the baby's transport and continued care at the mother's hospital.

Organ Donation

In October 1984, Loma Linda University Medical Center in California began performing human heart transplants in newborns stricken with a fatal congenital heart defect (anomaly) called hypoplastic left heart syndrome (HLHS). This syndrome affects 300 to 500 infants in the United States each year. Before transplantation became an option, a series of complex surgeries was the only hope for these children. These surgeries are high risk and have a high mortality rate; without intervention, however, this defect is always fatal.[3] Heart transplants have increased the number of infants who survive and thrive.

Hearts are not the only organs transplanted; livers, kidneys, blood vessels, and corneas have all been successfully utilized by infants and small children. Adults with glaucoma can also utilize corneas. Development of medications that reduce rejection of transplanted organs has greatly increased the success rate of transplants.

Rarely, infants who die in the NICU are eligible to become organ donors. There are no standard criteria for brain death in infants, as for older children and adults, but a paper published in 1989 describes clinical criteria that physicians can utilize.[4] Tests to determine brain death are performed in the NICU by a neonatologist and/or a pediatric neurologist. Brain death can be defined in several ways; however, it is commonly defined as an absence of brain stem reflexes such as breathing, sucking, gagging and blinking.[4] The criteria for organ donation are strict: The infant must be brain dead and infection free, and the organs that will be taken must be functioning normally. Specific tests—such as various blood tests, sonograms, and radiologic studies—are performed to evaluate each organ.

Brain death is a rare phenomenon. A study done at Loma Linda found that only 17 percent of neonatal deaths over a 14-year period carried the diagnosis of brain death. Of the 3.76 million live births in the United States per year, there are 40,000 neonatal deaths. Applying Loma Linda's 17 percent figure, about 400 infants per year in the United States might be brain dead and therefore possible organ donors.[4]

You may raise the possibility of organ donation, a physician or nurse involved in your baby's care may broach the subject, or someone you have never before met from hospital administration may bring it up. If your infant is dying and you would like to donate his organs, talk to the physician in charge of your baby's care.

Some states, such as New York, have laws under which all patients who have died or are dying are evaluated as possible organ donors.[5] If the patient meets the criteria, the physicians involved, a hospital administrator, or a transplant coordinator approaches the family. (A transplant coordinator works for a hospital that performs transplants or works for a local or national waiting list registry.)

If your infant is a suitable donor, organ donation will not rule out or delay a funeral.[3,6] Your baby will not be disfigured, so an open-casket service will still be possible. The surgeons, nurses, and staff who perform these proce-

"I felt lucky because we could donate our baby's organs to save another baby. At least there was some comfort in knowing our baby's death brought hope to someone else."

Message from a Grateful Parent

Dear Family,

It almost seems appropriate to think of you as family to us. You've done something for us that we could never have done for ourselves—given our son a second chance at life.

We gave him his first chance and have been struggling for 14 months to help him get by with his hopelessly inadequate little heart. It collapsed on him once and it took the doctors 30 minutes to revive him. Then you folks gave him a second chance.

As we were flying to the hospital holding him close to us with his older sister nearby, we had tears in our eyes thinking of you and your little girl. We're so thankful that good people like you can find the strength in their time of tragedy to think of others and remember that you have the power to give life to another. Your daughter has left a legacy during her short life that will live on and be a tribute to her. You are extraordinary people. To have the courage to donate your little girl's heart when I'm sure your hearts were broken is remarkable.

Our son is nearly 15 months old. He has battled courageously two heart surgeries (this transplant is his third cardiac surgery). His illness has crippled our family. He's been on oxygen the majority of his life, a tube placed in his stomach gives him nutrition, a probe attached to his toe constantly monitors whether his body is getting blood that is adequately oxygenated. Your daughter's heart may free him from all of this if he can pull through the tough transition period of adjusting to a new robust, healthy heart. His lungs have been damaged, but we're hoping and praying he'll pull through. He's a tough little guy.

You folks have been his only hope. I've become quite an emotional father and my eyes fill with tears even as I write this. Thank you. Thank you. Thank you. God bless you for rising above your grief to turn a tragedy into a saving act. Nothing can replace the loss of your sweet little girl, but a part of her lives on in a fellow human being. There can be no greater tribute to her. We give you our love and heartfelt sympathy at your loss. We are in your debt and can never possibly repay you. No one has done or can ever do anything greater for our family.

We love you,
Friends in need

Special thanks to Layne Kilpatrick, author of the preceding letter, and to Joyce Johnston, RN, CCRN, CCTC, Clinical Director/Cardiac Transplant, Loma Linda University Medical Center, Loma Linda, California. Reprinted by permission.

dures are sensitive and caring individuals who respect your infant as a person and who recognize your sorrow.

Neonatal organ donation is a very personal and emotional decision. Organ donation is not an alternative to life; only infants who are dead can be organ donors. There is no conflict of interest; the infant will die whether he is an organ donor or not. Ask as many questions as you have. Physicians, nurses, and social workers all serve as counselors for transplant programs. Transplant recipients may also work or volunteer for these programs, providing support, comfort, and information to families. Counselors who work with the registries are highly trained. They regularly deal with families wrestling with unexpected death and the decisions surrounding such circumstances. You may want to speak with family members and clergy; some religious beliefs preclude organ donation.

You may never have considered organ donation. But organ donation is a way of having something good come out of this terrible experience. Although it will not bring your child back to you, it may allow someone else's child to live. This is a very giving attitude—one you may have difficulty feeling fully in the acute stage of grief and loss. Looking back, however, parents who have donated their infant's organs have not regretted it. Again, this is a personal decision that parents should make as a team. But knowing that someone else was given a second chance at life may ease your sadness and grief at a later time.

"The doctors and nurses understand if you want to cry. I know this because they cried with me."

The Role of the NICU Staff

If the decision is made to let your infant die or to withdraw life-sustaining equipment, the physician caring for your child will discuss with you the details of how this will be done. Most often, babies on ventilators have their breathing tubes removed, or babies who depend on medications to maintain their circulation have the drugs stopped. When technologic support is withdrawn, babies are often sedated to prevent pain and suffering. If you have any questions or concerns about the procedure or pain relief, have them addressed before caregivers take any actions.

If a decision has been made to let your baby die, in most units the medical team will write something called a Do Not Resuscitate (DNR) order. These orders are most commonly utilized for older, terminally ill patients who wish to die peacefully. The DNR order prevents vigorous lifesaving measures from being carried out. If your baby is being supported with complex medical technology and you have made a decision that further treatment is futile, a DNR order allows the withdrawal of that technology so that the baby can die peacefully.

Education and personal coping strategies for managing death and dying influence how NICU staff members behave around the family of a dying baby. Most staff members are knowledgeable about the process and wonderfully supportive. Some team members, however, may seem to withdraw emotionally. Although they know that further treatment of your baby is futile, some physicians and nurses feel a great sense of failure when they realize there is nothing left "to do." If a staff member withdraws from you emotionally, do not interpret it as a criticism of your decision. The withdrawal probably reflects the staff member's own difficulty dealing with the many issues surrounding death in the NICU.

Naming the Baby

If you have not yet done so, name your child. Naming your baby will help you and others recognize that he was born and died, even though that life was very brief. It's up to you whether to use one of the names you may have selected before your baby's birth or to save those names for another child. If you cannot think of a name, ask your nurses, who would be privileged to make suggestions.

Baptism

Talk to your baby's nurses about the need for baptism or other important spiritual customs you wish to observe. Religious clergy are welcome in the NICU at your request, or ask for chaplaincy services if you wish clergy of a specific denomination. In most cases, nurses will baptize a dying baby if the parents' wishes are not known and a parent is not present.

Allowing the Baby to Die at Home

Not all infants with fatal anomalies or diseases require a lot of technologic support, and you may wish to take your baby home to die. If you decide to take your baby home, the NICU team will help you develop a home care plan, teach you what to expect as your baby's condition worsens, provide a contact person who will be available at all times to answer questions and give support, and provide an alternate plan in case home care becomes too difficult. If necessary, your baby can be readmitted to the hospital for supportive care (with a DNR order). Find out before discharge whether your baby would be readmitted to the NICU or to another unit.

Sending a baby home to die is unusual, and some units may have little or no experience with these circumstances. Speak with the nurse manager about what you would like to do and how you would like to do it. Some requests take time, so try to plan in advance and be flexible. Nurse managers and social workers can help you decipher rules and regulations, allow you to maintain control of the situation, and arrange events to your satisfaction.

The Gentle Good-Bye

While your infant is dying, the staff's main priority is the baby's comfort and companionship. If you are in the NICU, the staff will encourage you to hold your baby. He may still be attached to equipment or may be freed from most tubes and wires. If you are not in the unit and your infant's death is imminent and inevitable, your baby's nurse may hold your baby and make him comfortable. After your infant has died, most tubes and wires are disconnected, and you will be given the privacy you need to say good-bye to your child.

This may be the only time you are able to "parent" your baby, and it may be the only time you have been able to hold and care for your baby without wires and tubes getting in the way. You may hold your baby at any time during or following death. Some NICUs allow families to gather in a private hospital room to hold the baby and say good-bye. You may ask the nurse to stay with you or just to be available if you call her. Feel free to unwrap your baby's blanket and examine every inch. This is important parenting time, so do not feel pressured or hurried.

Remembering Your Baby

Most units have a camera and will offer to take pictures of your baby. There is an art to photographing a critically ill or deceased baby, and to some extent the expertise of the photographer will determine the quality and feeling of the photo. You may suggest that your baby be dressed or wrapped in a blanket and that your baby's arms and legs be supported with blanket rolls or your hands. You may wish to hold your baby for a family portrait. Some parents find these photos comforting: others are uncomfortable with them. If you do not want the photos, the staff will store them for you. Many parents request them some time after their baby's death.

Most units do not allow videotaping of critical events, but some may alter the rules if your baby's death is anticipated in a controlled setting—for example, when you are holding the baby in a private room. Pictures and videotapes are something you may put away and review on important dates, such as your baby's birthday, death date, and holidays.

The staff should also offer you the baby's belongings, such as blankets, clothing, footprints, crib card, and lock of hair if you request it. You may find all this comforting, but if you do not, at least hold onto these items. You may be glad to have them later on.

Seeing Your Baby Again

After your baby dies, he will be bathed. The nurses will do this, but you should be allowed to assist if you wish. Doing something comforting for your baby may help you say good-bye. After the bath, you may want to rock and hold your baby again. After you have said good-bye, your baby will be carried to the morgue.

If you wish to see your baby again, or if you were not present when your baby died, you may call the NICU and make arrangements to spend time with your baby. Most NICUs will provide a private place, wrap the baby in a warm blanket, and allow you to spend more time with your baby. Once your baby has left the NICU, ask how the hospital arranges for viewing and holding time.

After your baby has died, you will be asked to consider an autopsy. You will also need to make decisions about a funeral and burial or cremation, notify family and close friends about your baby's death, arrange for transport if your baby did not die at a hospital near your home, and perhaps

"A *year after Jessica's death,* I was ready to see the pictures the nurses had taken the day she died. I called the NICU *and her primary nurse sent them along with a lovely note about Jessie. Now I treasure these things.*"

Taking the Next Steps

253

deal with nursery furnishings and baby gifts. Again, take as much time as you need to sort out your choices. If you are having trouble, call on those who have helped and supported you up to now—your nurses, physicians, family, friends, social workers, and clergy.

Obtaining an Autopsy

Unless the cause of your baby's death is crystal clear, an autopsy may be one of the best things you can do for your child and for yourself. It may answer questions and provide explanations for what happened. There is no guarantee that it will answer all your questions, but an autopsy may be your best route to key information.

An autopsy will not significantly delay any funeral arrangements you may wish to make, so timing should not be a consideration in your decision. If other family members would like to see the baby before the autopsy, let everyone know when you give autopsy consent. In addition, an autopsy will not influence the type of wake or funeral you wish to have. An open casket is still possible, because pathologists are able to perform autopsies without disturbing the baby's face or hands.

Generally, the physician caring for your baby will obtain the autopsy consent. If you agree to an autopsy, make an appointment with your social worker and the infant's physician to review the results. The preliminary results may be known in a few days, but some lab results may take time. It's up to you when you want to learn the results. One month to six weeks after the death seems to be the time many parents are ready for this appointment; life has settled into a new routine, and you may be better able to handle the results. Usually, the physician and social worker who cared for your baby will meet with you and explain the results and, if you wish, give you a copy of the report. Any questions you may have can be answered at the meeting, but if you want more information at a later date, the physician should be a resource to you.

An autopsy will probably not provide all the information you wish to have. The cause of death sometimes remains unknown, and this can be frustrating. Although the autopsy may not identify the exact reason for your baby's death, it may reassure you that a number of possibilities—for example, genetic problems or suspected malformations—were not the cause.

Funeral Arrangements and Transport

A funeral allows you, your family, and close friends to say good-bye to your baby in a public way; it is a celebration of your baby's short life. It also allows public recognition that this person lived and had a profound influence on those lives he or she touched.

In the past, hospitals took care of a baby's body at the family's request. Today, parents or family members are financially responsible for these arrangements. Depending on the state in which you live, financial support may be available. If you are unclear about how to handle your baby's body, ask your nurse, social worker, or clergy about resources available to assist you.

Your social worker should be able to provide a list of reputable funeral homes and other available resources. Funeral homes sometimes donate the cost of a funeral for an infant.

Your beliefs may clearly define the type of funeral you will have, and a clergy member can assist you with the arrangements. Parents whose religious affiliation does not strictly prescribe funeral arrangements must make decisions about a traditional funeral and burial, a cremation and funeral service, or a simple memorial service with separate arrangements for the body.

If you have some definite ideas about how the wake and funeral should be handled, explain them to the funeral director. If you are having difficulty expressing your needs to a stranger, enlist the support of a resource person from the NICU (such as your nurse, clinical nurse specialist, social worker, or grief counselor) who can make phone calls with you. The funeral director is providing a service for you and should be able to meet your needs or, if something is absolutely impossible, to offer you acceptable alternatives. Do not feel shy or embarrassed about asking questions. Request an itemized list of the funeral home's charges and then consider cost-effective alternatives. For example, you may save a significant amount of money by dressing your baby yourself, before he is taken to the funeral home.

If your baby dies far from where you wish to bury him, the funeral home can arrange transport, or, if local laws allow, you may be able to transport the baby yourself. A knowledgeable funeral director or the hospital's grief counselor, social worker, or pastoral care personnel can help. Most are familiar with infants' and children's funerals. If you don't know how to proceed—for example, wake or no wake, open casket or closed, use of a cradle or bassinet for viewing, cremation or burial—ask your resource person to assist you.

Talking with Friends

As painful as it may be, you'll need to tell your close friends what has happened. If your baby's life was very short, friends may not be aware of the events surrounding the birth, and this may be your first chance to speak with them about your baby. Calling close friends helps mobilize support, validates your feelings of loss as they express their shock and grief, and helps make your baby's death more "real" for you. If you wish, ask a few close friends to pass the news to a list of other friends. This relieves you of endless phone calls. It may also prevent uncomfortable situations in which unknowing friends congratulate you on your baby's birth or bring gifts for the baby.

The Nursery and Baby Gifts

How you put away the baby's nursery is personal. You may wish to do it all yourself, a bit at a time or all at once. You may wish to do it with your partner or with other family members. Some parents request that family members or close friends put away the nursery for them. As grieving parents, you may need to communicate your needs clearly to well-meaning family members who would like to protect you from this painful task. Putting away the nursery may

"Most of our friends were there for us, helping out whenever they could, or just listening to us talk about our baby. But I was surprised and disappointed that some of my friends didn't call me after Joshua died. Really, what's so hard about saying, 'I'm so sorry this happened. Can I do anything to help?'"

be a form of healing closure, or you may decide that others would benefit more from this process. No one approach is correct. You will find your own way.

There are no rules of etiquette for managing baby gifts. You may choose to save some gifts in remembrance of your baby or for a special baby in your future.

Because returning baby gifts to friends and family can be painful and awkward, consider donating them to a shelter or other volunteer organization. Those who have given gifts are probably also those from whom you have or will receive sympathy. When you thank them for their support, let them know what happened to their gift.

If someone lent you furniture or made a major investment, however, offer to return the item. Make all these decisions at your own pace. You'll know when it's time.

Understanding Grief

Grief is an emotional response that occurs when someone close to you dies or when something else you value (such as a "perfect" birth experience) is lost. Grief is not an intellectual or rational response. Grief reactions differ from person to person, just as the depth and range of other emotions do. Grief is a strong emotion, marked by more intense feelings than those experienced in everyday life.[7] Because of its emotional nature, grief is very unsettling. A grieving person feels loss of control. He or she also feels overwhelmed, as well as all-consumed.[8] Some physical and behavioral signs of grief are given in the table on page 260.

Grief as a Process

Elisabeth Kübler-Ross first described the stages of grief in her book *On Death and Dying*.[9] Grief can be viewed as a process with different stages. It's important to recognize that no two people grieve the same way. Not everyone experiences all the stages of the grief process, and individuals experiencing the same loss may not experience the stages at the same time or in the same way. Partners may also grieve differently because their level of attachment to the lost child or the lost outcome is different. Most mothers attach earlier than fathers do because the reality of pregnancy is apparent earlier to the mother.[10]

Stage 1: Shock and Denial

The first stage of grief is shock and denial. This stage is characterized by disbelief and/or a refusal to accept your infant's death. At this stage, you may be unable to cope with usual life tasks and may need support people to assist you. Yet at this time, when you are least able to function, you may be responsible for making difficult decisions regarding organ donation, autopsy, and funeral arrangements.

If you know that your baby is going to die, you can make some of these decisions in a thoughtful manner with the assistance of family members, clergy, health care providers, and others you may wish to consult. If your baby dies suddenly, however, you may need time to absorb this reality before making decisions. If a baby has been transported to a different hospital than his mother and dies soon after, the father may be separated from the mother and too overwhelmed to speak up for himself or his partner. In any case, in this first stage of grief, you need time to gather support and information to make decisions.

Stage 2: Anger

The second stage of grief is anger, characterized by an awareness of the loss of your baby. You may be angry at health care providers for being unable to save your infant, at your infant for dying, or at other couples for having healthy, normal children. Anger can become destructive if partners blame each other for their infant's death or if the anger develops into guilt and self-blame. At this stage, you may analyze the situation endlessly, reviewing your behavior and thoughts in an effort to find a reason for the loss. The question "Why me?" is common. That question is often followed by "Is it because...?" questions addressed to the nurses, physician, social worker, or others involved in the care of your baby. Accurate information should help you resolve guilt for factors out of your control.

Stage 3: Bargaining

From early in life, most people bargain as a way to gain control of unpleasant situations. Bargaining parents try to make a deal with their supreme being—in fact, bargaining is sometimes considered a form of prayer. For example, "if you save my baby, I'll stop smoking and go to church more often." This stage may occur in conjunction with the shock and denial stage, as a way to delay recognition of the loss. Mostly, it is a beginning step in accepting that something terrible has occurred while still desperately trying to change the situation.

Stage 4: Withdrawal and Depression

The fourth stage of grief is withdrawal and depression. You accept your baby's death and realize you have reason to be sad. You may withdraw from other family members, from friends, and from medical personnel. This is a listless period. You may be too tired to interact or deal with others. Silence fills this time; the loss may still be too acutely painful to discuss, yet all other topics of conversation pale in comparison. Nothing is more important than this loss. This may be a very lonely time for parents, especially after the funeral, as others get on with their lives. This may also be the time when partnerships experience the most strain: You are barely able to help yourself and thus cannot help your partner. One partner may move on to the fifth stage of grief, acceptance, while the other needs more time to resolve the situation and to heal emotionally. It may seem as if this period takes a very long time; the days can be endless. Parent support groups can be helpful at this point. Knowing that others feel or have felt the same way and are or have been in the same situation can be a great comfort.

Stage 5: Acceptance of Loss

The last stage of the grieving process is acceptance of the loss. In the case of a child's death, this means accepting the loss of a life and its future. In the case of a serious disability, it means accepting the loss of the "perfect" child. Gradually, you resume a daily schedule, and the loss becomes less acutely painful. At this stage, you may be able to discuss your feelings with family members and friends. At this time or later you may decide to lead a support group for other parents who have experienced a loss, or you may become active in an organization that focuses on a particular disability or disease. As advocates for children, parents can have a profound impact on the health care system through lobbying or raising money for research.

Differences in How Men and Women Grieve

Expression of grief varies between the sexes. This is partly because of societal expectations of behaviors for each sex—that is, views of what is appropriate masculine and appropriate feminine behavior. Society expects men to be strong and unemotional in a crisis, while women are allowed to cry and "fall apart." Research has shown that women generally express grief outwardly, through crying, sadness, anger, and use of medications, while men tend to grieve inwardly, not expressing their feelings and remaining stoic through their loss.[11,12] Although the research describing these sex-based responses was done in the 1960s and 1970s, much appears still applicable today. Loss seems to provoke a return to traditional values.[10] Women feel as though they have to take care of their mate, both physically and emotionally. On the other hand, men may become distant and uncommunicative, unable to show emotions because it makes them too vulnerable. They may be too ashamed to show their partner how lost and sad they feel, believing that they have to be strong. A man may not want his partner to see him in this lost, vulnerable state.[10] Fathers have been ignored in the grieving process because of the erroneous belief that they do not experience the same loss as mothers.[10] Fortunately, popular culture has become far more accepting of masculine displays of emotion. Greater freedom to display their emotions and grieve openly may let men resolve their grief in a healthier manner.

Lack of communication between partners has been cited as one of the reasons for the high divorce rate among couples who have lost an infant to death, congenital anomalies, or mental retardation.[10] The loss of a child may well be the first major crisis a couple must face together. It can be frightening to see your partner lose control, and it may be difficult to deal with a crisis if both of you are lost, overwhelmed, and unable to support each other. The stress is great, and the potential for misunderstanding each other is high. Couples who communicate well are often able to deal with small misunderstandings before they become insurmountable problems.

Grief and Joy Together

A parent has written, "Grief is individual—and it is not so orderly... I think professionals and friends could be more supportive if they spent less time second-guessing where we are and more time dealing with how we are."[13] This is particularly true when one or more babies of a multiple pregnancy dies and one or more survives.

One mother has described this situation as "grieving and loving at the same time. But it's not like pulling and tugging. It's more like ripping and tearing. There are two violently different pulls."[14] Similar feelings occur when one child is healthy and the other is not. Your emotions are on a roller-coaster ride as you both celebrate the birth and life of a healthy child and grieve for what has been lost.

When one or more children from a multiple birth die in the NICU, it is not unusual for the grieving parents to wish that all their babies had died. In seeking relief from the turmoil, some parents may feel it would be easier just to grieve rather than to grieve while continuing to deal with ongoing NICU problems.[14] These are perfectly normal feelings. With time, the balance becomes easier. With time, you will learn to be happy for the surviving baby and develop the ability to deal with that child's problems while grieving for the baby who has died.

"Losing your baby changes your marriage. You both have to make an effort to stay close, and stay strong. It takes time and a whole lot of patience."

Coping with Grief

At this point in your life, it may seem that nothing will ever make you feel good again. No one can tell you exactly how to get through this experience, but you may find some of the following suggestions helpful.

If you have previously experienced a loss or have survived crises before, try to recall what helped you most in that situation. Falling back on old coping strategies may provide a way for you to get through this new experience. Also, try to maintain your usual daily habits, even if you are unable to sleep. A sense of "routine" may help you feel more normal and less "lost."[14]

During this time, you may find relief by expressing yourself artistically. This serves two purposes. First, it can help you sort through your emotions day by day. Second, when everything is over and for many years to come, your work will provide you with remembrances and memories of a bittersweet time. It is entirely up to you whether you share these outlets or keep them as your personal secret. Some parents have developed their journals into published books after their NICU experience has ended.[15,16] Some creative coping strategies include writing (a letter to your baby, poetry, a journal) or drawing, painting, pottery, or sculpture.

Others have found solace in activities such as exercising, throwing unbreakables at a wall, resting, and talking to supportive friends and family.

When they feel ready, many parents find it helps to plant a tree as a memorial to their baby, donate time or money to a children's charity, become a parent volunteer and lend support to other NICU parents, or become politically active for a children's cause.

Physical and Behavioral Signs of Grief

Physical Signs

Gastrointestinal System
Anorexia and weight loss
Overeating
Nausea and vomiting
Abdominal pain or feeling of
  emptiness
Diarrhea and constipation

Respiratory System
Sighing respiration
Choking or coughing
Shortness of breath
Hyperventilation

Cardiovascular System
Cardiac palpitations
  ("fluttering" in chest)
"Heavy" feeling in chest

Neuromuscular System
Headaches
Vertigo (dizziness)
Syncope (fainting)
Brissaud's disease (tics)
Muscular weakness or loss
  of strength

Behavioral Signs

Feelings of
Guilt
Sadness
Anger and hostility
Emptiness and apathy
Helplessness
Pain, desperation, and
  pessimism
Shame
Loneliness

**Preoccupation with the
Image of the Lost Infant**
Daydreams and fantasies
Nightmares
Longing

**Disturbed Interpersonal
Relationships**
Increased irritability and
  restlessness
Decreased sexual interest
  and drive
Withdrawal
Crying

**Inability to Return to Normal
Activities**
Fatigue and exhaustion or
  aimless overactivity
Insomnia or oversleeping
Short attention span
Slow speech, movement, and
  thought processes
Loss of concentration and
  motivation

From: Gardner SL, Merenstein GB, and Costello AJ. 1993. Grief and perinatal loss.
In *Handbook of Neonatal Intensive Care,* 3rd ed., Gardner SL, and Merenstein
GB, eds. St. Louis: Mosby-Year Book, 537–538. (Modified from Lindemann E.
1944. *American Journal of Psychiatry* 101:144–146. Copyright 1944, The
American Psychiatric Association; Marris P. 1974. *Loss and Change.* New York:
Pantheon; and Colgrove M. 1976. *How to Survive the Loss of a Love.* New York:
Lion Publishing.) Reprinted by permission.

Helping Others Cope with Their Grief

Coping with your own feelings may seem like all you can do right now. But as you move through the grieving process, you may find yourself supporting those around you.

Grandparents

Your baby's grandparents will grieve in their own ways for their own reasons. Like parents, they grieve the loss of the future. Grandparents develop their own fantasies about their grandchild—what the baby will look like, what they will do together, what they hope the child will become. When a grandchild dies or is severely disabled, grandparents also mourn the loss of that future.

In addition, grandparents hurt for you—their own children. They never stop being parents, and your pain compounds their grief. But don't overlook the support your parents offer. They may be separated from the situation enough to help you make plans and decisions.

Your Baby's Siblings

Sibling grief reactions vary depending upon the age of the sibling. Although younger children may not fully comprehend what has occurred, even the youngest child will sense the emotional turmoil surrounding the loss of the baby.[10]

Unlike adults, children do not grieve continuously; rather, they do so sporadically.[17] Much to your surprise, your children may be able to continue their daily routine and play and eat as usual. Then, when you least expect it, one of them may remember something about the baby and become sad.[17]

Some predictable grief reactions occur in children. They may feel guilty because they believe that they caused their sibling's death or disability by wishful thinking. They may have resented the baby and feel secretly relieved when the baby does not come home. They may misbehave as an attention-getting ploy and may regress in their behavior (go back to thumb-sucking or bed wetting, for example). They may experience frightening thoughts that others are going to die. They may also be frightened at the strong emotions they see from you for the first time.

Children are as unique as adults and may grieve in unique ways. An unconcerned attitude that continues without any change, however, may be a signal that your child is denying the situation or is unable to express his or her emotions.[18] Your child may benefit from professional counseling in dealing with the feelings; no child should be totally nonreactive to the loss of a sibling.

Even though it can be difficult while you are grieving, remember that your surviving children need you. Be as honest as possible with your children without going into too much detail. Answer questions concisely with as much explanation as you feel is appropriate. It's all right to admit that you don't have all the answers. Resources are available to assist you, but remember: You know your children best. Trust your instincts as you struggle with what to say.

When explaining death to children, use real words and express the problems honestly. Children may need reassurance that the same thing will not happen to them. Avoid likening death to sleep; doing so may result in sleeping problems. Be honest: "The baby was born too early, and she was too small," "The baby's heart didn't work right, and he couldn't make it," "The baby was born very sick, and she died," "The baby's problems are nobody's fault."

If you decide not to let your child see the baby, do not withhold knowledge of the infant. Even children as young as two or three years can sense a parent's turmoil and know that something very sad is occurring. Parents should honestly acknowledge what is happening and how they feel. Young children (generally those over the ages of six to eight years) can participate in a funeral or memorial service and may benefit from saying good-bye to their infant sibling.

A unique problem sometimes faces the sibling survivor(s) of a multiple pregnancy in which one or more of the babies have died. Survivors often feel a sense of missing something; they shared a womb with their sibling(s) yet do not share their lives. As soon as your child begins to ask questions about his birth, tell your surviving child or children their birth story, and address any fears and questions.[14] You may develop unique ways of celebrating events for the survivor(s) while remembering your lost infant(s).[14] Your family will decide the best way to celebrate and mourn simultaneously.

Friends

Friends may respond to your loss in a number of ways. Some who are sad and scared for you may withdraw simply because they do not know what to

---

The Concept of Death: Developmental Stages in Children's Understanding

Age	Concept of Death
Preschool	• See death as temporary, impersonal, and reversible • May think they can wish people dead when angry and have them back when it pleases them *Reaction:* Questioning, curiosity; will not be a closed subject
5–9 years	• Accept death as final and that all living things must die • Do not see death as a personal experience • Feel they can escape through their own efforts *Reaction:* Aggression, personification
9–11 years	• Begin to achieve a realistic view of death • Feel they are "invincible" and will not die until later in life *Reaction:* Anger, hostility
12+	• Have concept of death similar to adult concept • Do not accept meaning of personal death *Reaction:* May take unnecessary chances with own life

Adapted from: Trouy MB, and Larson C. 1987. Sibling grief. *Neonatal Network* 5(4): 35–40. Reprinted by permission.

do or say. Others may be more comfortable with your grief, stay close, and support you through this difficult time.

Many people have difficulty speaking to mourning parents and say nothing or the wrong thing. You will probably encounter many well-intentioned people with a knack for saying the wrong thing: "You're young, you can have others" and "This happened for the best."[14] You will probably also have dear, close friends who realize that "I'm sorry," "We're thinking of you," or just their presence is a great comfort to you.

Duration of Grief

Your life has now changed forever. Things are never the same after a child dies. But you will eventually find a new place of emotional peace where you feel comfortable and belong.

An Individual Timetable

Generally, the grief process takes two years.[19] Four factors influence its length, however:[7]
1. The nature of your loss
2. The level of significance of your loss
3. Your willingness to experience the intensity of your feelings about your loss
4. The quality of the support system available to you

People grieve at their own pace, depending on the variables just listed and on their personality. The first year is usually one of experiencing all the "firsts," living a full year of special dates (birthdays and holidays) and feeling the acute pain of your loss as these dates occur. Even though your baby's death may not affect how your family celebrates a particular event, you may feel your loss most at family gatherings.

The second year is usually spent looking toward the future, reorganizing your life without your baby in it. As time passes, your loss will feel less physically painful, and you'll learn to laugh again. Expect to experience occasional "blue" days, when some date or event causes you to re-experience your grief. If you feel you are too sad for too long, consider a support group or private therapy.

Chronic Sorrow

Grief may never completely resolve in the case of a disabled or chronically ill child. This may result in an ongoing process known as chronic sorrow. One woman describes its presence: mostly quiet, but occasionally erupting for different reasons. Chronic sorrow is not homogeneous—that is, it doesn't feel the same at all times. At times, the sorrow is strongly felt; in other situations, it is barely perceived. It is not a sorrow that can be cured, nor is it abnormal. It is an unresolved sorrow, because caring for or giving up a physically or mentally impaired child is an unresolvable situation.[13]

If you experience chronic sorrow, you are not alone. Of all children in the United States, 10 to 15 percent have some chronic health impairment; 1 to 2 percent of children have some severe chronic health conditions with special needs.[20]

Accepting help from others can help you conserve your strength, especially when your situation is ongoing. Respite care for you and your partner can help you recharge. Especially if your child is difficult to care for, you need to take breaks to avoid exhaustion. Don't be embarrassed to ask for help. Others, even close friends and relatives, may not realize how difficult your daily situation is. Community resources may also provide respite care and/or sponsor support groups. A social worker may be able to help you locate such resources. Support groups have been formed for almost every illness and disease (see Appendix D). Most parents find them helpful—as a source of information, if not emotionally.

At some point, you will accept your situation and be able to function and grow, albeit much differently than you may ever have imagined.

Questioning "Normalcy"

Throughout the grief process, be it for a lost child or a chronically ill child, you may question your "normalcy" again and again. "Is feeling this emotion normal?" "Have I been feeling sad, angry, or confused for too long?" Most people are able to negotiate the grief process with strong support from their partner, family members, friends, and coworkers. However, you may want to obtain help from a therapist, family counselor, social worker, or other professional if you feel you need it or if any of the following is occurring:[21]

- You are afraid you may physically harm yourself or someone else; you have thoughts of suicide.
- You are participating in activities that may damage your health (drug or alcohol abuse or overeating).
- The support of friends and family members is not enough.
- You sustain repeated losses.
- You suffer from low self-esteem, feel out of control, or feel "stressed out" all the time.

A Bittersweet Time

Few things in life are more difficult than making decisions for a disabled, chronically ill, or dying baby. Drawing on the love and support of family, friends, and the health care team will help you make the choices that will ultimately be best for you and your child. It may take time for your decisions to feel completely right. The choices facing you are complex and will awaken many new emotions. As time goes by, though, you'll be thankful that you were empowered to make these choices for your baby and grateful that you were able to control some aspects of this very overwhelming time in your life.

Chapter 14

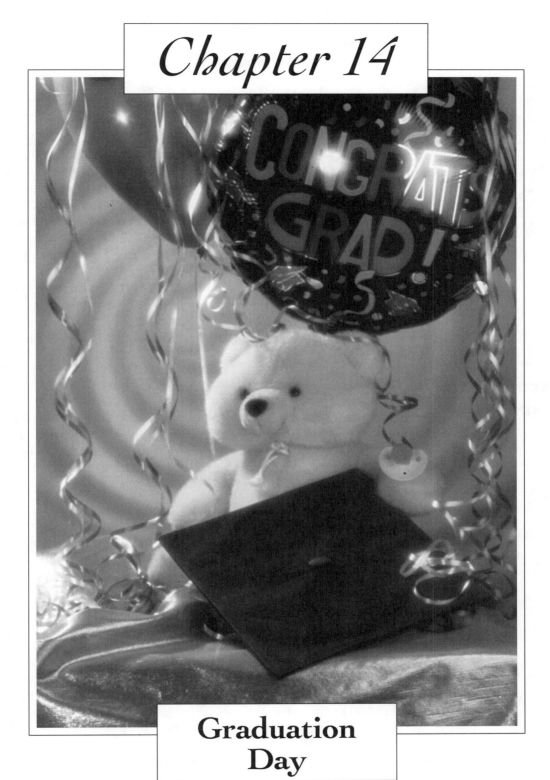

Graduation Day

Sharon Gregory, RNC, MN, CNNP

❝"All right," said Eeyore. "We're going. Only Don't Blame Me."❞

One day when you call to check on your baby, the nurse will tell you, "It's graduation day! Your baby will be leaving the NICU and going to the step-down unit." Graduation sounds like progress (and it is!), but what else changes? Being an NICU parent has meant dealing with daily changes, but by now you have developed a comfort level with the NICU staff, equipment, routines, and visiting procedures. Many things will be different in the new unit. This change means another period of adjustment.

This chapter explains what intermediate care is and what happens if this change in care means your baby must move to a new hospital. It also looks at ways in which you'll begin to play a more active role in your baby's care—and at a few complications that could delay your baby's progress toward discharge.

The Intermediate Care Experience

Some babies go home directly from the NICU, but most NICU babies are eventually transferred to a step-down unit for less intensive care before discharge. The step-down unit may be within the NICU itself or very nearby. Some NICUs transfer babies to a community hospital for continued convalescence. Knowing what to expect in the way of routines, staff members, and your role during this period of hospitalization will help alleviate your stress and enable you to participate in your baby's care more fully.

Intermediate Care Defined

The name of the step-down unit and the criteria for transfer to it vary from hospital to hospital. The unit may be called Intermediate Care, NICU Step-Down, Special Care, Growing Premie Unit, Level II Unit, or something else. Whatever the unit is called, your baby's transfer to it means that she has matured beyond the need for intensive life support. With a few rare exceptions, your baby is past the life-and-death crises and is on the road home. She has probably been weaned off the ventilator and possibly off oxygen. She has received feedings by tube and may have experimented with bottle or breast-feeding. Intravenous fluids have been discontinued or your baby is being weaned from them. If preterm, your baby probably weighs 2½ to 3 pounds (around 1,200 grams) when the transfer to intermediate care occurs.

As your NICU nurse prepares you for your baby's graduation, she may describe the intermediate care nursery as a quieter place, more able to work with your baby's sleep-wake cycles and abilities to interact with her surroundings. Because growing babies need lots of undisturbed rest, feeding time is usually the best time for interaction; therefore, your nurse may suggest that you begin to visit more frequently. Since your baby no longer requires frequent intensive nursing care, expect her nurse to have three to five other babies under her care. Some intermediate care settings keep the same nursing staff (your baby may even keep the same primary nurse) for the entire hospitalization. Or the RN in the intermediate care unit may supervise specially trained nursing assistants who help with feeding, vital signs, and other care tasks. Occupational or physical therapy personnel may be more visible in intermediate care as they work with you and your baby on feeding skills, positioning, comforting, and other behavioral and physical tasks. In intermediate care, there is generally a greater focus on parent involvement. Learning to care for your baby becomes the focal point of your visits.

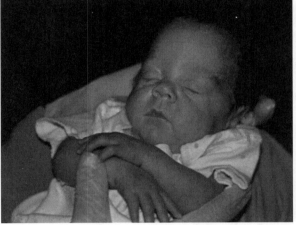

Ready for intermediate care.

With most of his medical crises behind him, this baby is now a "gainer and grower."

When you call to check on your baby in intermediate care, there will usually be less to report. Unless some complication occurs, your baby's condition will change much less often than in the NICU. Lab work, x-rays, and other tests are less frequent in intermediate care, and monitor alarms are heard less often. The staff focuses on your baby's progress and your plans for actively participating in care.

Emotional Changes

In the NICU, you may have been mostly an observer, watching nurses, respiratory therapists, doctors, and specialists care for your baby. You probably developed trusting relationships with members of the NICU staff—usually those staff who always discussed your baby's case openly and honestly and were willing to listen to your feelings and concerns. If your move to the intermediate care nursery means a change of personnel, you'll probably miss the comfortable working relationships you shared. You and your baby will need some time to get acquainted with a new team and to learn how to communicate well with that team. Eventually you will develop good communication and trusting relationships with staff members in the intermediate care nursery, just as you did with those in the NICU.

As things slow down, you may find that emotions from the past weeks are catching up with you. Your baby's major crises are over, but as you start to relax, you may also begin to feel the emotions that you've been too numb to acknowledge until now. You may have been too frightened or overwhelmed to express some of those feelings, but now they seem to come tumbling out at your partner, the nursery staff, and anyone else who is willing to listen. This outpouring will slow down eventually.

There are ways to gain control over these emotions. *Think* about what you are feeling. *See* your behavior as an expression of overwhelming emotion. *Talk* to a friend, your partner, or a counselor. *Write* in a journal or talk into a tape recorder. The length of time this process takes depends on the length of time your child was in the NICU, how early in your pregnancy your infant was born, how many life-and-death crises your baby experienced in the NICU, your support system, and your personal coping style. Ask your baby's nurse if the hospital has a support group, social worker, clinical nurse specialist, chaplain, or other person who supports the emotional needs of parents. Keep in mind that what you have been going through would be very stressful for any parent. Find coping skills that work for you.

By now, you're probably not the same passive, uninformed, and frightened parent who first visited the NICU. Now that you've observed and learned so much about NICU practices, your biggest challenge in adjusting to this new unit will be accepting that *different* is not necessarily *wrong*. Adjusting to new faces and new routines will take time. Your communication techniques (see Chapter 3) will need review and fine-tuning as you negotiate a new plan of care for your baby. If you're not given an orientation list for the intermediate care unit, review your original NICU orientation list (see Chapter 4) and investigate the plan for the remainder of your baby's hospital stay. This effort will communicate to staff that you're interested in how this new unit works. Most important, it will help you find out what you need to know about the unit to get comfortable so you can focus on learning to care for your baby before she is discharged.

Back Transport

If your baby was transferred to the NICU from a community hospital, the doctor may discuss transporting her back to your community hospital for continued convalescence and preparation for discharge. Back transport—also called return transport—is common in hospitals where acute-care beds, such as those in the NICU, are used for the sickest infants and less intensive care is done in community hospitals in the area.

Anxieties about Transfer

Feelings of anxiety as you face yet another change are normal. A tour of the community hospital special-care nursery can help allay many concerns about a transfer. Ask your social worker or primary nurse to call the nurse manager or clinical nurse specialist at the community hospital nursery and make an appointment for you to tour the nursery. Also check the financial aspects of back transport with a financial counselor or your insurance company to ensure that your coverage provides for back transport and transfer of hospital care.

Community hospitals with special-care nurseries are pleased and excited to care for your baby. Because basic care of a growing preterm or convalescing infant does not require the high level of vigilance and technology found in major medical centers, you may discover that you can learn to care for your baby in a more relaxed atmosphere and also receive more individual attention at the intermediate care nursery.

If your baby requires complex care—for a colostomy or a shunt, for example—you may need reassurance that the specialists involved in her care will still be available through the intermediate care nursery. Ask what access the community nursery has to specialty staff—such as ophthalmologists, audiologists, and pulmonologists—for consultations. Ask the nurse at the community hospital at what point it might be necessary to transport a baby with unanticipated difficulties back to the NICU and how this would be accomplished.

Your community hospital may be closer to home than the regional NICU and more convenient for visiting your baby. People who can help you as you and your baby make the transition to home are probably more available at the community hospital and are familiar with local support sources, such as medical equipment supply companies and community home health services.

With your questions answered, you should feel more secure about your baby's transfer to a community hospital intermediate care nursery. Most parents find this more peaceful atmosphere a welcome relief after the NICU.

If, however, you have serious reservations about the ability of the community hospital nursery to meet your baby's complicated care requirements or about follow-up services, make your concerns heard immediately to your discharge planner or neonatologist. You may not be able to make the ultimate decision, but a compromise may be reached that meets the needs of both your baby and the NICU. A delay in transfer or transfer to a different community hospital may be possible, but this will no doubt be a collaborative decision. Even though your feelings are running high, it's important to maintain some objectivity and present your case calmly and in a spirit of cooperation. You and the NICU staff have invested a lot to get your baby to the point where intermediate care is possible. Everyone shares your goal of a healthy baby at discharge.

Adjustments to This Change

As the transport incubator carrying your baby rolls into the intermediate care nursery at your community hospital, you may ask yourself just how you'll survive the stress of another adjustment. This may be a difficult transition. Many parents suffer separation anxiety and even feelings of abandonment as they leave the security of the NICU. Sometimes they transfer those angry feelings to the new nursery staff, delaying the development of good communication. But as you allow yourself to become comfortable with these new faces and routines, the sense of partnership will return.

Transport is stressful for babies, too. Yours may be sleepier or more irritable than usual or may not tolerate feedings well for the first 24 hours in the new environment. Some babies require a slight increase in supplemental oxygen following a transport or lose weight for the first few days. These temporary setbacks rarely reflect poor caregiving by the new nursery staff. Given an opportunity for quiet rest, your baby will quickly recover and adapt to this new environment. This is not the time to introduce new stressors, however, such as stepping up the bottle or breastfeeding schedule or quickly weaning your baby out of the incubator to a crib. As a parent, use this interim period to acquaint yourself with the staff and new routines.

"It was great to bring James back to our birth hospital. Some of those nurses had helped care for him the day he was born so sick, and we knew they would take good care of him now."

Unlike the parent whose baby convalesces in and is discharged from the same unit in the same hospital, you face the additional challenges of adjusting to and working with two hospital routines during this experience. It may help to know that the basic principles of intermediate care are the same in both community hospitals and hospitals with NICUs. The remainder of this chapter focuses on the intermediate care experience and what you may expect during this period of hospitalization.

Your Expanding Role in Care

Except in the unlikely case of complications, the intermediate care nursery is the gateway to home. In this environment suited for instruction and supervised practice, you and your baby will master the skills necessary for discharge. This is the time to take a more active role in your baby's care.

Negotiating the Schedule

You'll need to know your baby's schedule of activities to participate in care. Ask about the feeding schedule, bath time, and special treatments from respiratory therapy or physical therapy. Let the nurses know what you already feel comfortable doing (for example, changing a diaper) and what skills you're ready to tackle (such as giving vitamins). Nurses will gladly save a feeding or bath for parents or rearrange your baby's schedule to fit your visiting times. The intermediate care nursery also provides an excellent opportunity to begin or continue kangaroo care (see Chapter 4). Holding your baby in this special way gives you a chance to get to know her before homecoming.

Working with Your Baby's Cues Now

As an NICU parent, you've been taught about infant states and cues (see Chapter 4). As babies become more stable, they may develop distinct patterns of sleep and wakefulness. You may find your baby's states more predictable now. Use your observations as you work with your baby.

Your baby may take a few minutes to wake to the quiet alert state before feeding, for example. If you find your baby already awake or crying, you can use comforting techniques to re-establish a quiet alert state. If your baby is quietly looking at you, she is telling you to proceed. As you've already learned, be careful to introduce only one type of stimulation at a time. If your baby can look at your face, try speaking gently. Once your baby can handle both looking and listening, try rocking. Watch for new ways your baby has learned to cope with stimulation, such as finger-sucking, and encourage use of those coping tools. If the room is noisy or the lights are bright, your baby may become overstimulated. Be alert for signs of stress, and provide time-out periods when necessary. Because feeding time can be especially stressful for babies still perfecting their skills, ask the staff to help you control the environment as much as possible.

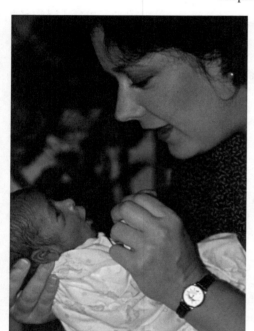

Clear invitation cues.

As your baby convalesces and matures, his periods of alertness are more sustained. This results in clear invitation cues from your baby.

Positioning Your Baby

The bigger your baby becomes, the more she will move around in bed. You have probably noticed positions she seems to prefer, however. Most babies prefer flexed positions and like boundaries around their bodies. You can help your baby get comfortable by making boundaries or nesting her with rolled blankets. The head of the bed may be tilted up if your baby tends to spit up after feeding.

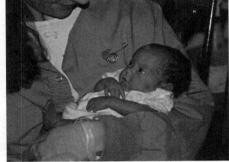

When holding your baby, position her so her arms, shoulders, and back flex forward. Preterm infants tend to extend backward because they did not have as much time in the flexed position while in the uterus as term babies did. Unless corrected, this backward extension can cause movement difficulties and delays in meeting developmental milestones.

Positioning for organization.
Your baby may still need help with positioning in order to organize herself. This baby is sprawled in the nurse's arms and has difficulty focusing on the nurse's voice.

When the nurse flexes the baby's legs, positions his arms in midline, and holds him close, the baby can concentrate and learn about his surroundings.

A baby's head movement must sometimes be limited to keep respiratory equipment in place. This can leave the baby's head temporarily flattened on the sides.[1] The look of this "premie head" concerns most families. Fortunately, head shape corrects with time, usually after your infant can hold her head up independently.

Diapering Your Baby

You probably changed your baby's diaper for the first time in the NICU. The diaper may simply have been lying under your baby, or you may have had to work with adhesive tabs or a diaper cover. Your baby's nurse showed you how to gently lift your baby's legs, clean the diaper area, and replace the diaper. This once-daunting task may have become routine by now; if not, it soon will. As you diaper your baby, be sure to examine the diaper area for rashes or redness and to note the consistency and color of the stool. You'll learn to recognize what amount is normal; the amount will increase as your baby grows.

You should notify your baby's nurse of any change in skin condition and then find out how to treat the problem. If the diaper area is red, a thin coat of clear ointment (such as A&D) will protect the area and help it heal. If a diaper rash develops, a zinc-based ointment (such as Desitin) may be applied, the skin may be left open to the air, or a heat lamp may be used to speed healing. A moist, bright red, solid-looking rash may indicate a yeast infection, which usually requires prescribed medication.

Performing Cord Care

Because many NICU babies stay in the hospital for more than two weeks, parents rarely need to concern themselves with caring for the umbilical cord site. The remainder of the umbilical cord dries up (often with the help of alcohol applied by the nurses) and falls off within two weeks. The cord site should be kept open to air, clean, and dry. Alcohol may be applied to the site for one or two days after the separation occurs. The baby should not have a tub bath until the cord has separated.[2]

Dressing Your Baby

Your first experience dressing your baby will probably involve putting on a hat or a pair of booties. Dressing your infant in real baby clothes may be scary at first. Those little arms and legs look very fragile. The staff is used to handling these little ones, and their confident movements may look harsh when you're still a bit afraid even to move your baby. But those little arms do fit in sleeves, and the legs go in the leg holes just like other children's. All parents are nervous at first, and your baby has been through a lot. Watch the nurses, and ask questions as they demonstrate dressing your baby. Take your time until you're comfortable. Before long, you'll be able to dress your baby completely, without a second thought.

Feeding Your Baby

Infants usually begin the transition from tube feedings to breastfeeding or bottle feeding by trying the breast or bottle once per shift or per day. At the same time, a plan is prepared for increasing the frequency of nipple feedings. As your infant is able, she will progress from one breast or bottle feeding per shift to the breast or bottle every other feeding and then, finally, to all nipple feedings. When bottle or breastfeeding frequency is increased, your infant may not gain weight for a time. In fact, some babies lose a little weight during this transition. After a few days, weight gain begins again.

Breastfeeding mothers sometimes find they must be assertive about their desire to introduce breast milk and breastfeeding as soon as possible. Some mothers worry that once introduced to bottle feeding, their baby will find breastfeeding more difficult. Breastfeeding and bottle feeding are different skills, but most babies are adaptable. Recent studies indicate that nipple confusion is more apt to occur when a baby is fed from a bottle only, for weeks before breastfeeding is attempted. If the two are introduced together or within days of each other, the baby rarely has problems switching to the breast from the bottle.[3] Chapter 5 has more information about this concern.

Caregivers base their feeding decisions on your baby's weight, gestational age, and general condition. The health care provider determines the plan for introducing what feeding in what concentration and by what route. Protocols often guide the nurse in advancing your baby's feeding. The earlier in gestation a baby is born, the slower feeding progresses.[4]

Feeding is a good time for parent-infant interaction. You can participate in feeding even before your baby is ready to tackle a complete bottle feeding or breastfeeding. Ask if you can hold your baby while the tube feeding goes in. Ask if the nurse will let you bottle feed the last few drops of the feeding.

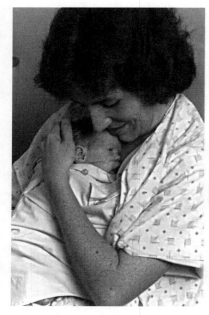

Time-out.

Your baby may need a quiet time-out to pull herself together, especially after feeding. Both breastfeeding and bottle feeding babies benefit from the restful snuggling provided during kangaroo care.

Once your baby begins breastfeeding or bottle feeding, you may hold and feed her. The nurse will stay nearby until you're comfortable and will offer tips if your baby is a slow feeder. Chapter 5 explains the basics of both breastfeeding and bottle feeding. Occupational therapists often work with babies and their parents to improve feeding skills. Feeding is quality time. You'll come to look forward to this special time with your baby.

Using the Bulb Syringe

A bulb syringe is used to remove secretions from a baby's mouth and nose. Until your baby can effectively clear her nose, the syringe will be used when she seems bothered by nasal stuffiness or discharge. To use a bulb syringe, first squeeze the bulb; then place the tip of the syringe gently into the baby's nostril (don't push it in). Releasing the bulb suctions the secretions. Don't hold the opposite nostril closed; this could cause painful pressure in the ear. Don't push the tip of the syringe too far into the nostril, because the tissue is easily damaged. Swelling as a result of tissue damage only complicates nasal stuffiness. To clean the bulb after use, force hot water through the bulb syringe, adding infant bath soap to the water if desired. Be sure to rinse any soap thoroughly from the bulb.

Massaging Your Baby

You may be able to massage your baby as part of caregiving in the intermediate unit. If you want to try massage, it's important to remember all the things you know about your baby's tolerance for stimulation. Vimala McClure's book *Infant Massage: A Handbook for Loving Parents* contains a helpful chapter on massaging premature babies.[5]

When you begin massage, the first step may simply be to "contain" your baby by putting a firm hand on her head or chest or by holding her arms and legs in a flexed position. Light massage tends to irritate very young preterm babies, but these infants enjoy small amounts of firm, gentle stroking.[5] The unit may have a nurse or occupational therapist who is a licensed massage instructor and who can teach you the skills.

Bathing Your Baby

Each hospital has different criteria and routines for tub-bathing infants, and even sponge-bathing may be postponed until the staff feels your baby is medically stable. You should be able to bathe your baby several times before discharge, however, so you can practice this care task with supervision.

Most babies do not require a bath more than two or three times per week.[6] Cleansing the diaper area and washing the baby's hands and face are all she will need on most days. When your baby's umbilical cord (and circumcision site if your baby boy has been circumcised) are healed, you may be taught tub-bathing.

"When Maria got to intermediate nursery and really started eating well, I couldn't pump enough breast milk to keep up. That's when the lactation specialist helped me most. Her encouragement kept me going, and in a few weeks, my milk supply caught up with Maria's appetite."

Just as dressing your baby can be frightening at first, giving your baby that first bath can be overwhelming. Your baby's nurse will teach you the components of a special-care bath—among them, removing electrode patches and protecting IV sites from water. When your baby can tolerate a tub bath, the nurse will provide a working surface, a warming light, a bathtub or basin, and the necessary linen and bath supplies. At first you'll probably serve as an assistant while the nurse gives most of the bath and demonstrates important points. As your confidence grows, you'll do more of the work, using the nurse as your resource.

Taking Your Baby's Temperature

Use of a thermometer is an important skill that every parent or caregiver should be comfortable with before the baby's discharge. A baby's "normal" temperature depends in part on age, weight, metabolism, and other health factors, but most NICU experts agree that a baby's normal axillary (armpit) temperature is in the range of 97.5° to 99°F (36.4° to 37.2°C).[7,8] Your baby's rectal temperature should be in the range of 98° to 100°F (36.7° to 37.8°C).[7,9] A rectal temperature higher than 100°F (37.8°C) usually indicates a fever.[9]

The most common methods for taking your baby's temperature are tympanic, skin, rectal, and axillary.

A tympanic thermometer measures temperature through a probe gently inserted into the baby's ear. This method is fast and easy, but the thermometer is expensive. Refer to the manufacturer's information about the thermometer's accuracy when used for infant temperature assessment.

To measure skin temperature, apply a fever strip to your baby's forehead. These strips are inexpensive, fast, and easy to use, but this approach is not as accurate as other methods. Fever strips may be used for general screening. If the strip indicates a high temperature, use a thermometer to obtain an exact reading.

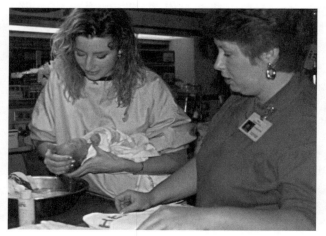

Gaining independence.

The nurse in intermediate care stands by to offer assistance but allows you to do as much caregiving as possible.

A rectal temperature is accurate, but it is also invasive, can cause injury, and is probably unpleasant for your baby. A rectal thermometer should be well lubricated (with petroleum jelly or a lubricating jelly like K-Y) before insertion. Depending on your baby's size, the thermometer should be inserted ½ to 1 inch into the rectum.[9] Never force a rectal thermometer. If you can't insert it gently, pull it back toward the rectum and gently probe in another direction. The recommended position for your baby is lying on her tummy over your legs. This lets you control your baby's movements and keep her from rolling onto the thermometer, which could cause an internal tear.

An axillary temperature—one taken in the armpit—is easy, it's more pleasant for your baby, and it's a perfectly acceptable way to assess temperature. This is probably the method the nurses will teach you. It's important to place the tip of the thermometer against skin in the center of the underarm. Hold the arm firmly while the temperature is registering. With an electronic thermometer, this method is quick. An accurate reading with a mercury glass thermometer takes approximately three minutes.[10]

Whether you take a tympanic, axillary, or rectal temperature, it's important to use the same method each time when monitoring your baby's temperature. Readings vary by as much as 2°F between axillary and rectal, so alternating methods makes it difficult to compare results. When reporting your baby's temperature to your health care provider, be sure you mention whether you used the axillary or the rectal method.

Giving Medications

If your baby will go home on medications, the nurses will teach you how to draw up the dose and give it to your baby. They should also teach you about the common side effects of any drugs your baby will be taking. Appendix B offers detailed information on many of the medications commonly given to babies. Chapter 16 gives tips on how to manage problems you may encounter with medicines at home.

Practice drawing up and administering your baby's medications before discharge. For many medications, you'll need to learn how to use a syringe to accurately measure the dose. Some medications should be mixed in a small amount of formula or breast milk to prevent stomach upset. Others need to be given directly into your baby's mouth. Breastfeeding mothers may be taught to give all medications directly into their baby's mouth just before nursing or halfway into the feeding. An alternative method is to express some breast milk into a bottle to be used for medication administration. Ask your nurse which method the hospital recommends. Your health care provider or specialist is usually responsible for adjusting dosages as your baby grows.

Ask why your baby is on each medication and how long she will need to take it. Drug levels or other tests may need to be run at certain intervals to assess the medication's effectiveness. In some cases (for example, with theophylline or phenobarbital), the baby may be allowed to outgrow the dose. The drug dose will be increased only if the baby shows the need—if, for example, apnea or seizures continue or recur. Ask all the questions you need of the intermediate care nurses and the neonatologist until you are comfortable with this part of your baby's plan. You need to know enough about your baby's medications to be a partner in her care after discharge. Once your baby is discharged, your health care provider is your resource, and you will be your child's primary case manager and advocate.

Learning Infant CPR

Every parent should know how to perform infant cardiopulmonary resuscitation (CPR). You can find a class through your local Red Cross or fire department. Many hospitals offer infant CPR classes as part of their parent education programs. Attend a class and learn this important skill now. Don't wait until the mad rush just before discharge. (See Appendix E for CPR information.)

Learning Special-Care Tasks

If your baby will be going home with special equipment for care, get involved in learning how to manage the equipment and do these tasks as soon as possible. Special-care tasks include gavage feeding; gastrostomy, colostomy, and tracheostomy care; and oxygen use for emergencies, during feedings, or by nasal cannula or ventilator. Chapter 16 contains more information on caring for babies with these special needs at home.

Have the nurses explain what they are doing as you watch. After a few times watching, do the task while a nurse talks you through it. Don't expect to perform the task as easily as the nurse does. (The nurse has had a lot more practice!) Gradually, the nurse will do less talking as you gain confidence. Don't wait until your baby's last week in the hospital to learn these skills. Give yourself plenty of time to practice and to get help if you need it.

Networking

Contact with the parents of other NICU graduates can be helpful—both before and after your baby's hospital discharge. Your baby's move to the intermediate nursery is a good time to begin making contacts. When available, support groups may be helpful. (The pros and cons of these groups are discussed in Chapter 6.) There may also be a support network of parents with previous NICU experience who can give you valuable insights and information. Call or meet with two or three other families. They can provide priceless guidance as you face decisions about a pediatrician or other health care provider and all the other choices you'll need to make as your baby's discharge date approaches. Appendix D lists many organizations that you can contact for information or support.

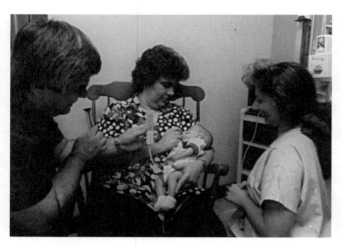

Special-care skills.

Now is the time to learn special skills you will need for your baby's care at home. This father gives the gastrostomy feeding, while the mother offers the baby a pacifier. The nurse provides teaching and reassurance to the family.

Watching for Complications

I t may seem as though your baby has balanced on a very thin wall between life and death since birth. When your baby is stable enough to graduate to intermediate care, however, the wall beneath her has widened considerably. In fact, most babies who graduate to a step-down unit are past real danger.

Because your baby was preterm or critically ill, however, she was also vulnerable to the hazards of the NICU environment. Technology kept your baby alive, but sometimes that technology can have side effects. Once your baby is in intermediate care, a few medical conditions can affect progress, but most cause only a temporary setback. Rarely, these conditions can mean readmission to the NICU.

Apnea and Bradycardia

Apnea and bradycardia (explained in Chapter 9) often occur in babies born at less than 32 weeks gestation, and episodes may continue in the intermediate care nursery. The staff will monitor the frequency, intensity, and duration of the episodes.

If your baby was not having apnea or bradycardia in the NICU or if the frequency or intensity of the episodes increases now, occurrences may be a sign of illness. If this happens, the physician or neonatal nurse practitioner will order tests to find the cause. If the apnea and bradycardia are because of immaturity, your baby may receive medication (aminophylline or caffeine) to decrease the episodes. If your baby is put on medication, drug levels in the blood may be checked periodically. As your infant grows, the doctor adjusts the dosage, or allows your baby to outgrow the dose if apnea and bradycardia resolve.

Unless they are a side effect of another illness, apnea and bradycardia often resolve around your baby's original due date. If your baby is ready to go home before that date, mild apnea and bradycardia may be the only factors preventing discharge. Management of the situation depends on the philosophy of your baby's neonatologists. In some units, your baby will have a pneumogram (explained in Chapter 15) to help determine the best course of action. Your baby may require continued monitoring in the hospital or may be a candidate for home monitoring and/or medication. If your baby goes home with a monitor, you'll be instructed in monitor use and infant CPR.[11]

Infections

Your recovering baby is prone to many kinds of infection. Despite the best precautions of staff and visitors, infections do occur. Some infections, such as thrush, are minor and respond to treatment rapidly. Others can be more serious.

Thrush

Your baby might get a yeast infection—called thrush—in her mouth. It looks like thick white patches on the tongue or gums. You cannot wipe these patches off. Infants with thrush often have feeding problems because of tenderness in the affected area. Thrush is usually treated with oral medication.[12]

Other Infections

Signs of other infections may include feeding difficulties (intolerance, vomiting, abdominal swelling, or poor feeding), decreased activity, increased frequency of apnea and bradycardia, an unstable temperature, and increased work of breathing. When the health care team becomes aware of these signs, your baby may have blood work, a spinal tap, a urine culture, or x-rays to identify the cause of infection. Intravenous antibiotics may be started, and your baby may be made NPO (no oral nutrition) as a precaution. In the occasional instance, your baby may be transferred back to the NICU for respiratory support, for increased monitoring, or simply for IV medications. Rarely, a baby overwhelmed by an infection may die. Most infections respond well to

"In the beginning, you expect complications and scary moments. In intermediate care, setbacks are more surprising, more disappointing, because you think those times are behind you."

treatment, and your infant will be back to normal in two or three days.[12] Chapters 9 and 10 provide more information on infections in newborns.

Hernias

Preterm infants are at risk for hernias—protrusion of a body part (such as a loop of intestine) through a muscle weakness or unusual opening inside the body. If your baby develops a hernia, it will eventually require surgical repair.[13]

Inguinal Hernia

The most common hernia is called an inguinal hernia. This condition occurs most often in males and usually presents as a bulge in the groin, especially after crying or straining during a bowel movement. Sometimes girls get inguinal hernias, which cause a bulge, or swelling, near the labia.

Usually, the boy's testicles stay in the inguinal canal (high in the groin, not down in the scrotal sac) until about 32 weeks gestation. At that time, the testicles descend into the scrotum, and the inguinal canal closes. But in preterm babies, the inguinal canal may not close after the testicles descend. This allows part of the intestine to push through this gap in the muscle wall into the scrotum. This may affect one or both sides and appears as a swelling in the scrotum.

As long as the hernia is reducible (the intestine can be easily and gently pushed back through the opening), immediate surgical correction is not necessary.[13] Surgery will usually be postponed until the child is older or requires other surgery. If the hernia becomes incarcerated (trapped in the scrotum), the scrotum will become blue and painful, and immediate surgery will be necessary.[13]

Umbilical Hernia

Another area where the muscle may not close properly is around the umbilical cord. An umbilical hernia causes the umbilical area, or belly button, to push outward when the baby cries.[14] As long as there is no marked discoloration, there is no cause for concern.[1] This condition usually corrects itself as your baby grows and the abdominal muscles strengthen and thicken.

Reflux

A condition known as gastroesophageal reflux occurs when the muscle at the entrance of the stomach has not matured and allows food to move back up the esophagus.[15] A variety of factors may contribute to the dysfunction of the valve. Respiratory distress that causes the diaphragm and abdominal muscles to work harder than they should, positioning of an infant on her back, and large volumes of food causing pressure on a weak valve may cause reflux. Feeding small amounts more frequently, feeding continuously by pump, raising the head of the bed, or placing the baby on her right side or on her tummy after feeding may help alleviate this condition. Reflux can lead to choking, aspiration, and/or apnea and bradycardia. If the condition is severe, treatment

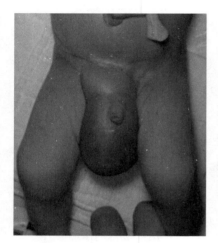

Inguinal hernia.

The bulge in this baby's groin is typical of an inguinal hernia.

Courtesy of Dr. David A. Clark, Louisiana State University Medical Center and Wyeth-Ayerst Laboratories, Philadelphia, Pennsylvania.

may include medication or surgery.[14] The surgery to correct reflux is called fundoplication (explained in Chapter 16).

Anemia

While your baby is in intermediate care, blood counts (hematocrit or hemoglobin) will be checked weekly or as the baby's situation requires. Preterm NICU babies are at risk for anemia (low red blood cell count) because their NICU stay required drawing of blood for testing and evaluation of treatment, and the body system that makes red blood cells is immature. (See Chapter 9 for more information.) Babies often cannot replenish their blood supply fast enough to keep up with the necessary blood tests in the NICU; therefore, blood transfusions may be given to correct anemia.

Anemia can cause low oxygen and glucose levels in the blood, which can cause the tissues and organs not to function properly. Infants with anemia may appear pale and lethargic, have an increase in apnea and/or bradycardia, and not eat well.[16] Infants on respiratory support may have regular transfusions. Keeping the blood count normal is important for keeping oxygen levels normal and allowing timely weaning from oxygen.

Most babies who have graduated to intermediate care are able to maintain their oxygen levels without help, so they shouldn't require many more transfusions. In intermediate care, blood levels are allowed to drop lower than in the NICU to stimulate the baby's own red blood cell production system. When an infant receives transfusions, the production of red blood cells in the bone marrow is not stimulated. A low red blood cell count is the necessary stimulus to trigger production. As with all immature systems, full functioning takes time.

When the hemoglobin and hematocrit drop, the system that produces red blood cells is stimulated to replenish the lost supply. A blood test called a reticulocyte ("retic") count shows the amount of developing red blood cells produced. If the retic count is within normal limits, transfusion will be postponed in the hope that the baby's system will do its job. In most infants, the process corrects itself without complication. Sometimes, babies are transfused the week before discharge. In that case, your health care provider's office may schedule follow-up lab work.

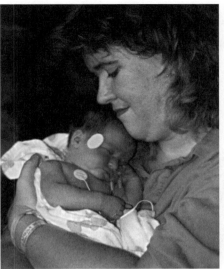

Being together.

The intermediate care setting is usually quieter than intensive care and offers more moments for just being together. Your feelings of belonging to each other can take awhile to develop, but time and patience result in a strong bond.

Your baby's graduation to the intermediate care unit is exciting and at the same time unsettling. As a student of your baby's behavior and special needs, you know you have much to learn. You'll begin to feel more like a parent as you assume much of your baby's caregiving. The more time you have to learn and practice your parenting skills in this more relaxed setting, the easier things will be in the long run. Go slowly, but don't procrastinate. Your baby will soon be homeward bound.

Moving Closer to Home

Chapter 15

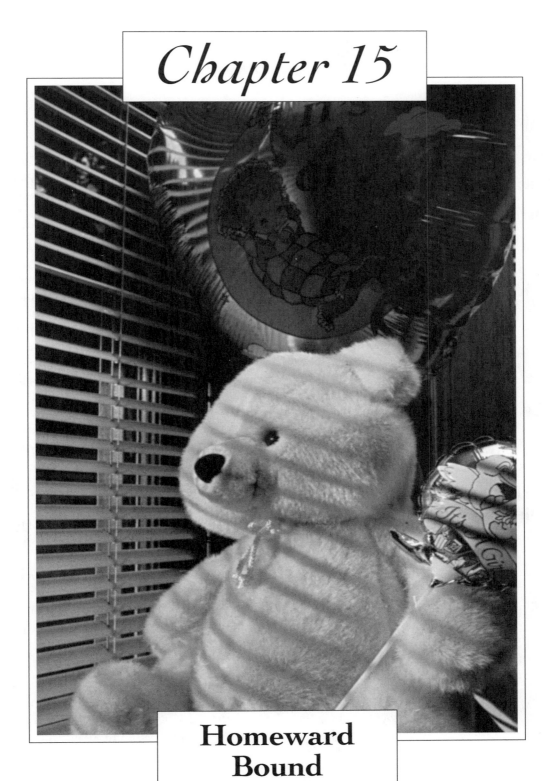

Homeward Bound

Sharon Gregory, RNC, MN, CNNP

❝"Think of all the possibilities, Piglet, before you settle down to enjoy yourselves."❞

Eeyore–

By the time your baby is eating well, gaining weight, and in an open crib, you should be very familiar with the process of discharge planning. When your preterm baby weighs about 4 pounds (about 1,800 grams), he may be almost ready for discharge. But discharge planning for all NICU babies begins long before these milestones are achieved. Soon after your baby stabilized in the NICU or was transferred to intermediate care, the health care team began work on a final discharge plan. Your baby's primary nurse, his nurse practitioner, a case manager, or a clinical nurse specialist may have been assigned to coordinate all aspects of the plan. The plan details teaching for parents, referrals that will need to be made to specialists or community services, and equipment that will be needed for home care. In many large facilities, you are invited to a meeting with representatives from all the departments that have helped care for your baby. Representatives from community agencies—such as public health, home health agencies, and equipment-supply companies—may also attend the meeting. Ask your baby's nurse about your hospital's process for discharge planning so that you can work with the staff to prepare your baby, yourself, your home, and your family and friends for this long-awaited event.

Signs of Progress Toward Discharge

Once your baby is in the intermediate unit, the signs of progress change. Even though your baby may go to intermediate care while still on oxygen or IV fluids, the primary focus now becomes your baby's ability to feed by bottle or breast, grow and gain weight, regulate body temperature, and organize behavior into meaningful patterns.

Because discharge depends on the interaction of many factors, your baby's caregiver may not be able to pinpoint an exact date far ahead of time. When the physician finally does set a date, it may be right around the corner. That's why it's important to begin learning care skills and preparing your home when you first notice signs of progress.

Graduation to a Crib

Maintaining body temperature involves calories and oxygen. The more energy your baby uses to keep warm, the less he will have for growing and healing. Your baby will progress from the incubator or radiant warmer to an open crib based on his ability to regulate body temperature. This ability depends, in part, on gestational age and weight. The transition is usually gradual, but your baby may be returned to the warmer environment at the first sign of inability to maintain temperature. It's not unusual for a baby's weight gain to slow, or even for weight to drop, for a day or so during the weaning process to an open crib.

Less Frequent Measurement of Vital Signs

Your baby's vital signs will probably be taken only before feeding and then, eventually, only before every other feeding. Some units will discontinue the cardiorespiratory monitor when the infant has had no apnea or bradycardia for a specific period of time. Routine measurements used to assess your baby's well-being—such as measurement of abdominal girth and daily urine dipstick screening—will be discontinued. Unless your baby has an ongoing cardiac or respiratory condition, frequent measurement of blood pressure and accurate measurement of intake and output may also be discontinued.

More Demands for Attention

Your baby is growing up and may begin demanding more attention. He may awaken before feeding time and move around or fuss. He may quietly watch a mobile or just enjoy the surrounding activity. He may even enjoy sitting up in an infant seat or swing for short periods.

Your baby may also seem irritable and inconsolable at times. The transition from an incubator to a crib, from tube feeding to breast- and/or bottle feeding, and from sick to well requires a lot of energy. Some babies get overwhelmed by all the activity. Others simply seem to be bored with hospitalization and ready to move on. In any case, this is a wonderful time to pay careful attention to your baby's cues and to experiment with kangaroo care (see Chapter 4), snuggling, rocking, walking, talking, and increasing or decreasing activity to find out how your baby responds to these actions.

Gaining and Growing

Your baby will gradually take more of his feedings in larger amounts from the breast or bottle and fewer feedings by feeding tube. This transition to the breast or bottle can be a slow process. (See Chapter 5 for more information.) Weight gain will usually average about ½ to 1 ounce (15 to 30 grams) per day. Don't worry if your baby doesn't gain weight every single day. After a day or two of little or no weight gain, he will probably gain well for the next few days. Look at the average weight gain over a several-day period, and you should see a good overall gaining trend. (See Chapter 9 for more information on weight gain and growth.)

Measurements of length and head circumference are also good indicators of overall growth. Many units measure these two parameters weekly; the baby's gestational age, degree of illness, ability to absorb nutrition, and hereditary factors must be considered. Depending on a baby's gestational age, head circumference increases about ½ to 1 centimeter per week on average during the first weeks after birth.[1] A growing baby's length increases about ½ centimeter per week, with an average length increase of about 10 to 12 inches (25 to 30 centimeters) in the first year.[2]

Giving Care Independently

As discharge nears, you're likely to need the unit staff less often for routine care procedures. Your baby's nurse may still talk you through the more complex tasks, but by now you should be fairly comfortable taking a temperature or changing a diaper. Use your nurse as a resource whenever you have questions or need assistance during this learning period.

Learning What's Normal For Your Baby

As nurses check vital signs, change diapers, and do other tasks, they constantly assess your baby. Assessment is noticing the baby's general condition and what is different from the baby's typical condition. An important part of learning to care for your baby is learning what is normal and understanding how to recognize a change.

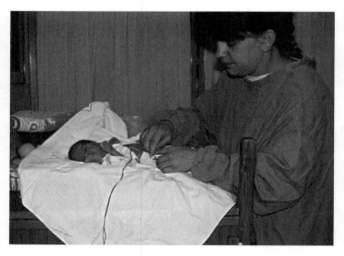

On your own.

You gain confidence as you do most of your baby's care independently now.

Corrected Age

If your baby was born early, he really has two birthdays. The day your baby was born is the official date of birth, but your original due date is also an important milestone for your baby.

When you measure your baby's development—that is, when you look at what is appropriate behavior for an infant of your baby's age—consider both of those dates. You'll need to determine your baby's corrected age, or postconceptional age (PCA), to know where he should be developmentally.

Calculating corrected age isn't difficult. You begin with your baby's actual age (number of weeks or months since the date of birth) and then subtract from it the number of weeks or months preterm your baby was at birth. This gives you your baby's corrected age. Here's the formula:

Actual age – Weeks or months preterm = Corrected age

A term pregnancy is 40 weeks gestation. To determine the number of weeks premature your baby was at birth, subtract his gestational age at birth from 40. For example, if your son was born at 28 weeks gestation, he was 12 weeks (3 months) premature. If he is now 6 months old, his corrected age is

Actual age	–	*Months premature*	=	*Corrected age*
6 months	–	*3 months*	=	*3 months*

In this case, even if your son is six months old, you should expect him to be at or near the developmental level of a three-month-old term baby. It would be unrealistic to expect your son to be physically ready to sit up with very little support or on his own—a skill that is frequently emerging in term babies around the age of six months. Your baby may just be beginning to roll over, which is developmentally normal for a term baby of three months and, therefore, for a baby whose age is three months corrected. Chapter 17 contains a useful table listing developmental milestones for infants and children of various ages.

Parents are often frustrated by well-meaning family and friends who express concerns about their baby's development. People may think your son is delayed for a six-month old for example, when in fact he is performing ahead of his corrected age of three months. Explaining corrected age and why your baby is so small can get tiresome after a while and many people continue to be confused. Don't worry—you'll only need to correct for prematurity until your child reaches the age of two to two and one-half years. Most of the catch-up growth and development take place by then.

Temperature

The nurses have probably already taught you how to take your baby's temperature. (If not, review the instructions in Chapter 14 and get help from your nurse.) Taking a temperature is an important skill for parents to master.

Check with your baby's caregivers to find out what temperature they consider normal for your baby. Most experts recommend that a baby's normal axillary (armpit) temperature is in the range of 97.5° to 99°F (36.4° to 37.2°C).[3,4] The range for a rectal temperature is 98° to 100°F (36.7° to 37.8°C).[3,5] The range may vary slightly depending on the region of the country in which you live.

Heart Rate

By watching your baby's cardiac monitor in the NICU, you probably became familiar with your baby's normal heart rate—and also with the fact that heart rate increases when a baby is active and awake and decreases during deep sleep. The resting heart rate for an infant is usually 120 to 160 beats per minute, but the normal range is broad—from 80 beats per minute during deep sleep for older infants to more than 200 beats per minute during crying. Unless your baby has a heart condition, you will probably not routinely check heart rate.

Breathing Rate

A baby's respiratory rate ranges from 32 to 60 breaths per minute. If your baby is working hard to breathe, the outline of the ribs is more visible, the respiratory rate may have increased, and your baby tires quickly when eating. If your baby will go home with a chronic respiratory condition, discuss with your nurses what is normal for your baby and what should be reported to your health care provider.

Color

By now, you probably know your baby's "normal" color. A change in color from a central pink (of lips, tongue, and gums) to pale, dusky, or yellow may indicate infection or a breathing or heart problem.

"Our nurse said she would not only wean Matthew's oxygen, but wean us from total dependence on the NICU."

Color changes also occur with apnea and bradycardia. If your baby has apneic and/or bradycardic episodes, it helps to know what kind of color changes your infant shows just before or when these episodes begin so that you can intervene quickly. Color is a primary indicator of your baby's health status. Learn what is normal for your baby and what changes should be reported to your care provider.

Cry

When your baby's breathing tube was removed, you probably heard him cry, perhaps for the first time. Over time, that first hoarse cry changed to what is now your baby's normal cry. Sometimes when a baby is sick, the cry becomes weaker or more high pitched. As your baby grows, you'll be able to tell the difference between hunger cries, tired cries, and sick cries.

Urine

Most babies have a wet diaper at least six times a day. If your baby has a chronic respiratory or cardiac condition, you'll want to note the number of diapers he wets in an average day. Ask your nurse or health care provider at what point you should report an increase or decrease in urine output. You may also wish to note the color and odor of your baby's urine, especially if he will take medications at home. Your baby's nurse or health care provider should tell you if his medications will affect urine frequency, odor, or appearance.

Stools

You'll also want to be aware of your baby's normal bowel patterns before he is discharged. As your baby progresses to full-strength feedings, bowel movements will change in consistency and color. A healthy baby has softly formed or mushy bowel movements without much odor. A constipated baby strains hard or cries during a bowel movement and produces small, hard, pelletlike feces. Notice how flat or round your baby's tummy is and whether it is soft or hard. If your baby does not have a bowel movement for several days, his tummy may become firm and distended. Notify your baby's nurse or doctor if you have concerns about changes from normal patterns.

Diarrhea is watery and foul smelling and demands immediate attention. Infants with diarrhea become dehydrated easily, and this can be life-threatening. Notify your baby's health care provider immediately any time your infant has more than one diarrhea stool.

Spit-up or Vomit

Spitting up is a common occurrence for most babies. Air bubbles from the stomach bring up a small amount of milk, which runs out of the baby's mouth. Vomit is ejected from the stomach with force and tends to come flying out of the baby's mouth. If your baby vomits more than one feeding or consistently spits up more than a tablespoon, let your baby's health care provider know about it.

Getting What Your Baby Will Need

While your baby is growing stronger and getting ready to go home, it's time to pull out all the baby care books that you hid away because they seemed so irrelevant to your NICU experience. Look over the baby supply and home preparation lists and start accumulating what you'll need. Now is also the time to cue eager friends or family members who have been waiting for the right moment to give you a baby shower.

Your baby will need many of the items on a basic newborn layette list. But as an NICU graduate, he may have some special needs as well. The information that follows should help answer many of your questions about baby supplies.

Clothing and Diapers

By the time they are ready for discharge, most preterm babies fit into newborn clothes. You may decide to purchase a few "going-out" items in premie size for special occasions, but keep in mind that your baby will quickly outgrow them and seldom use them.

Diapering Choices

Choice	Convenience	Health and Environmental Factors	Tips for Dealing with Diapers
Washing your own	• Time and effort required to launder • Diaper pail needed • Pins with pants or diaper covers required	• Feces are properly disposed of • Cloth diapers are reused, not thrown away • Water and energy are required to launder	• Rinse diaper in toilet to remove feces. • Put toilet-rinsed diaper into covered pail that has ½ cup of borax per gallon of water. • Machine wash in hot water using detergent. Adding ½ cup of white vinegar to rinse cycle may help eliminate urine and odor. • Dry on a hot cycle or line-dry thoroughly. • Clean empty pail carefully to reduce germ growth.
Diaper service	• Doorstep pick-up and delivery provided by service • Deodorized diaper pail usually provided by service • Pins with pants or diaper covers required	• Feces are properly disposed of • Cloth diapers are reused, not thrown away • Water and energy are required to launder	• Dump feces into toilet. It is not necessary to rinse soiled diaper. Serviced diapers are treated to slow growth of germs and odor. • Place diaper in pail provided by the service. • Set diapers at doorstep for pick-up service on assigned day.
Disposable diapers	• No laundering needed • No pins or covers needed to hold diaper in place • Must be purchased, brought home, and disposed of	• Feces left in diapers go to garbage as untreated waste • Diapers become litter when carelessly disposed of • Diapers increase garbage in landfills	• Dump feces into toilet. • Wrap diaper in its own plastic liner. • Do not flush diaper. • Place wrapped diaper into tightly covered trash can. This prevents the spread of germs by flies, animals, and children.

Adapted from: King County Nurses Association and the King County Solid Waste Division. *Diapering Baby: What's the Bottom Line?* Seattle, Washington. Reprinted by permission.

Sample Layette

Clothing
4–6 shirts
6–8 stretch suits
6 one-piece T-shirts with snaps at waist
4–6 gowns or kimonos
2 or 3 sweatshirts or sweaters
1 or 2 dressy outfits for special occasions
6 pairs booties or socks
12 fabric diaper covers or waterproof pants
5 dozen cloth diapers (also used as burp cloths)

Seasonal
Snowsuit
Warm hat
Warm booties
Cotton hat or bonnet
Cotton booties
Sunsuit or romper

Bedtime
6 receiving blankets
2 crib blankets
2–4 crib sheets
6–12 lap pads
2 waterproof pads
Crib bumper
Quilt
Baby intercom
Nightlight

Bath Time
2–4 bath towels
6–8 washcloths
Plastic bathtub
Foam bathtub liner (foam bath pillow)
Brush and comb set
Baby shampoo
Baby scissors

Health Care Supplies
Cool-mist humidifier
Thermometer and lubricant
Infant acetaminophen as recommended by your baby's health care provider
Medicine spoon

Plastic rolling cart or trays for special-care supplies
Bulletin board and calendar to keep track of appointments

Furniture
Bassinet or cradle
Crib and mattress
Chest of drawers
Laundry hamper
Baby laundry soap
Diaper pail
Baby swing
Rocking chair or recliner
Toy box

Outings
Diaper bag
Car seat
Padded head rest
Front carrier and/or backpack
Stroller

Breastfeeding
2 or 3 nursing bras
Nursing pads
Breast pump
Containers/bags for breast milk storage

Bottle Feeding
Disposable nurser kit
8 four-ounce or eight-ounce bottles
Baby formula as recommended by your baby's health care provider

Miscellaneous
2 or 3 pacifiers
Baby toys
Baby record book
Baby care books

For Later
High chair
Play yard
Bibs
Feeding spoons and cups
Portable crib
Childproofing supplies

Newborn diapers generally work fine for most preterm babies at discharge. Some hospitals send home a small supply of premie diapers at discharge. You might ask the nurse if your hospital does this. If not, consider getting a few weeks' supply before your baby's discharge. (See Appendix D for mail-order sources.)

Diapers will be part of your life for a long time, so give some thought to your choices. If you choose cloth diapers, should you use a diaper service or wash your own? You may begin with a preference for cloth or disposables and then change your mind as your baby grows, or you may decide to use a combination of cloth and disposable supplies.

Breastfeeding Aids

If you have been breastfeeding your baby, you will have the basic supplies already. You need two or three well-fitted nursing bras, containers for expressed milk, and perhaps a few bottles and nipples if your baby needs a supplemental bottle. Most breastfeeding mothers of NICU graduates also need an electric breast pump at home for a while after their baby's hospital discharge. (See Chapter 5 for breast pump information.) If your health care provider has recommended test weighing your baby after feeding, obtain a baby scale designed for this purpose by the time your baby comes home. (See Chapter 5 for information about this scale.)

Bottles and Formula

Your baby may require special formula. Your local pharmacy should be able to order it for you, or the hospital can give you information on other sources. Ask your social worker or nurse about the expense of special formula and if you should be aware of any other information. For example, is special formula considered a medication and therefore tax deductible or covered by insurance? Does the formula manufacturer provide formula for families under special circumstances? Investigate these possibilities and talk with the families of other NICU graduates. Special formula can be a major expense. Get all the cost-saving advice you can.

If your baby will be discharged on regular baby formula, he will no doubt make this transition before discharge. Find out which baby formula your caregiver recommends and why. Find out if the recommended brand is interchangeable with another brand. Differences in formula content may affect your infant's digestion.

Most hospitals use ready-to-feed (premixed) formula. At home, you may wish to buy a less expensive form of the recommended formula. You'll find ready-to-feed, concentrated-liquid, and powder formulas on your grocery's shelves. The powder type is usually the least expensive. Compare costs, and read the preparation instructions to decide which is most time- and cost-effective for you.

Water from most public water systems is acceptable for infant use. To be sure, however, ask your baby's health care provider about the necessity of boiling supplies when preparing formula, including the water used to dilute concentrate or powder formula. Most physicians are comfortable with a thorough washing of all supplies with hot soapy water and a bottle brush. Dishwashers are also efficient for bottle washing. If you have an alternate water source, such as a well, or if lead in the water is a concern, check with your baby's caregiver or the public health department for their recommendations.

Once your baby comes home, he will soon be eating regular baby portions, so special little bottles are rarely necessary. Many parents prefer the nursing systems that use plastic bags, feeling that their infant takes in less air during feeding. Other parents feel that washable plastic bottles are more environmentally responsible.

Thermometer and Acetaminophen

In case of illness, you'll need a reliable, easy-to-use thermometer. You may choose a digital model that can be used safely in your baby's armpit (a rectal or oral model works), or buy a rectal model for rectal use only. Glass mercury thermometers are reliable, but they break easily, putting a hazardous substance (mercury) in your home. Forehead strip thermometers (fever strips) are not as accurate as a true thermometer.

Acetaminophen may be given for fevers and for possible discomfort of immunizations. Acetaminophen drops (such as Tylenol and Tempra) are the easiest form of this medication to give to infants. Always keep a bottle available. You may need it for fevers, and later, for teething discomfort. Check with your health care provider for the proper dosage.

Car Seat

It's very important to place your baby in an approved car seat when you take him anywhere in a vehicle. Your lap is never a safe place for your baby in a moving vehicle. If your baby needs your attention and can't wait until you reach your destination, pull off the road and stop the car to help him. After all you and your baby have been through to get to this point, why take a chance with your baby's life by ignoring this basic safety rule of the road?

The American Academy of Pediatrics (AAP) publishes many brochures describing various car seat models and options. See Appendices C and D for car seat information and resources.

Stroller

First-time parents are usually amazed by all the baby paraphernalia necessary for a simple trip to the store. Strollers are invaluable for carrying not only your baby, but all the supplies and equipment your baby needs. If your baby requires a cardiac monitor or oxygen, purchase the best-manufactured stroller you can afford. Compare brands, and talk to other parents of special-care babies before deciding. Look for safety features, sturdiness, compartments and storage space, and ease in collapsing and setting up. Umbrella strollers do not give adequate head and back support for babies.

Nursery Monitor

Different from a cardiac monitor, a nursery monitor is an intercom that helps you hear your baby wherever you are in the house. When selecting a monitor, check range, power requirements, and ease of use. To keep your baby safe from accidental injury—for example, strangulation by the monitor cord or electrical shock from putting parts in his mouth—be sure to place the base of the monitor out of your baby's reach.

Humidifier

Ask your care provider about the likelihood that your baby will need a humidifier. A humidifier combats dryness in home air and may be recommended to keep respiratory secretions liquid and mobile and to help prevent infection.

Shop carefully for a humidifier. The most popular models are ultrasonic, which turn cold water into mist through high-frequency vibrations. You may wish to investigate demineralization filters or to use only distilled water in this unit. Another option is a warm-mist humidifier, which increases air humidity by boiling water like the old-fashioned steam vaporizers. Bear in mind that a humidifier containing hot water is hazardous around small children, tends to be noisy, and may overheat a small room.

Any humidifier must be kept scrupulously clean to prevent molds and bacteria from growing in the water reservoir. Check the manufacturer's recommendations for the best way to clean your model. As with any electrical equipment, the humidifier and its cord should be placed out of your baby's reach.

Bulletin Board and Calendar

A bulletin board and a calendar are not on most baby supply lists, but many parents of NICU graduates have a multitude of people and medical appointments to coordinate. Use the bulletin board to post each person's business card, or write each person's name, identification (pediatrician, lactation specialist, health insurance agent, and so on), telephone numbers, address, and other important information on a 3-by-5-inch card and put those on your board. Next to that health care team list, post a calendar on which to keep track of your baby's appointments, developmental milestones, and visitors; you may even post your bill payment schedule here. Some parents also post their baby's medication schedule and other information they refer to frequently, such as instructions from the physical therapist. This bulletin board will become your "communication station"—especially if your baby's care needs are complex. You may eventually outgrow the need for this organizational tool, but most parents find it helpful during the first few months at home.

Questions to Ask When Choosing a Pediatrician

1. To which hospital do you usually admit your pediatric patients? Why?

2. Are you board certified (Do you have training, have you taken an examination, and are you certified in a specialty?)

3. About how many children our child's age do you see each year?

4. What procedure do we follow if we need you on a weekend or at night?

5. How do you prefer we handle emergencies—that is, should we call you first or go directly to the emergency room?

6. Who covers for you when you are unavailable? Is that doctor board certified? Is he or she part of your practice, with easy access to your records?

7. What is the procedure for nonurgent calls—that is, should we make them at a certain time of day? Will you give advice on the telephone?

8. Do you have nurse practitioners or physician assistants who will provide care for our child? How do you use them? Can we meet them today?

9. Do you have a published fee schedule? If not, what are your fees for a well-baby visit, a school physical, and other relevant services? Do you charge for telephone consultations?

10. Do you have your own laboratory in the office? What types of tests do you perform there? Do you have a schedule of fees? Can our child's lab tests be performed outside if we request it?

11. What are your views on [breastfeeding, immunizations, or any other issues you—the parent—feel strongly about]? What importance do you place on preventive health measures?

12. Can we review our child's medical record during the course of care?

13. What patient education services do you offer?

14. Do you prescribe generic, rather than brand-name, drugs when comparable ones are available?

Questions for the Staff

1. Do you have a patient handbook? [If so, most if not all of the remaining questions are probably answered there.]

2. What is the usual waiting time to get a routine appointment?

3. How much time is allowed for a first-time physical? How much for a routine visit?

4. What is your procedure for prescription refills?

5. Do you accept our insurance plan?

6. Do you handle insurance-claim forms?

7. What payment terms are offered? Do you accept credit cards?

8. Do you call if the doctor is running behind schedule?

Adapted from: Inlander CC, and Dodson JL. 1992. *Take This Book to the Pediatrician with You: The Guide to Your Child's Health*. Allentown, Pennsylvania: People's Medical Society, 40–41. Reprinted by permission.

Welcome Home Sign

Last but not least, buy the biggest "Welcome Home!" sign you can find. Get an announcement ribbon, balloons, or whatever else will bring a sense of celebration to your baby's homecoming. When your baby's caregivers finally set a discharge date, consider planning a celebration dinner with your partner a few days before your baby is discharged. Once your baby comes homes, it may be a few weeks or more before you can find much quality couple time in your schedules.

Your baby is making good progress toward a homecoming date. You've purchased supplies and equipment, and you're comfortable with most of your baby's care tasks. What else needs to be done?

Arranging for Medical and Other Care After Discharge

Choosing Your Baby's Health Care Provider

Parents are sometimes caught the week before their baby's discharge without a clue as to who will provide their baby's care. As soon as you're able, begin the interviewing process and choose a health care provider. Finding a new caregiver can be an unsettling experience, especially after you've come to know and trust the hospital staff. Don't delay your search. As with any new relationship, expect a time of adjustment, uncertainty, and nervousness until trust is established. You need time to get acquainted.

Most neonatologists do not see infants outside the NICU or step-down unit, but depending on where you live, they may be able to recommend various health care professionals in your area. Your insurance program may have a list of health care providers; bring the list to the NICU for help in choosing a provider. Nurses, close friends, or parents of NICU graduates are other possible sources of recommendations. A healthy NICU graduate may not require the services of a pediatrician but may be cared for by a family physician or a qualified pediatric nurse practitioner. As you interview potential candidates, keep in mind that personality type and coping styles—both yours and the caregiver's—play into the decision. Health care professionals run the gamut from telling parents everything and involving them in all decisions to telling them as little as necessary and making most decisions themselves. Also consider at which hospital(s) the doctor has admitting privileges, the office location and hours, office policy on sick visits and phone calls, billing procedures, who takes calls when the health care provider is unavailable, and previous experience with NICU graduates. Make a list of questions ahead of time to take on your interviews. You may wish to interview more than one person.

Babies with special needs should have one doctor who is able to follow their progress. Choosing a pediatrician before your baby is discharged allows the neonatologist or primary physician caring for your baby to speak directly with the pediatrician or to send the doctor a written discharge summary of your baby's hospital course. If at all possible, your baby should be seen by a consistent caregiver rather than at a general health unit or clinic, where medical personnel change often. Many pediatricians accept patients on public assistance if you are without private insurance. In some states, Medicaid will also provide transportation for you to take your baby to the doctor.

Your pediatrician will become an important resource person as your special-care baby continues to grow and develop. The pediatrician you choose should be trained in the care of infants and children with special conditions, such as prematurity, or special needs, such as technology dependence.

Understanding Referrals

Certain specialists may continue to follow your baby after discharge. To help you, hospital staff will refer you to the appropriate health care agencies. Your baby's health care provider will be notified of the impending discharge. The neonatologist may call the physician and discuss your baby's hospital course or may arrange for a copy of the discharge summary to be sent to the office. Some health care professionals may prefer to see your baby at the hospital before discharge. Some neonatologists give parents a copy of the discharge summary. This is helpful in case you change doctors or have to see other specialists. When you receive this summary, make copies to distribute, and be sure to keep one for yourself. If you have questions about anything you read in the summary, ask your baby's nurse, or make an appointment with the neonatologist.

Your neonatologist should also give you the names of specialists who have served as consultants. If your baby had an intraventricular hemorrhage, for example, a neurologist may have been monitoring your baby's progress and will continue follow-up care after discharge. Some neonatal units have a pediatric developmentalist who specializes in treating babies with deficits common to preterm birth or prolonged hospitalization. Consulting physicians will usually meet with you or talk with you on the phone. They will indicate when and where follow-up exams should occur. Part of the work of parenting an NICU graduate is coordinating your baby's medical appointments.

To comply with legislation (Public Law 99-457), all states must have some mechanism for tracking preterm infants or those who are at risk for developmental delays or health problems. (See Chapter 17 for more information on Public Law 99-457.) After discharge, affiliated service providers will contact you at regular intervals to assess your baby and refer you to community resources as needed. These programs operate through the public health department. Some hospitals also have their own NICU follow-up clinic for developmental screening or appointments with specialists. Ask your discharge coordinator how this works in your region.

Preparing for an Emergency

Graduates of NICUs have a higher rate of rehospitalization than the average newborn population. Common reasons for readmission are dehydration because of vomiting or diarrhea, upper respiratory infections, and hernias or a shunt requiring repair.

Now is the time to prepare for an emergency in case one arises. Before your baby is discharged, go to the hospital where your baby is most likely to be readmitted. Know the fastest route from your house, and an alternate route, as well as the locations of the hospital's emergency entrance, parking, and admitting office. Be prepared to call the Emergency Medical Service system for an ambulance if you believe your baby's condition is critical, however. Post 9-1-1 or your community's EMS number on all your phones. Being ready will prevent panic in case of an emergency.

If you know your baby will come home with a cardiac monitor, a respirator, or oxygen, you also need to contact public services to ensure that you will receive priority help in community emergencies. The Emergency Medical Service system (or nearest fire station) and your utility providers (water, electric, and gas) should all be aware that you have a baby with special needs in your home. Ask your baby's nurse, case manager, or discharge planner for this letter to send to your utility companies. Be sure to notify them when your child is no longer technology dependent or if you move.

Deciding about Circumcision

Opinions vary regarding the necessity of circumcision (removal of the skin covering the tip of the penis in male infants). For some, circumcision is a religious requirement. For others, this decision is often more emotional than intellectual. You might want to go to your local library and read some articles explaining the pros and cons of circumcision. Ask the nurses in the newborn nursery about the percentage of parents in your region who opt for circumcision. As your son grows up, he will no doubt see a mix of circumcised and uncircumcised males. This is not an easy decision for many parents. Make sure you have enough information before you sign a consent.

The American Academy of Pediatrics states that routine circumcision of babies is not medically necessary.[6] Complications of circumcision are rare but include bleeding, pain, and infection. If you do decide to circumcise your son, it will usually be done right before discharge.

Some physicians prefer to perform circumcision in their office after your baby is older and larger. If your baby requires other surgery (hernia repair, or ostomy closure, for example), the procedure can be done at that time. Check with your insurance carrier to see if your insurance covers circumcision if it is not done in the hospital before discharge. If you decide to circumcise your baby, ask the doctor performing the circumcision about regional anesthesia and pain relief before and after circumcision.

Your baby's nurse or physician will instruct you in circumcision care. You'll be told to call the doctor if you notice bleeding, swelling, or bad-smelling drainage. In most cases, you will be instructed not to give your baby a tub bath until the circumcision is healed.

Thinking about Day Care

If you intend to use day care within two or three months of your infant's discharge, this is a good time to start your search. The early months at home will fly by. You'll be absorbed in your baby and in your family's adjustment to

"Rooming-in was the smartest thing we did during Latisha's NICU stay. I still had many questions after we got home, but spending the night with her in the hospital helped calm many of my fears about coming home."

this new addition. While your baby is still hospitalized, you'll have more time to explore the possibilities.

During your baby's first year, you may want to limit the number of children he is exposed to, because exposure increases the risk of illness. Not everyone can afford home care, and some families find it too invasive. Day care in someone's home offers a controlled environment with a low caretaker-to-children ratio. Look for a referral service, which can tell you ahead of time about age ranges, pets, smoking, training, years of experience, and hours. Personal referrals generally provide information from a parent's perspective on the personality of the care provider and the type of care given. Both large and small day care settings should offer informal visitation.

Babies who will need complex care require special consideration. Quality day care for special-needs infants is often hard to find, and you may face long waiting lists. For mothers who plan to return to work quickly (paid maternity leave may be used up during the NICU stay), the search for day care should begin as early as possible.

Predischarge Testing

While you're learning all you can about your baby's care, the discharge coordinator or case manager is planning your baby's final tests and making preparations for discharge. Common discharge tests are explained here, but not all NICU babies require all the tests discussed. Ask your baby's nurse what to expect as discharge draws near.

Sleep Study (Pneumocardiogram)

Infants with continuing apnea and bradycardia may have a special test to help determine the cause of these episodes. Depending on your region of the country, the test is called a sleep study, a pneumocardiogram (PCG), or a pneumogram. A pneumogram uses a monitor similar to your baby's cardio-respiratory monitor but with additional channels that record your baby's heart rate, respirations, air flow through the nose, and oxygen saturation. If gastroesophageal reflux is suspected as a cause of apnea and/or bradycardia, an additional probe is used to record the acidity of the baby's throat secretions. The baby uses this special monitor for a specified period of time, usually overnight, and specially trained personnel analyze the results. This may help determine the sequence of events that lead to, or trigger, an apneic/bradycardic episode.

Philosophies vary regarding the use of pneumograms, and not all NICUs use them. A pneumogram does not answer every question about the baby's apnea and bradycardia, and interpretations of the test vary regionally. Based on your baby's risk factors, history of apnea and bradycardia, and pneumogram results if used in your NICU, your health care team may recommend the use of a home monitor. You will be taught how to use the monitor before your baby goes home (see Chapter 16).

A home monitor can be a valuable tool, but it is also important to remember that the monitor does not provide a health guarantee for your baby. If a home monitor is optional for your baby, ask the doctor to explain the advantages and disadvantages of using it. You may also find it helpful to talk to other parents who have faced this decision. Use of the monitor may afford parents a greater feeling of security. However, over time the annoyance of the number of false alarms that need to be dealt with may cancel out the perceived benefit of having the monitor.

Eye Exam

If your baby was less than 32 weeks gestation at birth and required oxygen therapy, he will usually have an eye examination at between 5 and 7 weeks of age. Follow-up exams will be scheduled if the findings of the first exam warrant them.[7] The exam is to identify any changes in the eye tissue caused by retinopathy of prematurity (explained in Chapter 10).

Hearing Test

Hearing tests—also called audiology screenings—are done in many nurseries before discharge. Electronic sound and response monitoring determine if your baby can hear. Environmental conditions such as surrounding noise or a crying baby can cause inconclusive results, however. If this happens, a retest should be scheduled in a more controlled environment. If your baby responds to your voice or to noise-making toys held where he can't see them, there is usually no reason for concern. After discharge, your child's hearing should be monitored by your health care provider at periodic health exams. If you are concerned about your baby's hearing, don't hesitate to insist on a more extensive hearing examination. These are available in pediatric outpatient rehabilitation centers.

Blood Count

A final hematocrit or hemoglobin and reticulocyte level is usually done the week of discharge. Although it's unlikely, your baby might be anemic and need a transfusion at this time. (Chapter 9 has information about anemia.) If so, follow-up laboratory tests will usually be done in the pediatrician's office or an outpatient clinic.

Preparing Yourself, Your Home, and Your Family

If many miles have separated you from your baby, now is the time to use any available resources to spend as much time as possible with him before discharge. Ask your discharge planner for help with this very important aspect of parent education. But whether you're close to your baby's hospital or far away, you still need to make more decisions and preparations before your baby comes home.

Rooming-In

For various reasons, you may find the prospect of taking your baby home frightening. To decrease this anxiety, some hospitals offer rooming-in, an arrangement that allows parents to stay overnight at the hospital to care for

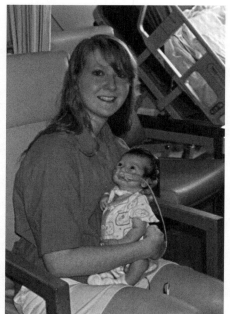

Rooming-in.

Spending a night or two in the hospital with your baby allows you to care for your baby as if you were at home. The nursery staff is immediately available if needed. Rooming-in is especially helpful if your baby's care is complex, as for this baby who is going home with a feeding tube and a tracheostomy.

their baby independently. Nursery staff is immediately available if needed during this time. Rooming-in validates parent learning and lets parents see for themselves what baby care will be like at home. Most parents feel that rooming-in builds their confidence and eases the transition to home.

Timing of the rooming-in experience is important. Ideally, rooming-in should take place as close to discharge as possible. To simulate the home environment, try to have any home monitoring equipment in place during rooming-in.

Think carefully about whether to room-in the night before discharge day, however. Spending the night with your baby in the hospital is exciting, but you may be exhausted in the morning. You may wish to room-in a day or two before your baby's discharge date instead. A good night's sleep the night before discharge may help ease some of the inevitable anxiety of your baby's homecoming.

Housecleaning

Many parents feel they must "sterilize" their home with industrial-type cleaning products to eliminate germs and dust before their baby's homecoming. The family pet may be permanently banished outdoors or given to a new owner. Although the intent behind these precautions is admirable, they often are not necessary and generally are impossible to keep up. Few families can maintain such high standards of cleanliness while giving baby care and normal living the priorities they must have.

Rely on common sense as you prepare—and maintain—your home. A thorough cleaning is enough. Harsh cleaning solutions and insecticidal sprays can leave residual odors that may irritate or even harm your baby.

Tobacco Smoke

Babies—especially those who have had or are having breathing difficulties—are at risk for a number of problems from exposure to tobacco smoke. The Committee on Environmental Hazards of the American Academy of Pediatrics has identified these problems: decreased lung growth, decreased lung function, and increased frequency of lower respiratory tract infections and respiratory symptoms.[8] Research also clearly shows that exposure to smoke can cause ear infections and related hearing problems, increased incidence of hospitalization related to bronchitis or pneumonia, and increased risk for sudden infant death syndrome (SIDS).[5,8] If you need more information or literature—for example, to convince family or close friends of the dangers of secondhand smoke to your baby—contact the American Lung Association or the American Academy of Pediatrics. (See Appendix D.)

Pets

Pets are important members of the family. Banishing a beloved companion may cause resentment. Instead, prepare your pet for your baby's arrival.

Bring home clothing or a blanket with your baby's scent on it. Siblings can help by spending extra time with the pet. Be alert for signs of aggression or jealousy when your baby comes home, and never leave your dog or cat unsupervised near your new baby. Extra attention and discipline will solve most problems.

Keeping your pet out of your baby's sleeping area may help reduce the risk of fur or dander irritating the baby's breathing passages. When your baby is developmentally mature enough to lie outside the crib, place a clean blanket or mat under the baby to keep fur, dander, dust, and carpet fibers from irritating the baby's airway during playtime.

Carefully assess all the factors involved in having a pet, and talk with your health care provider as you decide on a reasonable approach.

Siblings

Prepare your older children for what life may be like when their baby brother or sister comes home. Plan to spend special time alone with each of your other children a short time after your baby comes home. Encourage and allow them to talk about their feelings. This should reduce episodes of acting out. Most parenting books include information on helping siblings adjust to a new baby.

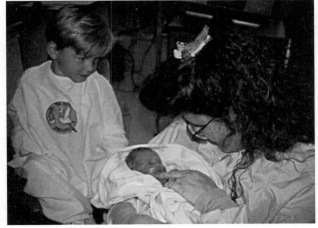

Sibling concerns.

As discharge day nears, your other children may have concerns about how life will change with a new baby at home.

Visitors

You'll need a traffic control plan for visitors. Start thinking about this before your baby's discharge, and set up a visiting schedule. Don't turn down offers of help, but use your calendar to keep track of who is planning to visit. Place limits on the number of visitors to your home. Your needs deserve top priority, and entertaining others is probably not at the top of your list right now. Let friends and extended family know that you'll need some time to adjust to this new baby at home and that you'll let them know when you're ready for visitors. Caring family and friends will respect your need for privacy and give you the time you need to make this adjustment. (Chapter 16 provides some suggestions for visitor control.)

Emotional Readiness

You're probably overwhelmed reading all of this, but believe it or not, in time you'll adjust. Start now by making sure that your expectations are realistic. When your baby comes home, you will experience times of great stress, nights when you'll be tempted to return your baby to the hospital, and moments when you'll wonder what you ever saw in your partner. Know that these feelings will pass. Before your baby comes home, think about your personal arsenal of coping mechanisms, focus on the positive, and enjoy your many good experiences with your baby. Above all, remember that you aren't the only one ever to endure this kind of turmoil or to wonder if you will survive.

Everyone develops individual coping mechanisms, but some general principles apply.

- Without an outlet, emotions take a toll on your body. Exercise; scream in the shower; scrub floors; talk to a counselor, pastor, or friend; lock yourself in the bathroom and have a good cry; or keep a journal—but do not lock in your feelings. If you are increasingly ill, accident-prone, fatigued, or depressed, try something different, or get help. These are red flags of emotions that need expression.

- You deserve a break. One person cannot carry the full responsibilities of a special-needs baby all the time. Even mothers of term infants need a break periodically: to sleep, to have some adult interaction, to exercise, or just to have a change of scenery. Couples need time alone together. Siblings need time with their parents. People cannot just "make do" indefinitely. Communication breakdowns and acting-out behavior should be clear signs of a need for attention. Have at least one support person trained to baby-sit. If you have home nurses, take an hour or so for yourself occasionally. Have an "at-home date" while someone else is responsible for the baby's care. Do not wait for spontaneous breaks in the chaos, or you will be too exhausted to enjoy them.

- Pay attention to self talk about your infant and his care. It is easy to become crisis-prone. The constant adrenaline rush is addictive and attention getting. Hypervigilance is a method of trying to decrease anxiety, but it is counterproductive. These behaviors are a sure course to burnout. On the other hand, do not stick your head in the clouds and act like your baby is just like every other baby. The letdown when illnesses arise or developmental milestones are not met will be as dramatic as your expectations are unrealistic. Be observant of changes in your baby's behavior, and develop methods of getting feedback (from a pediatrician, nurses, and friends) to help you assess without panic. All in all, be realistically optimistic.

- Develop a positive parenting image. If you have other children, draw from your experience. If not, give yourself a series of pats on the back for getting this far. Have confidence in your present level of competence and in your willingness and ability to continue to learn. Learn to trust your instincts as a parent.

- When overwhelmed, break things down into small steps. Sometimes all you can concentrate on is the next task, even if that task is a rest period. Feeling overwhelmed is a sure sign that you need help, a break, or a new plan. Making lists prevents anxiety-driven rumination over details. The lists may be of things to do or of feelings about something that is happening. Perhaps you could make a list of things others could help you do. Asking for help is sometimes difficult, but this is certainly the time to do so. When people ask, "Is there anything I can do?" do not politely insist, "We'll be okay." For those who truly want to help, you are doing them a service by letting them. Share your list with them and let them choose something that suits

"On the day our baby came home from the hospital, we showered most of the attention on his Big Sister. She wore her Big Sister shirt to day care and took cupcakes to celebrate. She had her dinner on a special new plate just for Big Sisters. She felt very important, and that helped her adjust to having a new baby in the house."

Factors to Consider when Choosing Professional Care Providers and Equipment Suppliers

Home Health Agency

- Availability of neonatal or pediatric nurses with at least one to two years of experience.
- Mechanism to ensure that the home care primary nurse or her supervisor becomes familiar with your baby's care needs before discharge. (Some hospitals include the nurse in discharge planning conferences or rounds. Others meet individually with your baby's home care primary nurse in the hospital.)
- Provision for 24-hour supervision by a nurse with pediatric ICU skills.
- Provision for inservice education for home nurses.
- Provision for planning conferences with parents and others providing family support.
- Staffing contingency plans for illness, emergencies, and tardiness.
- Mechanism for communication with physicians and families.
- Consistent, long-standing experience in providing a family-oriented approach to quality care.

Equipment Company

- 24-hour availability of trained professional staff.
- Pediatric experience and expertise.
- Appropriate range of equipment and supplies.
- Preventive maintenance of equipment.
- Written instructions for the operation and maintenance of equipment.
- Parent training in equipment operation, with plenty of opportunity for hands-on practice and instruction in troubleshooting.
- Prompt response to phone calls regarding problems.
- Reliable delivery of supplies to maintain home stock.
- Free loaner equipment if your equipment must be removed for repair or maintenance.
- Direct third-party billing services.
- Competitive pricing.
- Service to some patients without financial resources to pay.

From: McCarthy S. 1986. Discharge planning for medically fragile children. *Caring* 5(11): 38–39, 41. Reproduced by permission of The National Association for Home Care. Not for further reproduction.

them. Suggestions might include providing meals (freezable), shopping or running errands, doing laundry, helping at home—such as with cleaning or doing things with your other children so you can rest (or play), doing yard-work, and calling people with progress reports.

As your baby grows and heals in the intermediate care nursery, you will have a lot to do. It can be overwhelming at times. Make lists. Go slowly, but don't procrastinate. The closer you get to discharge, the more overwhelming all the loose ends will seem. The tasks discussed in this chapter are those that only you can do for your baby. Preparation gives you a chance to mobilize some of your anxious energy to make a difference in your child's future.

Investigating Professional Services

Parents of babies who will require special care at home have additional preparations to make. Chapter 16 explains how to manage the equipment and special treatments your baby may need after discharge. It may be helpful to read that chapter before you investigate home health agencies and equipment supply firms. There may be many companies providing equipment or nursing care in your area, or there may be very few.

In choosing a home health agency, you have many things to consider. First, check with your insurance carrier to find out exactly what is and what is not covered. Consider that some companies that provide nursing care may also provide equipment; others do not. You'll need to weigh the convenience of dealing with one company against the cost. Talking with other parents of NICU graduates can help. The hospital staff may also recommend companies (staff may call them "vendors"), but feel free to shop around.

Insurance companies acknowledge the cost-effectiveness of home care instead of prolonged hospitalization. They see the wisdom and cost savings of discharging a baby home as soon as possible. The ultimate goal of most insurers, however, is for parents to learn to assume the care of their infant themselves and to rely on the Emergency Medical Service system and hospital services when the child experiences illnesses or emergencies. Parents must therefore, realize that home-care nurses will usually not become permanent caretakers. The length of time they will be in your home will depend on your insurance company's policies. When an infant's care requires it, these policies may be challenged. In most instances, however, your child's condition will improve over time, and he will need less care. In more serious cases, exceptions will be made. But it's important that you understand the insurer's goal—for you to assume the care of your infant as quickly as possible. In cases where means permit and parents have other obligations, continued care may in some cases be negotiated privately with the home-care provider.

Discharge Day at Last!

Discharge day is a collage of excitement, fear, jangling nerves, and uncertainty. In spite of all the preparations—learning your baby's care needs and perhaps spending a night or two rooming-in—even the most competent parent feels nervous about assuming total responsibility for a baby at home.

Miscommunication often causes delays on discharge day. You may arrive first thing in the morning to be told that you'll have to wait for one more test, for the results of a previous test, or for a doctor or nurse practitioner to examine your baby or write an order. You may find this frustrating—or, if you are especially anxious, you may appreciate this short reprieve.

When everything is finally in order, make sure you get a copy of the doctor's discharge summary. Dress your baby in the special going-home clothes you've brought with you, and take a tour through the unit so that the nurses can say good-bye and celebrate with you.

Some parents want to do something special for the staff. Cookies and candy are always well received. If you want to give a small gift to an exceptional few, do so discreetly. Actually, thank you cards, a letter to the hospital administrator expressing appreciation of the NICU and nursery staffs, and letters and pictures from home are the most valuable gifts you can give the staff. They enjoy seeing the progress your special baby makes.

Now you're on your way out the door with reams of discharge instructions and bags of supplies, toys, and baby clothes. Don't forget your baby!

On Your Own

Since the birth of your baby, you've been on an emotional roller coaster. Homecoming is another adjustment—a time of shifting values, expectations, and priorities. Parents of NICU graduates have all the concerns of parents of healthy term infants, and then some. Don't isolate yourself and try to handle everything alone. You know people who can and will support you. Even though it's difficult to give up control, the more flexible you are, the easier homecoming will be. Lean on the counsel of others, your own spiritual resources, and any other support you're offered. You'll make it through, but you will be changed.

Like any other newborn's, your baby's homecoming is a big event. But for an NICU graduate, make it a gentler big event. Your family has a lot to celebrate. By all means, celebrate, but remember that you and your baby still have special needs.

Chapter 16

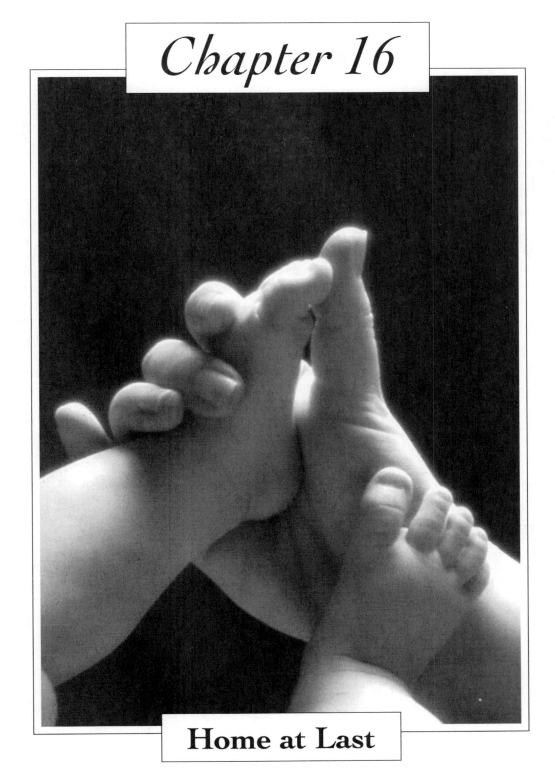

Home at Last

TrezMarie T. Zotkiewicz, RNC, MN

**"Pooh!" he whispered.
"Yes, Piglet?" "Nothing," said Piglet,
taking Pooh's paw. "I just wanted
to be sure of you."**

Welcome home! Your telephone is ringing, your baby is crying, your children are screaming, your dog is barking, your dishes and laundry are piling up—it all seems to be too much to handle. Bringing your baby home (finally) can be quite overwhelming. All of the other demands of everyday life will be waiting for you, along with your new baby and her special needs.

While your baby was in the hospital, your primary focus was on learning about her special-care needs, and by discharge, you had probably become quite competent in your baby's care. Now that you're home, though, everything seems to have turned into chaos. Relax! This is normal for anyone with a new baby in the house, even for experienced parents. It's especially true for parents of preterm babies or other infants with special needs.

Parenting any baby, especially one born at risk, demands an enormous amount of physical and psychological adjustment.[1] Most parents eagerly anticipate their baby's homecoming, but even the most experienced and prepared parents find the first few weeks an incredible challenge. This chapter offers practical suggestions and guidance for parents of preterm infants or of babies with special needs who are finally at home.

How Homecoming Affects You and Your Family

The transition from hospital to home is marked by moments of excitement, joy, anxiety, fear, uncertainty, and even depression. Parents who have spent time learning about their baby's care before discharge tend to feel less apprehensive about caring for their baby at home, but they too may experience a flood of new fears and face overwhelming responsibilities.[1–6]

Even though you're relieved that your baby is home, you may find that you miss the attention and support of the hospital staff. You may feel alone and abandoned as you make the adjustment to independent parenting. This is particularly true if family and other support is limited.[2,6,7,8] For some parents, the first days at home with their NICU graduate are as stressful as were the first days in the NICU.[9]

Feelings of Panic

You may feel panicked now that you have total responsibility for your baby's care. Until you're suddenly "cut off" at discharge, you may not realize just how much you have come to depend on the hospital staff for support. You may suddenly realize how much your baby's illness, the hustle-bustle of the NICU, and your continued concerns in intermediate care distracted your attention. You may feel as though you don't remember a single thing you were taught about caring for your baby.

It may help to realize that these feelings are common among most parents who bring home a new baby. In spite of all your preparations, expect this to be a stormy period as you and your family make the necessary adjustments. It may be of some consolation to know that you now share something with parents of healthy term babies: feelings of uncertainty and clumsiness with baby care at home. Although much of your anxiety may come from your baby's fragile beginnings and potential for future complications, you may be able to relate to the feelings expressed by this mother of a healthy term baby girl: "I finally had my baby home with me. I couldn't believe how tiny she was. She needed me for everything—she had to learn about me, about our family, and our home. After all our planning and expectation, I felt totally unprepared as her parent. That first week at home I checked on her every few hours to make sure she was breathing. I tried to prevent her from crying—yet she seemed to cry all the time. She fed every couple of hours at first, and we both had to learn how to breastfeed. I had so many questions about what to do with and for my baby. I felt constantly exhausted, worried and nervous. But she was mine...and I felt so happy and proud."[1]

Your feelings of panic should diminish as you find that you are indeed surviving. You may do things differently than they were done in the hospital, but as long as the decisions you make keep your baby warm and safe and thriving, you can have confidence in them.

Take advantage of any support you are offered because of your baby's NICU stay. A community health nurse making a home visit or an NICU home-visit nurse can reinforce your discharge teaching, validate your feelings, and help you to anticipate upcoming questions and concerns. If your NICU or intermediate care nursery does not provide a home visit, don't hesitate to call the unit for help during the first weeks at home.

Feelings of Grief and Guilt

When you first visited your baby in the NICU, you were probably assured that your baby's problems were not your fault and were, in fact, outside your control. Yet you may have felt guilty anyway and said to yourself many times, "If only I had...." Soon, though, the daily challenges of NICU survival overshadowed those feelings.

Now that your baby is home, feelings of sadness and guilt may resurface.[9] Your NICU graduate may not be the baby you envisioned during your pregnancy. Your NICU experience was probably very different from your fantasy of an uncomplicated birth, a short hospital stay, and an exciting homecoming for a healthy, predictable baby. Parents also feel guilty when they continue to grieve for what might have been instead of feeling grateful or accepting of the child they have.

This cycle of grief and guilt usually passes as you gain confidence caring for your baby and adjust to your role as a parent. Support from your family,

"When I visited Adam at the hospital he was always so quiet. The second I brought him home he started crying. Finally, I called his nurse and learned that he cried a lot for her, too. Adam kept crying, but at least I didn't take it so personally."

friends, and health care providers is important as you resolve these feelings and develop healthy parenting attitudes.

If your depression persists or if you continue to have upsetting memories of the NICU experience, seek help from a health care professional. Review your experience and feelings with someone familiar with your case; this may help you manage your feelings of loss and put them into proper perspective. Your focus has been on meeting the physical and emotional needs of your baby. Keep in mind that your own mental health goes hand in hand with your baby's healthy growth and development.

Feelings of Attachment

The bonds you established with your baby during hospitalization are very real. But development of true intimacy may have been difficult because of the lack of privacy and the distractions of hospital technology. Now that your baby is home, she may suddenly seem to be a little stranger. You may worry if you do not have strong feelings of love toward your baby.

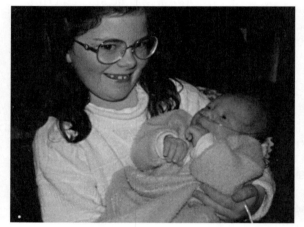

Big sister welcoming baby home.

Older children face many adjustments when your baby comes home. This is the time to involve them in the baby's care if they are interested.

Give yourself some time to get to know your baby—and to let your baby get to know you. At first, your baby will make incredible demands on your time and attention and seem to give back little. But as you gain confidence in meeting your baby's needs, she will begin to respond to your efforts with quiet alertness, more frequent eye contact, and that first amazing smile. All relationships take time to grow, and ultimately you will feel attached to and loving toward your baby.

It's a fact that NICU graduates are more at risk for abuse and neglect than are healthy term infants.[10,11] Some parents purposefully keep an emotional distance between themselves and their baby as protection in case the baby dies. Preterm, chronically ill, and technology-dependent infants tend to be more irritable than term infants. The additional stress parents feel because of these behavioral differences and their infant's special-care requirements may contribute to the alarming rate of child abuse and neglect in the population of NICU graduates.

Recognize when you have reached your limit and need a break from your baby. There is nothing bad or abnormal about feeling as though you are going to "lose it" with your baby. Walk away, calm down, and get help before you act on your out-of-control feelings. Call a family member, a friend, your pediatrician, your local social services department, your home health agency, or a parent support hotline. Talk about your feelings, and plan ahead so that someone can relieve you on very stressful days.

Impact on Your Older Children

The introduction of a new family member is traumatic for siblings—even when the baby is healthy. A baby who has had and may still have special needs causes repeated turmoil for your older children.

The NICU experience likely disrupted your family's routine, and in spite of your best efforts, older siblings may feel left out and less loved. During the NICU experience, your other children were probably aware of your tension and knew that the goal was to bring their new brother or sister home. Siblings who were involved in the baby's progress and who visited the baby in the hospital seem to make the homecoming adjustment more quickly than those who never interacted with the baby. But the reality of homecoming is still stressful for most siblings.[9]

Once the baby is home, your other children may be surprised that your attention is still focused so intensely on the baby. You can help children adjust to their new role as older brothers and sisters by suggesting activities appropriate to their age level. Before discharge day, arrange a special dinner or dessert just to celebrate this new status as an older sibling. Involve your children's teachers—perhaps by sending cookies to school along with a picture of the baby. One family's baby announcement gave the focus to the older sibling: "I'M A BIG SISTER!" was printed on the front of the card, and the baby's statistics were displayed in one column, with the sibling's age, weight, and height in the facing column. Another parent sent a balloon bouquet to her daughter at home and signed the card with the new baby's name. And a father showed sensitivity to both his partner's and his older child's feelings by setting up a surprise baby shower with the "secret" help of the older child—and including a few special gifts for the older sibling.

As your children now watch the baby take even more of your time, attention, and love, their reactions may be similar to those shown during your baby's NICU stay.[9] You may notice that they seem angry at you or the baby, regress to thumb-sucking or bed-wetting, act out to get your attention, anger easily, or have difficulty concentrating in school.

If older children are interested, involve them in the care of the new baby as much as possible, even though this may sometimes mean more work for you. Try not to criticize any "help" you receive, and praise a job well done. The more you can include older children in caregiving, the sooner they will adjust to the new baby's presence and be less frightened of any illness or disability.[12]

Spend some special time alone with each child, even if just for a few minutes of snuggling, reading a book, or taking a walk together. The addition of a new baby changes your relationship with your other children, and working through this adjustment together is an important part of your growth as a parent and as a family.

Coping As a Family

Your baby's homecoming will have an impact on the entire family. The stressors, as well as the solutions, will be unique to each family. Here are several recommendations from parents and professionals:[1-3,6,8,13,14]

- Talk honestly and openly with one another, share ideas, and listen to one another.
- Trust your instincts and your ability to adequately care for your baby.

"We not only learned to recognize Casey's cues, but each other's stress cues as well. My husband knew I needed a break when I started talking to myself. And I knew he was struggling when he started singing his old high school fight song. It may sound strange, but it worked for us."

- Acknowledge the fact that life will be different now that your baby is home, and talk about what this means to you and your family.
- Openly discuss feelings of isolation or lack of privacy and ways to actively cope with or change these stresses.
- Take time out for yourself, as a couple, or with other children and family, away from your baby—even if these periods are short.

Managing Visitors

When your baby comes home, your friends and neighbors may assume that the crisis is over and be less available for support. On the other hand, friends who were nowhere to be found during your NICU crisis may now knock on your door to see your new baby and expect to be treated as visitors.

Each family handles this transition differently, but most parents of NICU graduates will tell you to limit visitors. Your priority is to care for your baby and yourself. That may mean ignoring the doorbell at times and screening phone calls with an answering machine. Hang a sign on your door indicating your readiness (or unreadiness) for visitors: "Mom and Baby Are Sleeping Now." Or try a direct but humorous approach: "Welcome! Our Favorite Visitors Bring Snacks and Stay Thirty Minutes or Less!"

The more people your baby comes in contact with, the greater the risk of infection. Healthy visitors may be welcome, but anyone with a cold, cough, open sore (such as a fever blister), or communicable illness should not be allowed near the baby. Most people understand when you explain that a common illness picked up from an older child or adult can develop into a serious setback for an NICU graduate.

Try to limit how much visitors handle your baby. Remember, good hand washing is the best prevention against illness. Also, keep your baby from becoming overstimulated, which can occur from too much handling. A polite way to discourage holding is to secure your baby in an infant seat and see that she stays there.

You probably won't want to discourage all visitors, however, because you'll need help once your baby is home. Those friends who have seen you through your crisis will want you to be honest about your needs now that your baby is home. Now more than ever, you may need to devise a list of things people can do to help you, such as running errands, helping with laundry, or watching your children while you nap. Now is not the time to be Super Parent—ask for and accept help! For these first stressful weeks at home, allow yourself to put your family's needs first.

Financial Stress and Career Changes

Financial burdens may place added stress on your family. You may need to take an extended absence from work or even leave your job to care for your baby at home. If you did not do so before your baby's discharge, you may need to check with your social worker regarding your rights to a family leave of absence (see Chapter 7). Even under the best of circumstances, a loss of income may have far-reaching consequences on your family's future.

Maintaining your medical coverage often means a lack of freedom to move or change jobs—for fear that the baby will not be covered by a new insurance policy.[1-3,6,7,13,14] On the other hand, some parents may relocate so as to have access to medical care for their baby that would otherwise be unavailable or too far from home. Help is available for families of NICU graduates under financial stress. Work closely with your social worker and your hospital financial counselor to devise a plan (see Chapter 7).

Most NICU parents experience some degree of crisis as they adjust in the first four to six weeks after homecoming. Be patient. Give yourself some time to get off the emotional roller coaster before expecting to settle into some semblance of a normal life.

Babies are unique in the way they react to their surroundings and signal their needs. A large part of gaining confidence as a parent is feeling that you are adequately meeting your baby's needs. Parenting an NICU graduate can be challenging at first, especially if your baby does not signal those needs clearly or does not act predictably.

What to Expect from Your Baby— the Unexpected

Behavioral Differences Between Preterm and Term Babies

Compared with term infants of a similar chronologic age, many NICU graduates are challenging, difficult, and often frustrating for the first three to six months after arriving home. They tend to be more irritable and unpredictable in their behavior patterns than healthy term infants are. These patterns of behavioral disorganization are most noticeable in the areas of sleep, activity, and feeding. Most infants outgrow these differences by approximately six months of age.[1-3,15-22] Until that time, however, your baby may continue to try

---

Behavioral Differences between Preterm Infants and Term Infants in Their First Months at Home

Preterm infants are often different from full-term infants. Preterm infants usually:

- Spend less time awake.
- Are less alert and responsive when awake.
- Are less active but more fussy.
- Have shorter sleep-wake cycles.
- Arouse with fussing more frequently at night.
- Have a weaker suck; therefore, demand to be fed more often.
- Show delayed development of motor self-help skills, such as sitting without support.

Adapted from: Gorski PA. 1988. Fostering family development after preterm hospitalization. In *Pediatric Care of the ICN Graduate*, Ballard RA, ed. Philadelphia: WB Saunders, 27, 29. Reprinted by permission.

---

your patience. By understanding her behavior and helping her to become more organized, you'll find it easier to get into a routine.

Sleep Patterns

Many NICU graduates have spent months living in a bright and noisy environment. Although some quickly adjust to the peace and quiet of their new home, others appear to miss the bright lights and noise of the NICU. But no matter how peaceful or noisy your household, your baby will adjust in time. Try to be patient. Recognize that your baby needs time to learn about your home environment, just as you need time to develop your routine.[1,2,15,16]

Don't expect your preterm baby to sleep through the night for many months. Unlike a term baby, who might sleep a full six to eight hours at night by four months of age, your baby may not accomplish this task until six to eight months or later. During this transition period, play with your baby during daytime awake periods. Keep night feedings as quiet and as businesslike as possible, with minimal or soft lighting. This will help your baby learn the difference between day and night and may help you get much-needed sleep at appropriate hours.[1,2,15,16]

Babies vary in how easily they settle down to sleep. Following the same steps each time you put your baby down to sleep may help her learn a personal going-to-sleep routine. At first, you'll probably jump up and go to your baby at the first crying sound. But as you get to know each other and as you notice that your baby is developing self-comforting skills, you need to help your baby learn how to console herself and go back to sleep on her own. Self-comforting is an important skill for your baby. Beginning early to teach your baby to fall asleep on her own will ease you through the later developmental stage (at six to nine months corrected age) when sleep problems may emerge once again.

To help your baby rest, try playing the radio softly or placing a ticking clock in the room for those first few weeks at home. In addition, a soft night-light may be reassuring to you both. Remember to nest your baby with blankets to provide some boundaries. Let your baby suck on her fist or a pacifier if this seems calming.

Family Bed

Before you can establish a sleep routine with your baby, you need to decide on sleeping arrangements. Our culture has traditionally frowned upon parents sleeping with their infants and children, because we emphasize the development of independence and the importance of privacy. But behavioral specialists agree that sharing a bed with your infant is a personal and individual decision.[23–26] It may not be right for all parents, but if you feel that it's right for you, you should feel confident in your decision. The most important issue is not where your baby sleeps, but how responsive you are to her nighttime needs while also considering what's best for your family.

Parents of infants who require frequent nighttime feedings or who have special needs, such as medical treatments around the clock, may wish to keep their infant in the same room with them at night, even if not in the same bed, for a period after homecoming. In fact, it may not be possible for your baby to sleep in the same bed with you if she is on oxygen, has a tracheostomy tube for breathing, or requires an apnea monitor (all discussed later in this chapter). If your choice is not to share your bed with your baby, move her to a separate room as soon as the nighttime feedings decrease to an acceptable level for you to manage without too many sleep interruptions. Your baby (and you) will sleep better for it. The same is true for infants with special needs once your baby has adjusted to the transition home and you are comfortable managing care at home. The purchase of a nursery monitor (see Chapter 15) enables you to hear your baby from a different room in the house and may increase your peace of mind.

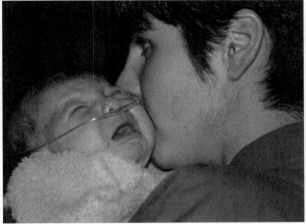

Crying.

Crying is stressful for babies and parents alike. Give yourself some time to figure out why your baby cries and what works best to calm him.

Fussing

Although your baby will sleep up to sixteen hours a day at first, her actual sleep intervals may be short. She may awaken and fuss every two to three hours until three to four months corrected age. These fussy periods may or may not coincide with hunger.

Your baby communicates some needs by fussing and crying. You'll learn to recognize the different cries your baby makes. If she is fed, is not too hot or too cold, has a clean and dry diaper, and is not uncomfortable or ill—but will not calm down with gentle holding, talking, or rocking—she may simply be tired or overstimulated. Put her down in a quiet place and let her try to pull herself together or go to sleep.

But what if your baby doesn't settle down and just keeps crying? You can try a variety of consoling techniques until you find what works best for your baby. Try rocking her, either in a rocking chair or in your arms. Some babies prefer an up-and-down motion to side-to-side movement, which may actually be stimulating. This is why some babies find a rocking swing comforting. Other babies like to be sung to or to hear music. Still others enjoy being gently stroked or patted, massaged, or swaddled snugly (but not too tightly) and surrounded by borders of blanket rolls for security and comfort. Make sure your baby can get at her hand or pacifier if sucking is comforting. Your baby may prefer a walk, either in your arms or in a stroller or a carriage. A warm bath has a calming effect on most babies but not all. For especially challenging little ones, more creative measures may be required: the sound of a vacuum cleaner or a fan, the smell of an article of your clothing in the crib, or a drive in the car.[2,15,23,25,27]

During your baby's first months at home, you'll be learning what she likes and doesn't like. The most frustrating thing for parents is that the same comfort measure doesn't work every time—and may not work two times in a row.

When you find something that works, stick with it until it doesn't work any longer. Babies like consistency and rituals, especially as they get older.

Baby-care experts Sears and Sears recommend "baby-wearing," not just as a response to crying, but to prevent crying and promote parent-infant attachment and the baby's development. You could place your baby in a front pouch and "wear" her around the house while you cook, clean, or even pay bills, for example. (If you're doing active chores, be sure to keep safety in mind.) This technique may make your baby cry less and enhance her learning.[25]

Some parents worry about spoiling their infant with too much holding. Don't worry. Experts agree that holding a baby in the early months meets the infant's basic need to feel safe. In fact, babies who are picked up as soon as they begin to cry tend to cry less often and for shorter periods than do babies whose parents don't respond quickly.[2,17,23–27]

This doesn't mean you have to pick your baby up with every peep you hear. As your baby grows, let her learn about and explore personal ways to self-comfort. She will discover that sucking her fist, holding her blanket, or clasping her hands together will help her feel better for a few moments.[1–3,16,17]

How long to let your baby cry remains controversial. Some baby-care experts feel that you should never let your baby cry it out alone. They recommend a quick response to your baby's cry, to satisfy the need for security and to let your baby know that she is important. These experts argue that by meeting your baby's dependence needs, you foster a more independent child.[25,26] Well-known pediatrician Dr. T. Berry Brazelton is in this group, arguing that letting your baby cry it out only teaches her that you've deserted her in this time of need, but that doesn't mean you must jump at the first whimper.[23]

Others feel that as long as your baby is in a safe place and her basic needs for safety, nourishment, and comfort are met, a few minutes of crying will not hurt her. Some babies seem to need to cry themselves to sleep—possibly because of fatigue or overstimulation or as a stress release—and will not be comforted by standard measures. If your baby is particularly demanding every day, make a plan for someone to relieve you periodically, even if only for an hour or so. You will need a break so that you can return to your baby in a more relaxed state of mind.

If your baby has special medical needs or turns blue with crying, you may not be able to let her cry even for a few minutes. And if your baby has a tracheostomy tube, you won't be able to hear her cry. You may need to purchase a bell to tie around an ankle to alert you that your baby is upset.

You'll probably find that as you adjust to your baby, you'll be less upset by her crying. This is not to say that you should become so desensitized to your baby's crying that you don't respond to basic needs. Whether you decide to respond to your baby's cry immediately or to wait a moment, the important thing is to do what you feel is right. Trust your instincts. Try a combination of approaches before you decide which one is right for you and your baby. It's important to balance a baby's need for your love and attention with the developmental need to learn self-consolation.[2,23,24,27]

"The medications, the breathing treatments, the special formula—it takes a lot out of you. Sometimes I would wonder how I could keep going, and then Rachel would look right at me and smile. That gorgeous toothless smile would revive me. She's worth every bit of hard work."

Now that your baby is home, you'll be making more independent decisions about when and how much your baby eats. Most parents discover things they didn't learn about their baby's eating habits while the baby was in the hospital and wonder if they are "doing it right" at home. Learning about feeding your baby takes time. But as you see your baby gaining and growing every day, you'll begin to feel more confident in your decisions.

Helping Your Baby Eat Well

Minimizing distractions during feeding time is important for all babies but especially for those who are easily overwhelmed and become stressed from too much stimulation. Monitor your baby's behavioral cues throughout the feeding. Does she frequently yawn, sneeze, hiccup, get frantic, or lose interest and fall asleep in the middle of feeding? Talking to and looking at your baby while she nipples or having the television on may be too much stimulation for your baby to handle.[19,20]

If your baby seems unusually stressed during feedings when there is a lot of activity around, you may want to turn her feeding period into a "quiet time" for the whole family. If you're lucky, younger children may imitate older ones who are relaxing with quiet activities while the baby eats. Sometimes another family member can keep siblings occupied while you feed the baby in a quieter area of the house.

Here are some suggestions for a successful feeding experience:[1,2,16,17]
- If you're bottle feeding, prepare the formula in advance.
- Minimize distractions in the room: Dim the lights, turn down the television or radio, and so on.
- Support your baby's head, neck, and hips, flexing them slightly.
- To help your baby anticipate the feeding, place your finger or a few drops of breast milk or formula in her mouth.
- If necessary, gently support your baby's jaw with your finger to keep the milk in her mouth.
- While making eye contact, talk softly or not at all.
- Monitor your baby's behavior for signs of stress, and give her a break when necessary.
- Allow for frequent rest breaks and burps.
- Give your baby time to recover after the feeding is over.

How Much and How Often to Feed

By the time your baby is ready to come home, she should be eating well enough to be gaining weight (usually about ½ to 1 ounce per day, or 3 to 8 ounces per week).[17] Before your baby's discharge, her health care provider probably gave you written guidelines for how much and how often to feed her. Some babies need to continue a specific feeding schedule and fluid restrictions after discharge. Your health care provider may adjust that schedule only after weighing and examining your baby in the office. Other infants may be able to

Concerns about Feeding

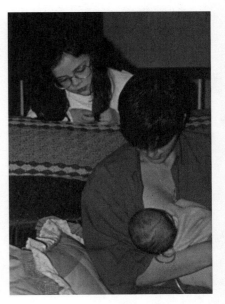

Breastfeeding at home.
Making the transition to breastfeeding at home can be challenging. Your older child may feel left out of this part of baby care, and you may miss the support of the hospital staff. Call upon all available community resources to help ensure your success.

feed on demand—meaning that the baby determines how much and how often to eat.

The doctor should have told you before discharge whether to feed your baby on demand or to follow a feeding schedule (for example, 2 ounces every three hours) for the first few weeks to ensure continued weight gain. Allowing your baby to feed on demand encourages behavioral development, which may produce better weight gain and encourage establishment of sleep patterns. Until she is more mature, she may not have a predictable sleeping or feeding schedule. She may wake up hungry every two to three hours, may sleep for four hours, or may wake up hungry and then fall asleep halfway through a feeding.[1,2,16,17]

If you'll be feeding your baby on demand at home, you should begin to feed her this way before discharge. This will give you an opportunity to learn the behavioral cues your infant uses to signal readiness to eat.[28] A breastfed baby needs six to eight and possibly more feedings per day.[28,29] A bottle fed baby may need at least six feedings per day.[17]

Your health care provider may suggest that you consider a modified demand schedule for breastfeeding a preterm infant who is 35 to 36 weeks gestation at the time of discharge. This is because a preterm infant's need for sleep may override the desire to feed, resulting in poor weight gain or dehydration. Your health care provider may suggest feeding your baby every two to five hours, with a minimum of six feedings per day.[28] You may need to continue to use a breast pump with this approach to ensure an adequate milk supply. Still other health care providers may recommend breastfeeding at least eight times per day.[28,29] Clearly, feeding schedules need to be individualized. A visit from a home health nurse or lactation specialist during the first week or two after discharge can help to resolve breastfeeding issues.

As your baby grows, so should her appetite. If your baby takes less than what she needs at a feeding, she may wake up earlier or take more at the next feeding. If she takes in too much or eats too quickly, she may spit up. Once she is able to take in more at each feeding, the time between feedings may lengthen. It's particularly nice when your baby starts lengthening the time between feedings at night, letting you get more sleep.

If you are breastfeeding and your baby is working hard to nurse, or if it is unclear how much milk your baby is getting, you may be instructed to supplement the amount your baby takes at the breast. Your health care provider will ask you to provide either breast milk or formula by using a bottle, a supplemental nursing device, finger feeding, or cup feeding so your baby will receive enough calories for growth (see Chapter 5). If a bottle is used, Dad or another caregiver may at times give the supplement so you can get some rest. Usually, once your baby is sucking and swallowing for at least 15 minutes at the breast and is growing and gaining weight, the health care provider will discontinue supplementation.[29]

Some health care providers now recommend test weighing the baby on a scale designed especially for this purpose (see Chapter 5 for more information about test weighing). By weighing your baby before and after breastfeeding, you can accurately calculate how much milk she is receiving at each feeding. The Medela BabyWeigh scale ([800] TELL-YOU) provides an easy and accurate method for monitoring breast milk intake. As you see your baby's intake increasing, you decrease the amount of supplementation. This ends the guessing and insecurity about how much your baby is eating and may increase your confidence in your ability to breastfeed.

How Long to Feed

Feeding length varies, depending on how frequently your baby wants to eat and how easily she tires while feeding. Breastfed infants may begin nursing only a few minutes on each side and may require more frequent feedings. You should hear sucking and swallowing, along with some pauses. Gradually, your baby may work up to nursing 20 minutes or more on each side. The usual length of time it takes a breastfed infant to complete a feeding is 20 to 40 minutes.[29] Breastfed infants tend to take twice as long as bottle fed infants to eat.[30] But as long as your baby seems content after feeding and is gaining weight (weight checks may need to be done at home or in the doctor's office), there's no reason to limit feeding time. In fact, your baby may become frustrated if you end the feeding too soon. Babies nurse not only to satisfy hunger, but also to satisfy their needs for sucking, security, and comfort. Falling asleep or ceasing to suck are the usual indicators that a feeding is over.[28–30]

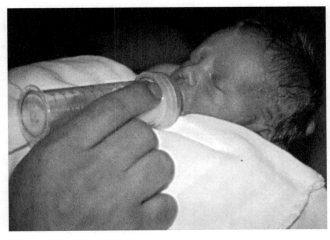

Bottle feeding at home.

Practice the basics of bottle feeding once you get home: positioning properly, watching cues, providing rest periods, and stopping when your baby signals that he has had enough.

In general, a feeding for a bottle fed baby should not last longer than 30 minutes.[17] Most babies will finish much sooner than that, in 10 to 20 minutes. If your baby is unable to take everything by nipple and requires supplementation by gavage (a feeding tube), you should still try to limit the total feeding time to 30 minutes. Your baby will have more difficulty gaining weight if she uses all her calories to get through long, perhaps stressful, feeding periods.

Weight Gain

As you settle into a feeding routine, you may wonder whether your baby is gaining enough weight. Typical weight gain is ½ to 1 ounce (15 to 30 grams) per day, or about 3 to 8 ounces per week.[17]

Your health care provider may recommend weekly weight checks at the office to check for adequate weight gain or by the home health nurse for the first few weeks after discharge or longer. It's important that your baby be weighed on the same scale each time to accurately assess weight gain. Once your baby demonstrates good growth at home, everyone (including you) will relax a bit.

Feeding Challenges

Some babies are more challenging to feed than others. Before your baby is discharged home from the hospital, you should know if she is a gulper, a spitter, a breath holder, or a pokey eater.

Your nurse talked to you before discharge about any feeding problems your baby has. She probably helped you practice feeding your baby when you visited. The nurse, the lactation consultant, or an occupational therapist may have worked with you on specific feeding and positioning techniques that work best for your baby. If you roomed-in before discharge, you had the chance to practice feeding your baby several times in a row. Now you'll put all that practice to good use at home.

A bottle feeding infant who gulps rapidly and then spits everything up may need a nipple that delivers the formula slowly. You might need to try a few different types of standard bottle nipples before you find the one that works best. You may need to regulate the length of time the nipple is in your baby's mouth as well. Frequent burping and feeding the baby in a more upright position may also help prevent spitting up.

Breastfeeding babies are usually able to adjust to the fast flow of milk that accompanies the mother's let-down reflex. Sometimes, babies who are just learning to breastfeed have difficulty with a moment of faster milk flow and may become apneic, choke, or spit up.[28,30,31] One solution to this problem is to pump for a few minutes before the baby begins to nurse. This will decrease the surge of milk entering your baby's mouth as your milk lets down. Another technique is to get the baby latched on well, then slowly recline (in a reclining chair or against pillows behind you) so that the baby is positioned nearly on top of your breast. Then when the milk lets down, your reclining position lessens the force of the milk spray into the baby's mouth, and any overflowing breast milk can easily dribble forward out of the baby's mouth.

If your baby is a breath holder, she may have been discharged with an apnea monitor (discussed later in this chapter) to alert you to severe episodes of apnea (pauses in breathing) or bradycardia (slowing of the heart rate). If your baby tends to hold her breath (common also with gulpers), watch her breathing pattern and color during feedings. If you notice breath holding or a color change (to pale, dusky, or blue) at any time during a feeding, take the nipple out of your baby's mouth. Try gentle stimulation—rubbing or patting your baby's back, for example—to wake your baby up and remind her to breathe. The rubbing or patting may also bring up a burp. If you find you need frequent vigorous stimulation to keep your baby breathing during feedings, call your health care provider at once.

Some babies work hard to suck. Whether it's because their oral-motor development is still immature for their corrected age or because of unresolved breathing problems, they may need a special nipple made for premature infants, which is softer and allows more milk to come out with less effort. Take care when feeding with this nipple to keep your baby from choking if the milk comes out too rapidly. These nipples are not sold commercially and should be used at home only on recommendation of your health care provider. Because the nipples can be washed in hot soapy water and reused, you don't need too many of them. If your baby needs this type of nipple, the nursery may have provided you with a supply at discharge, or you may have to special-order the nipples.

Babies typically outgrow the need for a premie nipple within the first month after they're home. By that time, they are usually approaching the weight of a term newborn and are able to make the switch to a commercial nipple. If your baby begins to cough and sputter on the milk as her suck gets stronger, she may be ready for a standard nipple. You may need to try several nipples before you find the one that works best for your baby.

If you have difficulty feeding your baby after discharge, contact your health care professional. Frequently, all you need is a phone call to the NICU or inter-mediate care nursery for some advice and reassurance from a nurse who is familiar with your baby's eating habits. If not, an outpatient referral to a lacta-tion specialist or an occupational therapist may be in order.

A Feeding Log

Whether your baby is breastfeeding or bottle feeding, you may want to keep a log of each feeding for the first few weeks or month at home. Use a notebook to document:

1. Feeding times
2. Feedings missed (for example, when your baby begins to sleep longer at night)
3. Time at breast or amount per bottle
4. Any spitting up and approximately how much
5. Wet and dirty diapers
6. Special comments (for example: Is your baby satisfied after a feeding, or does she cry a lot? Does your baby fall asleep in the middle of the feeding? Does your baby need to be awakened for feedings?)

All these observations are worth noting. Bring this information with you when you take your baby to your health care provider. It will help your health care provider decide if your baby is taking in enough calories to grow. You may be concerned that your baby frequently spits up 1 to 2 teaspoons after each feeding, for example. As long as your baby is gaining weight adequately, your health care provider may advise you just to continue monitoring the amounts and to practice reflux precautions, such as holding the baby more upright dur-ing feedings, burping frequently, and elevating the head of the bed.

On the other hand, you may report that your baby is irritable, cries all the time, and needs to be bundled or dressed warmly to maintain her tempera-ture. This history will help your health care provider determine why your infant isn't gaining weight despite a healthy appetite. Your baby is most likely burning up calories crying, working to breathe, or keeping warm. An increase in the amount and/or frequency of feedings is usually all that your baby needs. Occasionally, special additives to breast milk or formula or specially

"It helps if you are confident with your baby's care before you leave the hospital so you can go home and train other people to help you. You need two or three people, whether they be family or friends, to help."

prepared high calorie formula may be necessary to promote adequate growth and development.

Keeping a log is a simple and valuable way to work in partnership with your baby's health care team. Appointments at the health care provider's office are often only 15 to 30 minutes long, giving you little time to organize your questions. If you come prepared with your questions and information log, you will be able to make the most of your office visit. Once your baby has established a consistent pattern of feeding and gaining weight for you at home, you can comfortably retire your feeding log as part of your baby book.

Other Common Homecoming Concerns

It may have seemed like an eternity until you were able to take your baby home. Now, at last, you have control over your baby and your family life—or do you? The normal elements of baby care may not be so routine for you. The first few days, weeks, and even months at home may in fact be chaotic. This section addresses some common concerns, with the goal of helping you to organize your family life once again.

Bathing at Home

You can bathe your baby any time it's convenient for you. Don't feel you must stay with the hospital schedule, although knowing the logic behind that schedule is helpful. Typically, it's better to bathe before feeding, because a bath involves a lot of handling, which may cause spitting up if your baby has a full stomach. On the other hand, a bath followed immediately by a feeding may exhaust your baby. If your baby feeds poorly after a bath, you may need to allow time for a rest before feeding.[2,16,17]

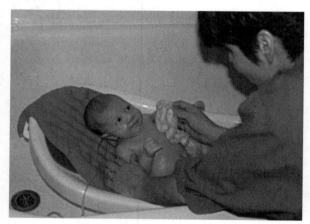

Tub-bathing.

Bath time will become play time as your baby grows older. A sponge insert helps support this slippery baby and allows him to feel more secure.

As long as you keep your baby's face, neck, skin folds, and diaper area clean, you don't have to bathe her every day. A sponge bath will suffice until your baby can tolerate a tub bath without undue stress. On the other hand, a tub bath can be a relaxing and rewarding time for both you and your baby. For many babies, it may be less stressful than a sponge bath. Some parents get into the tub with their baby to hold and snuggle as they wash. This provides skin-to-skin contact for you and your baby. Remember to hold your baby securely and be sure the bath water isn't too hot for your baby.

With practice, you'll find the tub-bathing method that works best for you. There are only a few rules for tub-bathing your baby: Don't let your baby get too cold, and keep your baby safe. Never leave your baby unattended in the tub. If the phone or doorbell rings and you must answer it, wrap the baby in a towel and take her with you. If you must reach for something or turn away, keep one hand securely on your baby.

Bathe your baby in the warmest area of the house—preferably one free from drafts. You'll need only a few inches of water that feels comfortably warm to your wrist or elbow. Your baby will be slippery when wet; try placing a soft towel in the bottom of the tub, or buy a preformed sponge insert for the tub. Use a mild soap (ask your health care provider for a recommendation) to wash your baby's body. No soap is needed on your baby's face. Avoid using lotions; they may irritate your baby's skin. Most health care providers also advise against powder, which can irritate your baby's breathing passages.[2,16,17]

If your son was circumcised shortly before discharge, you were probably instructed not to tub-bathe him until the circumcision is healed. If you chose not to have your baby circumcised, you simply need to wash the penis at bath time. Don't try to pull back the foreskin. It will naturally separate from the penis over several years, and as your son grows, you'll teach him to wash carefully as part of his daily routine.

Keeping Your Baby Warm Enough

Before discharge, you learned how to take your baby's temperature. Unless you've been instructed to check your baby's temperature routinely, you'll probably take it only when you suspect illness. But how can you tell if your baby is maintaining a comfortable body temperature?

It's not necessary to turn your heat up to a sweltering level to keep your baby warm; a normal household temperature is fine for most babies. If you have special concerns, ask your health care provider for advice. In the first few days at home, you may wish to check your baby's axillary (armpit) temperature randomly to see how she is adjusting to the temperature of your home.

Because most of your baby's heat loss occurs from the surface of the head, your health care provider may recommend that your baby wear a soft cotton hat, day and night, until she weighs more than about 2,250 grams (about 5 pounds). Aside from this recommendation, most baby-care experts recommend dressing a baby in the same layers of clothing that you would wear to be comfortable.[2,15–17] If you're comfortable in a T-shirt and shorts, for example, your baby probably needs a footed jumper suit. On a cooler day, when you need a shirt and a pullover sweater, dress your baby in a jumper suit and a sweater. Avoid the temptation to overdress your baby.

The most reliable way to determine temperature is to take your baby's temperature with a thermometer. But when you don't suspect illness, your baby's appearance or behavior may give clues to her temperature status. Usually, a baby who is dressed too warmly will fuss, turn red, and possibly sweat. A cool baby may also fuss but will not turn red and may have cool, pale, or marbled-looking hands and/or feet. The temperature of a baby's hands or feet may not be reliable, but if her tummy feels cool, add a layer of clothing and check her temperature in an hour or so. If your baby seems consistently cool or isn't gaining weight despite eating well and being otherwise healthy, try adding a comfortable cotton hat to conserve heat so that your baby can use calories for growth.

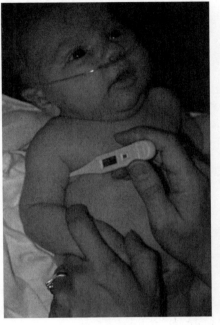

Taking a temperature.

Taking an axillary temperature is safer, easier, and less stressful than taking a rectal temperature. Remember to tell your health care professional what method you have used when you report your baby's temperature.

Outings

Use common sense when deciding about outings. There's probably no reason why your baby can't sit outside in the shade with you on a nice spring

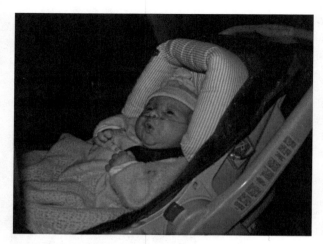

Going for a ride.

Learn safe and proper use of your baby's car seat. (See Appendix C for information on car seat use.)

day or go with you to a friend's house for lunch. If you're debating over whether it's wise to take your baby someplace with you, ask yourself about chances for exposure to illness.

Although their recommendations vary, most health care providers suggest limiting your baby's public outings for the first one to two months at home. Fall and winter months are particularly bad for respiratory and flu viruses that could put your preterm or special-needs infant back into the hospital. If you do take your baby out, avoid crowded places like shopping malls, grocery stores, and religious services. Many parents find these places frustrating anyway, because well-meaning people continually stop them to inquire about the baby.[2,3,17] One mother of triplets stated, "You get tired of people stopping you at every corner to look at the babies. Once someone said to me, 'I'm glad they're yours and not mine,' and I said, 'I'm glad they're mine and not yours, too!' "

Sudden Infant Death Syndrome

Many parents worry about their baby's chances of death from sudden infant death syndrome (SIDS). This syndrome accounts for more than 6,000 infant deaths in the United States each year. With an average of 1 to 3 SIDS-related deaths per 1,000 live births, however, the incidence in this country and Canada is actually low.[32]

The media have played an important role in keeping parents informed of the latest scientific theories about SIDS. But at this time, no one theory explains these infant deaths. A panel from the National Institute of Child Health and Human Development (NICHD) modified the definition of SIDS in 1992, saying that it is "the sudden death of an infant under 1 year of age which remains unexplained after a thorough case investigation, including performance of a complete autopsy, examination of the death scene, and review of the clinical history."[32]

Many countries throughout the world have been involved in the study of SIDS. Several factors appear to be associated with an increased relative risk for SIDS. They include:[32]

- Low birth weight. The risk of SIDS is higher among infants born weighing less than 5 pounds, 8 ounces (2,500 grams), with an even higher relative risk if birth weight is less than 3 pounds, 5 ounces (1,500 grams).
- Gender. Male infants have a 50 percent higher incidence of SIDS death than do female infants.
- Race and ethnicity. The highest SIDS rates have been found in Native American and African American populations (2.5 to 6 per 1,000 live births), whereas Asians, Caucasians, and Hispanics have lower rates (1 to 2.5 per 1,000).

- Geography. Australia, New Zealand, and Northern Ireland generally have the highest incidence of SIDS (3 to 7 per 1,000 live births), whereas Hong Kong, Japan, and Sweden have the lowest rates (0.5 to 1 per 1,000). The United States, along with several other countries, falls in between (1 to 3 per 1,000 live births).
- Season and climate. Some studies have identified an increased incidence of SIDS during cold months, but other factors may also contribute to this increased risk. They include infection (colds and flu are more common in winter months), temperature of the baby's room (too warm), nutrition or metabolic processes, infant care practices, and lifestyle.
- Cigarette smoking during pregnancy and in the household.
- Substance abuse by the mother.
- Lack of prenatal care.
- Low socioeconomic status.
- An unmarried mother.
- Young maternal age (teenage).
- Short interval between pregnancies.
- Prior SIDS death. There is an average fivefold (or 1 percent) increase in the risk of SIDS above the baseline for subsequent siblings when an earlier sibling has died of SIDS.
- Prematurity and intrauterine growth retardation. These factors contribute significantly to an increased risk of SIDS, but apnea of prematurity does not. Up to 18 percent of all SIDS cases occur in preterm infants. But preterm infants diagnosed with apnea of prematurity do not have a higher incidence of SIDS than do other premature infants.
- History of illness preceding death.

Other factors related to SIDS are also being investigated at this time. One of them is age: SIDS generally occurs in infants less than six months of age. The peak incidence of SIDS occurs between two and four months of age, and SIDS does not appear to occur before the age of one month.[32,33] Breastfeeding has been associated with a decreased incidence of SIDS. Immunizations, such as the combination diphtheria-pertussis-tetanus (DPT) vaccine and the polio vaccine, have *not* been associated with a higher risk of SIDS. The DPT immunization may even offer a small degree of protection against SIDS.[32,34]

The most recent theory to receive widespread media coverage addresses sleep position and SIDS. Following an extensive review of data from other countries, the American Academy of Pediatrics (AAP), in 1992, recommended that healthy infants be positioned for sleep on their side or back instead of prone (tummy-down).[32–34] The side-lying or back-lying sleeping position is recommended only for *healthy* infants, however. For premature infants with respiratory distress and for infants with certain upper airway problems, gastroesophageal reflux, or other medical problems, the prone position may well be the sleep position of choice.[34] Check with your health care provider to determine what sleep position is best for your baby.

The side-lying position is not as risky as the prone position but does have some risk because of its unstable nature. Infants put down in a side-lying position frequently end up prone at some point during the night.[33] Support cushions that help keep babies in the side-lying position are now available commercially.

Because factors other than sleep position may contribute to SIDS, the AAP also recommends the following:[34,35]

- Don't overdress or overbundle your baby or overheat your baby's room. Avoid heavy bedding that could lead to thermal stress and SIDS, especially if your baby's head is covered while lying prone. (The infant's movements during sleep could inadvertently throw the covers over her head.)
- Place your baby on a firm mattress covered only with a sheet. Avoid soft sleep surfaces, such as fluffy bedding, pillows, beanbags, or water beds, which may increase your baby's risk of suffocation from rebreathing exhaled carbon dioxide.
- Avoid maternal and household smoking.

More studies need to be done in the area of SIDS and sleep position. Some still criticize the theory that prone positioning contributes to SIDS.[36] Remember that sleeping on the tummy does not cause SIDS—and that a side-lying or a back-lying position does not necessarily *prevent* SIDS. As noted earlier, many other factors increase the relative risk of SIDS. In countries that have organized public campaigns to encourage parents to avoid the prone position, however, the incidence of SIDS has decreased by 20 to 67 percent.[32-36]

If you or someone you know has lost an infant to SIDS, ask your health care provider about grief counseling or SIDS support groups in your area. Appendix D provides names and addresses of many national SIDS organizations.

Managing Advice

The phrase "If I were you..." may already make your cheeks burn. As they did when you were pregnant, well-meaning individuals will continue to give you advice, only this time about your baby. Only you can decide what will work for you.

Your health care team has also given you recommendations for care of your baby at home. A bulletin board and calendar (see Chapter 15) may help you organize the instructional information you received from the hospital. Trust your instincts. You will soon know what needs to be done now and what can wait. Above all, let yourself enjoy the time you spend with your baby now that she is finally home and you're becoming a family.

Parent or Paramedic?

Most parents feel like paramedics-in-training throughout their children's lives. The first fever, the first rash, the first fall off the tricycle—all present new experiences in assessment and treatment. Most parents learn, through experience, the difference between serious and minor problems.

Protecting Your Baby from Family Illnesses

It's too bad that we can't wave a magic wand and protect our babies from illness and injury once they're home. The possibility of illness is especially frightening for parents of preterm infants or infants with special needs, who have already had to overcome many obstacles just to get home.

You know to limit visitors soon after your baby's arrival home and to ask that friends or family with illnesses not visit. But what if you or someone in your household gets sick? How do you keep your baby from getting the illness?

Good hand washing is the best way to prevent the spread of infection. This includes washing your hands after you blow your nose, after you sneeze or cough into your hands, and before you pick up your baby. Good hand washing is a *must* if you or someone in your family has the flu or other stomach illness. Avoid kissing or getting too close to your baby's face, especially if you have a respiratory illness or cold sore (herpes simplex virus).

It may help protect your baby during the more acute phase of your illness if another caregiver is available to provide most (but not necessarily all) of your baby's care. Some parents request a box of face masks from the hospital to take home with them in the event of a family illness. This is really not helpful, because once the mask is moistened from breathing, it doesn't provide much protection.

Keeping ill siblings away from their baby sister or brother can be difficult; it may be easier to keep the baby away from them. A careful explanation may help if the ill child is old enough to understand cause-and-effect relationships. Washing the sibling's hands periodically may help, but young children often do not cover their nose and mouth when they cough or sneeze. In addition to good hand washing, common sense helps prevent the spread of family illnesses.

Working with Your Baby's Health Care Provider

Babies with special needs usually require more vigilant watching for illness, because for these infants, a simple respiratory infection can be life-threatening. Balance this vigilance with common sense and a dose of reality. Your baby's health care providers probably explained the risks illness may present for your baby before her discharge.

If your baby is a healthy NICU graduate with few or no complications, most illnesses will run their course without problems. If your baby has special needs, illness may represent a greater threat. Communicate well with your health care provider to find out when you should call about a suspected illness and to discuss plans for home treatment, examination, or rehospitalization. You need to feel that your health care provider listens to you and takes the time to answer your questions. Seeing your health care provider on a regular basis for the first few months gives you the opportunity to get answers to your questions and concerns about baby care and parenting. The health care provider also closely monitors your baby's weight gain, medical status, and development. Anticipatory guidance in the office often prevents emergency telephone calls, unnecessary trips to the office, or emergency room visits during times of anxiety.[1-3]

"I was trying to be a good mom, but how would I know if I was doing everything right? Then the pediatrician told me that Adam was doing well because of my 'strong mothering skills.' Wow! That one comment was a turning point for me— I could do this!"

Signs and Symptoms of Illness

Knowing how much care and monitoring your baby required in the NICU, you may be concerned that you won't be able to tell when your baby is getting sick at home. You'll quickly learn, though, what is and what is not normal behavior for your baby. You'll be the best person to determine when something is not right. Trust your instincts. All babies get sick, but not every illness is life-threatening.

Some signs and symptoms of illness include:[17,37]

- Fever (a temperature higher than 99°F [37.2°C] axillary or 100°F [37.8°C] rectally) or a low temperature (less than 97°F [36.1°C] axillary) that does not respond to warming efforts or is accompanied by other symptoms of illness.
- Lack of interest in eating, or not feeding as well as usual.
- Vomiting of most or all feedings.
- Frequent watery stools (usually more than five per day) that soak into the diaper.
- A decrease in wet diapers.
- Behavior that is "just not right"—for example, less activity than usual, more sleeping, or more difficulty awakening.
- Difficulty breathing (breathing may be faster and harder, and your baby may draw in the chest muscles [called retractions] with each breath) or noisy breathing.
- More crying and irritability than usual (normal means of calming and comforting don't work). Refusal to sleep.
- Change in color: Pale, bluish, or marbled-looking (mottled) appearance.

It's important to be able to recognize when your baby is not acting like herself, but you aren't expected to play doctor. When you have concerns about illness, call your health care provider. Most offices expect calls from concerned parents and have experienced nurses to help you. Don't be shy, but be ready to supply the following information:

- Baby's name, age, and last appointment date and any concerns noted at that time.
- Why you suspect that your baby is ill.
- Baby's temperature and your method of measurement (axillary or rectal).
- Current medications. Also, any new medications or recently discontinued medications. Recent immunizations.
- Anything else your doctor should know—for example, illnesses in the family or at day care; whether your baby has shown these symptoms before, and what seemed to work last time.

Giving Medications: Missed or Vomited Doses

If your baby must continue on one or more medications at home, you need to know the name, the purpose, the dose (how much), the possible side effects, when to give, and how to administer each medication to your baby. The nurse should have given you this information in writing at discharge. Tack it to your bulletin board for handy reference.

Give all medications as directed by your baby's health care provider. Most medications work best when a specific level is maintained in the body. Missing one dose of a medication is usually not a problem, however. If you do forget a dose or if your baby vomits shortly after you give a dose, give the normal dose of the medication at the next regularly scheduled time. Some health care providers instruct you to repeat the dose once if your baby vomits within 15 minutes after receiving it. If you did not do so before discharge, check with your baby's doctor or nurse before repeating a dose, because *some medications should not be repeated under any circumstances. Never* try to make up for a missed or vomited dose by doubling or increasing the next dose.[17]

Vomiting is a common potential side effect of many of the medications given to babies. It's a sign that there may be too much of the medication in the baby's body or in the blood. Vomiting may also occur if the baby is ill with a stomach virus. Call your health care provider if your baby misses or vomits two regularly scheduled doses or if she begins to vomit more feedings than usual. A blood test to check the level of the medication in your baby's body may be needed. Also notify your doctor if your baby experiences any of the potential adverse side effects associated with a medication.[17] Appendix B contains information about common medications prescribed for infants, including potential side effects.

Don't forget these basic rules about medications:

- Keep all medications out of the reach of children.
- Use a standard pharmaceutical measuring spoon, cup, or dropper to measure medications. Do not use your regular silverware or household measuring spoons to estimate a dosage.
- Do not give your baby nonprescription medicines without consulting your baby's health care provider.
- Do not use old prescription medicines or another child's prescription medicine.
- Find out how to store the medication. For example, some medicines require refrigeration.
- Do not administer medications in the dark. Be sure you have enough light to read the label, measure the dose, and see that your baby actually receives the medication.

The Biggest Adjustment of Your Life

Having your baby home at last can seem overwhelming. Trying to establish a home routine while at the same time meeting the unpredictable demands of your baby can be exhausting. There just don't seem to be enough hours in the day.

Amid caring for your baby, making time for your other children, and attending to your partner, it's easy to forget your own basic care needs. Remember that you need to get a haircut once in a while, visit the dentist, and get some exercise. Take advantage of trustworthy volunteers who are willing to watch your baby occasionally so that you can take care of your personal needs.

Even though time alone may be short, partners also need to make time for each other if they are to successfully meet the challenge of caring for an NICU graduate. Unfortunately, the divorce rate among parents of NICU graduates is 30 percent above the average.[1,7,13] One father of an NICU graduate with special needs offers this advice: "Communication is the most important thing between parents. Talk to each other, ask questions, and above all, listen to each other. Share everything and trust your instincts. This will help you get through even the most difficult times."

Special Care for Technology-Dependent Infants

Studies have shown that the discharge of a healthy preterm infant is extremely stressful for most families. The added demands of a chronically ill or technology-dependent infant can intensify this stress and even permanently change the family structure. Parents who wanted to keep their families intact spearheaded the movement to care for infants with special needs at home. But the trade-offs for these families are many.[1–3,6–8,13,14]

Infants who are technology dependent most commonly require cardio-respiratory monitoring, respiratory support, or nutritional support in the home. The homecoming of a technology-dependent baby can produce mixed emotions in parents. It's exciting to have your baby home at last and your family reunited. It's also frightening and fatiguing to have to constantly attend to your baby's complex needs.[7,13,38,39]

You may feel overwhelmed, isolated, and exhausted. Not only do you need to manage your baby's care, but you have to understand the equipment, deal with the many people involved in your baby's care, perhaps care for other children, manage career demands, and try to restore some semblance of a normal life.[38]

You cannot do this all alone. Your hospital discharge planning team should have identified community resources available to you and helped you contact them. (See also Appendix D.) Use all the resources available to you. They may provide financial assistance, social services, and personal support.[38]

This section explains some of the devices commonly used in home care. Although the information provided here was current at the time of publication, home-care technology is constantly changing. To stay up-to-date on what is available for your baby, continue to ask questions of your baby's health care providers.

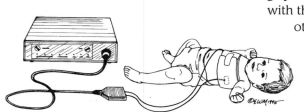

Home apnea monitor.

Use your baby's apnea monitor whenever the baby is sleeping or when you are busy. The soft belt fits over the two leads and around the baby's chest and is connected by a cable to the apnea monitor. The monitor can be removed when you are playing with your baby and at bath time.

Apnea Monitor

Infants may require apnea monitoring in the home for a variety of problems that affect breathing. They include apnea, oxygen dependence because of bronchopulmonary dysplasia (BPD), tracheostomy or ventilator use, family history of apnea or sudden infant death syndrome (SIDS), and neuromuscular diseases that compromise respiratory effort. Because apnea is relatively common in preterm infants, it is the focus of this section.

Apnea is any pause in breathing (respirations) of 20 or more seconds or of less than 20 seconds if it is accompanied by cyanosis (blue color), bradycardia (slowing of the heart rate below what's normal for the baby's age), or oxygen desaturation (too little oxygen available to the tissues). Before discharge, the doctor will have ruled out other physiologic causes for your baby's apnea, such as anemia, gastroesophageal reflux, bronchospasm related to underlying BPD, or seizures.[3,17,38,40]

Babies diagnosed with apnea of prematurity are often treated with medications such as theophylline or caffeine, which help stimulate the respiratory center in the brain. Babies who have frequent episodes of apnea and bradycardia are not discharged, even with an apnea monitor, until the episodes resolve or become less severe. In most cases, babies outgrow apnea and bradycardia. Clinical observation usually determines whether your baby is breathing well enough on her own to be discharged safely. Some units also perform a pneumocardiogram (PCG) before discharge to monitor your baby's breathing and heart rate more closely. Also called a sleep study, a PCG is sensitive to periodic breathing, apnea, poor oxygenation, or slowing of the heart rate that may not trigger the alarms of traditional monitors. Institutions vary in their use and interpretation of PCGs (see Chapter 15). Many hospitals do not use them at all but rely heavily on your baby's clinical history (recent episodes) to determine the need for home apnea monitoring.[3,17,40]

Most hospitals do not provide apnea monitors for home use. Instead, the monitor is ordered from an outside company (sometimes referred to as a vendor or a durable medical equipment [DME] company) and is delivered to the hospital before your baby's discharge. Your discharge planner, case manager, or social worker coordinates this process. The vendor instructs parents in the use of the apnea monitor before the baby's discharge. The DME company also provides an instruction manual and a phone number for monitor problems once you are home. The vendor should encourage parents to ask questions.

Some hospitals require that parents spend a night rooming-in with their baby before discharge to ensure that the monitor is working properly and that the parents feel comfortable and competent in its operation. Rooming-in is also excellent for practicing the routine care, feedings, and other specialty care (such as medication administration) your baby may need (see Chapter 15). You will learn how to respond to monitor alarms and when to notify your doctor about unusual events. You will also have a chance to get to know your baby's behavior on a 24-hour basis, with nurses and doctors nearby to answer questions.

If your baby has come home with an apnea monitor, you'll want to use it whenever you or your baby is sleeping and when you are busy. It's acceptable to take the monitor off when you're playing with your baby during more alert periods and when you're bathing your baby. This gives her skin a break from the belt that secures the monitor. The belt can irritate her skin, especially when the weather is warm.

Parents are often relieved that their baby has been discharged home on a monitor. It makes them feel more secure. After about a week, though, they're

"I went back to work two weeks after Katie's birth. I finished my maternity leave two months later, when Katie came home from the hospital. That's when we really needed our time together."

ready to throw the monitor out the window, because false alarms are driving them crazy. False alarms are usually set off by abdominal breathing or by loose or incorrectly placed monitor electrodes (leads). The frequency of false alarms tends to increase as a baby grows older and becomes more active. Ignoring the alarms or assuming them to be false can be potentially dangerous.[3,40]

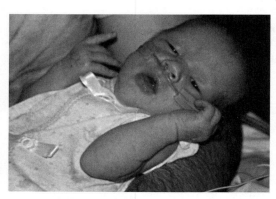

Nasal cannula.

You will learn how to secure your baby's nasal cannula. Techniques vary from place to place. You will discover what works best for you and your baby.

Health care providers will ask you to keep a log (record) of alarms at home to help them determine when to discontinue monitoring and/or medications. Most babies who come home on both monitor and medications are allowed to outgrow the dose of medication provided the apnea and bradycardia episodes diminish and then stop. When your baby has been free of apnea and bradycardia for a designated period, your health care provider will stop the medication. A home PCG may be ordered a few days later. The apnea monitor is frequently continued for another month or two. If no episodes of apnea or bradycardia are recorded, the monitor may then be discontinued. A second home PCG may be done immediately before monitor use is stopped.[3,40]

An apnea monitor usually has three alarms: for apnea, slow heart rate, and fast heart rate. Your health care provider tells the equipment company what alarm settings to use for your baby. Typically, the apnea alarm is set at 15 seconds; slow heart rate, at 80 beats per minute; and fast heart rate, at 210 beats per minute. The alarm limits are lowered as your baby gets older.

As with anything electrical, you need to take certain precautions if your infant has a home apnea monitor. Your baby should not be left unsupervised with other children. Infants have been electrocuted by older siblings placing their lead wires into a wall socket. Most monitors today have a protective covering over the lead wires to prevent this from occurring. If your baby's monitor does not have this safety feature, ask for a newer model. Even with a protective design, older children should be specifically warned not to handle the monitor.[3,40] Letters from your health care provider will be given to you to send to your telephone company, electric company, and local Emergency Medical Service (EMS) system alerting them that you have an infant with special needs in your home.

Oxygen

Babies who are medically stable on supplemental oxygen may go home on oxygen, provided that parents learn the necessary care before discharge. Bronchopulmonary dysplasia (BPD) is the most common condition of babies discharged home on oxygen. With BPD, the lungs are damaged and scarred from long periods on a ventilator and on oxygen. Smaller babies and those born earlier than 32 weeks gestation are at the greatest risk for developing this complication. The heart and lungs of a baby with BPD must work particularly hard. Fortunately, as the baby grows, so does new lung tissue—and the damaged lung may heal.[17,40,41]

Other reasons for sending a baby home with supplemental oxygen include:[3,17,40,41]

- Evidence of oxygen desaturation when breathing room air while awake, at rest, with activity, or with feedings.
- Poor nippling caused by "air hunger" (baby seems to have difficulty catching her breath).
- Apnea or bradycardia that responds to supplemental oxygen.
- Poor weight gain.
- Airway problems, tracheostomy, or ventilator use.

Supplemental oxygen is usually delivered through a nasal cannula—a small tube that fits under your baby's nose and around the head.[3,17,40,41] Three types of oxygen delivery systems are used in the home:

1. Compressed gas: Oxygen in the gaseous state is pressurized into cylinders, or tanks. A small, portable tank is delivered to the hospital, and a very large, nonportable tank is sent directly to your home. A respiratory therapist from the equipment supply company will show you how to read the gauges to determine when you need to refill your tanks. The length of time between tank refillings depends on how much oxygen your baby uses and on the size of the tank. A portable E cylinder set at ½ liter of oxygen per minute by nasal cannula, for example, lasts about 20 hours. A smaller D cylinder lasts about 12 hours. The larger H cylinder backup tank at the same setting lasts approximately 175 hours.[17] Larger backup tanks come in a few different sizes as well. Usually the company exchanges your large tank with a full one when the pressure in it reaches 500 pounds per square inch (psi).[3,17,40]

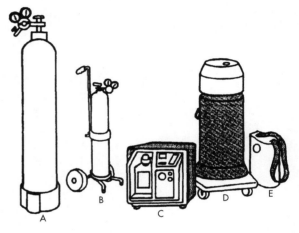

Types of oxygen systems.

(A) H cylinder compressed oxygen tank (backup oxygen tank).
(B) E cylinder with portable carrier.
(C) Oxygen concentrator.
(D) Liquid oxygen tank.
(E) Liquid oxygen portable tank.

From: Parker L, and Richardson C. 1990. Ochsner NICU Babybook: Parent Edition. New Orleans: Alton Ochsner Medical Foundation. Reprinted by permission.

2. Oxygen concentrator: An oxygen concentrator is a device that separates oxygen out of the air and gives it to your baby. Because a concentrator runs on electricity, a portable backup oxygen tank is necessary when your baby is not near an electrical outlet and in the event of a power outage.

3. Liquid oxygen: Oxygen that has been cooled to a liquid state is called liquid oxygen. It changes to a gas as your baby breathes it. A liquid oxygen tank takes up considerably less space than a large compressed oxygen tank, which contains oxygen in the gaseous form and is used as a backup oxygen tank. As with a compressed oxygen system, a small, portable tank is delivered to the hospital, and a larger, nonportable tank is sent directly to your home. One drawback of liquid oxygen is that it evaporates when not in use. It's also expensive and may not be covered under insurance provisions.[3,17,40] A portable liquid oxygen tank set at ½ liter of oxygen per minute via nasal cannula lasts approximately 8 hours. The larger backup tank at the same setting lasts approximately 500 hours.[17]

Regardless of the type of oxygen system in your home, certain safety precautions must be followed. Because oxygen is a highly flammable substance, there should be no smoking in a room where oxygen equipment is located.

When your baby is receiving oxygen, keep her at least 6 feet away from open flames, such as heaters, fireplaces, or gas appliances with pilot lights. Oxygen tanks themselves should also be kept at least 6 feet away from an open flame, radiator, or heater. Do not use rubbing alcohol, petroleum jelly, or spray cans near a baby on oxygen. Keep the door to your baby's room open so the room is well ventilated and not stuffy.[17] Finally, make sure the smoke detectors in your home work well, and periodically review your home fire escape plan with your family.

Your instruction in home oxygen use should have begun well before discharge to give you ample opportunity to ask questions and practice operating the equipment. Rooming-in with your baby and the oxygen equipment is an excellent way to achieve these goals (see Chapter 15). Infants who are oxygen dependent sometimes need chest physiotherapy (CPT, which is percussion on the chest to help loosen secretions [phlegm]; see Chapter 10), periodic aerosol breathing treatments (medication inhaled directly into the lungs to open breathing passages), and systemic oral medications at home. Rooming-in also provides the opportunity to learn these aspects of your baby's care.

After discharge, babies on oxygen will receive home health nursing visits or private-duty nursing if medically necessary. The amount and type of home nursing follow-up is determined by your baby's physician, your individual needs, and your health care coverage.

The decision to begin weaning a baby from oxygen depends on many factors. Some physicians begin weaning when the baby's respiratory effort decreases and oxygen saturation stabilizes. Other physicians keep the baby on oxygen to ensure continued weight gain and attainment of developmental milestones. Studies report fewer respiratory infections in infants on oxygen than in those whose oxygen saturation levels are borderline.[42] Your doctor will take into account these and other factors unique to your baby. Weaning is usually gradual and is accompanied by physical examinations, chest x-rays, and frequent oxygenation measurements (which can be done in your home by a respiratory therapist). If at any time your baby fails to progress in the weaning schedule, she will be evaluated to determine the cause. Your baby will be assessed frequently throughout the weaning process to determine her tolerance for increasingly lower levels of oxygen, until the oxygen is finally discontinued.[3,40,41]

Feeding Tubes

Although most infants are able to take in adequate nutrition by mouth before discharge, a few cannot. Babies who have problems with their heart, lungs, brain, muscle coordination, esophagus (food pipe), or mouth (such as cleft lip and/or palate) may not be able to suck and/or swallow well. A variety of feeding tubes is available to make sure your infant receives the proper nourishment for growth and development.

Nasogastric and Orogastric Tubes

Use of a nasogastric (NG) tube is generally a temporary measure to supplement your baby's oral intake. An NG tube is often used for infants who are able to nipple some of their feeding but not enough to get adequate calories for growth and development. It is inserted into one nostril of your baby's nose and passed through the esophagus into the stomach, then taped in place for a period of time. When it's changed, the tube is inserted through the other nostril.

The most common problem with NG tubes is that they can cause nasal irritation and/or bleeding. If this occurs, change the NG tube to the other side until the irritated nostril heals. Rarely, if used for extended periods (usually several months), NG tubes can also cause esophageal irritation and/or erosions. If you note blood when checking residuals or in your baby's vomit, notify the doctor immediately.

If your baby has an NG tube, you may let her nipple as much as possible by mouth first. Then you'll attach a syringe filled with the remainder of the milk to the NG tube and feed the milk to your baby slowly by gravity flow. If your baby has not fallen asleep and is not too stressed, you may want to offer a pacifier during the gavage portion of the feeding. This helps your baby to associate sucking with the feeling of getting a full stomach.[3,17,40]

Some babies can't tolerate an NG tube because it blocks part of one nostril and may interfere with breathing. An orogastric (OG) tube, which is inserted into the baby's mouth, may be used instead. Parents who do not wish to have anything taped to their baby's face may prefer the OG tube, which is usually inserted before each feeding and removed afterward. Frequent insertion of an OG tube can stress some babies, however, and an NG tube that remains taped in place is more convenient for a baby who requires frequent gavage feedings. Both NG and OG tubes can cause gagging and vomiting on insertion and removal.

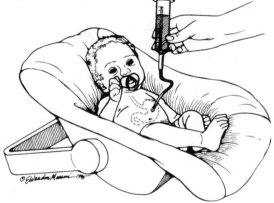

Gastrostomy tube feeding.

Your baby's gastrostomy tube ensures that she receives adequate nutrition. A feeding syringe attaches to the gastrostomy tube, and the formula flows into the baby's stomach by gravity. Most health care professionals recommend offering the baby a pacifier to suck during the feeding so that she learns to associate sucking with the feeling of a full stomach.

If your baby has an OG tube, you may insert the OG tube and gavage feed your baby first, then remove the tube and let her finish the feeding by sucking. If the OG tube is inserted after feeding, the baby may gag and vomit everything she worked so hard to eat. As your baby's feeding abilities improve, you will gavage feed less and allow your baby to suck more. It's preferable to end your baby's feeding with the pleasant association of sucking.

Before discharge, your baby's health care providers should have given you written instructions for gavage feedings. The instructions should cover gathering equipment, measuring and inserting the tube, checking for correct placement of the tube, checking any residual from the previous feeding, feeding your baby, removing the tube, and cleaning the equipment.[3,17,40]

Gastrostomy Tube

An ostomy is formed by surgically creating an artificial opening in the gastrointestinal tract. This opening in the stomach (gastrostomy) or the intestine (jejunostomy, ileostomy, or colostomy) is attached to the skin covering the abdominal wall.[43,44]

When health care providers anticipate that your infant will have long-term feeding difficulties, your baby will go to surgery for placement of a gastrostomy tube (GT). A rubber tube is inserted into your baby's stomach through a hole made in the stomach by a surgeon. You can then feed the prescribed amount of formula through the tube directly into your baby's stomach. If your baby has problems with gastroesophageal reflux (spitting up; see Chapter 14), a surgical procedure called a fundoplication is sometimes done at the same time the GT is placed. A fundoplication tightens the valve between the esophagus (food pipe) and the stomach. This prevents food from moving back up into the baby's esophagus. Feedings are usually started slowly, using the gastrostomy tube, two to three days after surgery. [3,17,40,43,44]

Your baby may also eat by mouth if she can and if there are no other medical reasons not to. A GT, like a nasogastric (NG) tube, may be used to supply what your baby cannot take by mouth. You attach a syringe filled with the remaining formula to the GT and feed the milk to your baby slowly by gravity flow. It's beneficial to give your baby a pacifier during the GT feeding so that she learns to associate sucking with the feeling of getting a full stomach. This technique, called nonnutritive sucking, is particularly important for babies who cannot nipple feed at all but will accept a pacifier.[3,17,40,43,44] When your baby's nippling ability improves to the point that she is getting adequate nutrition orally, the GT may be removed.

Button gastrostomy tube: If you and your doctor feel your baby may have difficulty feeding over a longer period of time, the GT may be converted to a button gastrostomy after two to three months or once your baby reaches a certain weight (usually about 4,530 grams, or 10 pounds). This procedure can usually be done in your doctor's office.

A button gastrostomy allows you to remove the feeding-tube attachment after the feeding. A flap, which looks similar to a valve on a beach ball when it's pushed in, then closes the area over the stoma (the opening in the abdominal wall). Button gastrostomies are less obvious under shirts and are easy to care for. You can even submerge a button underwater during a bath.

Percutaneous endoscopic gastrostomy tube: If your baby has no problems with reflux and does not require surgery for a fundoplication but is a weak feeder, she may have a percutaneous endoscopic gastrostomy (PEG) tube. A PEG is a type of gastrostomy tube that can be inserted without surgery. Percutaneous means "through the skin." An endoscope is a floppy tube with a light on the end that is used to place the PEG tube properly in the stomach. When a PEG tube is inserted, the baby's throat is numbed and then the endoscope is used to pass the tube through the baby's mouth and into the stomach. The tube is then advanced up out of the stomach through a small hole made through the skin of the abdomen. A PEG tube requires only a small opening (stoma) in the stomach; local anesthesia is used to numb the abdominal skin. If long-term feeding problems are anticipated, a PEG tube may be replaced

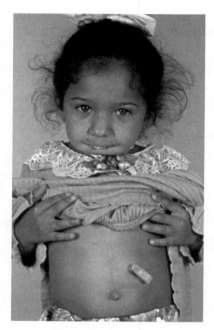

Button gastrostomy.

A button gastrostomy allows removal of the feeding tube attachment after feeding. A button is not obvious under clothing and can even be submerged at bath time.

with a button gastrostomy after two to three months or when your baby weighs about 4,530 grams, or 10 pounds.

The procedures for feeding with and care of a PEG tube are similar to those for a GT. They include gathering equipment, checking for any residual from the previous feeding, feeding your baby, removing the syringe, and cleaning the equipment. Gastrostomy, button, and PEG tube care also includes routine cleaning around the stoma (insertion site). Your doctor may order cleaning once or twice a day and as needed. You may be instructed to clean the site with a mild soap and water and/or half-strength hydrogen peroxide (hydrogen peroxide can dry and irritate the skin). You should have received written instructions before discharge. Local skin irritation and drainage from the stoma site are the most common complications of gastrostomy tubes. If either occurs, your doctor may recommend a topical antibiotic ointment or a drying powder. Accidental removal of the tube and tube movement within the stomach are rare complications.[3,17,40,43–45] Accidental removal of your baby's gastrostomy tube is not a medical emergency. You will be taught how to replace it or instructed to call your baby's doctor if this occurs.

Continuous Feedings

Infants unable to nipple feed or handle bolus feedings (the entire feeding given at once instead of over a long period of time) may require continuous feedings using a feeding pump. Continuous feedings may be given through any of the feeding tubes just discussed. You should have received instruction in the use of the equipment before your baby's discharge. Equipment and supplies for home tube feedings, as well as home nursing follow-up, are also arranged before discharge based on your baby's medical condition, your individual needs, and your health care coverage.

Ileostomy and Colostomy

An ileostomy or a colostomy is most commonly performed after surgical removal of a portion of the small or large intestine, respectively. One of these procedures may have been necessary if your baby had necrotizing enterocolitis (NEC; see Chapter 10), an imperforate anus (or anal atresia), Hirschsprung's disease, an intestinal obstruction, or some other problem with the gastrointestinal tract. In both of these procedures, an opening (stoma) is made in the abdominal wall, and a portion of the intestine is brought to the surface and attached to the skin. Your baby's bowel movements will come through this hole instead of from her rectum. The stoma is covered with a bag or pouch to collect the stool, which is more liquid than what you would find in a diaper. Ostomies are often temporary. When your baby is big enough and the intestines are healed enough, the cut sections may be surgically put back together again.[3,17,43]

Before discharge, you were taught how to empty and change your baby's ostomy bag and do skin care. Post the written instructions you were given on your bulletin board for reference. Basic care is reviewed here. Hold the opened bottom of the ostomy bag over a container to empty the stool, or use a large

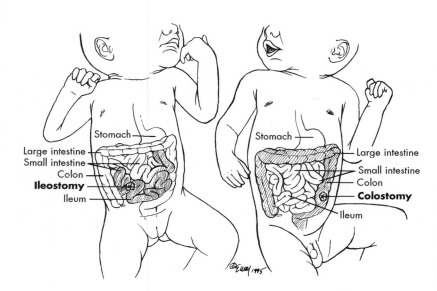

Ileostomy.

A portion of the small intestine is brought to the surface and attached to the skin. The baby's bowel movements will come through this hole instead of through her rectum. A plastic bag fits over the stoma and collects the stool.

Colostomy.

A portion of the large intestine is brought to the surface and attached to the skin. As with an ileostomy, the stoma of the colostomy is covered by a disposable plastic bag that collects the baby's bowel movements.

syringe to empty stool that is more liquid. Use a squeeze bottle or large syringe filled with cool water to rinse the stool out of the bag. Then dry the bottom of the bag and close it with the twist tie provided or with a rubber band. Ostomy bags need to be changed routinely every few days or if leaking occurs. Once the old bag is removed, wash the skin with a mild soap and water, rinse and pat dry, and inspect the skin for redness or sores. Antibiotic ointments or adhesive powders and pastes are sometimes needed to remedy problems of skin irritation, bleeding, or leakage of stool. Call your health care provider if these problems persist. Ostomy bags are attached to adhesive backings cut to fit around your baby's stoma. The new bag fits over the stoma and sticks with adhesive backing onto the skin.[3,17,43]

Equipment and supplies for home ostomy care and home nursing follow-up are arranged before discharge based on your baby's medical condition, your individual needs, and your health care coverage.

Tracheostomy

A tracheostomy is a surgical opening made through your baby's neck and into the windpipe (trachea). Your baby then breathes through a tube inserted in this artificial opening instead of through the nose or mouth. The most common reasons babies require a tracheostomy include:[3,17,40,46]

- Birth defects that affect the airway.
- Upper airway obstructions, such as tracheomalacia (a soft airway that collapses with respirations) or subglottic stenosis (a narrowing of the trachea caused by prolonged ventilation or repeated intubations).
- The need for continued ventilation (ventilator dependence).
- Neuromuscular disorders that affect the ability to swallow and handle saliva, thus interfering with breathing.

A tracheostomy is not always permanent. The tube may be removed once the underlying problem is corrected or your baby grows big enough and no longer needs help breathing.[3,17,40,46]

Home care for a baby with a tracheostomy (or trach, pronounced trake) is quite involved and requires a significant commitment to learning on the family's part. Having more than one family member learn tracheostomy care helps to ensure that the primary caregiver will get much-needed relief and support. This is not always possible, however, and the issue is generally addressed with your doctors, nurses, and social workers during discharge planning.

Home tracheostomy care includes:

- Routine suctioning of the tracheostomy tube to clear the artificial airway of secretions (mucus).
- Use of an oxygen bag and saline (a sterile saltwater solution) to assist with breathing and secretion removal. An oxygen bag is a device that when squeezed delivers air and/or oxygen like a breath to the baby through the tracheostomy tube (or face mask, if the tracheostomy tube is not functioning in an emergency).
- Daily cleaning of the skin around the tracheostomy opening (stoma) with either mild soap and water or half-strength hydrogen peroxide (as recommended by your doctor) and assessment of the skin for irritation.
- Daily changing of the tracheostomy ties or tracheostomy tube holder.
- Routine changing of the tracheostomy tube itself (usually recommended every one to four weeks) or daily changing and cleaning of the inner cannula (inner cannulas are used with larger tracheostomies in older children).
- Operation and cleaning of equipment and supplies.
- Special attention to general baby care and safety, because a baby with a tracheostomy cannot make any crying or cooing sounds.

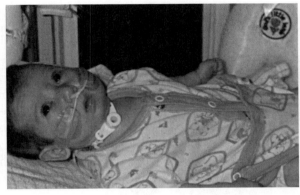

Tracheostomy.

A tracheostomy is a surgical opening made through the baby's neck and into the windpipe (trachea). The baby breathes through a tube inserted into this opening instead of through her nose or mouth.

Babies discharged home with a tracheostomy tube also often require some type of humidification; an apnea monitor to alert parents to potential problems, such as plugging of the tube; aerosol or breathing treatments; and medications.[3,17,40,46]

At discharge, parents of babies with a tracheostomy tube learn what is normal breathing for their baby by observing and participating in the baby's care. This knowledge helps you watch for signs of breathing problems, which may include:

- Irritability, restlessness, and/or sweating.
- Increased respiratory rate.
- Noisy respirations (grunting, gurgling, or whistling from the tracheostomy).
- Nasal flaring.
- Retractions (sinking in of the chest and skin, making the breastbone and ribs visible).
- Color change (to pale, dusky, or blue).

Problems with a tracheostomy tube can be life-threatening. You need to be able to identify potential problems right away and then immediately contact your physician, Emergency Medical Service system, or ambulance service. Plugging of the tracheostomy with mucus, vomit, or blood requires quick thinking and fast action by the parent to prevent a life-threatening event. Before discharge, care providers should have discussed actions to take in emergencies, and you may even have been asked to play-act your responses. It's also important that you know how to ventilate your baby using an oxygen bag or by mouth-to-tracheostomy-tube ventilations. For acute emergencies, parents should also know how to perform infant cardiopulmonary

"No matter what happens to your baby at home, you have enough time to make a plan. Stop and think things through in an emergency. Don't run, walk. Don't panic, direct someone to help. When you use the first moments of an emergency to get organized, you save precious seconds when they matter the most."

resuscitation (CPR) modified for a baby with a tracheostomy.[3,40,46,47] Post your emergency instructions on a kitchen cupboard or closet door or at the head of your baby's bed.

The more you learned about your baby's tracheostomy care and other needs through rooming-in and independent caretaking during your infant's hospital stay, the smoother the transition to home will be.

Your pediatrician will work closely with the specialist who placed your baby's tracheostomy tube to determine the timing of weaning and decannulation (removal of the tube). Once your baby is big enough or the problem that necessitated the tracheostomy is corrected, the weaning process may begin. Frequently, your baby will be weaned to a tube that is a size smaller than the one in place or allowed to outgrow the tube in place without changing to a larger size. If she is able to tolerate the smaller tube for the designated trial period (weeks or months), then she may be weaned to the next smaller size, if necessary. As your baby gradually begins to breathe around the smaller tube, you may be able to hear her make sounds. Before decannulation occurs, your baby's tracheostomy may be capped to see if she can tolerate the full work of breathing on her own. Capping is often done in the hospital overnight so that your baby's respiratory rate, heart rate, and oxygen saturation can be monitored. A blood gas analysis of your baby's oxygenation and carbon dioxide levels may also be performed. If all parameters remain within normal limits for your baby, the tracheostomy tube will be removed. The hole in the neck is usually left to heal gradually on its own without surgical repair. It will leave a small scar.[3,40,46]

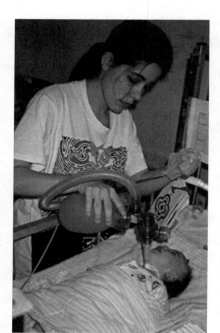

Suctioning the tracheostomy at home.

This baby's mother hand-bags through his tracheostomy during suctioning. When she is finished, she re-attaches his tracheostomy to a home ventilator. Care of a ventilator-dependent baby requires help from many community services and a tremendous commitment on the part of the baby's family.

Home Ventilator

In some instances, infants who need long-term ventilatory support can be cared for at home. As is the case with any technology-dependent infant, there are several important factors to consider regarding the practicality of home ventilation.

First, other than being unable to wean from the ventilator, is your baby basically stable? That is, is the disease or condition that is causing the need for ventilation under control? Your baby's doctor will determine the answer to this question.

Second, what are your own feelings? A 24-hour-per-day, 7-day-per-week commitment can place a tremendous strain on even the best-functioning families. Sometimes, the decision must be made in the best interest of the family as a whole, not necessarily in the best interest of one member. You should not feel pressured into taking your ventilator-dependent infant home. Centers for intermediate care may be available in your area.

Third, is your home environment appropriate for ventilator care? Do you have enough space to handle all of the equipment and supplies? Are there enough electrical outlets? The company supplying the ventilator and supplies can assess your home's electrical capability.

A Night in the Life of a Special Child

Somewhere in a far-off place, people sleep through the night and wake to a ringing alarm clock. In our house, the alarm can ring or buzz loudly no matter what the clock says.

Our little one, and I do mean little, has wriggled free of his monitor's leads again.

I sleepily push the wrong button on the monitor, and the intermittent sound changes to a never-ending wail. Oops! My spouse squints open one eye. I smile sorrowfully, shaking my head with guilt, and with open hands pantomime what stupidity it took to set the whole thing off. She squints and covers her ears, burrowing under the covers.

I walk the few steps to David's crib and check wires, leads, baby. The sound continues...it may never stop..... Then there is silence. But I turn to see my wife holding the monitor's buttons to still the alarm.

My "Sorry, Honey" follows her back to bed, and I am left standing alone.

I touch the lamp to read the daily log sheet, and bright light fills the room, causing me to wince. Even my son turns and covers his head with his blanket. Now I have two of them, mother and son, "night-burrowing light eschewers," and I have to ask myself, "Why am I not in bed?" I read the log and it says why. It's time to feed David.

I lean heavily on the rail going downstairs to the kitchen, finding that late-night stiffness, as usual, ends with the last step downward. I think of mixing the formula, but after checking the refrigerator, I am rewarded with a prepared bottle. This means a quick heating, and I am back upstairs. But did I turn off the lights? Back down I go, and up. Did I make sure the refrigerator was closed? This time I check everything and then thump back up the stairs with the bottle.... "Bottle? Where's the bottle?" Up from the kitchen again, I am now a proven competitor in Late-Night Stair Aerobics. Leaning on the crib for support as I gasp for oxygen, I find the angelic David asleep, making cute little facial expressions while his daddy wonders why the room seems so warm.

In any event, little David must be fed. "Come on, Son, try the bottle this time!" But David only opens his mouth to voice his refusal. One look from my wife, now "the frown that lives under the covers," and I realize that David must be fed by his feeding tube. His doctors want him to conserve energy and sleep at night, saving his nippling attempts for the daylight hours.

Actually, tube feeding a child is an easy task, taking only a little dexterity and planning. Once the feeding tube syringe is attached, maneuvering the already-uncapped bottle and pouring is simple. At night and with only a few hours sleep, I find myself in a slow-motion comedy of errors culminating with the ever-present where-did-I-put-the-feeding-tube-cap routine. Five minutes later, I find the cap just where I left it, only slightly hidden by the written log papers.

continued...

I don't spill any this time, and David takes it all. Usually, the last 5 to 10 milliliters just won't go in. But that's when I am allowed to "plunge" the formula slowly into the baby. Another concern is that a cough, burp, or some other stomach motion can "refill" the feeding syringe, and then I must begin the feeding again. We who have mastered the feeding tube find that a little pinch to the tube will hold back the flood, much as the little Dutch boy with the dike.

Feeding is over. David is breathing fine, and his skin color is good. His little face nuzzles his blanket. I pause and try to memorize the picture. David is quite a resilient little guy, and that's the key. Without resilience, David would not be home, would not be growing or getting better. Sure, he struggles, but life is a struggle. Together, though, we try to make it better. We try, we fail, we succeed, and the process repeats itself. It's like breathing. You don't think about it a lot. You just do it.

I yawn and smile. David's okay, and I'm tired. I try not to trip over anything, and I crawl beneath the very welcome bedcovers. I roll onto my back, and as my head touches the pillow, I wonder, "Did I turn the monitor back on?" I throw back the covers, march to the crib, and press the button. The buzzer sounds, David starts crying, and I can't shut it off. I pick up the baby to quiet him, and then there is abrupt silence again. My wife breathes heavily, with her hand on the silenced monitor. She pats David gently and signals me to return to bed. The next feeding will be her turn.

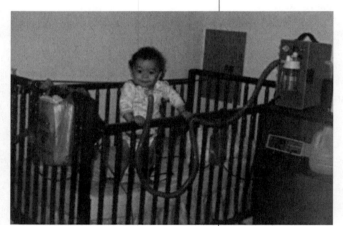

Home setup for a tracheostomy dependent baby.

Home care for a technology-dependent baby is not easy but is well worth the effort for many families.

Feeding tubes, syringes, nebulizers, monitors and alarms, treatments, therapy, operations, doctors, nurses, social workers, insurance, bills, government programs, etcetera. Nothing seems to end. But then there are wonderful little milestones every day. David is born, he can breathe, he survives the operation, another operation, he can smile, he can suck, he can lift his head, he can even eat and wet, and these go on. I remember every day that we have been given hope, and every day that our hopes have been crushed. The memories of those earlier days fade as each day with David fills our lives with new hopes and love. I mentioned earlier that resilience was the key to David's survival, and really it's the key for us all. A lot of our resilience comes from the humor that we find even in the struggles of everyday life.

Special thanks to Penn Hendler for contributing this story about a typical night feeding with his son, David.

Finally, what community support systems are available in your area? These may include appropriately trained home nurses, 24-hour servicing of equipment and supplies, emergency medical services, other support persons to provide backup or respite care, early intervention programs, and financial resources.[3,7,40,41,46,48]

If your infant is ventilator dependent, you'll have been trained in use of a home ventilator (which is different from the NICU ventilator), but you'll also need to know about tracheostomy care, use of an apnea monitor, home oxygen therapy (possibly), and if your baby has a feeding problem, gastrostomy care. This specialized training is usually provided through your NICU or at a transitional care facility that has a home ventilator program. Training usually takes several weeks, during which you room-in with your baby to learn the necessary care.[3,40,41,46,48]

After discharge, you and your baby will be closely followed by a variety of services. A home health nurse may visit daily to assess your baby, or private-duty nurses may be in your home to monitor your baby up to 24 hours a day. A respiratory therapist from the equipment supply company will do periodic ventilator checks and assist you with other equipment and supply needs. An education specialist from the early-intervention program (explained in Chapter 17) may visit to do an individual family service plan.

Several doctors may follow your baby closely. Often a pediatric pulmonologist manages the ventilator care. If weaning from the ventilator becomes possible as your baby grows, it will be done in small increments as your baby can tolerate it. You, the respiratory therapist, and your baby's nurses will need to monitor your baby closely as she is weaned from the ventilator. Frequent visits to doctors' offices and an occasional readmission to the hospital for pulmonary function tests may also be required.[3,40,41,46,48]

The Key: Coordination

For a technology-dependent infant, it's crucial that coordination of care continues after discharge. As a parent, you need to identify one person who will coordinate your infant's medical care now that you are home. That person most often is your primary health care provider. Teamwork is essential in caring for your special baby. Work closely with your health care professionals, and stay in close touch with your insurance case manager or social worker.

Pulling It All Together

Now that you're home at last, your feelings and family structure may be changing. The anxiety and fear about making it through each day of hospitalization are replaced by exhaustion and perhaps sleepless nights. You may be about ready to send back the baby you couldn't wait to bring home.

Have confidence in what you've learned about your baby's care. Identify helpful resources and use them. The challenge of establishing a home routine remains yours, however. As one mother put it, "My life has never been in such chaos, and yet it's never been more rewarding!"

Chapter 17

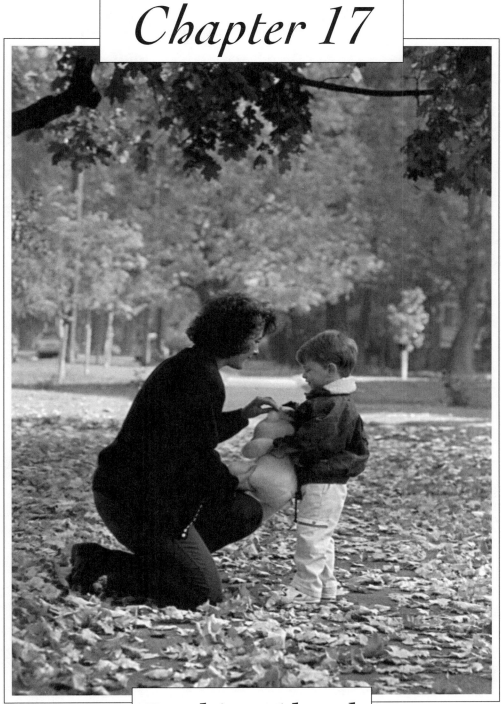

Looking Ahead

TrezMarie T. Zotkiewicz, RNC, MN

"Piglet sighed with happiness, and began to think about himself. He was BRAVE..."

The NICU experience doesn't end at discharge. Many parents describe their baby's first year of life as the longest roller-coaster ride of their lives. The first weeks at home are filled with mixed emotions, new challenges, and changes within your family. Now that you're home and settling into a routine, you'll begin looking to the future.

Developing Normally

Having a baby in the NICU is frightening. Your initial concern is survival. Once your baby is medically stable, though, it's only natural to wonder, "Will my baby be normal?" This section addresses medical and environmental risk factors that can affect your child's development and also looks at the potential for behavioral and learning problems.

Neonatal Risk Factors

Although it's difficult to talk in absolutes about developmental outcome among NICU graduates, it's safe to say that most NICU infants do not have significant disabilities.[1-5] Even so, many parents worry about their baby's risk of having physical and/or developmental delays, cerebral palsy, or visual or hearing losses. Usually, the more complicated the hospital course, the greater the risk of problems. Neonatal factors—that is, factors related to your baby's experience in the uterus, during labor and birth, and in the early days of life—that predispose infants to developmental, physical, visual, or auditory challenges include:[1-5]

- Prematurity and low birth weight of less than 3 pounds, 5 ounces (1,500 grams). The lower an infant's birth weight, the higher the risk of future problems
- Intraventricular hemorrhage (IVH) and periventricular leukomalacia (PVL)
- Perinatal asphyxia, with or without seizures and brain damage
- Bronchopulmonary dysplasia (BPD) and long-term mechanical ventilation with prolonged need for supplemental oxygen
- Other chronic illnesses, such as short bowel or short gut syndrome
- Significant intrauterine growth retardation (IUGR)
- Multiple birth defects and known genetic syndromes, especially defects of the head and neck
- Neonatal infections (cytomegalovirus, herpes, Group B Streptococcus, and others)
- Significant hyperbilirubinemia (jaundice) requiring exchange transfusion

344

- Receiving an ototoxic medication (one with side effects that can negatively affect hearing, such as certain antibiotics) for more than five days
- An extended NICU stay

You'll find more information on most of these factors in Chapters 8 through 10.

Environmental Risk Factors

A baby's medical problems are not the only factors that play a role in determining his developmental outcome. The family's socioeconomic status also influences childhood development. The risk of developmental delays and other health problems is greater for both term and preterm infants on the lower rungs of the socioeconomic ladder than for those from more affluent families. The significant financial pressures and other stressors that less-advantaged families must face can affect the development of their children.[6-8]

The caregiver's educational level and the quality of the care given also influence a baby's development. The amount of attention and stimulation a baby receives at home and the types of opportunities a baby has to learn new skills all play a part in developmental outcome.[1-5]

The impact of your baby's environment on his development can't be emphasized enough. Infants with known developmental risk factors, such as an intraventricular hemorrhage (IVH), may develop normally with early intervention and appropriate stimulation at home. Conversely, babies discharged as "well premies" may return to follow-up clinics with significant delays, in part because of lack of learning opportunities at home. An environment rich in learning opportunities is of utmost importance to your baby's developmental progress.

Developmental tests are often used to measure a child's mental, social, speech and language, and physical skills. Activities such as playing pat-a-cake, using a spoon to stir pretend coffee, pointing to body parts on a doll, drawing, and playing with simple puzzles are used to elicit responses that help testers determine a child's developmental progress. But children who have never played pat-a-cake or put together a puzzle may fail these parts of developmental tests because they have never had the opportunity to learn these skills. This type of developmental delay is related to lack of learning opportunities provided by parents and other caregivers—and is preventable.[1-5]

Potential for Behavior Problems

Behavior problems may be evident in early infancy. Infants who are preterm or chronically ill are often irritable and show unpredictable feeding, crying, and sleeping patterns. They are less responsive than their well, term counterparts and therefore require understanding of their behavioral cues to prevent overstimulation.

Not all premature or chronically ill babies have behavior problems in childhood, but some do. Behavior problems seen in early childhood include frequent temper tantrums, overaggressivness in play, hyperactivity, and exaggerated separation anxiety. As these children reach school age, their behaviors may worsen, or improve with maturity. Some may have discipline problems because of a short attention span, hyperactivity, and aggressive or disorganized behavior. Others may show more introverted behavior marked by extreme shyness and passivity, anxiety, or depression.[1-3,6,9-11] Close follow-up and teamwork with your child's teachers, counselors, and health care provider is important if your child is to reach his full potential.

"Why must parents use their children's growth and development for comparison and competition? My child is her own person, and her achievements belong to her, not to me, and not to anyone else."

Potential for Learning Problems

Few NICU graduates experience learning problems, but very low birth weight (less than 1,500 grams at birth), neonatal complications, and the environment may contribute to later learning deficits at school. Some children may have problems with eye-hand coordination—and therefore may have difficulty drawing or writing, especially writing numbers for math. Language disorders may show themselves as lack of fluency and inability to follow directions. Poor reading comprehension may result in avoidance of classroom participation. Finally, limited mental functioning may be characterized by memory deficits, poor decision-making ability, and difficulty in processing new information. Children who experience problems such as these in school may require special education classes to facilitate learning.[1-3,6]

You play an important role in determining your child's potential. Knowing what resources are available and using them is just as important for enhancing your child's development as for preventing medical complications. Your child also needs to be loved, nurtured, and made to feel important. You don't have to purchase every developmental toy on the market. Children can learn a lot from the people around them and from an environment that's naturally rich with learning opportunities for a curious mind.

Potential for Cerebral Palsy

Cerebral palsy (CP) is a diagnosis that many parents of premature infants fear. The actual incidence of CP is between 3 and 6 percent for infants born prematurely. "CP is defined as an abnormality of posture or movement generated from nonprogressive damage to the brain."[3]

The diagnosis of CP is generally not made until the premature infant is 12 to 18 months corrected age unless the child's problems are severe. The characteristics of CP can range from mild muscle tone abnormalities with normal or above-average intelligence to severe physical disability and mental retardation.[3] Chapter 10 also includes information about CP.

Close developmental follow-up and early-intervention programs (discussed later in this chapter) are essential in identifying and/or minimizing the effects of CP and other developmental delays.

K nowing what to expect in the way of follow-up for your NICU graduate and how you can contribute to your baby's progress are important and rewarding aspects of parenting an NICU graduate. You play a vital role in your baby's growth and development.

Developmental Follow-Up

Infants with any of the neonatal factors listed earlier in this chapter may be at risk for developmental delay. At discharge from the NICU, you and your baby may be referred to a developmental follow-up clinic, often in conjunction with a referral to your community early-intervention program. If your hospital does not have an infant high-risk clinic, your health care provider will be responsible for monitoring your child's development and making any necessary referrals.

Your baby's follow-up should include basic monitoring of hearing, vision, and growth, including height, weight, and head circumference. If your baby weighed less than 3 pounds, 5 ounces (1,500 grams) or had a difficult hospital course, you should expect additional developmental screening tests.

Many screening tests are available, and health care professionals have individual preferences as to which they use. You may hear any of these names: the Neonatal Neurodevelopmental Examination (NNE), the Denver Developmental Screening Test (DDST), the Early Screening Inventory (ESI), the Bayley Scales of Infant Development, and the McCarthy Scales of Children's Abilities. Screening-test results that suggest problems indicate a need for further evaluation and assessment.[12]

Some of the specialists your baby may need to see include a developmental and/or educational specialist, physical and/or occupational therapist, neurologist, psychologist, ophthalmologist, audiologist, nutritionist, orthopedist, otolaryngologist (ear, nose, and throat [ENT] doctor), and surgeon, to name a few. Your knowledge of what is normal for your baby, both medically and developmentally, will assist these professionals in enhancing your baby's health, growth, and development.

Early-Intervention Programs and Public Law 99-457

The foundation for learning begins in early infancy. Therefore, every infant identified as at risk for developmental delay should receive intervention as early as possible. Early-intervention programs appear to influence developmental outcome by helping not only the infant, but the baby's family as well.

Public Law (PL) 94-142, the Education for All Handicapped Children Act, is a federal law passed in 1975 that mandated special education programs for all disabled children from 6 to 21 years of age. Public Law 99-457, part H, the Education of the Handicapped Amendments, is a federal law passed in 1986 that was designed to provide early-intervention programs for disabled or at-risk infants and toddlers (birth through age 2) who needed special services. It also created incentives for states to expand services for disabled children from the ages of 3 to 5. These services are provided free through the public school system and may include physical therapy, occupational therapy, speech therapy, audiology, special education, and individual and family counseling. The goal of PL 99-457, part H, is to prevent developmental delay in the at-risk population and to optimize the development of those infants and toddlers already experiencing disabilities.[1,13–16]

Your baby may be eligible for services if he is experiencing any difficulties with physical, mental, language, social, hearing, visual, behavior, or emotional skills. You may have received a referral to your local early-intervention program before your baby was discharged from the hospital. Your social worker may have filled out a multidisciplinary evaluation form, which would have also been signed by you and by your baby's physician or nurse. Your health care provider may make a referral if any developmental concerns arise during office visits. Finally, you may request a referral if you feel your infant or child needs help. To do so, contact your local school system or your state department of education. You may need to ask specifically for the person in charge of the special education programs. Some states have toll-free telephone numbers to call for information about services in your area. Services vary from state to state.[1,13–16]

Once a referral is made, a team of professionals will gather information about your baby and family for an assessment of needs. If the team determines that your infant needs services, an individualized family service plan (IFSP) will be developed. The IFSP is based on the information from the assessment and on your perception of intervention needs.

Services may be provided to your baby and family in your home or at a center. Location of services and the type of instruction (individual or group) provided varies from area to area and from state to state. The quality of available services also varies from area to area, which can be a source of frustration for parents.

You are the most valuable member of your baby's team. You are your child's advocate and know your infant better than anyone else. It's important that you become actively involved in your baby's growth and development. A good-quality program helps both parents and baby. Some parents think that early intervention is the sole responsibility of trained professionals; but in reality, parents can make the biggest difference in a child's life. Professionals can instruct you in developmentally appropriate activities to include as you play with your baby. They may teach you special exercises to strengthen your baby's muscles or positioning techniques if your child has any physical disabilities. Enjoy working with your child, and take pride in knowing that you are making a difference in his development.[1,13–16]

Developmental Milestones and Your Baby

As you monitor your baby's development, bear in mind that children do not all learn the same things at the same times. Even healthy term babies achieve the developmental milestones over a range of ages. The chart on the following pages lists developmental milestones and the average ages when they occur. An additional chart entitled, "Watch Your Baby for These Signs" lists developmental problems that you should call to the attention of your health care provider. Remember that every baby is different—some babies are walking by 9 months; others, not until 15 months. Some babies are more assertive, more active, and quicker to learn—and therefore may develop at a faster pace than babies who are content to observe and socialize. These temperament differences may also be evident later in life in children's behavior.[1–3,6]

Another important factor in developmental progress is the presence of chronic illness. Even if brain development is normal, children with severe lung disease, heart disease, or intestinal problems may have delays because they cannot physically handle some activities. This is especially apparent in the baby's gross motor (large muscle movement) development.

Infants who receive more frequent attention and more sensitive social responses achieve developmental milestones more rapidly. Studies have shown this to be true in both the term and preterm populations. Quality care from loving, attentive parents can help infants born preterm, at risk, or with certain neonatal problems achieve optimum development.[6]

Dr. Kathryn Barnard, a professor of nursing at the University of Washington, directed the development of important assessment tools to measure "the health and caregiving environments of infants and young children."[17] Specially trained health care professionals use this system to help parents and other health care professionals identify strengths and problem areas in parent-child interaction that research has found to be predictive of a child's later development. By observing the child's environment and noting behavioral components of the interaction between parent and child during a home visit, a feeding session, and a "teaching" session, the health care professional is able to identify areas of parent strength, problem areas to work on, and areas of concern that may require further assessment. Originally designed for use with term infants and their families, these scales have also shown positive correlations with the intellectual and behavioral development of preterm infants and their families.[17]

Not everyone has the advantage of a visiting nurse who has the special training required to use these tools for home care and follow-up. Therefore, selected components of the scales are shown on pages 354 and 355 to guide you in areas over which you may have some control. If many of the suggestions in these tables seem to you like simple common sense, know that you are already on the right track to optimizing your baby's development.

As your baby grows, you'll have many opportunities to teach different skills. You are your child's most important teacher. You'll learn to couple realistic expectations of your child's abilities with support and inspiration for your child to stretch those abilities to their greatest potential.

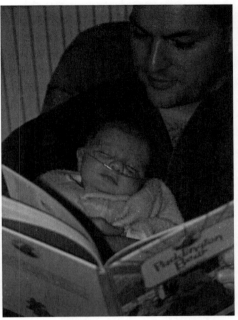

Story time.

It is never too soon to begin reading aloud to your baby.

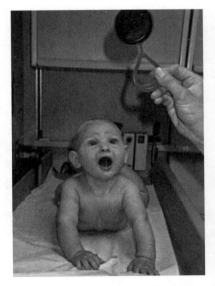

Developmental checkup.

Delighted with the rattle, this six-month-old baby shows appropriate growth and development.

Average Age	Developmental Milestones	Ways to Optimize Your Baby's Development
0-1 Month	Lifts head Briefly watches and follows face or object with eyes Responds to sounds Smiles spontaneously Vocalizes ("talks")	Talk to your baby. Place your face or a bright/shiny object 8–12 inches in front of your baby's face. Provide bells or rattles. Hang mobiles. Position baby on stomach for play.
2 Months	Holds head erect, bobbing when supported in sitting position Follows face or object with eyes as it moves to left or right over midline Smiles responsively Coos, laughs, squeals	Talk to your baby. Get your baby to follow your face or an object (a colorful puppet is nice) by moving left, right, up, and down. Smile and make happy sounds. Sing songs. Give your baby different textures (stuffed animals, plastic toys, terry cloth) to feel.
3 Months	Lifts head and chest when lying on stomach, supports self on arms Has improved control of head Shows vigorous body movements Recognizes bottle or breast Plays with rattle Reaches for objects Glances from one object to another Coos, laughs, squeals	Position on stomach for play; support in sitting position. Offer toys/objects that baby has to reach for or work to get at. Offer rattle or small toy that baby can grasp. Shake rattle in baby's hand if baby doesn't do it by himself (babies learn by doing). Talk, smile, socialize with baby.
4 Months	Has good head control Rolls over Reaches for and may grasp rattle or plastic rod if held near hand Pulls to sitting position without head lagging behind When held in sitting position, follows moving object Turns to sounds Laughs aloud Enjoys play	Change positions during play—sitting, lying on back or stomach. Encourage rolling over by offering toys on side opposite baby's position. Bring baby's hands together to center of body; let baby bring hands to mouth. Shake rattle or bell to elicit response.

Average Age	Developmental Milestones	Ways to Optimize Your Baby's Development
6 Months	Sits briefly with no support Rolls over from back to stomach Transfers objects from hand to hand and from hand to mouth Bangs toys Babbles	Position on back and place toys out of reach to one side to encourage rolling over onto stomach. Let baby explore the environment by placing toys and objects into his mouth (as long as they are clean and safe). Encourage banging and sound production. Continue talking, singing, smiling, and laughing with baby.
9 Months	Waves bye-bye Plays pat-a-cake Says "Ma Ma" and "Da Da" Indicates wants Sits alone, pulls to stand, changes positions without falling Plays with two toys at same time	Play social games with baby. Name objects to encourage vocabulary development. Place infant on floor with several toys to play with.
12 Months (1 Year)	Jabbers expressively; may say two or three words Drinks from cup Can pick up toys using thumb and forefinger Likes to imitate Turns pages in book Stands and walks alone, although may be somewhat unsteady Gives affection Follows simple directions accompanied by gestures	Continue to name objects. Offer cup with a lid or partly filled standard cup. Praise efforts to imitate. Read to child and let him turn pages (children's books with thick pages work best). Give simple directions ("Give Mommy the book") and praise if request is followed.

Average Age	Developmental Milestones	Ways to Optimize Your Baby's Development
15 Months	Vocalizes with pitch, as in conversation May say four or five words Walks steadily without support Runs Throws ball Helps feed and dress self (can probably only remove garments); "helps" with housework Scribbles	Have conversations with child. Offer finger foods; let child try to feed and dress self with your help. Praise efforts to help with housework. Let child color with crayons or use soap-based finger paints with supervision.
18 Months	May say five to ten words Walks, runs, climbs up and downstairs with help Likes pull toys Likes being read to Continues to try to feed, dress, and wash self Points to body parts when asked Stacks blocks	Encourage conversation. Play ball: throwing and kicking. Offer blocks. Read books together. Encourage and praise attempts to feed, dress, and wash (including to brush teeth).
24 Months (2 Years)	Uses two or three words together to communicate needs ("more milk") Recognizes familiar pictures; can point to and name pictures or objects in a book May ask for items by name: ball, doll, cup Can tell the difference between objects Improving at feeding, dressing, washing, and imitating housework skills Beginning to play with two- or three-piece puzzles	Encourage child to vocalize needs instead of pointing. Read together—have child point to and name pictures in a book (doggie, kitty cat, ball, house, and so on). Continue to praise attempts at dressing, washing, feeding, and housework. Encourage use of spoon and fork. Offer simple puzzles to encourage size and shape differentiation. Play games that encourage large-muscle development and interactive skills (tag, hide-and-seek, ball). Encourage cooperation with other children. Plan outings (to the store or zoo, for example) for more learning experiences.

Adapted from: Hanson MJ, and VandenBerg KA. 1993. *Homecoming for Babies After the Intensive Care Nursery: A Guide for Parents in Supporting Their Baby's Early Development*. Austin, Texas: Pro-Ed, 19–25; Parker L, and Richard C. 1990. Growth and development. In *Ochsner NICU Babybook*. New Orleans: Alton Ochsner Medical Foundation, 1–8; Frankenburg WK, et al. 1990. *Denver II Screening Manual*. Denver: Denver Developmental Materials, 1–48; and Bayley N. 1993. *Bayley Scales of Infant Development Manual,* 2nd ed. San Antonio, Texas: Psychological Corp., Harcourt, Brace & Co., 328–349.

Note: If your baby was born preterm, calculate corrected age (see Chapter 15). Use that number to monitor development.

Watch Your Baby for These Signs:

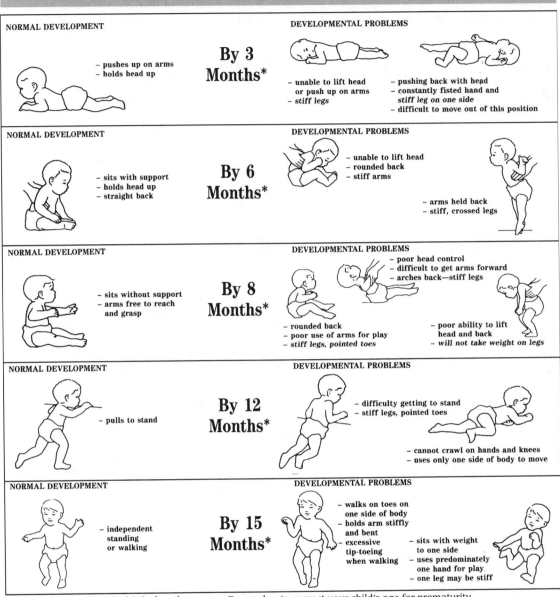

NORMAL DEVELOPMENT

– pushes up on arms
– holds head up

By 3 Months*

DEVELOPMENTAL PROBLEMS

– unable to lift head or push up on arms
– stiff legs

– pushing back with head
– constantly fisted hand and *stiff leg on one side*
– difficult to move out of this position

NORMAL DEVELOPMENT

– sits with support
– holds head up
– straight back

By 6 Months*

DEVELOPMENTAL PROBLEMS

– unable to lift head
– rounded back
– stiff arms

– arms held back
– stiff, crossed legs

NORMAL DEVELOPMENT

– sits without support
– arms free to reach and grasp

By 8 Months*

DEVELOPMENTAL PROBLEMS

– poor head control
– difficult to get arms forward
– arches back—stiff legs

– rounded back
– poor use of arms for play
– stiff legs, pointed toes

– poor ability to lift head and back
– will *not* take weight on legs

NORMAL DEVELOPMENT

– pulls to stand

By 12 Months*

DEVELOPMENTAL PROBLEMS

– difficulty getting to stand
– stiff legs, pointed toes

– cannot crawl on hands and knees
– uses only one side of body to move

NORMAL DEVELOPMENT

– independent standing or walking

By 15 Months*

DEVELOPMENTAL PROBLEMS

– walks on toes on one side of body
– holds arm stiffly and bent
– excessive tip-toeing when walking

– sits with weight to one side
– uses predominately one hand for play
– one leg may be stiff

* 90 percent of babies do this before these ages. Remember to correct your child's age for prematurity.

From: Pathways Awareness Foundation. 1993. *Parents...If You See Any of These Warnings Signs...Don't Delay.* Chicago: Illinois Chapter American Academy of Pediatrics. Reprinted by permission.

Your Home Environment

You foster your child's physical, emotional, and intellectual growth when you:

- Provide a safe, hazard-free play area.
- Provide age-appropriate toys and toys that challenge continuing development (mobile, push or pull toy, table and chairs, fit-together toys, blocks or nesting toys).
- Provide children's books and music.
- Provide opportunities for "messy" types of play ("feeling" the food, wading in mud puddles).
- Provide a special place for your child to keep toys and "treasures."
- Provide opportunities for your child to get out of the house frequently for grocery shopping, family activities, visits with relatives, and so on.
- Speak to your child spontaneously in a clear and audible voice and occasionally praise your child's qualities or behavior.
- Respond to your child's vocalizations ("talking").
- Caress or kiss your child often and appropriately.
- Show positive emotional response when others praise your child.
- Do not show hostility to your child, slap or spank him, or speak negatively about him.
- Talk to your child while doing activities that do not include him (housework, visiting with friends).
- Tend to keep your child where you can see him and look at him often.
- Read to your child often.
- Allow your child to eat at least one meal a day with the family or be present at a family meal.
- Spend some time each day playing with your child; teaching him about new toys, objects, and people; and challenging your child's development appropriately.
- Try to provide a regular baby-sitter rather than a different person each time.
- Provide for your child's health care needs.

Adapted from: Caldwell BE. 1978. Home observation for measurement of the environment (birth to three years). In *Nursing Child Assessment Home Inventory*. Seattle: NCAST Publications. Reprinted by permission of the author.

Feeding Your Baby

You provide your baby with an opportunity for socializing and learning during feeding when you make sure that:

- Your baby feels safe and comfortable.
- Your baby's head is higher than his hips.
- Your baby's trunk is touching yours for at least half the feeding.
- The two of you can make eye contact.
- Your face is at least 7–8 inches away from your baby's face except during kissing, caressing, or burping.
- Your baby can move his arms.
- You pay more attention to your baby during the feeding than to other people or things around you.
- You smile and gently touch your baby during the feeding.
- You let your baby touch and explore your breast or the bottle.
- You talk to your baby about the feeding. ("Are you ready to eat?" "Do you need a break?" "This is nice warm milk!" "Are you feeling full?")
- You also talk to your baby about things other than the feeding ("It's so warm and sunny today!" "Do you hear that dog barking?") and do not use baby talk.
- You respond to your baby's smile or "talking" with your own smile, touch, or voice.

Your baby learns that feeding is safe and enjoyable when you:

- Pause the feeding when your baby shows distress.
- Do not interrupt your baby's sucking by removing or jiggling the nipple.
- Comfort your baby in response to distress with a gentle voice and touch, a position change, and general soothing.
- Stop the feeding when your baby falls asleep, pushes the food away, or turns his head away and your attempts to continue the feeding (repositioning, burping, waiting) prove unsuccessful.

Adapted from: Barnard KE. 1987. Feeding scale (birth to one year). In *Nursing Child Assessment Feeding Scale*. Seattle: NCAST Publications. Reprinted by permission of the author.

Teaching Your Child

Your child understands that you are a loving and supportive teacher and feels good about testing his abilities when you

- Position and support your child so that he can reach toys and make eye contact with you.
- Provide a learning area that is free from distractions.
- Let your child touch and play with toys before you start to give instructions.
- Describe toys to your child before beginning. ("Look at this smooth red block.")
- Have your child's attention before you begin a lesson. ("Matthew, are you ready to start?")
- Are relaxed and laugh and smile with your child while teaching.
- Make encouraging statements and gently pat, stroke, hug, or kiss your child during the lesson.
- Give clear instructions as you demonstrate a task. For example, "See how the green block stacks on top of the red block?" is more helpful than, "Put this one up here."
- Give your child at least five seconds to try a skill before you help.
- Praise your child for effort and improved performance by commenting, smiling, and/or nodding.
- Respond to your child's smiles and "talking," but do not interrupt his vocalizing.
- Change your child's position or the position of the toys after an unsuccessful try.
- Do not force your child to complete a task or make your child perform a task repeatedly after successfully completing it once.
- Respond to your child's distress by stopping, soothing, or diverting attention to a different task.
- Let your child know when the "teaching session" is over.
- Spend no more than five minutes and no less than one minute teaching your child.

Adapted from: Barnard KE. 1987. Teaching scale (birth to three years). In *Nursing Child Assessment Teaching Scale*. Seattle: NCAST Publications. Reprinted by permission of the author.

Chances of Hospital Readmission

Technologic advances in perinatal and neonatal medicine are creating a growing population of infants with special medical needs, both in the hospital and at home. Babies are going home sicker and quicker than ever before. Despite parental training in special care and close medical follow-up, these infants are at significant risk for rehospitalization. A baby born weighing less than 3 pounds, 5 ounces (1,500 grams) has a 30 to 50 percent greater chance of being rehospitalized during the first year of life than does a term infant of normal birth weight. Depending on the underlying disease, statistics are similar for chronically ill or technology-dependent infants.[1,18–21]

These statistics are not meant to frighten you. Rather, they are to remind you that your baby may still have special health needs at discharge and that going home, in reality, is just the beginning of a whole new set of challenges for you and your family.[18-23]

Common Reasons for Rehospitalization

"Tommy was rehospitalized three times during his first year at home. Each time was discouraging and exhausting for the whole family. But now that he's two years old, and he gets sick less often, I think we've turned the corner."

Common childhood diseases can be potentially life-threatening for very low birth weight infants, those with BPD or other chronic illnesses, and technology-dependent infants. Immunizing your NICU graduate (discussed later in this chapter) is an important step in preventing many potentially serious diseases.

Respiratory infections are the most frequent cause of hospital readmission among NICU graduates. They may result in continued need for supplemental oxygen, ventilator support, respiratory treatments, and/or medications for reactive airway disease (similar to asthma). The common cold, which is an upper respiratory infection, may cause your baby significant respiratory distress. Ear infections, accompanied by fever, may also stress your baby and increase the work of breathing. Infections of the lower respiratory tract, such as pneumonia, can have the greatest impact on your baby, possibly requiring an extended hospital readmission.[1,9,20,21,23,24] Researchers are investigating the effectiveness of monthly infusions of intravenous immunoglobulin throughout the respiratory virus season in preventing infection with respiratory syncytial virus (RSV), a common cause of upper and lower respiratory tract infections in high-risk infants (for example, babies with bronchopulmonary dysplasia).[25] Ask your health care provider about the status of this promising therapy if your baby is at risk for RSV infection.

Feeding difficulties and unmet nutrition needs may also lead to repeated hospital admissions. Your baby may not be meeting his nutritional requirements if he is nippling poorly, burning up too many calories working to breathe, or experiencing gastroesophageal reflux (spitting up; see Chapter 14). When conventional treatment methods for increasing nutritional intake fail, your baby may be readmitted for evaluation and/or for a surgical procedure called a fundoplication (see Chapter 16) if reflux is severe. Optimal nutrition and weight gain are necessary to help your baby fight infections, decrease the work of breathing, lower oxygen requirements, and attain developmental milestones.[1,9,20,21,23,24]

If your NICU graduate is on an apnea monitor at home, you may at some point notice more frequent or intense episodes of apnea and bradycardia. Report this trend to your pediatrician immediately. In some cases, a test to check the theophylline or caffeine level in your baby's blood may be done in your doctor's office. If the episodes of apnea and bradycardia are severe or are accompanied by other signs of illness, your baby may need to be readmitted to the hospital for closer monitoring, further evaluation, and/or medication adjustments.[1,9,20,21,23,24]

Neurodevelopmental problems, vision and hearing impairments, and cosmetic surgeries may also require hospital readmission, especially when your child is older.[1,9,20,21,23,24] A child with cerebral palsy may require orthopedic surgeries to release tight tendons. A child with a blocked tear duct may need a minor surgical procedure to open it up. If your baby has scars from NICU procedures (chest tubes or major line placement), you may want to consider cosmetic surgery when he is older.

Your Part in Preventing Rehospitalization

You can't necessarily control the progress of your baby's medical recovery, but you can take steps to reduce the risks for rehospitalization. Here are some suggestions.

Providing Adequate Care

Prevention of rehospitalization actually begins before discharge as you learn about your baby's special-care needs. Ask questions and practice until you feel comfortable with and competent at providing your baby's care. Speak up if you have questions or feel that you are being hurried out the door. It's normal to feel somewhat apprehensive when your baby first comes home, but it helps to know that you are familiar with your baby's care and understand how to monitor for potential problems.[20,21,23]

Working with Your Health Care Provider

Selecting a health care provider who understands the complex needs of an NICU graduate also helps prevent rehospitalization. Weekly visits to the office may be necessary for the first month to monitor your baby's weight gain and general progress and to address your questions and concerns. Early identification of illness and good communication with your health care provider can prevent a minor illness from turning into a major hospitalization.[1,9,10,21,26]

Hand Washing

Good hand washing is the easiest and most effective way to prevent the spread of infection. Wash your hands after changing diapers and before preparing food. Make it a habit to wash when you return from work or running errands, and encourage siblings to wash when they come home from school, day care, or a friend's house. Hand washing is not only important for family and visitors, though. Wash your baby's hands after an outing, before he eats finger foods, and when common sense tells you it is a good idea.

Immunizations

Another important measure in preventing infection and rehospitalization is making sure that your baby is immunized on schedule and that he receives boosters as appropriate. An immunization chart can be found on page 358. The immunization schedule for preterm infants is the same as that for term babies. You don't have to correct for age.

You may have heard horror stories about possible side effects of immunization or been given other reasons not to immunize your baby. What is truly horrible is that measles, polio, and pertussis (whooping cough) are

"Because of our baby's disabilities, we measure her progress in small steps. We won't worry about when she'll walk until we celebrate the fact that she can crawl."

Vaccinations: What and When

Vaccines are listed under the routinely recommended ages. Bars indicate range of acceptable ages for vaccination. Shaded bars indicate catch-up vaccination: at 11–12 years of age, hepatitis B vaccine should be administered to children not previously vaccinated, and Varicella Zoster Virus vaccine should be administered to children not previously vaccinated who lack a reliable history of chickenpox.

Age ▶ Vaccine ▼	Birth	1 mo	2 mos	4 mos	6 mos	12 mos	15 mos	18 mos	4–6 yrs	11–12 yrs	14–16 yrs
Hepatitis B	Hep B-1										
		Hep B-2			Hep B-3					Hep B-3	
Diphtheria, Tetanus, Pertussis			DTP	DTP	DTP	DTP (DTaP at 15+ mo)			DTP or DTaP	Td	
H. influenzae type b			Hib	Hib	Hib	Hib					
Polio			OPV	OPV	OPV				OPV		
Measles, Mumps, Rubella						MMR			MMR or MMR		
Varicella Zoster Virus Vaccine						Var				Var	

Note: This immunization schedule, prepared by the Centers for Disease Control, part of the U.S. Public Health Service, is revised occasionally. Ask for updated information when you visit your health care provider.

reappearing after being nearly eliminated decades ago. The benefit of preventing these diseases through immunizations usually far outweighs the risks of any dangerous, yet uncommon side effects of the immunizations.[27–30]

Your health care provider will give you written information about each immunization your baby should receive. This information will include the pros and cons of receiving the immunization so that you can make an informed decision regarding consent.[31–34]

A vaccine for chickenpox is now available commercially in the United States for individuals ages 12 months and up. Please consult your health care provider about its availability in your area, as well as for concerns about potential side effects, transmission of the disease following vaccination, and concerns about lifelong immunity.

Coping with Rehospitalization

If your baby's rehospitalization is planned and anticipated (a hernia repair, for example), you may consider it a milestone and look forward to continued progress at home. If your baby is rehospitalized with an illness or emergency, though, you may feel angry, guilty, frustrated, and inadequate as a parent. Even when forewarned, parents often blame themselves when their baby has to be rehospitalized. They feel as if they have failed to provide adequate care for their baby at home. "If only I had..." is a familiar phrase. It may help to realize that rehospitalization often occurs despite all your good care and precautions. It is not an indication that you did something wrong. Recognize that your NICU graduate has the potential for many medical problems beyond your scope of caregiving and that hospitalization is sometimes necessary to get him back on the road to progress.

If your baby's rehospitalization is unanticipated, take this opportunity to examine your management of the events leading up to the readmission. Instead of asking yourself, "What did I do wrong?" ask yourself, "How did I manage this crisis?" Here are some questions to consider:

- Did I have enough information to know what signs and symptoms to report?
- Did I know who to talk to about my concerns? Did that person really listen to me?
- Did I report my concerns to my health care provider in a timely manner?
- Did everyone involved in this hospitalization (myself and the health care professionals) communicate well to define the problem and decide on treatment?
- Did I learn something from this experience?
- What aspects of this experience did I manage well?
- What, if anything, would I do differently next time?

Your answers to these questions may reveal that you need more support and information to monitor your baby's special-care needs. You may want to discuss your need for better communication with your baby's health care professionals. Or you may discover, as is true for most parents, that you did everything you knew to do.

Before discharge, you may not have known what you didn't know—and that made it difficult to ask questions. It's often after you get home or after an unanticipated rehospitalization that your learning needs become clear.

Every parenting crisis presents an opportunity to learn. Even though rehospitalization is not an experience you'd deliberately seek, try to look at it as a chance to manage a difficult situation, advocate your baby's needs, and grow as a responsible and caring parent.

Working With Your Baby's Health Care Providers

Learning to communicate and negotiate effectively was important to your survival and involvement in the NICU (see Chapter 3). Communication skills will continue to serve you well as you meet and work with numerous health care providers in your community. Because you and members of your baby's caregiving team may have different expectations, it's important to create the best possible working relationship.

Developing a Partnership

Give yourself time to develop a trusting relationship with your baby's health care providers. Begin by being honest and expressing your needs and expectations. Your health care providers will appreciate the fact that you value and depend on their experience and advice, but they should also realize that you have experience and information that will influence your child's health care. Over time, you will work out a relationship that allows for negotiation

Considerations When Choosing a New Health Care Provider

1. Be wary of anyone who promises a quick or guaranteed cure for a major illness. Most such claims are fraudulent, as are many patient testimonials of cures. (The American Medical Association's guidelines for ethical physician advertising restrict the use of testimonials.)

2. If claims are made, ask for copies of published research in reputable journals, documenting the claims.

3. Consult public-interest groups specializing in the disease or condition your child is being treated for to request information on up-to-date therapies. (See Appendix D for the names and addresses of many such groups.)

4. Ask for a written explanation of a proposed new therapy so you and others involved in your baby's care can thoughtfully review it.

5. If the proposed therapy is part of a research project, you are entitled to a copy of the protocol (the research guidelines) along with a full explanation of the risks and benefits. All institutions that carry out legitimate research must have an institutional review board or similar committee to oversee the program; the board must approve the research protocol before patients are enrolled. If, after you have reviewed the risks and benefits, your questions are not answered to your satisfaction or you have concerns about the benefits to your child, you are free to refuse to participate in the research, without jeopardizing your child's continuing care.

6. Legitimate research studies rarely charge patients for study-related treatments and tests; charlatans always do.

7. Remember that the Food and Drug Administration will study new drugs for many years before granting approval for use, so the availability of a drug for research purposes does not necessarily mean it has cleared the FDA approval process.

8. If your baby is currently undergoing traditional therapy, don't stop that therapy to begin an unproven or experimental one. Perhaps the saddest aspect of medical fraud is the thousands who suffer needlessly and even die because they turned away from traditional therapy before its effectiveness could be shown in their case. Most legitimate research projects continue the conventional therapy while applying the unproven treatment to some patients.

9. Finally, before beginning any therapy—whether accepted or experimental—that involves substantial risk, cost, or time, get a second opinion from someone you respect and trust.

Adapted from: Inlander CB, and Dodson JL. 1992. *Take This Book to the Pediatrician with You: The Guide to Your Child's Health.* Allentown, Pennsylvania: People's Medical Society, 28–29. Reprinted by permission.

and polite disagreement. You should be able to trust one another enough so that it is acceptable for either of you to say "I don't know" or "You were right." Your relationship will grow strong enough to survive small disagreements if you also remember to express your appreciation when your health care provider's expertise has been especially helpful. Everyone likes to feel successful. Your acknowledgment of a job well done helps inspire future problem solving and keeps your partnership strong.[35]

Changing Health Care Providers

At some point in your child's care, you may find yourself thinking about switching health care providers. To stay in control, plan ahead and try to avoid an abrupt termination of this important relationship.

Laying the Groundwork

Before switching health care providers, try to discuss your concerns. Unmet expectations are the source of many problems, and honest communication may help resolve the situation. Be specific about your concerns, and look for a respectful and courteous response. Be prepared to participate in mutual problem solving. Most problems have two sides. Just as you expect the health care provider to consider your side of the story, you need to give the professional's perspective equal consideration. Most health care providers prefer to discuss concerns in person; however, if this seems impossible for you, write your health care provider a letter stating why you are dissatisfied.

There is rarely a reason for hostility when terminating a relationship with a health care professional. Also, despite the fact that the health care provider has been an authority figure in your situation, there is no reason to feel intimidated in this process.

Before you end your relationship with your current caregiver, find another. You don't want to be caught in the awkward situation of needing care and not having someone familiar with your baby.

Making a Wise Choice

Choose your new health care professional with care. In your efforts to find answers to your baby's complex needs, it's possible to be taken in by the promise of a fast cure. Review the basic rules of interviewing and selection (see Chapter 15), and this time focus some of your questions on the areas in which you are having problems with your current health care professional. Additional factors to consider are listed on page 360.

Graduates of an NICU may come home with nursing support, equipment, supplies, medications, and a long list of caregiving requirements. You've been given a list of dos and don'ts for your baby's care and warned of the potential for rehospitalization. It's no wonder that at first you tend to overprotect your baby. In some cases, though, this sheltering continues well past the point of necessity and beyond what is healthy for you and your child. The

"Loving enough but not too much, caring but not interfering, helping when help is needed but respecting the value of struggle and enterprise, requiring the right amount of cooperation without overloading the child with excessive demands—how in the world are parents supposed to do all that?... And yet, over time, through a process of trial and error, with great efforts at empathy and a few flashes of inspiration, that's what we strive to learn and to do. And we carry out our very complex task without much in the way of preparation."

From: Williams LH, Berman HS, and Rose L. 1987. Learning to be a not too precious parent. In *The Too Precious Child: The Perils of Being a Superparent and How to Avoid Them*. New York: Atheneum, 192. Reprinted by permission.

The Overprotective Parent

psychologic damage of overprotecting a child can be more limiting than any diagnosed disability.[1,10,36–40]

Vulnerable Child Syndrome

When parents continue to view their child as sickly despite healthy findings on physical examinations, professionals describe this attitude as vulnerable child syndrome. When the child reaches school age, he is not allowed to participate in sports or special events. The parents don't encourage high academic standards, and so their healthy, mentally normal child performs below his potential.[1,10,21,36,40]

The psychologic impact of overprotection can be devastating to children. Overprotection stunts children's efforts to develop skills appropriate for their age. They may continue to experience separation anxiety. They may have temper tantrums whenever they do not get their way. They may have difficulty playing with or participating in social games with other children. They may bite or hit other children during outbursts of anger. School grades tend to be below average, possibly because of frequent absences from school with real or imagined illness to blame. Children may actually feed into parental overprotection by complaining of nonspecific symptoms or of a problem with one organ to focus the parents' anxiety on a specific area.[1,10,40]

Children who are severely overprotected by their parents are more likely than not to have had special medical needs as infants—for example, a medical history of prematurity, apnea and bradycardia, failure to thrive, or another chronic illness. Professional intervention is often necessary to help parents recognize and accept that the illness event, which took place years earlier, is now over. Only then can these parents begin to view their child as a healthy individual and encourage his social development.[1,10,40]

A Difficult Balance

Because your baby spent time in the NICU, he is at risk for overprotection. Close watchfulness may be necessary and appropriate early in life because of continued medical problems. Listen to your health care provider and to other child-care specialists when they tell you that your baby is medically stable and developmentally ready for new challenges, however. They can educate you about normal infant behavior and basic parenting. The authors of the book *The Too Precious Child* recommend that parents ask their health care professional the following questions to avoid becoming overprotective parents:[41]

1. Does the fact that my baby has had this problem mean that he is in any way worse off than a baby born without any problems?
2. If my baby is more at risk, what can I do to reduce the risk? What signs and symptoms should I watch for? For how long will my baby continue to be "at risk"?
3. Is my baby fully recovered?

Share your anxiety with your health care provider. She may be in the best position to alleviate your fears and help prevent you from sheltering your child

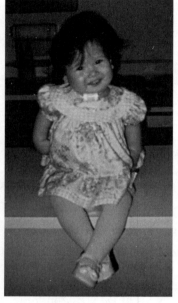

Successful NICU graduate.

Babies with special needs require close follow-up but usually show steady progress and appropriate development. This child also appears on page 298 and 337.

for longer than is necessary. Don't hesitate to call or visit your health care provider more frequently than usual if you're experiencing undue stress over your child's health. You may also benefit from speaking with other parents of NICU graduates. Getting involved with people and/or support groups who have experienced or are feeling similar fears can help you learn to cope with these feelings in a positive way.[1,10,21,36,40]

Caring for and protecting your baby without providing *too* much care and protection is indeed a tricky balancing act. You've worked hard to get to this point, and it's only natural to want to safeguard your special baby. But part of being a parent is growing with your child and realizing when it's time to loosen your grip in some areas and to expect your child's cooperation in others.

As your child explores the world, fights his own battles, and begins to feel accomplished as an individual, he will grow healthier. You'll find your own way as you give your child's potential abilities a chance to unfold. Through trial and error, you'll learn how much to expect from your child and when the time is right to stretch your expectations a bit further. Every child's needs are different, but most benefit from parents who expect socially acceptable behavior and accomplishments that reflect their child's fullest abilities.

Planning Another Baby

The decision to have another baby is very personal and usually involves emotion more than logic. As you think about the future, look closely at your reasons for wanting another baby.

The birth of a preterm or sick baby may change the way you look at future pregnancies. A complicated pregnancy or a baby's prolonged NICU stay is enough to make some women decide against additional pregnancies. This is especially true for women who have had more than one complicated or premature birth. On the other hand, some women feel as if they've "failed" in this pregnancy and want another pregnancy as a chance to "do it right." Families of an NICU graduate with special needs sometimes find that having other children makes their life more normal and that a healthy child makes them more aware of healthy aspects of their ill child.[35]

Questions to Ask Yourself

Do you truly want another child, or are you trying to make up for a pregnancy and birth that did not proceed quite as you planned? Does your partner want another child? What about your family, including your other children? Will you be able to keep up with the stressful caregiving demands of your NICU graduate while you're pregnant?

Also consider your personal finances, home environment, and employment situation before deciding to become pregnant again. If you are restricted to home or put on bed rest during your next pregnancy, will employment disability insurance be necessary or available to you? What child-care arrangements will you make if you must be hospitalized or are restricted to bed during your pregnancy? Is your partner willing to make some sacrifices for another pregnancy?[9] Perhaps the most important question to ask is this one:

Are you ready for another pregnancy knowing that you may face complications and another NICU experience?

Every pregnancy is different. All the anticipatory planning in the world will not prevent unexpected events from occurring. A woman with no obvious risk factors may experience a complicated pregnancy and birth, and a woman with previous pregnancy and birth complications may later deliver a healthy, term baby. In any case, if you decide to have another baby, plan your pregnancy; seek early prenatal care; and follow the basic guidelines of a healthy diet, moderate exercise, rest, and relaxation to give your baby the best chance for a healthy beginning.

Believing In Yourself

Many parents of NICU graduates are a bit frightened to look far ahead. In fact, fear of the unknown contributes to chronic stress in many families. The potential for rehospitalization, future health problems, and overprotection of your baby is very real.

The NICU experience does not make for an easy transition to parenthood. As your baby grows, you'll continue to discover important parenting resources within yourself—for managing stress, for advocating your baby's needs, and for seeking support and lending it to those around you. For you, parenthood has brought with it unique changes—different from those felt by parents whose baby was born healthy. It's given you opportunities for strengthening relationships, uncovering hidden strengths, and reordering priorities.

On those occasions when you are coping well, take a moment to congratulate yourself for a job well done. You may face many challenges ahead. But you can feel good about your abilities as a parent as long as you continue to ask questions and actively participate on the health care team as your baby's advocate.

Your baby's growth and development will reflect not only his medical legacy, but the way you bring him up as well. A parent's most difficult task is knowing when to offer a helping hand—and when to provide a gentle push forward. Your job is to inspire achievement and independence, while realizing that some of life's most valuable lessons come from disappointment. Your success as a parent depends on your ability to trust yourself to make a positive impact on your child's life.

Your child's success will depend largely on your outlook on life—and what you teach your child about achieving his personal best.

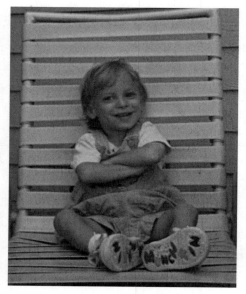

Enjoying life.

This NICU graduate is doing well at two years of age—thanks to good NICU care, excellent parenting, and her own fighting spirit. This little girl appears as a baby numerous times in this book, as on page 62 and 117.

Appendices

Appendix A
Weights and Measures: Conversion Charts

❝"There you are," said Piglet.
"Inside as well as outside," said Pooh proudly.❞

Conversion of Pounds and Ounces to Grams

Ounces

	0	1	2	3	4	5	6	7	**8**	9	10	11	12	13	14	15
0	—	28	57	85	113	142	170	198	227	255	283	312	340	369	397	425
1	454	482	510	539	567	595	624	652	680	709	737	765	794	822	850	879
2	907	936	964	992	1,021	1,049	1,077	1,106	1,134	1,162	1,191	1,219	1,247	1,276	1,304	1,332
3	1,361	1,389	1,417	1,446	1,474	1,502	1,531	1,559	**1,588**	1,616	1,644	1,673	1,701	1,729	1,758	1,786
4	1,814	1,843	1,871	1,899	1,928	1,956	1,984	2,013	2,041	2,070	2,098	2,126	2,155	2,183	2,211	2,240
5	2,268	2,296	2,325	2,353	2,381	2,410	2,438	2,466	2,495	2,523	2,551	2,580	2,608	2,637	2,665	2,693
6	2,722	2,750	2,778	2,807	2,835	2,863	2,892	2,920	2,948	2,977	3,005	3,033	3,062	3,090	3,118	3,147
7	3,175	3,203	3,232	3,260	3,289	3,317	3,345	3,374	3,402	3,430	3,459	3,487	3,515	3,544	3,572	3,600
8	3,629	3,657	3,685	3,714	3,742	3,770	3,799	3,827	3,856	3,884	3,912	3,941	3,969	3,997	4,026	4,054
9	4,082	4,111	4,139	4,167	4,196	4,224	4,252	4,281	4,309	4,337	4,366	4,394	4,423	4,451	4,479	4,508
10	4,536	4,564	4,593	4,621	4,649	4,678	4,706	4,734	4,763	4,791	4,819	4,848	4,876	4,904	4,933	4,961
11	4,990	5,018	5,046	5,075	5103	5,131	5,160	5,188	5,216	5,245	5,273	5,301	5,330	5,358	5,386	5,415
12	5,443	5,471	5,500	5,528	5,557	5,585	5,613	5,642	5,670	5,698	5,727	5,755	5,783	5,812	5,840	5,868

(Left axis: Pounds)

To Convert Pounds and Ounces to Grams:

Find the baby's weight in pounds down the left side of the table. Find the ounces across the top of the table. The intersection of the two measurements equals the equivalent weight in grams. For example, **3** pounds, **8** ounces equals **1,588** grams.

To Convert Grams to Pounds and Ounces:

Find the baby's weight in grams on the chart. Look to the far left line for the pound measurement and to the top of the gram column for the ounces.

Conversion of Centimeters to Inches

Centimeters	Inches	Centimeters	Inches	Centimeters	Inches
25.4	10	43.2	17	61.0	24
26.7	10½	44.4	17½	62.2	24½
27.9	11	45.7	18	63.5	25
29.2	11½	47.0	18½	64.8	25½
30.5	12	48.3	19	66.1	26
31.8	12½	49.5	19½	67.4	26½
33.0	13	50.8	20	68.7	27
34.3	13½	52.1	20½	69.9	27½
35.6	14	53.3	21	71.2	28
36.8	14½	54.6	21½	72.5	28½
38.1	15	55.9	22	73.8	29
39.4	15½	57.2	22½	75.1	29½
40.6	16	58.4	23	76.4	30
41.9	16½	59.7	23½	77.6	30½

Conversion of Temperature (Fahrenheit and Centigrade)

To convert degrees Fahrenheit to degrees centigrade, subtract 32, multiply by 5, and divide by 9. To convert degrees centigrade to degrees Fahrenheit, multiply by 9, divide by 5, and add 32.

Fahrenheit	Centigrade
96.1	35.6
96.4	35.8
96.8	36.0
97.7	36.5
98.6	37.0
99.5	37.5
100.4	38.0
101.3	38.5
102.2	39.0
103.1	39.5
104.0	40.0
104.9	40.5
105.8	41.0
106.7	41.5
107.6	42.0

Appendix B
Medications and Your Baby

Debbie Fraser Askin, RNC, MN

❝"To make you grow big and strong, dear. You don't want to grow up small and weak like Piglet, do you?"❞

Kanga—

Many drugs are used in the treatment of sick or premature infants. Some have been used for many years. Others have been developed more recently. All have undergone careful testing before use.

Reasons for Giving Medications

Your baby may receive medications in the NICU for many reasons. Some drugs, such as phenobarbital or vitamin K, may be given to keep your baby from developing certain conditions or complications. Others, such as theophylline or antibiotics, are given to treat a problem that your baby has developed. Drugs such as vitamins and iron are given as supplements to breast milk or formula. Certain drugs—antibiotics, for example—may be given for a short time, whereas others, such as theophylline and phenobarbital, may be needed for many weeks or months.

The decision to give medication to an infant comes after careful thought. Your baby's doctor will weigh the benefits of giving a drug against any risks or possible side effects the drug may produce.

All drugs have a *desired effect*—that is, a reason for which they are given. Desired effects may include fighting infection, increasing blood pressure, or relieving pain.

Many drugs also have possible *side effects*. That means that in addition to the action they are intended to produce, they can cause changes—ranging from minor to major—in other body functions. Minor side effects of some drugs may include nausea or rash. Major side effects—such as depression of breathing or lowering of the blood pressure—can be serious enough in some infants that the drug must be discontinued. Potential major side effects are especially of concern in ill or very premature babies. Note, though, that each baby reacts differently to a given medication. Some experience no side effects from a specific drug; others show some of the side effects described for the drug in the listing later in this appendix.

Finally, some drugs can have *toxic effects*. They can poison the body if given in too large a dose (an overdose) or if the concentration of the drug in the blood becomes unexpectedly high. When drugs with potentially toxic effects are given, levels in the blood are monitored closely to guard against toxicity.

Methods of Giving Medications

Various methods (routes of administration) are used to give drugs to infants in the NICU. The route used may depend both on the drug being given and on the infant's condition.

Intravenous

In sick infants, many drugs are given directly into a vein through an intravenous (IV) infusion. This route allows the baby's body to quickly begin to use the medication.

Oral

Some drugs are easily absorbed by the baby's digestive system and are well tolerated by the stomach; these drugs may be given orally (by mouth). Others cannot be given orally because the baby's digestive system cannot absorb them or because they will upset the stomach or the bowel. In some cases, very ill infants may not receive any fluid or medication orally because of concerns about their digestive system.

Inhalation

Drugs given by inhalation—those that are breathed in—are usually intended to treat lung problems. One such drug is albuterol. Medication given directly into the lungs may produce fewer side effects than if it were given intravenously. The lungs have a rich blood supply and therefore can absorb some medications quite well. Inhalatory drugs may be given by face mask, by nebulizer (puffer), or through the endotracheal tube.

Rectal

In some cases, drugs may be given through a thin tube or a suppository (specially prepared capsule) placed in the baby's rectum. This may be done if an oral drug is desirable but cannot be given because of surgery or feeding problems.

Intramuscular

Intramuscular (IM) drugs—those given by needle—are often poorly absorbed by babies because of their immature muscle mass and poor circulation. Drugs that may be given IM include vitamin K (given routinely to newborn infants) and some drugs needed in emergency situations when an IV route may not be available.

Transdermal

The transdermal route—literally, "across or through the skin"—involves the use of skin patches. This route is becoming more popular in adults. Because infants have thin skin, drugs cross into the bloodstream quite readily. At this time, few drugs are available in patches for use in the NICU; therefore, this route is not frequently used.

Safety of Medications

Most drugs given to newborn babies have been used for a number of years. During that time, their effects and side effects have been carefully studied. New drugs are also being developed and tested. Most of these drugs are used in adults for some time before they are given to babies.

All new medications used in the United States and Canada must be approved by these federal governments before they become available. Manufacturers of drugs must complete a series of steps before this approval is given. In the United States, manufacturers submit information and animal study results for each new drug to the Food and Drug Administration (FDA), which then grants the drug investigational status. At that time, the drug is tested on healthy adults and then on small numbers of patients for whom it is intended. Finally, clinical trials occur, in which the new drug is tested on larger groups of patients. In Canada, this process is handled by the Health Protection Branch of Health and Welfare Canada. If your baby's doctor would like your infant to receive an investigational drug, the doctor will explain the situation to you and obtain your permission.

Monitoring of Drug Levels

When certain drugs are given, it's necessary to monitor the amount of the drug that is present in your baby's blood (called the serum drug level). Drugs requiring monitoring of levels are those with a narrow range between desired effects and toxic side effects. Levels are monitored to ensure that an adequate amount of the drug is present to achieve the desired effect but that the level is not so high as to cause side effects.

Discontinuation of a Baby's Medication

The decision to stop a medication depends on a number of things. For some drugs, such as an antibiotic, the medication is stopped when your baby is free of infection. Other drugs may be given for a certain number of doses. Still others may be given over a period of weeks or months, depending on the problem being treated. Some drugs can be stopped at any time, while others cannot be stopped all at once. Instead, the baby must be slowly weaned from the medication. The amount given or the frequency with which the drug is given is reduced over time—so that the baby's body becomes used to being without the drug. With some medications the baby is weaned by being allowed to outgrow the dose. Be sure your baby's caregiver explains your baby's medication plan to you.

Common Drugs in the NICU

This section lists some of the drugs that may be given to babies who are sick or premature. The drugs are arranged alphabetically by common (generic) name. Trade or brand names follow the common name in parentheses. The entry for each drug describes what the drug is used for; what side effects it might produce; contraindications, if any, for its administration (medical conditions a health care provider considers when weighing the risks and benefits of a particular drug); information about monitoring, if available; and special notes. The information provided here is general and every baby's medication needs are unique. Be sure to discuss your baby's medications with the doctors and nurses caring for him or her.

Antibiotics: Agents that inhibit or stop the growth of microorganisms—usually bacteria. The best-known antibiotics are members of the penicillin family. Broad-spectrum antibiotics are those that are effective against a wide range of bacteria. Cefotaxime is one of these.

Anticonvulsants: Agents that prevent, control, or relieve convulsions (involuntary muscle contractions). Generally sedative-type drugs, anticonvulsants include diazepam, lorazepam, phenobarbital, and phenytoin.

Diuretics: Agents that help the kidneys get rid of excess water in the body by increasing urine excretion. Two examples are aldactazide and furosemide.

Narcotics: Agents that relieve pain. Narcotics also dull the senses, bring on a stuporous state, and affect the central nervous system. Medical personnel may refer to them as opioid analgesics. They include fentanyl, meperidine, and morphine sulfate.

Sedatives: Agents that calm by reducing nervousness, excitement, and activity. They work by depressing the activity of tissue in the central nervous system. Called sedative-hypnotics by medical personnel, these agents do not directly reduce pain. They include chloral hydrate, midazolam, and phenobarbital, as well as the anticonvulsant agents diazepam and lorazepam.

Steroids: Agents that decrease inflammation. Dexamethasone is one of these.

Stimulants: Agents that increase the functional activity or efficiency of an organ or system. They act on the tissue of the nervous system to increase tension in the muscles, thus increasing stimulation to the tissue. Caffeine and epinephrine are included in this category. Many stimulants target their effect to a specific organ or body system.

Acetaminophen (Tempra, Tylenol)

Use: A mild pain reliever that also reduces fever; available as an oral medication or as a suppository.
Side effects: Rash.

Acetazolamide (Diamox)

Use: A drug used to slow the development of hydrocephalus (water on the brain) by reducing production of cerebrospinal fluid (CSF).
Side effects: Vomiting, diarrhea, drowsiness, irritability, chemical imbalances in the blood (acidosis).
Contraindications: Cannot be given to some babies who have chemical imbalances in the blood.

Acyclovir (Zovirax)

Use: A medication that helps babies fight infections caused by some viruses; in particular, may be used to treat herpes or chickenpox.
Side effects: Irritation at the IV site; temporary decrease in kidney function.

Albuterol (Salbutamol, Ventolin)

Use: A drug used to treat airway problems such as those that occur in some babies with bronchopulmonary dysplasia (BPD). Ventolin works by relaxing, or "opening up," the breathing tubes in the lungs.

Indications: Wheezing or airway spasms.

Side effects: Increased heart rate, increased blood pressure, headache, tremors, hyperglycemia.

Aldactazide.

See Hydrochlorothiazide/Spironolactone

Amikacin

Use: An antibiotic used to treat infections caused by organisms sensitive to it.

Side effects: Can damage kidneys and hearing at high blood levels.

Monitoring: Blood levels of this drug are monitored.

Aminophylline (IV) and Theophylline (Oral)

Use: These medications are used in two groups of infants: those with apnea and those with bronchopulmonary dysplasia (BPD). Older infants or children with asthma may also receive theophylline. Used in the treatment of apnea of prematurity, theophylline stimulates the baby's breathing center to make breathing more regular. In BPD and asthma, theophylline helps to dilate the breathing tubes (bronchi) in the lungs and relieve muscle spasms in the bronchi.

Side effects: Diuresis (increased urine production), increased heart rate, vomiting, increased activity, irritability.

Monitoring: Blood levels of these drugs are monitored.

Amoxicillin

Use: A member of the penicillin family; an oral antibiotic used against infection caused by an organism sensitive to it.

Side effects: Allergic reaction (very uncommon in young babies because their immune system is not fully developed), vomiting, diarrhea, occasional rash.

Ampicillin

Use: An antibiotic from the penicillin family; effective against a number of bacteria that cause infection in infants.

Side effects: Allergy (rare in newborns), rash, diarrhea.

Ativan. See Lorazepam

Bactrim. See Co-Trimoxazole

Caffeine

Use: A stimulant that acts on the baby's breathing center and is used to treat apnea of prematurity.

Side effects: Restlessness, vomiting, high heart rate.

Monitoring: Blood levels of this drug are monitored.

Capoten. See Captopril

Captopril (Capoten)

Use: A medication used to treat high blood pressure and in the management of congestive heart failure.

Side effects: Low blood pressure, increased heart rate, chemical imbalances in the blood.

Contraindications: Usually not given to babies with kidney failure.

Cefotaxime Sodium (Claforan)

Use: A cephalosporin antibiotic used to treat suspected sepsis (infection in the blood).

Side effects: Rash, diarrhea.

Chloral Hydrate (Noctec)

Use: A sedative that can be given for restlessness or agitation; not used to relieve pain. Only given orally or rectally.

Side effects: Nausea, diarrhea, drowsiness, respiratory depression.

Contraindications: Only given orally or rectally; can't be used if these routes aren't available. Usually not given to infants with severe liver or kidney disease.

Claforan. See Cefotaxime Sodium

Cloxacillin

Use: An oral antibiotic from the penicillin family used to fight infection caused by an organism sensitive to it.

Side effects: Allergic reaction (uncommon in young babies), vomiting, diarrhea, occasional rash.

Co-Trimoxazole (Septra, Bactrim)

Use: An oral antibiotic used to treat susceptible bacteria—in particular, those that cause many ear and urinary tract infections.

Side effects: Rash, nausea, diarrhea.

Contraindications: Usually not given to infants less than one month of age.

Decadron. See Dexamethasone

Demerol. See Meperidine

Dexamethasone (Decadron)

Use: A form of steroid with anti-inflammatory properties; has been shown to improve lung function of some infants with bronchopulmonary dysplasia (BPD). Dexamethasone may be started as early as two weeks of age in very low birth weight infants or infants with severe lung disease. In the treatment of BPD, dexamethasone may be given over long periods of time, ranging from several weeks to two months. Also used to treat tracheal edema. Following placement of an endotracheal tube, some infants develop swelling of the vocal cords, which makes breathing after extubation more difficult. Dexamethasone is used in these infants to reduce swelling around the cords. This course of dexamethasone is short, lasting 24 to 48 hours.

Side effects: High blood pressure, high blood sugar, suppression of growth, fluid and blood chemistry imbalances, increased risk of infection.

Note: The benefits and risks of this drug must be considered in infants with infection or high blood pressure.

Diamox. See Acetazolamide

Diazepam (Valium)

Use: A medication given either as a sedative or as treatment for neonatal seizures.

Side effects: Low blood pressure, drowsiness, slowed breathing efforts.

Digoxin

Use: A medication used to help strengthen the muscle of the heart; used in the treatment of congestive heart failure (CHF).

Side effects: Low heart rate, changes in the rhythm of the heart, nausea and vomiting.

Contraindications: Cannot be used in infants with low potassium levels in the blood or with severe kidney or liver disease; should not be given to babies with a low heart rate.

Monitoring: Blood levels of this drug are monitored. The amount of drug the baby is receiving may need to be adjusted often in the first week to two weeks of treatment until drug blood levels stabilize.

Note: If your baby is going home on this drug, you will be taught how to watch for signs that he or she is receiving too much medication.

Dilantin. See Phenytoin

Dobutamine/Dopamine

Use: Two drugs used to improve low blood pressure and low urine output; given intravenously (IV) in a continuous infusion. Both drugs have similar uses and side effects; dopamine is more commonly used than dobutamine, however.

Side effects: Increased heart rate, changes in heart rhythm. When given through an IV in the limbs, can cause problems with circulation around the IV site.

Monitoring: Heart rate, blood pressure, and urine output are monitored carefully.

Dopram. See Doxapram

Doxapram (Dopram)

Use: A drug used to treat apnea of prematurity in infants whose apnea does not resolve with theophylline alone.

Side effects: High blood pressure, increased heart rate, feeding problems, increased crying.

Contraindications: Cannot be given to infants with swelling or pressure in the brain, seizures, or high blood pressure.

Epinephrine

Use: A powerful heart stimulant used to help strengthen the heart muscle and/or to treat cardiac failure and low blood pressure.

Side effects: Heart rhythm changes, high blood pressure, local irritation at the IV site.

Monitoring: Heart rate and blood pressure are monitored closely.

Erythromycin

Use: Erythromycin ointment may be used in the newborn's eyes just after delivery to prevent possible eye infections. An antibiotic used to treat infections caused by organisms sensitive to it.

Side effects: Vomiting, diarrhea, discomfort at site if given by injection.

Fentanyl (Sublimaze)

Use: A narcotic used for pain relief, sedation, or anesthesia; may be used in the nursery or in the operating room during surgery.

Side effects: Decreased breathing efforts, muscle rigidity, some risk of lowered blood pressure. Withdrawal symptoms can occur if the drug is discontinued abruptly after several days of use. Gradual weaning of the drug is recommended.

Note: Fentanyl is usually used only in infants receiving mechanical ventilation because it can produce respiratory depression (decreased breathing efforts).

Fer-In-Sol. See Ferrous Sulfate

Ferrous Sulfate (Fer-In-Sol)

Use: A mineral that helps to overcome anemia. As premature infants approach six to eight weeks of age, their iron stores become depleted as their bodies begin to produce hemoglobin and they need extra iron.

Side effects: Constipation, black stools, nausea.

Folic Acid

Use: One of the B vitamins; a deficiency, common in premature infants, results in a type of anemia.

Side effects: Skin redness or rash (rare).

Furosemide (Lasix)

Use: A diuretic that helps the kidneys get rid of excess water; used to treat conditions such as congestive heart failure (CHF), patent ductus arteriosus (PDA), fluid in the lungs, bronchopulmonary dysplasia (BPD), and some kidney diseases.

Side effects: Chemical imbalances in the blood, kidney stones (with prolonged use). If given with other potentially ear-damaging drugs, hearing damage may occur.

Gentamicin

Use: An antibiotic that is effective against most kinds of bacteria that occur in babies; used when infection is suspected or when infection with a bacterium sensitive to it is identified.

Side effects: At high blood levels, damage to the kidneys and hearing.

Monitoring: Blood levels of this drug are monitored.

Hydralazine

Use: A medication used to treat high blood pressure.

Side effects: Low blood pressure, stomach irritation and bleeding.

Hydrochlorothiazide/Spironolactone (Aldactazide)

Use: An oral diuretic that helps the kidneys to remove extra water from the body; used in longer-term treatment of conditions such as bronchopulmonary dysplasia (BPD), edema, and congestive heart failure (CHF).

Side effects: Diarrhea, lethargy, chemical imbalances.

Contraindications: Cannot be given to some babies with kidney problems.

Indocin. See Indomethacin

Indomethacin (Indocin)

Use: A medication used to close a patent ductus arteriosus (PDA).

Side effects: Temporary decrease in urine production resulting in swelling (edema) and fluid imbalances.

Contraindications: Cannot be given to babies with active kidney problems, bleeding problems, high bilirubin, or necrotizing enterocolitis (NEC).

Insulin

Use: A drug used to treat high blood sugar. Premature infants frequently develop imbalances in their blood sugar. This is a temporary problem related to immaturity and is not a sign of diabetes.

Side effects: Possible high or low blood sugar levels as the medication level is adjusted or when the medication is stopped.

Monitoring: Frequent blood sampling needed when insulin is started or adjusted to monitor blood sugar levels.

Iron. See Ferrous Sulfate

Lasix. See Furosemide

Lorazepam (Ativan)

Use: A medication given either as a sedative or as a treatment for neonatal seizures.

Side effects: Low blood pressure, nausea and vomiting, drowsiness, slowed breathing efforts.

Contraindications: Cannot be given to some babies with kidney or liver disease.

Meperidine (Demerol)

Use: A narcotic used to provide pain relief—often after surgical procedures.

Side effects: Respiratory depression (slowed breathing).

Midazolam (Versed)

Use: A short-acting sedative used especially before major procedures for its calming effects.

Side effects: Apnea, increased heart rate, drowsiness, cough, low blood pressure.

Morphine Sulfate

Use: A narcotic used for pain relief and sedation. It may be given as a continuous intravenous infusion or intermittently (IV).

Side effects: Low blood pressure, respiratory depression (slowed breathing), urine retention, physical tolerance and dependence possible after prolonged use.

Mycostatin. See Nystatin

Naloxone (Narcan)

Use: A drug that reverses the effects of narcotic agents such as morphine or meperidine. It may be given after delivery to newborns with decreased breathing efforts whose mothers received meperidine shortly before delivery. It may also be used to reverse the effects of narcotics given to infants for sedation or pain relief.

Side effects: Tremors, rapid breathing.

Narcan. See Naloxone

Noctec. See Chloral Hydrate

Nystatin (Mycostatin)

Use: A medication used in a cream or oral form to treat yeast (Candida) infections. These infections appear as a pebbly rash, usually in the diaper area, or as white patches in the mouth (thrush).

Side effects: Nausea, diarrhea, local irritation.

Pancuronium Bromide (Pavulon)

Use: A medication that causes temporary paralysis of muscles; used to keep critically ill babies from breathing against, or "fighting" the ventilator, thereby helping to improve oxygen levels in the blood.

Side effects: Increased heart rate, swelling (edema) of the limbs, increased saliva production, low blood pressure.

Note: Because pancuronium keeps infants from making any breathing efforts, it is only given to infants on mechanical ventilation. Babies receiving pancuronium cannot move, but they can hear your voice and feel your touch.

Pavulon. See Pancuronium

Penicillin

Use: An antibiotic used to treat susceptible bacteria, especially Group B ß-hemolytic Streptococcus (ß-strep).

Side effects: Diarrhea.

Phenobarbital, or Phenobarb

Use: An anticonvulsant used to treat neonatal seizures; also used as a sedative in some instances.

Side effects: Drowsiness, lethargy, low blood pressure, depressed respirations, nausea.

Monitoring: Blood levels of this drug are monitored.

Phenytoin (Dilantin)

Use: An anticonvulsant used to treat seizures; usually added if phenobarbital does not control the seizures.

Side effects: Low blood pressure, nausea, constipation, jaundice, rash, drowsiness.

Contraindications: Cannot be given to babies with severe liver or kidney disease.

Monitoring: Blood levels of this drug are monitored.

Prostaglandin E$_1$ (PGE$_1$)

Use: A medication used to improve oxygenation and circulation of newborns with cyanotic congenital heart disease. Maintains blood flow through the ductus arteriosus until surgery can be performed.

Side effects: Elevated temperature, apnea, low blood pressure, skin flushing, bradycardia, tachycardia.

Salbutamol. See Albuterol

Septra. See Co-Trimoxazole

Spironolactone.
See Hydrochlorothiazide/Spironolactone

Sublimaze. See Fentanyl

Sufentanil (Sufenta)

Use: A synthetic narcotic approximately ten times more potent than fentanyl. Used most often as anesthesia for cardiovascular surgery.

Side effects: Decreased breathing efforts, muscle rigidity.

Tempra. See Acetaminophen

Theophylline. See Aminophylline

Tri-Vi-Sol

Indications: A combination of Vitamins A, C, and D that comes in liquid drops used to supplement the formula or breast milk that your baby is receiving.

Tylenol. See Acetaminophen

Valium. See Diazepam

Vancomycin

Use: An antibiotic used to treat suspected or confirmed neonatal infections.

Side effects: Diarrhea, vomiting; at high blood levels, possible kidney or hearing damage.

Monitoring: Blood levels of this drug are monitored.

Vecuronium Bromide

Use: A drug used to cause temporary paralysis of muscles and to keep critically ill babies from breathing against, or "fighting," the ventilator; also helps to improve oxygen levels in the blood.

Side effects: Increased heart rate, swelling (edema) of the limbs, increased saliva production, low blood pressure.

Note: Because vecuronium keeps infants from making any breathing efforts, it is only given to infants on mechanical ventilation. Babies receiving vecuronium cannot move, but they can hear your voice and feel your touch.

Ventolin. See Albuterol

Versed. See Midazolam

Vitamins. See also Folic Acid, Tri-Vi-Sol

Use: Various combinations of vitamins may be prescribed for your infant. Vitamin solutions may or may not be prescribed for your baby after discharge. Discuss this with your health care provider.

Vitamin D

Indications: Liquid drops given to premature infants to supplement the vitamin D in breast milk or formula. A shortage of vitamin D in the body may lead to weakening of the bones.

Vitamin K

Indications: Injection is routinely given to all newborns soon after birth to help the body form clotting substances that help prevent bleeding.

Side effects: Pain or swelling at the injection site.

Zovirax. See Acyclovir

Appendix C
Car Seat Safety

Jeanette Zaichkin, RNC, MN

❝"I must move about more. I must come and go."❞

Eeyore–

When your baby is in the hospital, her safety depends largely on the vigilance and expertise of the nurses, physicians, and other professionals who care for her. When she leaves the hospital and comes home, her safety depends on the steps you take to protect her from harm. This safekeeping begins on discharge day when you buckle your baby into her car seat for a safe trip home.

A car seat is also called a child safety seat or child restraint (CR). It doesn't matter what term you use—the fact remains that using a car seat every time your baby is in the car is one of the most important things you can do to protect her. Many parents convince their children when they are very young that the car engine will not start until every person is buckled up. This routine may also offer an opportunity to convince other family members of the importance of using seat belts.

This appendix provides car seat information that will be helpful as you prepare for your baby's hospital discharge. The following list gives questions to ask the NICU team about car seats and suggestions for how to learn to use your baby's car seat before the baby's discharge. The remainder of this appendix provides important information about car seat use and safety.

For more resources about travel safety for babies, see Appendix D (Parent Resources) under "Travel and Car Seat Information."

Prepare Ahead for Your Baby's Ride Home

- If you cannot afford to purchase a car seat, ask your baby's nurse or your social worker about resources for car seat loan or rental.

- Ask the NICU team if your baby has any special needs that will influence your selection of a car seat. Some babies need a car seat that allows the baby to lie flat.

- Ask NICU team members if they recommend a car seat "trial." This is important if your baby has cardiac or respiratory problems at discharge. During a car seat trial, your baby sits in her car seat in the NICU while her nurse monitors her color, heart rate, breathing, and oxygen saturation. If the trial indicates that she cannot tolerate the upright position because she slumps down or her head falls forward, the nurse will teach you how to position your baby correctly or will suggest a different type of car seat.

- Ask the NICU team and other parents of NICU graduates for their recommendations about car seat purchase. Models change from year to year, and some car seats are easier to use than others. The American Academy of Pediatrics offers a helpful pamphlet for parents entitled "The Family Shopping Guide to Car Seats" (see Appendix D under "Travel and Car Seat Information").

- If you decide to use a previously owned or used car seat check the car seat for strength and stability. It is best to use seats less than 10 years old. Be sure it has never been in an automobile accident. Try to obtain the manufacturer's instruction booklet. Call the manufacturer to be sure that it has not been recalled. (Major car seat manufacturers are listed at the end of this appendix.)

- Read your automobile owner's manual for special instructions regarding car seat use. Every make and model has specifications for proper car seat installation. Some models require that the dealer install special adapters to secure a car seat safely. Some seat belts require the use of a locking clip (Table C-1). Some seat belts are not compatible with car seats at all.

- Read the car seat instructions before it is time to buckle your baby into the car. Practice securing your car seat in the car and taking it out again. If necessary, learn how to secure special-care items such as your baby's oxygen cylinder or apnea monitor. Decide where to position the baby and other passengers so that the baby is supervised and safely placed in the car.

- If possible, take your car seat to the NICU a day or two before your baby's discharge. With the nurse's help, position your baby safely and buckle her into the car seat. Learning how to use the car seat is easy when you have time and help in the NICU. You will have a more difficult time if you wait until you are nervous and rushed in the hospital driveway on discharge day.

Table of Contents

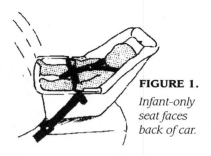

FIGURE 1.

Infant-only seat faces back of car.

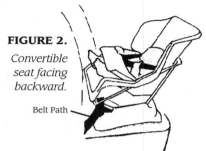

FIGURE 2.

Convertible seat facing backward.

Belt Path

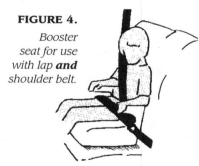

FIGURE 3.

Convertible seat facing forward.

Retainer Clip holds harness in place

Belt Path

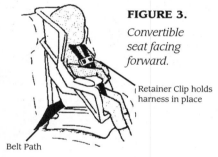

FIGURE 4.

*Booster seat for use with lap **and** shoulder belt.*

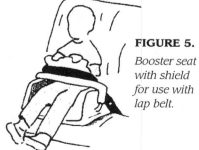

FIGURE 5.

Booster seat with shield for use with lap belt.

American Academy of Pediatrics One-Minute Safety Checkup

Using a car seat correctly makes a big difference. Even the "safest" seat may not protect your child in a crash, so take a minute to check to be sure...

Do you have the instructions?

- Follow them and keep them with your seat for use as your child grows older.
- Use your vehicle owner's manual for help in fastening the seat in securely.

Is your child facing the right way for her height, weight, and age?

- If you use a seat made only for infants (Figure 1), always face it backward.
- A baby up to 20 pounds should ride facing the back of the car (Figure 2).
- A child over 20 pounds faces forward (Figure 3).
- The impact from an air bag can seriously injure or kill a baby riding in front in a rear-facing safety seat. Carry your baby in back, facing the rear.

Is the auto safety belt in the right place and pulled tight?

- The belt must go in the correct, marked path to hold the seat in place.
- A convertible seat faces backward for an infant (Figure 2) and forward for a toddler (Figure 3). It has two different belt paths, one for each direction.

Is the harness snug? Does it stay on the child's shoulders?

- Shoulder straps go in the lowest slots for babies riding backward and in the top slots for children facing forward.
- The retainer clip at armpit level (Figure 3) holds harness straps on the shoulders.

Does your child use a booster seat if she is over 40 pounds and has outgrown her convertible seat?

- A booster seat helps the safety belt protect a child until the child grows big enough to fit the belt alone.
- A booster seat with no shield is used only with a lap and shoulder belt (Figure 4).
- If your car has only lap belts, use a booster with a shield (Figure 5).

Have you fixed your child's car seat if it has been recalled?

For a list of recalled seats that need repair, ask your pediatrician, local safety group, or The Washington State Safety Restraint Coalition (800) 282-5587.

FACT SHEET from Safe Ride News Publications, 117 East Louisa Street, Box 290, Seattle, WA 98102, (originally published by AAP, revised 1996 by *Safe Ride News*). This information should not be used as a substitute for the medical care and advice of your pediatrician. There may be variations in treatment that your pediatrician may recommend based on the individual facts and circumstances. Reprinted by permission of the American Academy of Pediatrics.

Car Seat Safety for Low Birthweight Infants and Children with Special Needs

Every Baby Deserves to Be Protected in the Car!

All newborn infants need special attention to be comfortable and safe in the car. To function properly, the safety restraint must fit the infant's body. The restraint must be installed securely, and the infant must be buckled in with adequate padding.

Some infants have special transportation needs at discharge. These can be met with planning, parent education, and availability of suitable child restraint devices.

Correct selection of a restraint device is particularly important for newborn infants who:

- are preterm or weigh less than 5½ pounds (2,500 grams)
- have certain other congenital conditions such as spina bifida, hydrocephalus, Pierre Robin syndrome, and neuromuscular disorders.

In some cases, the use of some or all conventional infant/child safety seats may be unsuitable. Devices are available to accommodate virtually all special needs.

FIGURE C-1a and b.

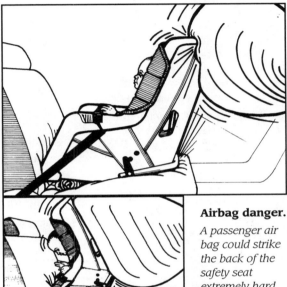

Airbag danger.

A passenger air bag could strike the back of the safety seat extremely hard. This could seriously injure a baby's head.

After the impact, the air bag could throw the safety seat up and into the headrest or between the seats.

The Basics of Protection

- The safety seat must be the right size for the baby.
- Household carriers or feeding seats are not strong enough to protect a baby in a crash.
- The seat must meet current federal motor vehicle safety standards and have been made after January 1, 1981—check the label.
- It must be used correctly, with the baby fastened into the car seat or car bed and the device fastened into the car.
- The baby should ride where an adult can see the baby.
- Infants riding in rear-facing safety seats must never ride in the front seat of a vehicle with a passenger-side frontal air bag. In a crash, the air bag would hit the back of the safety seat very hard and could seriously injure the infant (See Figure C-1a and C-1b). The Dream Ride Ultra (see drawing on page 381) in the flat car bed position can be used in front with an air bag. Both bed and baby would be below the frontal air bag if it were to deploy. (However, the Dream Ride Ultra does not fit well on most bucket seats.)

Selecting the Seat

- If you already own a car seat, you may be able to use it, depending on how it fits your baby. Many models can be adapted with padding, as long as they don't have a shield.

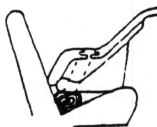

FIGURE C-2
Safety seat dimensions.

Infant safety seat showing maximum recommended dimensions for correct harness fit on a very small baby.

• Car seats with shields in front should not be used for very small babies, because the baby's face or chest could hit the shield in a crash.
• Car seats with a space of 5½ inches or less between the crotch strap and the seat back will keep your baby from slouching too much. Seat harnesses with shoulder strap slots located 10 inches or less above the seat bottom will work best to hold your baby in place (Figure C-2).
• Child safety seats with a five-point harness (at both shoulders, both hips, and between the legs), can be adjusted to provide good upper torso support for many children with special needs. Infant-only car seats with recline capabilities are useful for many infants with medical problems, especially respiratory conditions.
• Children with tracheostomies should avoid using child restraint systems with a harness-tray/shield combination or an armrest. Upon sudden impact, the child could fall forward and cause the tracheostomy to contact the shield or armrest, possibly resulting in injury and a blocked airway.[1] A child safety seat with a five-point harness should be selected for children with tracheostomies.
• Some babies may have trouble breathing when they sit in a semireclined seat, such as a car seat, feeding seat, or swing. If this is the case, your baby should ride lying flat in a special bed made for use in the car. (See more information on car beds on page 384.)

Positioning the Baby in the Car Seat

• An infant under 20 pounds should always ride facing the back of the vehicle.
• The safety seat should recline halfway back, at a 45 degree tilt, so the infant's head stays upright. If the vehicle seat slopes so that the infant's head falls forward, the safety seat should be tipped back so the base of the seat is horizontal. (Some infant safety seats have tilt indicators.) To tilt the seat, wedge a firm roll of cloth or newspaper under the base below the infant's feet (Figure C-3). The safety seat should never be reclined beyond 45 degrees.
• The infant's buttocks and back should be flat against the back of the safety seat. Rolled-up diapers or small blankets can make the seat fit better (Figure C-4).
• Shoulder straps must be in the lowest slots, the harness snug, and the harness retainer clip at armpit level.
• Any blankets used must be put over the infant after the harness has been adjusted snugly.
• If an add-on safety seat pad is used, it must have slits for harness straps to be pulled through. It must not have thick padding behind the infant's back.

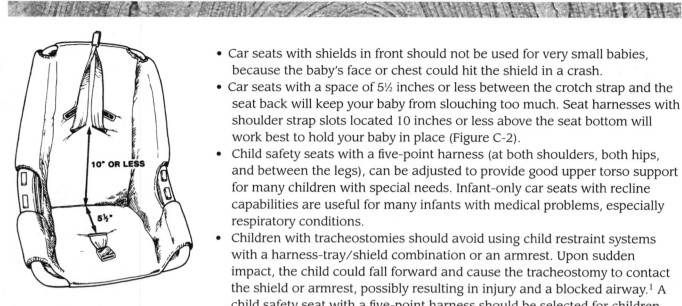

FIGURE C-3
Wedge to tilt safety seat.

A firm roll is wedged under the safety seat below the infant's feet to make the base of the seat horizontal.

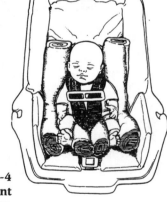

FIGURE C-4
Padding placement for a small baby.

Padding beside head, torso, and in crotch of newborn infant in infant-only safety seat. No padding should be placed under the infant's buttocks.

From: Transporting Newborn Infants Including Low Birthweight Infants: What Health Care Providers Need to Know. Safe Ride News Insert, Summer 1995.

- If an infant has been demonstrated to be at risk for potential breathing problems, she should ride lying flat in a special bed made for use in the car. Position the baby's head as far as possible from the side of the vehicle. The baby's health care provider will indicate whether the baby should lie on her back or tummy.

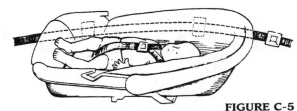

FIGURE C-5
Seat belt placement for a car bed.

Dream Ride used as a car bed, with harness holding infant. Seat belt threads through loops on the back side of the bed.

From: What Every Premature or Small Baby Needs to Know. Safe Ride News, *Spring 1992.*

Securing the Car Seat and Medical Equipment in the Vehicle

- Safety seats should be used only with safety belts that lock tightly and hold the seat firmly in place.
- Users must check their auto owner's manual and safety seat instructions for guidance when securing the car seat into the vehicle.
- Locking clips that come with all new safety seats will lock one common type of lap-shoulder belt (Table C-1). Some vehicles have belts that can be switched to lock around child safety seats. Others have auxiliary belts or buckles (available from the vehicle dealer) for anchoring safety seats.
- If your baby is riding flat in a car bed that uses a harness, it should be snug (Figure C-5). Unfortunately, many vehicles have contoured seats on which a flat car bed does not rest securely.
- An apnea monitor, portable oxygen tank, or other equipment must be anchored to the floor of the car or under the seat so it won't fly around in a crash and injure you or someone else.

Restraints for Older Children with Special Needs

- Use a safety-tested and federally approved child restraint system whenever possible. Standard child restraint devices may be used for some children with special medical problems. Use of a "special" car seat for a child with medical problems may be postponed until a child exceeds the limits of a standard car seat.
- For children who have poor head control and weigh more than 20 pounds, use a convertible seat that can be semireclined when facing forward. Soft padding may be positioned behind the neck and on either side of the head to promote anatomical alignment. This padding should not be placed behind the head itself or behind the trunk (Figure C-6). Do not use head bands to restrain the child's head separately from the torso.
- Only firm padding, such as a single folded sheet, should be used behind a child's back. No compressible padding should be placed behind or under the child in the seat. Soft padding (such as blankets, pillows, or soft foam) compress on impact and can prevent harness straps from maintaining a secure and tight fit on a child's body. A dangerous slack in the harness system on impact could result from the use of soft padding behind or underneath the child.[2]

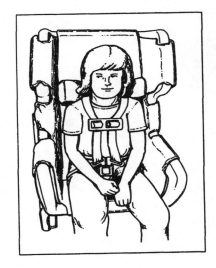

FIGURE C-6
Padding for an older child.

Child in convertible seat, with soft padding positioned behind the neck and on either side of the head to promote anatomical alignment.

From: Policy Statement: Transporting Children with Special Needs. Safe Ride News Insert, *Winter 1993.*

TABLE C-1 What is a Locking Clip, and How Do I Know If I Need One?

A child safety seat that is installed and used correctly provides optimum crash protection for your child. If the child safety seat you own doesn't fit into your car, don't try to "make" it work through makeshift measures. Incorrect use of a child safety seat can drastically reduce its effectiveness.

FIGURE A.

To assure that you properly install the child safety seat in your car, carefully read and follow the manufacturer's instructions. Also check your automobile owner's manual for installation instructions.

With some seat belt systems, a locking clip (Figure A) is needed to "lock" the lap-shoulder style automobile seat belt tightly around a child safety seat.

- *Do not* use a locking clip on "lap only" seat belts.
- *Do not* use a locking clip on lap-shoulder belts that have a "locking latchplate" (Figure B).
- *Do not* use a locking clip with lap-shoulder belts having a sewn-on latchplate (Figure C). This belt style cannot secure a child safety seat unless it has a combination retractor (consult your automobile owner's manual).
- *Do use* a locking clip on a continuous loop lap–shoulder belt with a latchplate that slides freely along the belt (Figure D). These belts have a retractor that does not lock until the impact of a collision.

Locking Bar

FIGURE B.

FIGURE C.

To attach the locking clip:

1. Buckle the seat belt around or through the safety seat according to the manufacturer's instructions.
2. Tighten—as snugly as you can—the lap portion of the belt by pulling on the shoulder portion and feeding the excess into the retractor. It is helpful to place your knee in the child safety seat and press it down into the car seat while tightening the belt.
3. When the belt is tight, pinch the belt webbing together behind the sliding latchplate and unbuckle the belt while still holding the webbing so it won't loosen.
4. Thread the belt webbing onto the clip, one side at a time. Keep the clip close to the sliding latchplate, no farther than ½ inch (Figure E).
5. Rethread the seat belt correctly around or through the safety seat and fasten the buckle. Pull the lap portion and the shoulder portion of the belt separately to be sure that the clip is securely in place. Tug the seat forward and side to side. If the seat still is not secure, unbuckle, remove the locking clip, and repeat steps 1 through 5.

The locking clip will stay in place until you remove it. If the child safety seat is removed, the locking clip must also be detached before the lap-shoulder belt is used by any passenger.

Where Can I Get a Locking Clip If I Need One?

FIGURE D.

Child safety seat manufacturers provide a clip with every seat. If you need a locking clip and cannot obtain one from a store in your area, call the manufacturer of your child's seat to obtain one.

Washington State Safety Restraint Coalition. *What is a Locking Clip and How Do I Know If I Need One?* Reprinted by permission.

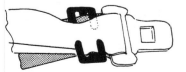

FIGURE E.

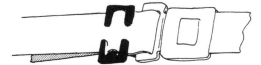

- Lateral support may be provided with rolled blankets, towels, or foam rolls (Figure C-7).
- A foam roll or rolled blanket may be placed under a child's knees to inhibit hypertonicity or opisthotonic positioning (Figure C-8).
- Crotch rolls may be added between the child's legs and the crotch strap to keep the hips against the back of the seat and the child positioned upright (Figure C-9).
- For prone positioning in a restraint system, the child's height and weight must be evaluated. For instance, infants with Pierre Robin syndrome who must lie prone to maintain an open airway may be placed prone in the Dyn-O-Mite infant car seat by Evenflo (Piqua, Ohio) with specific modifications, or the Dream Ride from Cosco (Columbus, Indiana).[3] Use of these two restraints in this manner, however, is limited to infants under approximately 10 pounds in order to be able to achieve a comfortable fit, although both restraints provide a fit for supine infants up to 17 pounds. Care must be taken, however, to evaluate the height of the child and the added space taken up by a cast or any other ancillary medical apparatus before determining if these can effectively secure the child.

Padding placement for body support.

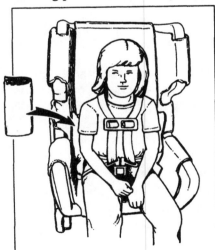

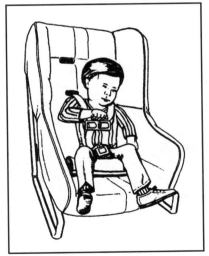

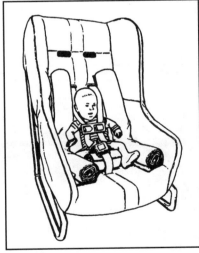

FIGURE C-7

Child in convertible seat; rolled blankets, towels, or foam rolls can provide lateral support.

From: Policy Statement: Transporting Children with Special Needs. Safe Ride News Insert, Winter 1993.

FIGURE C-8

Child in convertible seat; foam roll or rolled blanket placed under knees can inhibit hypertonicity or opisthotonic positioning.

From: Policy Statement: Transporting Children with Special Needs. Safe Ride News Insert, Winter 1993.

FIGURE C-9

Infant in convertible seat, with rolls added between the legs and the crotch strap to ensure proper positioning.

From: Policy Statement: Transporting Children with Special Needs. Safe Ride News Insert, Winter 1993.

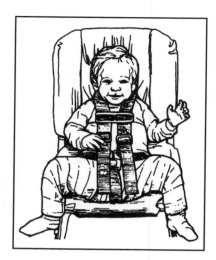

FIGURE C-10
Safety seat for spica cast.

Child with spica cast seated in modified seat with cut-away sides and seat bottom.

From: Policy Statement: Transporting Children with Special Needs. Safe Ride News Insert, *Winter 1993.*

- For children with spica casts, a specially modified Evenflo 410 convertible safety seat (Spelcast) has cut-away sides and seat bottom that provide room for a comfortable and snug fit into the restraint system (Figure C-10).
- Many toddlers, preschool, and school-aged children in body or hip spica casts have limited resources available to them for safe transport in motor vehicles. One resource, the modified E-Z-On Vest, has performed satisfactorily during dynamic crash-testing with a test dummy weighted to 105 pounds and is available commercially. The E-Z-On Vest has been altered by adding double loops on both sides of the vest. Two sets of seat belts are used to secure the child at the side against the vehicle seat. An ancillary belt loops around the casted leg or legs at the knees and is routed through the other seat belt (Figure C-11). When it is not possible to fit a child onto a vehicle seat, use of an ambulance for transport is recommended. For lateral positioning on the vehicle seat (e.g. as required by car bed restraint on the modified E-Z-On Vest), position the child's head as far as possible from the side of the vehicle.
- When in transit, ancillary medical equipment (walkers, crutches, oxygen tanks, monitors, and so on) should be positioned and secured on the vehicle floor; positioned and secured underneath a vehicle seat or wheelchair; or secured to the bus seat, bus floor, or bus wall below the window line.
- Electrical equipment to be used during transit should have portable self-contained power for twice the expected transport duration. For improved safety, lead acid batteries on electrically powered wheelchairs or other mobile seating devices and respiratory systems should be converted, whenever possible, to gel-cell or dry-cell batteries. To house and protect batteries during everyday use, transportation, and collision, external battery boxes are recommended.

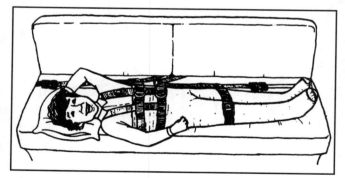

FIGURE C-11
Safety restraint for body cast.

Child with modified E-Z-On Vest.

From: Policy Statement: Transporting Children with Special Needs. Safe Ride News Insert, *Winter 1993.*

- Once a child has outgrown a car safety seat, there are other choices available for proper and secure occupant restraint, depending upon the needs of the child for support. Some systems—such as the Britax (the Special Car Seat), the Orthopaedics Positioning Seat, the Carrie Car Seat, the Carrie Bus Seat, and the Snug Seat—provide for full support for the child's head, neck, and back. Others, such as the conventional E-Z-On Vest, can be used to provide additional trunk support for a child who already has stable neck control.

- Travel chair restraint systems are another choice for restraint that should be evaluated against the nature of the child's disability, individual positioning requirements, and types of motor vehicles used for transport. Willingness of the user to install tethers, add additional lap seat belts, or obtain appropriate tie-down systems for some of these devices should be a consideration for selection and proper use.

- Some older children with disabilities can also be transferred to a conventional belt-positioning booster car seat for trunk support. A belt-positioning booster seat has a removable shield. The shoulder and lap belt are positioned across the child's chest and pelvis and secured through side arms on the booster seat. Older children with hyperactivity, autism, or emotional disturbances may require a restraint that is more difficult to release. Booster car seats with seat belts routed underneath the seat base may be helpful in reducing the child's likelihood of evacuating the restraint during travel.

- In addition, use of conventional lap-shoulder systems may also be useful in providing for trunk restraint of some children with special needs. Lap-shoulder belts should be used properly. If a shoulder belt rests on a child's face, position the child toward the middle of the vehicle seat to lower the shoulder belt onto the chest. Do not place the shoulder belt underneath the child's arm or behind the vehicle seat back. Use of a belt-positioning booster seat may also help assure proper placement of the shoulder belt on the child's chest.

- The recommendations in this publication do not indicate an exclusive course of treatment or serve as a standard of medical care. Variations, taking into account individual circumstances, may be appropriate.

References

1. Stroup KB, Wylie P, and Bull MJ. 1987. Car seats for children with mechanically assisted ventilation. *Pediatrics* 80(2): 290–292.

2. Bull MJ, et al. 1990. Establishing a special needs car seat loan program. *Pediatrics* 85(4): 540–547.

3. Stroup KB, Weber K, and Bull MJ. 1987. Safe transportation solutions for children with special needs. In *31st Proceedings of the American Association for Automotive Medicine* (September 28–30: New Orleans, 297–307.

Information Compiled from:

American Academy of Pediatrics and Safe Ride News Publications. What Every Premature or Small Baby Needs to Know... Before Riding in the Car. *Safe Ride News,* Spring 1995; AAP Policy statement: Transporting Children with Special Needs. *Safe Ride News,* Winter 1993; Infants and Air Bags Don't Mix. *Safe Ride News*, Spring 1993 (revised 1995); Transporting Newborn Infants Including Low Birthweight Infants and Those with Special Needs. Safe Ride News, Summer, 1995. Reprinted by permission.

To request updates or reproducable copies of the materials used above. Please contact *Safe Ride News*, 117 East Louisa Street, Box 290, Seattle, WA 98102.

Child Restraints and Automobiles: An Uneasy Union

by Annemarie Shelness

Many belt systems found in today's cars are incompatible with child restraints (CRs), but with the necessary know-how and a little effort, most obstacles can be overcome. This is not so with the newest problem to come to light. Recent changes in the design of vehicle seats and seat belt anchorages make secure installation of some CRs at best questionable and in some vehicles virtually impossible. Solutions are being worked on in many countries and a number of approaches are on the drawing board.

The Problem

Safety belts are being anchored forward of the intersection between the seat cushion and the seat back, known as the "bight" (Figure 1). Two of the "Big Three" U.S. automakers, Ford and General Motors, and many foreign manufacturers are installing forward-anchored belts in the rear seats in a growing number of their models. Chrysler is not doing so, for now.*

The farther the belt anchorage is forward of the bight, the less secure CR installation becomes (Figure 2). Even where the distance is no greater than 2 or 3 inches, this location, added to the "reel-out" and belt stretch that normally occur, could allow the CR to move forward a considerable distance in a crash. This could place the child's head at risk of striking the interior of the vehicle. In some instances, especially in small, two-door cars, where rear seat cushions are scooped out and belt anchorages are as much as 8 or even 10 inches forward of the bight, correct CR installation becomes impossible.

The Reasons

Automakers have sound reasons for making this change in belt geometry, which benefits children who have outgrown CRs as well as adults. Where belts are anchored behind the bight, there is a serious risk that occupants will slide down, feetfirst, under the belt, a phenomenon known as "submarining." This causes the lap belt to ride up over the abdomen. "Loading" soft tissue in this manner can cause spinal and other internal injuries.

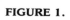

FIGURE 1.

Rear seat of current GM model, showing belts anchored forward of bight.

FIGURE 2.

Infant restraint, convertible and small shield booster, comparing installation with forward-anchored belt (light) and belt anchored behind the seat bight (dark). The latter holds the restraints back as well as down. (Illustrations by Kathleen Richards.)

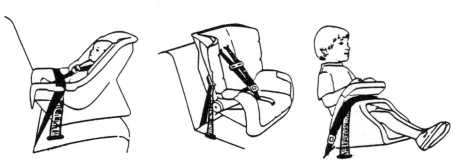

* A few sporty, two-door imports sold under the Chrystler name have had such belts.

With belt anchorages placed forward of the bight, the lap portion of the belt is routed over the upper thighs, below the pelvic bones, allowing the upper torso to move forward into the shoulder belt.

Using child restraints with these belt configurations presents a problem. Where belts are only two or three inches forward of the bight, some CRs may feel secure when hand pressure is applied. But head excursion, that is, the distance the child's head moves forward, could increase significantly.[1]

Recommendations Differ

Numerous discussions with safety engineers have pointed up the fact that major auto manufacturers do not agree on whether forward-anchored belts are, in fact, detrimental for children in CRs.

The prospect of returning to CRs with tethers is of grave concern to many safety advocates. First, only one CR manufacturer, Evenflo, advertises the availability of tethers for its convertible CRs in this country. Cosco and Renolux will supply them on request for their own products. Second, tethers are usable only for forward-facing CRs, although rear-facing CRs also may be affected. Third, in the seventies and early eighties, when tether seats were on the market in the U.S., it was found that 85 percent of tethers were either not used at all or installed incorrectly.[2] In Canada, tethers have been used on forward-facing CRs for the past decade to meet stringent head excursion requirements. A recent, extensive Transport Canada study found the tether misuse rate was over 60 percent.

One Expert's View

Richard Stalnaker, PhD, is uniquely qualified to comment: In the seventies, as research scientist at the University of Michigan Highway Safety Research Institute (now The University of Michigan Transportation Research Institute, or UMTRI), he was involved in the dynamic testing of child restraints. Now a professor at Ohio State University, specializing in accident investigation and reconstruction, he frequently serves as an expert witness in product liability cases involving child restraints.

Dr. Stalnaker explains: "Where belt anchor points have been moved forward, the lap belt attaches to the restraint in an almost vertical direction, instead of coming up from behind and securing the CR at an angle. In a serious crash, a CR may not perform as designed." He expressed particular concern about shield boosters and those convertible restraints that are secured through the front, beneath the child's feet, when rear-facing. The farther forward the belt is anchored, the more questionable performance will be, he added.

A Promising "Fix"

In Europe, automakers and child restraint manufacturers have long been aware of the problem. The International Standards Organization (ISO) Working Group on Child Restraint Systems has been trying to find a solution that would allow the installation of CRs independent of vehicle seat belts. The first such system was demonstrated at an ISO meeting in 1990 by the Swedish

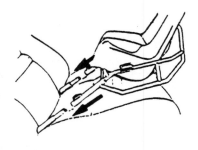

FIGURE 3.

Original ISOFIX concept, with extensions of CR plugging into sockets secured to the vehicle through the seat.

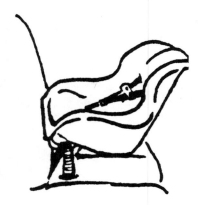

FIGURE 4.

Avoid CRs with the belt path under the feet, close to the vehicle seat.

delegation. Named ISOFIX, it consisted of two sockets mounted in the bight, into which extensions on the CR "plugged in," locking the CR tightly in place (Figure 3).

Since this first demonstration took place, the British have pursued a somewhat different approach. The latest concept calls for three anchor points: two in the bight and one at the center front below the seat cushion. The CR would have projections terminating in spring-loaded "jaws" that would snap onto steel rods embedded in the vehicle seat. The locking mechanism would be similar to that of an automobile trunk latch.

How far are we in the U.S. from making some type of universal "fix" a reality? It has been discussed at the Society of Automotive Engineers (SAE) Children's Restraint System Task Force meetings, but the major thrust is coming from Europe. Howard Willson, chairman of the task force, believes that once Europe requires an independent CR attachment method, U.S. automakers will follow suit.

Once the final version of ISOFIX has been agreed on, one more step remains. CR manufacturers will have to do their part in providing models with corresponding connectors. ISOFIX would take care of the many interface problems that now make CR use so difficult at times and ensure that all CRs are tightly secured—provided, of course, that ISOFIX itself can be fail-safe.

There is little hard information on which to base guidance for parents at this time (see "CRs and Forward-Anchored Belts"). They should be warned to take a close look at rear seat belt configurations and try a child restraint before purchasing a new or used car.

CRs and Forward-Anchored Belts

Unfortunately, there is not much parents can do to counteract the effect of these safety belts, and real-world experience and test data are still limited. Here are a few tips on selection of vehicles and restraints:

1. When purchasing a vehicle, consider the anchorage placement of rear seat belts.
2. Note features of CRs for use in a car with belts anchored forward of the bight:
   - For infants riding facing the rear, avoid CRs with the belt path under the feet, close to the vehicle seat (Figure 4).
   - For forward-facing convertibles, a correctly installed tether will help anchor the device at the top (Figure 2).
   - In seating positions with lap-shoulder belts, a belt positioning booster will work better than boosters with shields.

References

1. Weber K (UM), and Radowich VG (NHTSA). 1987. Performance evaluation of child restraints relative to vehicle lap-belt anchorage locations. *SP-690, Society of Automotive Engineers* (February 23–27), 105–110.

2. Shelness A, and Jewett J. 1983. Observed misuse of child restraints. *SAE Child Injury and Restraint Conference Proceedings* (November).

Annemarie Shelness was executive director of Physicians for Automotive Safety for 18 years and is a member of both the SAE Children's Restraint Systems Task Force and the ISO Working Group on Child Restraint Systems.

American Academy of Pediatrics. 1993. *Safe Ride News* 12(3): 3–4. Reprinted by permission.

Guide to Transportation Safety Products for Children with Special Needs

Vehicle restraints are now available for children with all kinds of special health care needs. Many children under 50 pounds can use standard car seats.

This list is adapted from materials of the National Easter Seal Society and the Automotive Safety for Children Program, Riley Hospital, Indianapolis. It is not intended to be all-inclusive; inclusion does not imply product endorsement. Prices are subject to change.

Note: Products for children under 50 pounds are certified by manufacturers to meet FMVSS (federal motor vehicle safety standard) 213. Those for children over 50 pounds are not subject to any federal motor vehicle safety standard. Manufacturers of those listed here claim that their products pass tests similar to those for standard 213.

Low Birth Weight Infants

Standard Safety Seats: Models without shields only

From:	Retail outlets
Cost:	$35–$70
Weight:	Up to 20 pounds
Height:	Up to 26 inches
Comments:	Blanket rolls at sides and between legs provide positioning support. Small harness dimensions recommended: 10 inches from buttocks to shoulder strap slots, 5½ inches from crotch strap to buttocks.

Dream Ride, DR Ultra

From:	Cosco
Cost:	$40
Weight:	Up to 20 pounds
Height:	Up to 26 inches
Comments:	Car bed converts to rear-facing infant safety seat.

Dyn-O-Mite

From:	Evenflo Products
Cost:	$21–$24.40
Weight:	Up to 20 pounds
Height:	Up to 20 inches
Comments:	Two positions*, two harness positions accommodate growth, one-piece harness tie belt.

*In fully reclined position, use Dyn-O-Mite only with lap-shoulder belt wrapped around the back of the safety seat for added stability.

Infant/Child Must Lie Prone or Supine

Dream Ride, DR Ultra

(See under "Low Birth Weight Babies"; use horizontal for preterm infant with potential breathing problems)

Modified E-Z-On Vest

From:	E-Z-On Products, Inc.
Cost:	$80
Weight:	Up to 100 pounds
Height:	Determined by length of vehicle seat
Size:	Hips 22–32 inches
Comments:	Must have hip measurement to order vest. Shoulder strap length adjustable on new models.

Orthopedic Needs Requiring Casting

Spelcast Restraint

From: Snug Seat, Inc.
Cost: $250
Weight: Up to 50 pounds, including cast
Height: Up to 40 inches
Comments: Appropriate for hip spica cast position. Convertible for rear or forward facing. Top tether recommended in forward facing position.

Behavior Problems

Regular E-Z-On Vest

From: E-Z-On Products, Inc.
Cost: $74.75
Weight: Up to 164 pounds
Height: Determined by height of vehicle seat
Size: Waist 22–43 inches
Comments: Top tether or Cam Wrap (mounting strap used on school buses) required. New styles with "adjustable" zippers and shoulder straps now available.

Poor Trunk and/or Head Control

Regular E-Z-On Vest

(see under "Behavior Problems," head control needed)

Besi Restraining Harness

(see under "Behavior Problems," head control needed)

Little Cargo Vest

From: Little Cargo, Inc.
Cost: $39.95
Weight: 25–40 pounds
Height: Up to 40 inches
Comments: Head control needed.

Standard Child Safety Seat

From: Retail outlets
Cost: Varies by product
Weight: Up to 40 pounds
Height: Up to 40 inches
Comments: Blanket rolls at sides and between legs provide positioning, support. Choose models with three recline positions (use middle position for forward-facing child with poor head control).

Columbia Positioning Seat

From: Columbia Medical
Cost: $599
Weight: 20–102 pounds
Height: Up to 60 inches
Comments: Top tether strap (free) should be used for children over 60 pounds.

Modified E-Z-On Vest

From: E-Z-On Products, Inc.
Cost: $70
Weight: Up to 100 pounds
Height: Determined by height and length of vehicle seat
Comments: Modified vest for child who must lie flat requires full-width bench seat.

Besi Restraining Harness

From: Besi Manufacturing
Cost: $65
Size: Waist 22–44 inches
Comments: Zipper inserts adjust sizes. School bus use only, with Cam Wrap. *(Note: another Besi product, Little People Restraint System, is not suitable.)*

Ortho-Kinetics Travel Chair

From: Ortho-Kinetics
Cost: Varies with options
Weight: 15–90 pounds
Height: 30–54 inches
Comments: Can be used in a bus with a Q-Straint or Kinedyne System tie-down system.

Carrie Car Seat

From: JA Preston
Cost: $932–$1,225
Weight: 20–130 pounds
Height: 30–68 inches
Comments: Be sure model is approved for use in a motor vehicle. Tether required.

Snug Seat I and II

From: Snug Seat, Inc.
Cost: Snug I: $750
            Snug II: $595
Weight: Snug I: 15–40 pounds
            Snug II: 20–70 pounds
Height: Snug I: Child's head not to extend above seat back
            Snug II: Up to 60 inches
Comments: Snug I: Heavy Duty Mobility Base is crash tested for vehicle use. Both seats for use facing forward only.

Gorilla

From:	Snug Seat, Inc.
Cost:	$495
Weight:	20–105 pounds
Height:	Child's head not to extend above seat back height
Comments:	Side pads and seat extension.

Mulholland

From:	Positioning Systems, Inc.
Cost:	$2,500–$3,000
Weight:	6–50 pounds
Height:	Customized for client
Comments:	Used as a car seat for only up to 50 pounds. Car seat passed van and bus crash testing but base has not passed.

Technology Dependent

Standard Safety Seats (with Harness Only)

From:	Retail outlets
Cost:	Varies by product
Comments:	Seats with shields not recommended, could interfere with equipment. Secure ancillary equipment in motor vehicle.

Bus Transport

Carrie Bus Seat

From:	JA Preston	
Cost:	Small: $348.87;	Large: $464.14
Weight:	20–100 pounds	60–100 pounds
Height:	30–58 inches	
Comments:	For use on the school bus seat. Lap belt and tether required.	

Cruiser Transport

From:	Convaid Products, Inc.
Cost:	$808–$1,066
Comments:	For children ages 1–5. Crash tested facing forward with Q-Straint with positive lock. Accessories available.

Sit'N'Stroll

From:	Safeline Products
Cost:	$149
Weight:	5–40 pounds
Height:	None stated
Comments:	Rear facing for infants up to 32 pounds, preferred position. Converts to stroller.

Kid EZB (Bus Transport Model 4JB)

From:	Kid-Care Mobility Products
Cost:	$1,300–$1,900
Weight:	Up to 35 pounds
Age:	Infant to age 7
Comments:	Tested with base in rear facing position for infant to 20 pounds and forward facing for toddlers. Recline shell for infant use. Tested with Q-Straint 4-point tie-down and with 3-point restraint in forward facing.

Kid-E-X (Kid Kart Model EX05)

From:	Kid-Care Mobility Products
Cost:	$1,400–$1,800
Weight:	50–90 pounds
Height:	35–60 inches
Comments:	Crash tested with Q-Straint with positive lock and three-point restraint system.

Manufacturers

Besi Manufacturing
9445 Sutton Place
Hamilton, OH 45011
(800) 543-8222

Columbia Medical
PO Box 633
Pacific Palisades, CA 90272
(310) 454-6612

Convaid Products, Inc.
PO Box 4209
Rancho Palos Verde, CA 90274
(800) 552-1020

Cosco
2525 State Street
Columbus, IN 47201
(800) 544-1108
(812) 372-0141

Evenflo Products
1801 Commerce Drive
Piqua, OH 45356
(800) 233-5921
(513) 773-3971

E-Z-On Products, Inc.
500 Commerce Way West, Suite 3
Jupiter, FL 33458
(407) 747-6920

Gunnell
8440 State Street
Millington, MI 48746
(800) 551-0055

JA Preston
4 Sammons Court
Bolingbrook, IL 60440
(800) 631-7277

Kid-Care Mobility Products
732 Cruiser Lane
Belgrade, MT 59714
(800) 388-5278

Little Cargo, Inc.
100 North Broadway, Suite 2000
St. Louis, MO 63102
(800) 933-8580

Ortho-Kinetics
PO Box 1647
Waukesha, WI 53187
(800) 824-1068

Positioning Systems, Inc.
215 North 12th Street
PO Box 391
Santa Paula, CA 93060
(805) 525-7165

Safeline Products
Writters Center One
1777 South Belaire, Suite 3330
Denver, CO 80222
(800) 829-1625

Snug Seat, Inc.
PO Box 1739
Matthews, NC 28106
(800) 336-SNUG

This material was originally published in January 1995. It was updated in March 1996 for this publication. Please contact *Safe Ride News*/American Academy of Pediatrics for further updates (847) 228-5005. American Academy of Pediatrics. 1995. *Safe Ride News*. Reprinted by permission.

Appendix D
Parent Resources

Denise Merrill

❝"Hallo!" said Tigger. "I've found somebody just like me. I thought I was the only one of them."❞

Resources abound for families of sick and preterm babies. The trick is finding the help that is right for you. Here, many organizations are listed that you may investigate as potential sources of information and support. Often, one organization will lead you to others that you will also find valuable. We've also included suggestions for further reading, and mail-order sources of special supplies.

Information and Support Organizations

Apnea

National Association of Apnea Professionals (NAAP)
PO Box 4031
Waianae, HI 96792
(800) 392-2514

Asthma and Lung Disorders

Allergy and Asthma Network/ Mothers of Asthmatics, Inc.
3554 Chain Bridge Road, Suite 200
Fairfax, VA 22030
(703) 385-4403

American Lung Association
1740 Broadway
New York, NY 10019-4374
(212) 315-8700

Lung Line
1400 Jackson Street
Denver, CO 80206
(800) 222-LUNG [222-5864]
(303) 355-LUNG [355-5864]

Birth Defects

Arizona Poison and Drug Information Center
1501 North Campbell Avenue
Room 1156
Tucson, AZ 85724
(800) 362-0101
(602) 626-6016

Association of Birth Defect Children
827 Irma Avenue
Orlando, FL 32803
(800) 313-2232—Information line only
(407) 245-7035

California Teratogen Registry
University of California Medical Center at San Diego
225 West Dickinson Street
Room H8124B
San Diego, CA 92103-1990
(800) 532-3749
(619) 294-6084

DES Action USA
1615 Broadway, Suite 510
Oakland, CA 94612
(510) 465-4011

Iowa Teratogen Information Services
Department of Pediatrics
Division of Medical Genetics
University of Iowa
200 Hawkins Drive
Iowa City, IA 52242
(319) 356-2674

Magee Women's Hospital
Department of Reproductive Genetics
300 Halket Street
Pittsburgh, PA 15213
(412) 641-1000

393

March of Dimes Birth Defects Foundation
1275 Mamaroneck Avenue
White Plains, NY 10605
(914) 428-7100

National Clearinghouse for Alcohol and Drug Information
11426 Rockville Pike
Rockville, MD 20852
(800) 729-6686—Direct to office services
(800) 662-4357—24-hour recorded line
(301) 468-2600

National Institute of Environmental Health Services
Public Affairs Office
Research Triangle Park, NC 27709
(919) 541-3345

Pregnancy Healthline of Pennsylvania Hospital
907 Pine Street
Philadelphia, PA 19107
(215) 829-5437

Teratology Hotline of Children's Hospital of Wisconsin
Birth Defects Center
PO Box 1997
Milwaukee, WI 53201
(414) 266-2000—University of Wisconsin main number

Blood Disorders

American Society of Pediatric Hematology
Wyler Children's Hospital
5841 South Maryland Avenue
MC4060
Chicago, IL 60637
(312) 702-6808

Canadian Hemophilia Society
62 St. Clair Avenue East, Suite 308
Toronto, ON M4T 1N5
Canada
(416) 972-0641

Children's Blood Foundation
333 East 38th Street
New York, NY 10016
(212) 297-4336

Cooley's Anemia Foundation, Inc.
(Thalassemia)
129-09 26th Avenue, Suite 203
Flushing, NY 11354-1131
(800) 522-7222—In New York only
(718) 321-2873

Hemochromatosis Research Foundation, Inc.
PO Box 8569
Albany, NY 12208
(518) 489-0972

Hereditary Hemorrhagic Telangiectasia Foundation, Inc. (HHT Foundation International, Inc.)
PO Box 8087
New Haven, CT 06530
(800) HHT-NETW [448-6389]
(313) 561-2537

Histiocytosis–X Association of America
302 North Broadway
Pitman, NJ 08071
(800) 548-2758

Iron Overload Diseases Association, Inc.
433 Westwind Drive
Palm Beach, FL 33408
(407) 840-8512

National Association for Sickle Cell Disease, Inc.
200 Corporate Pointe, Suite 495
Culver City, CA 90230-7633
(800) 421-8453
(213) 936-7205

National Hemophilia Foundation
The Soho Building
110 Greene Street, Suite 303
New York, NY 10012
(212) 219-8180

Sickle Cell Disease Branch
6701 Rockledge Drive, MSC 7950
Bethesda, MD 20892-7950
(301) 435-0055

Thrombocytopenia Absent Radius Syndrome Association (TARSA)
212 Sherwood Drive
Egharbor Township, NJ 08234
(609) 927-0418

Bone Disorders

American Academy of Orthopedic Surgeons
6300 North River Road
Rosemont, IL 60018-4262
(800) 346-AAOS [346-2267]
(708) 823-7186

Conservative Orthopedics International Association
1811 Monroe
Dearborn, MI 48124
(313) 563-0360—Phone and FAX

Freeman-Sheldon Syndrome Parent Support Group
509 East Northmont Way
Salt Lake City, UT 84103
(801) 364-7060

National Support Group for Arthrogryposis Multiplex Congenita
PO Box 5192
Sonora, CA 95370
(209) 928-3688

Pediatric Orthopedic Society of North America
6300 North River Road, Suite 727
Rosemont, IL 60018-4226
(708) 698-1692

Breastfeeding. See Nutrition

Cancer

AMC Cancer Information and Counseling Line
(800) 525-3777

American Brain Tumor Association
2720 River Road, Suite 146
Des Plaines, IL 60018
(708) 827-9910

American Cancer Society
1599 Clifton Road NE
Atlanta, GA 30329
(404) 320-3333

Canadian Cancer Society
10 Alcorn Avenue
Toronto, ON M4V 3B1
Canada
(416) 961-7223

Leukemia Society of America, Inc.
600 Third Avenue
New York, NY 10016
(212) 573-8484

National Brain Tumor Foundation
785 Market Street, Suite 1600
San Francisco, CA 94103
(415) 284-0208

National Cancer Care Foundation
1180 Avenue of the Americas
New York, NY 10036
(212) 221-3300

National Cancer Institute
Office of Cancer Communications
31 Center Drive, MSC 2580
Building 31, Room 10A07
Bethesda, MD 20892-2580
(800) 4-CANCER [422-6237]—Cancer information service
(301) 496-5583

National Foundation for Cancer Research
7315 Wisconsin Avenue, Suite 500W
Bethesda, MD 20814
(800) 321-CURE [321-2873]

Parents of Kids with Cancer/ Parents' Advocacy for Kids with Cancer
81 Eastside Circle
Petaluma, CA 94954
(707) 763-7967

Cardiovascular Disease

American College of Cardiology
9111 Old Georgetown Road
Bethesda, MD 20814-1699
(301) 897-5400

American Heart Association
7272 Greenville Avenue
Dallas, TX 75231-4596
(214) 706-1179—Public information line

Council on Cardiovascular Disease in the Young
American Heart Association National Center
7272 Greenville Avenue
Dallas, TX 75231
(214) 373-6300

ECMO Moms and Dads
(International Parent Support)
c/o Blair and Gayle Willson
PO Box 53848
Lubbock, TX 79453
(806) 794-0259

The Mended Hearts, Inc.
7320 Greenville Avenue
Dallas, TX 75231
(214) 706-1179—Public information line

National Heart, Lung, Blood Information Center
PO Box 30105
Bethesda, MD 20824-0105
(301) 251-1222

Cesarean Birth

Cesareans/Support Education and Concern (C/SEC)
22 Forest Road
Framingham, MA 01701
(508) 877-8266

Childbirth. See High Risk Pregnancy and Birth; Pregnancy and Childbirth

Chromosomal Abnormalities

5p Minus Society
(Cri-Du-Chat Syndrome)
11609 Oakmont
Overland Park, KS 66210
(913) 469-8900
(913) 469-5246—FAX

Association for Children with Down Syndrome, Inc.
2616 Martin Avenue
Bellmore, NY 11710
(516) 221-4700

National Association for Down Syndrome
(Chicago Metropolitan Area Only)
PO Box 4542
Oak Brook, IL 60522
(708) 325-9112

National Down Syndrome Congress
1605 Chantilly Drive, Suite 250
Atlanta, GA 30324
(800) 232-NDSC [232-6372]
(404) 633-1555

National Down Syndrome Society
666 Broadway
New York, NY 10012
(800) 221-4602
(212) 460-9330

National Fragile X Foundation
1441 York Street, Suite 303
Denver, CO 80206
(800) 688-8765
(303) 333-6155

Parents of Down Syndrome Children
c/o Montgomery County Association
for Retarded Citizens
11600 Nebel Street
Rockville, MD 20852
(301) 984-5792

Support Group for Monosomy 9P
43304 Kipton Nickle Plate Road
La Grange, OH 44050
(216) 775-4255

Support Organization for Trisomy 18, 13, and Related Disorders
5030 Cole
Pocatello, ID 83202
(208) 237-8782

Turner's Syndrome Society
7777 Keele Street, Second Floor
Concord, ON L4K IY7
Canada
(800) 465-6744
(905) 660-7766
(905) 660-7450—FAX

Craniofacial Disorders

AboutFace—The Craniofacial Family Society
99 Crowns Lane, Fourth Floor
Toronto, ON M5R 3P4
Canada
(800) 665-3223
(416) 944-3223

American Cleft Palate–Craniofacial Association
1218 Grandview Avenue
Pittsburgh, PA 15211
(800) 24-CLEFT [242-5338]
(800) 23-CLEFT [232-5338]—In
Pennsylvania only
(412) 481-1376

Cleft Palate Parents' Council
28 Cambria Road
Syosset, NY 11791
(516) 931-4252

Let's Face It
PO Box 29972
Bellingham, WA 98228-1972
(360) 676-7325

National Association for the Craniofacially Handicapped
PO Box 11082
Chattanooga, TN 37401
(615) 266-1632

National Foundation for Facial Reconstruction
317 East 34th Street, #901
New York, NY 10016
(212) 263-6656

Prescription Parents, Inc.
66 Vine Street
Newton, MA 02167
(617) 527-0878

Digestive Disorders

Celiac Sprue Association/United States of America, Inc.
PO Box 31700
Omaha, NE 68131-0700
(402) 558-0600

Digestive Disease National Coalition (DDNC)
711 Second Street NE, Suite 200
Washington, DC 20002
(202) 544-7497

Gluten Intolerance Group of North America
PO Box 23053
Seattle, WA 98102-0353
(206) 325-6980

National Digestive Diseases Information Clearinghouse
2 Information Way
Bethesda, MD 20892-3570
(301) 654-3810

National Foundation for Ileitis and Colitis, Inc.
386 Park Avenue South, 17th Floor
New York, NY 10016
(800) 932-2423
(212) 685-3440

Disabilities

Federation for Children with Special Needs
95 Berkeley Street, Suite 104
Boston, MA 02116
(617) 482-2915

National Information Center for Children and Youth with Disabilities
PO Box 1492
Washington, DC 20013-1492
(800) 695-0285

National Lekotek Center
(Provides information regarding play for children with disabilities)
2100 Ridge Avenue
Evanston, IL 60201
(708) 328-0001
(800) 366-7529

National Parent Network on Disabilities
1600 Prince Street, Suite 115
Alexandria, VA 22314
(703) 684-6763

Fetal Alcohol Syndrome

Fetal Alcohol Syndrome Network
158 Rosemont Avenue
Coatesville, PA 19320-3727
(610) 384-1133

Formula. See Nutrition

Hearing Impairments

Alexander Graham Bell Association for the Deaf
3417 Volta Place NW
Washington, DC 20007-2778
(202) 337-5220—TDD same number

American Society for Deaf Children
814 Thayer Street
Silver Spring, MD 20910
(301) 588-6545

Department of Speech and Hearing
St. Christopher's Hospital for Children
Erie Avenue at Front Street
Philadelphia, PA 19134
(215) 427-5469
(215) 427-5305—TDD

Hear Center
301 East Del Mar Boulevard
Pasadena, CA 91101
(213) 681-4641

National Association of the Deaf (NAD)
814 Thayer Avenue
Silver Spring, MD 20910
(301) 587-1788

National Information Center on Deafness
Gallaudet University
800 Florida Avenue NE
Washington, DC 20002-3695
(202) 651-5051
(202) 651-5052—TDD

Heart Diseases. See Cardiovascular Disease

High Risk Pregnancy and Birth

Center for Study of Multiple Births
333 East Superior Street, Room 464
Chicago, IL 60611
(312) 266-9093

National Perinatal Association (NPA), Inc.
3500 East Fletcher Avenue, Suite 209
Tampa, FL 33613
(813) 971-1008

National Perinatal Information Center (NPIC)
1 State Street, Suite 102
Providence, RI 02908
(401) 274-0650

Parent Care, Inc.
(Makes referrals to local support groups whenever possible.)
9041 Colgate Street
Indianapolis, IN 46268-1210
(317) 872-9913
(317) 872-0795—FAX

Partners in Intensive Care
PO Box 41043
Bethesda, MD 20824-1043
(301) 681-2708

Sidelines
Candace Hurley, Director
PO Box 1808
Laguna Beach, CA 92652
(714) 497-2265
(714) 497-5722—FAX

Immunologic Disorders

American Association of Immunologists
9650 Rockville Pike
Bethesda, MD 20814-3994
(301) 530-7178

Athletes and Entertainers for Kids
381 Van Ness Avenue
Torrance, CA 90501
(800) 933-KIDS [933-5437]
(310) 783-0575
(310) 783-0585—FAX

Dissatisfied Parents Together
512 West Maple Avenue, #206
Vienna, VA 22180
(703) 938-3783

National Pediatric HIV Resource Center
15 South Ninth Street
Newark, NJ 07107
(201) 268-8251

Pediatric AIDS Foundation
1311 Colorado Avenue
Santa Monica, CA 90404
(310) 395-9051—California
(202) 434-1170—Washington, DC

Joint Disorders

American Juvenile Arthritis Organization/Arthritis Foundation
1314 Spring Street NW
Atlanta, GA 30309
(404) 872-7100

National Arthritis and Musculoskeletal and Skin Diseases
NAMSIC
1 AMS Circle
Bethesda, MD 20892-3675
(301) 495-4484

Kidney Disorders

American Association of Kidney Patients
100 South Ashley Drive, Suite 280
Tampa, FL 33602
(813) 223-7099

National Institute of Diabetes and Digestive and Kidney Diseases
National Institute of Health
31 Center Drive
Building 31, Room 9A04
Bethesda, MD 20892
(301) 496-3583

National Kidney and Urological Diseases Information Clearinghouse
3 Information Way
Bethesda, MD 20892-3580
(301) 654-4415

National Kidney Foundation
30 East 33rd Street
New York, NY 10016
(800) 622-9010
(212) 889-2210

Polycystic Kidney Research Foundation
4901 Main Street, Suite 320
Kansas City, MO 64112
(816) 931-2600

Learning Disabilities

Children with Attention Deficit Disorder
499 Northwest 70th Avenue
Suite 101
Plantation, FL 33317
(305) 587-3700

Council for Learning Disabilities (CLD)
PO Box 40303
Overland Park, KS 66204
(913) 492-8755

Learning Disabilities Association of America (LDA)
4156 Library Road
Pittsburgh, PA 15234
(412) 341-8077

Learning Disabilities Network
72 Sharp Street, Suite A-2
Hingham, MA 02043
(617) 340-5605

National Attention Deficit Disorders Association
2620 Ivy Place
Toledo, OH 43613
(800) 487-2282

National Center for Learning Disabilities (NCLD)
381 Park Avenue South, Suite 1420
New York, NY 10016
(212) 545-7510

Orton Dyslexia Society
8600 LaSalle Road
Chester House, Suite 382
Baltimore, MD 21286
(410) 296-0232

Legal Issues

American Bar Association Center on Children and the Law
1800 M Street NW, Suite 300
Washington, DC 20036
(202) 662-1720

Brazelton Center for Mental Health Law
1101 15th Street NW, Suite 1212
Washington, DC 20005
(202) 467-5730

Disability Rights Education and Defense Fund
2212 Sixth Street
Berkeley, CA 94710
(510) 644-2555

National Center for Law and the Deaf
Gallaudet University
800 Florida Avenue NE
Washington, DC 20002
(202) 651-5373—Voice and TDD

Liver Disorders

American Liver Foundation
1425 Pompton Avenue
Cedar Grove, NY 07009-1000
(800) 223-0179
(201) 857-2626

Loss of a Child

Aiding Mothers and Fathers Experiencing Neonatal Death (AMEND)
4324 Berrywick Terrace
St. Louis, MO 63128
(314) 487-7582

Compassionate Friends
PO Box 3696
Oak Brook, IL 60522
(708) 990-0010

Good Grief
North 3919 Maple Street
Spokane, WA 99205
(509) 624-3182

Good Grief Program
Judge Baker Children's Center
295 Longwood Avenue
Boston, MA 02115
(617) 232-2111

Grief Recovery Institute
8306 Wilshire Boulevard, Suite 21A
Beverly Hills, CA 90211
(800) 445-4808—Help line
(213) 650-1234

Help House—Women's Resource Center
190 Blydenburg Road
Islandia, NY 11722
(516) 342-9401

Helping Other Parents in Normal Grieving (HOPING)
Edward W. Sparrow Hospital
1215 East Michigan Avenue
Lansing, MI 48909-7980
(517) 483-3873

Partners in Intensive Care
PO Box 41043
Bethesda, MD 20824-1043
(301) 681-2708

Pen-Parents
PO Box 8738
Reno, NV 89507
(702) 826-7332—Phone and FAX

Pregnancy and Infant Loss Center
1421 East Wayzata Boulevard, #30
Wayzata, MN 55391
(612) 473-9372

RTS Bereavement Services
1910 South Avenue
La Crosse, WI 54601
(608) 791-4747

Unite, Inc.
c/o Jeanes Hospital
7600 Central Avenue
Philadelphia, PA 19111
(215) 728-2082

Lung Disorders. See Asthma and Lung Disorders

Metabolic Disorders

American Diabetes Association, Inc.
1660 Duke Street
Alexandria, VA 22314
(800) 232-3472
(703) 549-1500

Association for Glycogen Storage Diseases
Box 896
Durant, IA 52747
(319) 785-6038

Cystic Fibrosis Foundation
6931 Arlington Road
Bethesda, MD 20814
(800) 344-4823
(301) 951-4422

Cystinosis Foundation
1212 Broadway, Suite 830
Oakland, CA 94612
(510) 834-7897

Dysautonomia Foundation, Inc.
20 East 46th Street, Room 302
New York, NY 10017
(212) 949-6644

Inherited Metabolic Disease (IMD) Clinic
Children's Hospital
1056 East 19th Avenue
Box 153
Denver, CO 80218
(303) 861-6847

Joslin Diabetes Center
1 Joslin Place
Boston, MA 02215
(617) 732-2400

Juvenile Diabetes Foundation International
120 Wall Street, 19th Floor
New York, NY 10005
(800) 223-1138
(212) 889-7575

Lowe's Syndrome Association
222 Lincoln Street
West Lafayette, IN 47906
(317) 743-3634

National Diabetes Information Clearinghouse
1 Information Way
Bethesda, MD 20892-3560
(301) 496-3583

National Institute of Diabetes and Digestive and Kidney Diseases
31 Center Drive
Building 31, Room 9A04
Bethesda, MD 20892
(301) 496-3583

National Mucopolysaccharidosis (MPS) Society
17 Kraemer Street
Hicksville, NY 11801
(516) 931-6338

National Organization for Albinism and Hypopigmentation (NOAH)
1530 Locust Street, #29
Philadelphia, PA 19102
(800) 473-2310
(215) 545-2322

National Tay-Sachs and Allied Diseases Association
2001 Beacon Street
Brookline, MA 02146
(617) 277-4463

Organic Acidemia Association
2287 Cypress Avenue
San Pablo, CA 94806
(510) 724-0297

United Leukodystrophy Foundation
2304 Highland Drive
Sycamore, IL 60178
(815) 895-3211

Williams Syndrome Association
PO Box 297
Clawson, MI 48017
(810) 541-3630

Wilson's Disease Association
PO Box 75324
Washington, DC 20013
(800) 399-0266
(703) 743-1415

Neurologic Disorders

American Academy for Cerebral Palsy and Developmental Medicine (AACPDM)
6300 North River Road, Suite 727
Rosemont, IL 60018-4226
(708) 698-1635

Angelman Syndrome Foundation
PO Box 12437
Gainesville, FL 32604
(904) 332-3303

Children's Brain Diseases Foundation
350 Parnassus Avenue, Suite 900
San Francisco, CA 94117
(415) 565-6259

Epilepsy Foundation of America
4351 Garden City Drive
Landover, MD 20785
(800) 332-1000
(301) 459-3700

Guardians of Hydrocephalus Research Foundation
2618 Avenue Z
Brooklyn, NY 11235
(718) 743-4473
(718) 934-4090

Hydrocephalus Association
870 Market Street, Suite 955
San Francisco, CA 94102
(415) 776-4713

International Joseph Diseases Foundation, Inc.
PO Box 2550
Livermore, CA 94551-2550
(510) 371-1287
(510) 371-1288—FAX

Intraventricular Hemorrhage
(IVH Parents)
PO Box 56-1111
Miami, FL 33256-1111
(305) 232-0381

National Ataxia Foundation
750 Twelve Oaks Center
15500 Wayzata Boulevard
Wayzata, MN 55391
(612) 473-7666

National Hydrocephalus Foundation
1670 Green Oak Circle
Lawrenceville, GA 30243
(815) 467-6548
(800) 431-8093—General information

National Neurofibromatosis Foundation, Inc.
95 Pine Street, 16th Floor
New York, NY 10005
(800) 323-7938
(212) 344-6633

National Reye's Syndrome Foundation
PO Box 829
Bryan, OH 43506
(419) 636-2679
(800) 233-7393—24-hour hotline

National Spasmodic Torticollis Association
PO Box 873
Royal Oak, MI 48068-0873
(800) 487-8385

National Tuberous Sclerosis Association
8181 Professional Place, Suite 110
Landover, MD 20785
(800) 942-6825
(301) 459-9888
(301) 577-0016—FAX

Neurofibromatosis, Inc.
8855 Annapolis Road, Suite 110
Lanham, MD 20706
(800) 942-6825
(301) 577-8984
(301) 577-0016—FAX

Ontario Cerebral Palsy Association (OCPA)
40 Dundas Street West, Suite 222
Toronto, ON M5G 2C2
Canada
(416) 426-7190

Reflex Sympathetic Dystrophy Syndrome
116 Haddon Avenue, Suite D
Haddonfield, NJ 08033
(609) 795-8845

Rett's Syndrome Association
9121 Piscataway Road, Suite 2B
Clinton, MD 20735
(301) 856-3334

Spina Bifida Association of America
4590 MacArthur Boulevard NW
Suite 250
Washington, DC 20007-4226
(800) 621-3141

Spina Bifida Association of Canada
388 Donald Street, Suite 220
Winnipeg, MB R3B 2J4
Canada
(204) 957-1784

Sturge-Weber Foundation
PO Box 418
Mount Freedom, NJ 07970
(800) 627-5482

Threshold: Intractable Seizure Disorder Support Group
26 Stavola Road
Middletown, NJ 07748
(908) 957-0714

United Cerebral Palsy
1660 L Street NW, Suite 700
Washington, DC 20036
(202) 842-1266

Neuromuscular Disorders

Amyotrophic Lateral Sclerosis Association
21021 Ventura Boulevard, Suite 321
Woodland Hills, CA 91364
(800) 340-2060
(818) 340-7500

Benign Essential Blepharospasm Research Foundation, Inc.
PO Box 12468
Beaumont, TX 77726-2468
(409) 832-0788

Charcot-Marie Tooth Association
c/o Crozer Mills Enterprise Center
601 Upland Avenue
Upland, PA 19015
(610) 499-7486

Charcot-Marie Tooth Disease International
1 Springbank Drive
St. Catharines, ON L2S 2K1
Canada
(905) 687-3630

Families of Spinal Muscular Atrophy
PO Box 196
Libertyville, IL 60048
(800) 886-1762
(708) 367-7620
(708) 367-7623—FAX

Muscular Dystrophy Association
1111 Sheet Road
South Hampton, PA 18966
(215) 322-7120

Myasthenia Gravis Foundation
222 South Riverside Plaza
Suite 1540
Chicago, IL 60606
(800) 541-5454

Nursing

American Academy of Nurse Practitioners
Capitol Station, LBJ Building
PO Box 12846
Austin, TX 78711
(512) 442-4262

The Association of Women's Health, Obstetric, and Neonatal Nurses (AWHONN)
700 14th Street NW, Suite 600
Washington, DC 20005-2019
(202) 662-1600

National Association of Neonatal Nurses
1304 Southpoint Boulevard, Suite 280
Petaluma, CA 94954-6861
(800) 451-3795

National Association of Pediatric Nurse Associates and Practitioners
1101 Kings Highway North, Suite 206
Cherry Hill, NJ 08034-1912
(609) 667-1773

Nutrition: Breastfeeding and Formula

Ameda-Egnell
(breastfeeding support, education, equipment rental information)
755 Industrial Drive
Cary, IL 60013
(800) 323-8750

Formula, Inc.
1815 North Hartford Street
Arlington, VA 22201
(703) 527-7171

Human Lactation Center
666 Sturges Highway
Westport, CT 06880
(203) 259-5995

Infant Formula Council
5775 Peachtree-Dunwoody Road
Suite 500-G
Atlanta, GA 30342
(404) 252-3663

Lact-Aid International
PO Box 1066
Athens, TN 37371
(615) 744-9090

La Leche League International
9616 Minneapolis Avenue
PO Box 1209
Franklin Park, IL 60131-8209
(800) 525-3243
(708) 519-7730

Medela, Inc.
(breastfeeding support, education, equipment rental information)
4610 Prime Parkway
McHenry, IL 60050
(800) TELL-YOU [835-5968]

Wellstart, San Diego Lactation Program
4062 First Avenue
San Diego, CA 92103
(619) 295-5193

Parenting

Active Parenting, Inc.
810 Franklin Court, Suite B
Marietta, GA 30067
(800) 826-0060
(404) 429-0565

American Academy of Pediatrics
PO Box 927
Elk Grove Village, IL 60009-0927
(847) 228-5005

Association for the Care of Children's Health (ACCH)
7910 Woodmont Avenue, Suite 300
Bethesda, MD 20814
(301) 654-6549
(301) 986-4553—FAX

Fatherhood Project
Families at Work Institute
330 Seventh Avenue
New York, NY 10001
(212) 465-2044

Gay and Lesbian Advocates and Defenders (GLAD)
PO Box 218
Boston, MA 02112
(617) 426-1350

Grandparents—Grandchildren
3851 Centraloma Drive
San Diego, CA 92107
(619) 223-0344

National Fathers' Network
The Merrywood School
16120 Northeast Eighth Street
Bellevue, WA 98008
(206) 747-4004

National Foster Parent Association
Information and Services Office
9 Dartmoor Drive
Crystal Lake, IL 60014
(815) 455-2527

Parental Stress Services
600 South Federal, Suite 205
Chicago, IL 60605
(312) 427-1161

Parents without Partners
401 North Michigan Avenue
Chicago, IL 60611-4267
(800) 637-7974—International PWP

Single Mothers by Choice
PO Box 1642
Gracie Square Station
New York, NY 10028
(212) 988-0993

Single Parent Resource Center
31 East 28th Street, Second Floor
New York, NY 10016
(212) 951-7030
(212) 951-7037—FAX

Women on Their Own
PO Box 1026
Willingboro, NJ 08046
(609) 871-1499

Pregnancy and Childbirth

American College of Nurse-Midwives
818 Connecticut Avenue NW
Suite 900
Washington, DC 20006
(202) 728-9860

American College of Obstetricians and Gynecologists
409 12th Street SW
Washington, DC 20024
(202) 863-2518

American College of Obstetricians and Gynecologists Publications
ACOG Distribution
PO Box 4500
Kearneysville, WV 25430-4500
(800) 762-2264

American Society for Psychoprophylaxis in Obstetrics
(ASPO/Lamaze)
1200 19th Street NW, Suite 300
Washington, DC 20036
(800) 368-4404
(202) 857-1128

Childbirth Education Association, Inc.
PO Box 1609
Springfield, VA 22151
(703) 941-7183

Childbirth Education Foundation
PO Box 5
Richboro, PA 18954
(215) 357-2792

Couple to Couple League, International
PO Box 111184
Cincinnati, OH 45211
(513) 471-2000

Healthy Mothers, Healthy Babies Coalition
409 12th Street SW
Washington, DC 20024-2188
(202) 863-2458

Maternity Center Association
48 East 92nd Street
New York, NY 10128
(212) 369-7300

Mothers' Center Development Project
336 Fulton Avenue
Hempstead, NY 11550
(800) 645-3828
(516) 486-6614

National Women's Health Network
514 Tenth Street NW, Suite 400
Washington, DC 20004
(202) 347-1140

The Pregnancy Healthline
455 St. Antoine Street West
Room 601
Montreal, QU A2Z 1G1
Canada
(514) 876-4564

Rare Disorders

Information Services Vancouver
(Provides listing of community services in Vancouver)
3102 Main Street, Suite 202
Vancouver, BC V5T 3G7
Canada
(604) 875-6381

Lethbridge Society for Rare Disorders (LSRD)
Box 35
Lethbridge, AB T1J 3Y3
Canada
(403) 329-0665

National Information Center for Children and Youth with Disabilities
PO Box 1492
Washington, DC 20013-1492
(202) 884-8200

Rehabilitation

National Rehabilitation Information Center
8455 Colesville Road, Suite 935
Silver Spring, MD 20910
(800) 346-2742
(301) 588-9284

World Rehabilitation Fund
Room 500
386 Park Avenue South,
New York, NY 10016-4901
(212) 725-7875

Siblings

Sibling Support Project
Children's Hospital and Medical Center
4800 Sand Point Way NE
Seattle, WA 98105
(206) 368-4911

Skin Disorders

Dystrophic Epidermolysis Bullosa Research Association of America, Inc.
40 Rector Street, Eighth Floor
New York, NY 10006
(212) 693-6610

Foundation for Ichthyosis and Related Skin Types
PO Box 20921
Raleigh, NC 27619
(919) 782-5728

Scleroderma Federation
Peabody Building
1 Newberry Street
Peabody, MA 01960
(508) 535-6600

Sudden Infant Death Syndrome

Association of SIDS Program Professionals
Massachusetts Center for SIDS
Boston City Hospital
818 Harrison Avenue
Boston, MA 02118
(617) 534-7437

Back to Sleep
(Provides information about SIDS and sleep position)
PO Box 29111
Washington, DC 20040
(800) 505-CRIB [505-2742]

Canadian Foundation for the Study of Infant Deaths
586 Eglinton Avenue East, Suite 308
Toronto, ON M4P 1P2
Canada
(416) 488-3260

Colorado SIDS Program, Inc.
6825 East Tennessee Avenue
Denver, CO 80224-1628
(800) 332-1018—In Colorado only
(303) 320-7771

Guild for Infant Survival
PO Box 17432
Irving, CA 92713-7432
(800) 247-4370

Minnesota Sudden Infant Death Center
Children's Health Center
2525 Chicago Avenue South
Minneapolis, MN 55404
(612) 813-6285

National Center for the Prevention of Sudden Infant Death Syndrome
1314 Bedford Avenue, Suite 210
Baltimore, MD 21208
(800) 221-7437
(410) 653-8709

Travel and Car Seat Information

AAP 1995 Family Shopping Guide to Car Seats
Send SASE to American Academy of Pediatrics
Department C (Shopping Guide)
PO Box 927
Elk Grove Village, IL 60009-0927
(847) 228-5005

Dana Foundation
PO Box 1050
Germantown, MD 20875
(301) 540-7295

Mobility International
PO Box 10767
Eugene, OR 97440
(503) 343-1284—Voice and TDD

Riley Hospital for Children
Automotive Safety for Children Program
702 Barnhill Drive, Room 1603
Indianapolis, IN 46202
(317) 274-2977

Safe Ride News Publications
726 Belmont Place East
Seattle, WA 98102

SafetyBeltSafe USA
123 West Manchester Blvd.
Englewood, CA 90301
1-800-745-SAFE
(for Spanish language service, call 1-800-747-SANO)

Safety Restraint Coalition
PO Box 70277
Bellevue, WA 98007
(206) 828-8975

Travelin' Talk Network
PO Box 3534
Clarksville, TN 37043-3534
(615) 552-6670

Twins and Multiples

MOST (Mothers of Super Twins)
PO Box 951
Brentwood, NY 11717-0627
(516) 434-MOST [434-6678]

National Organization of Mothers of Twins Clubs, Inc.
12404 Princess Jeanne NE
Albuquerque, NM 87112-4640
(505) 275-0955

Triplet Connection
PO Box 99571
Stockton, CA 95209
(209) 474-3073

Twin Services
PO Box 10066
Berkeley, CA 94709
(510) 524-0863

Vaccination

National Vaccine Information Center
512 West Maple Drive, #206
Vienna, VA 22180
(703) 938-3783

Visual Impairments

American Council of the Blind (ACB)
1155 15th Street NW, Suite 720
Washington, DC 20005
(800) 424-8666
(202) 467-5081

American Foundation for the Blind
11 Penn Plaza, Suite 300
New York, NY 10001
(800) 232-5463
(212) 502-7600

Association for Macular Diseases
210 East 64th Street
New York, NY 10021
(212) 605-3719

Blind Children's Center
4120 Marathon Street
Los Angeles, CA 90029
(800) 222-3566
(800) 222-3567—In California only

Braille Institute
741 North Vermont Avenue
Los Angeles, CA 90029
(213) 663-1111

Hadley School for the Blind
700 Elm Street
Winnetka, IL 60093
(708) 446-8111

Helen Keller National Center for Deaf-Blind Youths and Adults
111 Middle Neck Road
Sands Point, NY 11050
(516) 944-8900

National Association for Parents of the Visually Impaired
PO Box 317
Watertown, MA 02272
(800) 562-6265
(315) 245-3442

National Association for the Visually Handicapped
22 West 21st Street
New York, NY 10010
(212) 889-3141

Retinitis Pigmentosa International Society for Degenerative Eye Diseases
PO Box 900
Woodland Hills, CA 91365
(800) 344-4877
(818) 992-0500

RP Foundation Fighting Blindness
11350 McCormick Road
Executive Plaza 1, Suite 800
Hunt Valley, MD 21031-1014
(410) 785-1414

Vision Foundation, Inc.
818 Mount Auburn Street
Watertown, MA 02172
(800) 852-3029—In MA only
(617) 926-4232

Additional Resources

Books

Breastfeeding

Boston Association for Childbirth Education, Nursing Mother's Council Staff, Walker M, and Driscoll J. 1991. *Breastfeeding Your Baby.* Garden City Park, New York: Avery.

Gotsch G. 1990. *Breastfeeding Your Premature Baby* (booklet). Schaumburg, Illinois: La Leche League International.

Gotsch G. 1994. *Breastfeeding Pure and Simple.* Schaumburg, Illinois: La Leche League International.

Huggins K. 1995. *The Nursing Mother's Companion.* Boston: Harvard Common Press.

Jones C, and Lawrence R. 1993. *Breastfeeding Your Baby: A Guide for the Contemporary Family.* New York: Simon & Schuster.

Kitzinger S. 1989. *Breastfeeding Your Baby.* New York: Alfred A. Knopf.

Olds S, and Eiger M. 1986. *The Complete Book of Breastfeeding.* New York: Workman.

Price A, and Dana N. 1987. *Working Woman's Guide to Breastfeeding.* New York: Simon & Schuster.

Pryor K. 1991. *Nursing Your Baby.* New York: Pocket Books.

Torgus J. 1991. *The Womanly Art of Breastfeeding: 35th Anniversary Edition.* Schaumburg, Illinois: La Leche League International.

From Childbirth Graphics

PO Box 21207, Waco, TX 76702-1207,
(800) 299-3366, ext. 287

1994. *Nursing Your Baby with a Cleft Palate or Cleft Lip*
1990. *Nursing Your Baby with Down Syndrome*
1995. *Nursing Your Neurologically Impaired Baby*
1993. *Nursing Your Premature Baby*

Grief and Loss

Bernstein J. 1983. *Books to Help Children Cope with Separation and Loss: An Annotated Bibliography.* New York: Bowker.

Davis DL. 1990. *Empty Cradle, Broken Heart: Surviving the Death of Your Baby.* Golden, Colorado: Fulcrum.

Dodge N. 1985. *Thumpy's Story: A Story of Love and Grief Shared.* Springfield, Illinois: Prairie Lark Press. (For children.)

Fitzgerald H. 1992. *The Grieving Child: A Parent's Guide.* New York: Simon & Schuster (Fireside).

Friedman R. 1982. *Surviving Pregnancy Loss.* Boston: Little, Brown.

Jennings J. 1995. *Big George: The Autobiography of an Angel.* Carson, California: Hay House, Inc.

Kohn I, and Moffit P. 1993. *A Silent Sorrow: Pregnancy Loss Guidance and Support for You and Your Family.* New York: Delacorte Press.

Kushner HS. 1983. *When Bad Things Happen to Good People.* New York: Avon.

Lasker J, and Borg S. 1989. *When Pregnancy Fails: Families Coping with Miscarriage, Stillbirth, and Infant Death.* New York: Bantam.

Limbo RK, and Wheeler SR. 1986. *When a Baby Dies: A Handbook for Healing and Helping.* La Crosse, Wisconsin: RTS Bereavement Services.

Rogoff M. 1995. *Sylvie's Life.* Berkeley, California: Zenobia Press.

Viorst J. 1971. *The Tenth Good Thing about Barney.* New York: Atheneum. (For children.)

From the Centering Corporation

1531 North Saddle Creek Road, Omaha, NE 68104
(402) 553-1200

1990. *For Bereaved Grandparents*
1989. *Given in Love: For Mothers Releasing a Baby for Adoption*
1991. *Healing Together*
1990. *Making Loving Memories: A Gentle Guide to What You Can Do When Your Baby Dies*
1988. *No New Baby* (for children)
1992. *Not Just Another Day: Families, Grief, and Special Days*
1982. *Where's Jess?* (for children)

Growth and Development

Auckett A, and Field T. 1988. *Baby Massage: Parent-Child Bonding through Touch.* New York: Newmarket Press.

Brazelton TB. 1992. *Touchpoints: Your Child's Emotional and Behavioral Development.* Reading, Massachusetts: Addison-Wesley.

Heinl T. 1991. *Baby Massage: Shared Growth through the Hands.* Boston: Sigo Press.

Leach P. 1990. *Your Baby and Child From Birth to Age 5.* New York: Alfred A. Knopf.

Munger E, and Bowdon SJ. 1993. *The New Beyond Peek-a-Boo and Pat-a-Cake: Activities for Baby's First 24 Months.* Clinton, New Jersey: New Win

Oppenheim J, and Oppenheim S. 1995. *The Best Toys, Books, and Videos for Kids: The 1996 Guide to 1,000 Plus Kid-Tested Classic and New Products for Ages 0 to 10.* New York: HarperCollins.

Schneider V. 1989. *Infant Massage: A Handbook for Loving Parents.* New York: Bantam.

Trelease J. 1995. *The Read-Aloud Handbook,* 4th ed. New York: Penguin.

Walker M, and Lansdown R. 1994. *Your Child's Development from Birth through Adolescence: A Complete Guide for Parents.* New York: Random House.

Welch M. 1989. *Holding Time.* New York: Simon & Schuster.

White B. 1988. *Educating the Infant and Toddler.* New York: The Free Press.

Health Care and Children

American Heart Association. 1991. *If Your Child Has a Congenital Heart Defect.* Dallas, Texas: American Heart Association. (Call your local American Heart Association office to request this booklet.)

Bindler R, et al. 1996. *Your Child's Medicines: Advice for Families of Children with Special Needs.* Spokane, Washington: Intercollegiate Center for Nursing Education. (Call Vicki Christenson to request information about this booklet: (509) 326-7270.

Brill M. 1993. *Keys to Parenting a Child with Down Syndrome.* Hauppauge, New York: Barron's Educational Series.

Fancher VW. 1991. *Safe Kids: A Complete Child Safety Handbook and Resource Guide for Parents.* New York: John Wiley & Sons.

Featherstone H. 1981. *A Difference in the Family: Living with a Disabled Child.* New York: Basic Books.

Finston P. 1990. *Parenting Plus: Raising Children with Special Health Needs.* New York: Dutton.

Hanson MJ. 1987. *Teaching the Infant with Down Syndrome: A Guide for Parents and Professionals.* Austin, Texas: Pro-Ed.

Inlander C. 1992. *Take This Book to the Pediatrician with You.* Allentown, Pennsylvania: People's Medical Society.

Jones ML. 1985. *Home Care for the Chronically Ill or Disabled Child.* New York: Harper & Row.

Kumin L. 1994. *Communication Skills in Children with Down Syndrome: A Guide for Parents.* Rockville, Maryland: Woodbine House.

Luterman DM. 1991. *When Your Child is Deaf.* Parkton, Maryland: York Press.

Moynihan P. 1989. *Whole Parent, Whole Child: A Parents' Guide to Raising a Child with a Chronic Illness.* Minnetonka, Minnesota: Chronimed.

Neifert M. 1991. *Dr. Mom's Parenting Guide: Commonsense Guidance for the Life of Your Child.* New York: Dutton.

Register C. 1987. *Living with Chronic Illness: Days of Patience and Passion.* New York: Free Press/Macmillan.

Scully T, and Scully C. 1987. *Playing God: The New World of Medical Choices.* New York: Simon & Schuster.

Scully T, and Scully C. 1989. *Making Medical Decisions,* 2nd ed. New York: Simon & Schuster.

Sears W. 1995. *SIDS: A Parent's Guide to Understanding and Preventing Sudden Infant Death Syndrome.* Boston: Little, Brown.

Segal M. 1988. *In Time and with Love: Caring for the Special Needs Baby.* New York: Newmarket Press.

Seligman M, and Darling RB. 1989. *Ordinary Families, Special Children: A Systems Approach to Childhood Disability.* New York: Guilford Press.

Shelov SP, et al. 1991. *The American Academy of Pediatrics: Caring for Your Baby and Young Child—Birth to Age 5—The Complete and Authoritative Guide.* New York: Bantam.

Simons R. 1987. *After the Tears: Parents Talk about Raising a Child with a Disability.* Orlando: Harcourt Brace.

Stray-Gunderson K, ed. 1986. *Babies with Down Syndrome.* Bethesda: Woodbine House.

Thompson CE. 1991. *Raising a Handicapped Child.* New York: Ballantine.

Turnbull HR, et al. 1989. *Disability and the Family: A Guide to Decisions for Adulthood.* Baltimore: Paul H. Brookes Co.

Williams LH, Berman HS, and Rose L. 1987. *The Too Precious Child: The Perils of Being a Superparent and How to Avoid Them.* New York: Atheneum.

Parenting

Albi L, et al. 1993. *Mothering Twins: From Hearing the News to Beyond the Terrible Twos.* New York: Simon & Schuster.

Barnett N. 1990. *I Wish Someone Had Told Me: Comfort, Support, and Advice for New Moms from More than 60 Real-Life Mothers.* New York: Simon & Schuster.

Brazelton TB. 1989. *Families: Crisis and Caring.* Reading, Pennsylvania: Addison-Wesley.

Brazelton TB. 1992. *Working and Caring.* Reading, Pennsylvania: Addison-Wesley.

Bryan EM. 1992. *Twins, Triplets, and More: From Pre-Birth Through High School—What Every Parent Needs to Know When Raising Two or More.* New York: St. Martin's Press.

Greene DS. 1988. *79 Ways to Calm a Crying Baby.* New York: Simon & Schuster.

Gromada K. 1986. *Mothering Multiples.* Schaumburg, Illinois: La Leche League International.

Huntley R. 1991. *The Sleep Book for Tired Parents: A Practical Guide to Solving Children's Sleep Problems.* Seattle, Washington: Parenting Press.

Jones S. 1992. *Crying Baby, Sleepless Nights. Why Your Baby is Crying and What You Can Do About It.* Boston: Harvard Common Press.

Kitzinger S. 1989. *The Crying Baby.* New York: Viking Penguin.

Lazear J, and Lazear W. 1993. *Meditations for Parents Who Do Too Much.* (A Fireside Parkside Meditation Book accompanied by CD or cassette tape by composer Jim Oliver.) New York: Simon & Schuster.

Lewis D, and Lewis G. 1992. *Motherhood Stress.* Grand Rapids: Zondervan.

Lindsey JW. 1993. *Teen Dads: Rights, Responsibilities and Joys.* Buena Park, California: Morning Glory Press.

Martin A. 1993. *The Lesbian and Gay Parenting Handbook: Creating and Raising Our Families.* New York: HarperCollins.

Mayer A. 1992. *How to Stay Lovers While Raising Your Children.* New York: St. Martin's Press.

Newman S. 1990. *Parenting an Only Child: The Joys and Challenges of Raising Your One and Only.* New York: Doubleday.

Noble E. 1991. *Having Twins: A Parent's Guide to Pregnancy, Birth and Early Childhood.* Boston: Houghton Mifflin Co.

Price A, Neifert M, and Dana N. 1987. *Dr. Mom.* New York: Dutton.

Rolfe R. 1990. *You Can Postpone Anything but Love: Expanding Our Potential As Parents.* New York: Warner.

Salk L. 1992. *Familyhood: Nurturing the Values That Matter.* New York: Simon & Schuster.

Sammons W. 1989. *Self-Calmed Baby: A Liberating New Approach to Parenting Your Infant.* New York: Little, Brown & Co.

Sears W. 1986. *Becoming a Father.* Bristol, Pennsylvania: Taylor & Francis.

Sullivan SA. 1992. *Father's Almanac.* New York: Doubleday.

Thevenin T. 1993. *Mothering and Fathering: The Gender Differences in Child Rearing.* Garden City Park, New York: Avery.

Todd L. 1993. *You and Your Newborn Baby: A Guide to the First Months After Birth.* Boston: Harvard Common Press.

Weston DC, and Weston MS. 1993. *Playful Parenting: Turning the Dilemma of Discipline into Fun and Games.* Los Angeles: Jeremy P. Tarcher.

Pregnancy and Childbirth

Eisenberg A, Murkoff HE, and Hathaway SE. 1991. *What to Expect When You're Expecting.* New York: Workman.

Hales D. 1990. *Intensive Caring: New Hope for High Risk Pregnancy.* New York: Crown.

Heinowitz J. 1995. *Pregnant Fathers: Entering Parenthood Together.* San Diego, California: Parents As Partners Press.

Johnston S. 1990. *Pregnancy Bedrest: A Guide for the Pregnant Woman and Her Family.* New York: Henry Holt.

Katz M. 1988. *Preventing Preterm Birth: A Parent's Guide.* Burlingame, California: Psychological and Educational Publications.

Kitzinger S. 1989. *The Complete Book of Pregnancy and Childbirth.* New York: Alfred A. Knopf.

Rich L. 1993. *When Pregnancy Isn't Perfect: A Layperson's Guide to Complications in Pregnancy.* New York: Dutton.

Shapiro J. 1993. *When Men Are Pregnant: Needs and Concerns of Expectant Fathers.* San Luis Obispo, California: Impact Publishers.

Simkin P, Whalley J, and Keppler A. 1991. *Pregnancy, Childbirth, and the Newborn: The Complete Guide.* New York: Simon & Schuster.

Premature Babies

DiGeronimo T, and Manginello F. 1991. *Your Premature Baby: Everything You Need to Know about Childbirth, Treatment, and Parenting of Premature Infants.* New York: John Wiley & Sons.

Flushman B, et al. 1991. *My Special Start: A Guide for Parents in the Neonatal Intensive Care Unit.* Palo Alto, California: VORT Corporation.

Harrison H. 1983. *The Premature Baby Book: A Parent's Guide to Coping and Caring in the First Years.* New York: St. Martin's Press.

Hynan MT. 1987. *The Pain of Premature Parents: A Psychological Guide for Coping.* Lanham, Massachusetts: University Press of America.

Ludington-Hoe SM, and Golant SK. 1993. *Kangaroo Care: The Best You Can Do to Help Your Preterm Infant.* New York: Bantam.

VandenBerg KA, and Hanson MJ. 1993. *Homecoming for Babies After the Neonatal Intensive Care Nursery: A Guide for Parents in Supporting Baby's Early Development.* Austin, Texas: Pro-Ed.

Siblings/Children Books

Falswell C. 1993. *We Have a Baby.* New York: Clarion Books.

Frasier D. 1991. *On the Day You Were Born.* San Diego: Harcourt Brace Jovanovich.

Lafferty L, and Flood B. 1995. *Born Early: A Premature Baby's Story for Children.* Grand Junction, Colorado: Songbird Publishing.

Pankow V. 1987. *No Bigger Than My Teddy Bear.* Nashville: Abingdon Press.

Powell T, and Gallagher PA. 1993. *Brothers and Sisters: A Special Part of Exceptional Families,* 2nd ed. Baltimore: Paul H. Brookes Co.

Rogers F. 1985. *The New Baby.* New York: Putnam.

Scott A. 1992. *On Mother's Lap.* New York: Clarion Books.

Magazines

Exceptional Parent. (800) 247-8080.

Growing Child. (800) 927-7289.

Healthy Kids. Available free from your child's pediatrician, or subscribe from the American Academy of Pediatrics. (847) 981-7944.

Neonatal and Pediatric ICU Parenting Magazine. (412) 863-6641.

Twins. (800) 821-5533.

Videotapes

Breastfeeding: A Special Relationship. 1990. Tully MR, and Overfield M.

Caring for Your NICU Baby (2 booklets included). Newborn Transitional Project of the Kansas Early Childhood Research Institute. Paul H. Brookes Co.

Diapers and Delirium. Driscoll J.

Expect More Than a Baby. Beam Productions.

The Gift of Baby Massage. Klinger R.

Hey, What about Me? (for siblings). Kidvidz.

Introduction to the NICU (2 booklets included). Newborn Transitional Project of the Kansas Early Childhood Research Institute. Paul H. Brookes Co.

You Can Breastfeed Your Preterm Baby. 1989. O'Leary MJ. (3 videotapes and accompanying brochures). Health Sciences Center for Educational Resources, Distribution Center, SB-56, University of Washington, Seattle, WA 98195, (206) 685-1186.

Endorsed/approved videotapes from the American Academy of Pediatrics

Write to the American Academy of Pediatrics or call for the Parent Resource Guide pamphlet at (847) 981-6771.

Baby Alive (infant and child safety).

Baby Talk (new baby care).

Breastfeeding: The Art of Mothering (information about breastfeeding).

Child Safety Outdoors (prevention of childhood injuries).

Infant and Toddler Emergency First Aid (series of two videos).

Injoy Videos

Write or call for a comprehensive catalog of videos for childbirth and parenting education:

3970 Broadway, Suite B4
Boulder, CO 80304
(800) 326-2082

Mail Order

Books

Barnes & Noble. *Special Needs Selection Catalogue.* Boston, Massachusetts, (617) 236-7442.

Birth and Life Bookstore. *Imprints Catalog.* Salem, Oregon, (503) 371-4445.

Clothing and Baby Supplies

Mainly Multiples. (800) 388-TWIN [388-8946].
One Step Ahead. (800) 274-8440.
Premie Store. (800) O-SO-TINY [676-8469].

Premie Wear. (800) 992-TINY [992-8469].
The Right Start. (800) LITTLE 1 [548-8531].
TLC. (800) 755-4TLC [755-4852].

Diapers

Commonwealth Premature Pampers. (800) 543-4932 or, in Ohio, (800) 582-2623.

Toys and Other Items

Dolly Downs dolls (cloth doll with Down Syndrome, story, tape). (800) 682-3714.

Kapable Kids catalog (toys for children with disabilities). (800) 356-1564.

Oppenheim Toy Portfolio (toys for children with special needs). (212) 598-0502.

Resources for Children with Special Needs. (212) 677-4650.

Toys "R" Us Toy Guide for Differently-Abled Kids! (catalog). Call the store nearest you or write for a catalog: PO Box 8501, Nevada, IA 50201-9968.

Appendix E
Cardiopulmonary Resuscitation
for an Infant (Younger Than One Year)

Objectives	Critical Performance	Reason
Assessment: Determine un-responsiveness. Shout for help.	Tap or gently shake victim's shoulder. Call out "Help!" If help arrives, send someone to activate the EMS system.	You do not want to begin CPR unnecessarily if the infant is sleeping. A call for help will summon persons nearby but allow you to begin CPR if necessary.

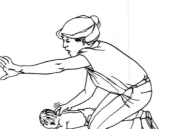

Action: Position the infant on his or her back.	Turn the infant as a unit, supporting head and neck. Place the infant on a firm surface. If the infant's head or neck has possibly been injured, turn the infant carefully, holding the head and neck as a unit to avoid bending or turning the neck.	For CPR to be effective, the infant must be flat on his or her back on a firm surface. CPR cannot be performed if the infant is face down.

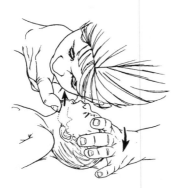

Action: Open the airway (head tilt–chin lift).	Lift the chin up and out gently with one hand while pushing down on the forehead with the other to tilt the head back into a neutral position. Don't close the mouth. If trauma is suspected, use the jaw thrust to open the airway.	The airway must be opened to determine whether the infant is breathing. Infants may be unable to breathe because the tongue is obstructing the airway.
Assessment: Determine breath-lessness.	Maintain an open airway. Turn your head toward the infant's chest with your ear directly over and close to the infant's mouth. *Look* at the chest for movement. *Listen* for the sounds of breathing. *Feel* for breath on your cheek.	Hearing and feeling are the only true ways of determining the presence of effective breathing. If there is chest movement but you cannot feel or hear air, the airway may still be obstructed. Rescue breathing should not be performed on someone who is breathing effectively.

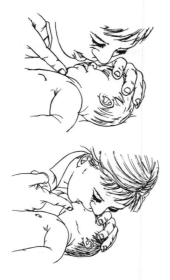

Objectives

Action: If the victim is not breathing, provide rescue breathing. Give 2 slow rescue breaths (1 to 1½ seconds per breath). Observe the rise of the chest with each breath.

Critical Performance

Maintain pressure on the infant's forehead to keep the head tilted. With the other hand lift the chin; open your mouth wide and take a deep breath. Cover the infant's mouth and nose with your mouth, making a tight seal. Breathe into the infant's mouth and nose twice, completely refilling your lungs between breaths. Watch for the infant's chest to rise.

Each rescue breath is given over 1 to 1½ seconds, allowing the infant's lungs to deflate between breaths. If the rescue breaths do not cause the infant's chest to rise, the airway is obstructed. Reposition the head, lift the chin, and try again. If the chest still does not rise with the rescue breath, take necessary steps to clear the obstructed airway.

Reason

It is important to get as much oxygen as possible into the infant. If your rescue breathing is effective, you will:
- Feel air going in as you blow
- Feel the air leaving your own lungs
- See the infant's chest rise and fall

The most common cause of an obstructed airway is that the airway has not been properly opened.

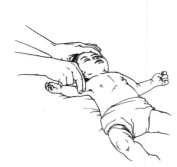

Assessment:
Determine pulse-lessness.

Place 2 or 3 fingers on the inside of the infant's upper arm, between the elbow and shoulder. Press gently on the inside of the arm with your index and middle fingers. Maintain head tilt with the other hand. Feel for the brachial pulse.

- If pulse is present and breathing has not resumed, breathe for the infant at the rate of 20 times per minute.

- If there is no pulse, start chest compressions.

This step should not take more than a few seconds. If the heart is beating effectively, you should be able to feel a strong, rapid pulse within a few seconds. If you do not feel a pulse, begin chest compressions.

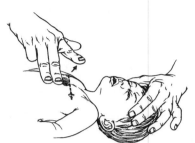

Objectives

Action: Begin the first cycle of chest compressions.

Critical Performance

To begin the first cycle, imagine a line drawn between the infant's nipples. Place 2 or 3 fingers on the breastbone (sternum) about 1 finger's width below that line. Because of wide variations in the relative sizes of rescuers' hands and infants' chests, these instructions are only guidelines. After finding the position for compressions, make sure your fingers are not over the bottom of the sternum (xiphoid). Compress the infant's chest downward approximately one-third to one-half the depth of the chest (about ½ to 1 inch, but these measurements are not precise) at least 100 times per minute.

Compress smoothly and evenly, and release pressure between compressions to allow the chest to return to its normal position. Do not lift your fingers off the chest.

To achieve a proper rate and ratio, count aloud: "one-two-three-four-five-breathe..."

Reason

Proper finger placement is important to maximize the effectiveness of compressions and minimize the risk of injury to the infant.

With each compression, you want to squeeze the heart and increase pressure within the chest so that blood moves to the vital organs.

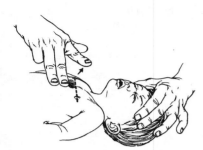

Objectives

Action: Give **5** compressions and **1** breath.

Critical Performance

Ventilate properly. After every **5** compressions, deliver **1** rescue breath. Pause briefly after each 5th compression to deliver the 1 breath.

Reason

Adequate oxygenation must be maintained.

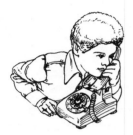

Action: Activate the EMS system at the end of 20 cycles or 20 rescue breaths (approximately 1 minute).

After EMS notification, resume CPR, beginning with chest compressions. Check every few minutes for return of pulse.

Know your local EMS telephone number. If a second person is available, he or she should telephone the local EMS immediately while you continue CPR. If you are alone, perform CPR for approximately 1 minute *before* activating the EMS system.

• If the pulse returns, check for spontaneous breathing.
—If there is no breathing, give 1 rescue breath every 3 seconds (20 breaths per minute) and monitor the pulse.
—If breathing resumes, maintain an open airway and monitor breathing and pulse.

• If pulse *and* breathing resume and are regular and there is no evidence of trauma, turn the infant on his or her side, continue to monitor breathing and pulse, and await rescue personnel.

Notification of the EMS system at this time allows the caller to give complete information about the infant's condition.

From: American Academy of Pediatrics. 1994. The performance guidelines and how to use them. In *Pediatric Basic Life Support*. Dallas, Texas: American Heart Association, 32–39. Reprinted by permission.

References

Chapter 1

1. Main DM, and Main EK. 1991. Preterm birth. In *Obstetrics: Normal and Problem Pregnancies*, 2nd ed., Gabbe SG, Niebyl JR, and Simpson JL, eds. New York: Churchill Livingstone, 829–880.

2. May KA, and Mahlmeister LR. 1994. Monitoring the at-risk fetus. In *Maternal and Neonatal Nursing: Family-Centered Care*, 3rd ed. Philadelphia: JB Lippincott, 547–568.

3. Freeman RK, and Garite TJ. 1981. The physiologic basis of fetal monitoring. In *Fetal Heart Rate Monitoring*. Baltimore: Williams & Wilkins, 7–18.

4. Freeman RK, and Garite TJ. 1981. Management of fetal distress. In *Fetal Heart Rate Monitoring*. Baltimore: Williams & Wilkins, 89–112.

5. American Academy of Pediatrics and American College of Obstetricians and Gynecologists. 1992. Antepartum and intrapartum care. In *Guidelines for Perinatal Care*, 3rd ed., Freeman RK, and Poland RL, eds. Elk Grove Village, Illinois: American Academy of Pediatrics, 81.

6. Chestnut DH, and Dailey PA. 1993. Anesthesia for preterm labor and delivery. In *Anesthesia for Obstetrics*, 3rd ed., Shnider SM, and Levinson G, eds. Baltimore: Williams & Wilkins, 337–364.

7. May KA, and Mahlmeister LR. 1994. Modifying labor patterns and mode of delivery. In *Maternal and Neonatal Nursing: Family-Centered Care*, 3rd ed. Philadelphia: JB Lippincott, 569–598.

8. Blackburn ST, and Loper DL. 1992. Parturition and uterine physiology. In *Maternal, Fetal, and Neonatal Physiology: A Clinical Perspective*. Philadelphia: WB Saunders, 126.

9. Auvenshine MA, and Enriquez MG. 1985. Maternal physiologic adaptation. In *Maternity Nursing: Dimensions of Change*. Monterey, California: Wadsworth (Health Sciences Division), 383.

10. May KA, and Mahlmeister LR. 1994. Managing pain during the intrapartum and postpartum periods. In *Maternal and Neonatal Nursing: Family-Centered Care*, 3rd ed. Philadelphia: JB Lippincott, 599–635.

Chapter 2

1. Bloom RS, and Cropley C. 1995. *Textbook of Newborn Resuscitation*. Elk Grove Village, Illinois: American Heart Association, 3B-37–38.

2. Korones SB. 1986. Evaluation and management of the infant immediately after birth. In *High-Risk Newborn Infants: The Basis for Intensive Nursing Care*, 4th ed. St. Louis: Mosby-Year Book, 78–80.

3. American Academy of Pediatrics and American College of Obstetricians and Gynecologists. 1992. Postpartum and follow-up care. In *Guidelines for Perinatal Care*, 3rd ed., Freeman RK, and Poland RL, eds. Elk Grove Village, Illinois: American Academy of Pediatrics, 94, 96.

4. Theorell CJ. 1993. Diagnostic imaging. In *Comprehensive Neonatal Nursing: A Physiologic Perspective*, Kenner C, Brueggemeyer A, and Gunderson LP, eds. Philadelphia: WB Saunders, 859.

5. Korones SB. 1986. Basic principles and clinical significance of acid-base, fluid, and electrolyte disturbances. In *High-Risk Newborn Infants: The Basis for Intensive Nursing Care*, 4th ed. St. Louis: Mosby-Year Book, 183.

6. DiGiacomo JE, Hagedorn MI, and Hay WW. 1989. Glucose homeostasis. In *Handbook of Neonatal Intensive Care*, 2nd ed., Merenstein GB, and Gardner SL, eds. St. Louis: Mosby-Year Book, 230.

7. Merenstein GB, Gardner SL, and Blake WW. 1989. Heat balance. In *Handbook of Neonatal Intensive Care*, 2nd ed., Merenstein GB, and Gardner SL, eds. St. Louis: Mosby-Year Book, 111–125.

8. Pierce JR, and Turner BS. 1989. Physiologic monitoring. In *Handbook of Neonatal Intensive Care*, 2nd ed., Merenstein GB, and Gardner SL, eds. St. Louis: Mosby-Year Book, 127.

9. Portman R, Browder S, and Distefano SM. 1989. Neonatal nephrology. In *Handbook of Neonatal Intensive Care*, 2nd ed., Merenstein GB, and Gardner SL, eds. St. Louis: Mosby-Year Book, 486–488.

10. Adcock EW, and Consolvo CA. 1989. Fluid and electrolyte management. In *Handbook of Neonatal Intensive Care*, 2nd ed., Merenstein GB, and Gardner SL, eds. St. Louis: Mosby-Year Book, 219.

11. American Academy of Pediatrics and American College of Obstetricians and Gynecologists. 1992. Special considerations. In *Guidelines for Perinatal Care*, 3rd ed., Freeman RK, and Poland RL, eds. Elk Grove Village, Illinois: American Academy of Pediatrics, 201.

12. Hagedorn MI, Gardner SL, and Abman SH. 1989. Respiratory diseases. In *Handbook of Neonatal Intensive Care*, 2nd ed., Merenstein GB, and Gardner SL, eds. St. Louis: Mosby-Year Book, 365–426.

13. American Academy of Pediatrics and American College of Obstetricians and Gynecologists. 1992. Interhospital care of the perinatal patient. In *Guidelines for Perinatal Care*, 3rd ed., Freeman RK, and Poland RL, eds. Elk Grove Village, Illinois: American Academy of Pediatrics, 35–47.

Chapter 4

1. Gorski PA. 1991. Behavioral assessment in the newborn. In *Diseases of the Newborn*, 6th ed., Taeusch HW, Ballard RA, and Avery ME, eds. Philadelphia: WB Saunders, 225–235.

2. Moore KL. 1982. The eye and the ear. In *The Developing Human*, 3rd ed. Philadelphia: WB Saunders, 413–431.

3. Blackburn S, and Kang R. 1991. *Early Parent-Infant Relationships*, 2nd ed., Raff BS, and Fiore E, eds. New York: March of Dimes Birth Defects Foundation, 26.

4. Moore KL. 1982. The nervous system. In *The Developing Human*, 3rd ed. Philadelphia: WB Saunders, 375–412.

5. Gardner SL, et al. 1989. The neonate and the environment: Impact on development. In *Handbook of Neonatal Intensive Care*, 2nd ed., Merenstein GB, and Gardner SL, eds. St. Louis: Mosby-Year Book, 628–676.

6. Montagu A. 1978. Culture and contact. In *Touching: The Human Significance of the Skin*, 2nd ed. New York: Harper & Row, 231–316.

7. Ponsonby AL, et al. 1993. Factors potentiating the risk of sudden infant death syndrome associated with the prone position. *New England Journal of Medicine* 329(6): 377–382.

8. United States Government Product Safety Commission. 1994. *Consumer product safety alert: Soft bedding products and sleep position contribute to infant suffocation deaths*. Washington, DC: U.S. Government Printing Office.

9. Blackburn S, and Kang R. 1991. *Early Parent-Infant Relationships*, 2nd ed., Raff BS, and Fiore E, eds. New York: March of Dimes Birth Defects Foundation, 22.

10. Brazelton TB. 1984. The manual. In *Neonatal Behavioral Assessment Scale*, 2nd ed. London: Spastics International Medical Publications, 19.

11. Hatcher D, and Lehman K. 1985. *Baby Talk for Parents Who Are Getting to Know Their Special Care Baby*. Omaha, Nebraska: Centering Corporation.

12. VandenBerg KA. 1993. *Reading Your Baby's Cues and State*. Austin, Texas: Pro-Ed.

13. Als H. 1986. A synactive model of neonatal behavioral organization: Framework for the assessment of neurobehavioral development in the premature infant and for the support of infants and

parents in the neonatal intensive care environment. *Physical and Occupational Therapy in Pediatrics* 6: 3–53.

14. Ludington-Hoe SM, and Golant SK. 1993. Why you should use kangaroo care. In *Kangaroo Care: The Best You Can Do to Help Your Preterm Infant.* New York: Bantam, 67.

15. Ludington-Hoe SM, and Golant SK. 1993. The best times to use kangaroo care. In *Kangaroo Care: The Best You Can Do to Help Your Preterm Infant.* New York: Bantam, 107.

Chapter 5

1. Bu'Lock F, Woolridge MW, and Baum JD. 1990. Development of coordination of sucking, swallowing and breathing: Ultrasound study of term and preterm infants. *Developmental Medicine and Child Neurology* 32(8): 669–678.

2. Lucas A. 1993. Enteral nutrition. In *Nutritional Needs of the Preterm Infant: Scientific Basis and Practical Guidelines,* Tsang RC, et al., eds. Baltimore: Williams & Wilkins, 208–223.

3. Lawrence PB. 1994. Breast milk. Best source of nutrition for term and preterm infants. *Pediatric Clinics of North America* 41(5): 925–941.

4. Lawrence R. 1994. Host-resistance factors and immunologic significance of human milk. In *Breastfeeding: A Guide for the Medical Profession,* 4th ed. St. Louis: Mosby-Year Book, 149–180.

5. Davis DW, and Bell PA. 1991. Infant feeding practices and occlusal outcomes: A longitudinal study. *Journal/Canadian Dental Association* 57(7): 593–594.

6. Verge CF, et al. 1994. Environmental factors in childhood IDDM. A population-based, case-control study. *Diabetes Care* 17(12): 1381–1389.

7. Mathur GP, et al. 1993. Breastfeeding and childhood cancer. *Indian Pediatrics* 30(5): 651–657.

8. Rigas A, et al. 1993. Breast-feeding and maternal smoking in the etiology of Crohn's disease and ulcerative colitis in childhood. *Annals of Epidemiology* 3(4): 387–392.

9. Anderson GC. 1991. Current knowledge about skin-to-skin (kangaroo) care for preterm infants. *Journal of Perinatology* 11(3): 216–226.

10. Anderson GH. 1984. The effect of prematurity on milk composition and its physiological basis. *Federation Proceedings* 43(9): 2438–2442.

11. Lucas A, and Cole TJ. 1990. Breast milk and neonatal necrotizing enterocolitis. *Lancet* 336(8730): 1519–1523.

12. Lucas A, et al. 1992. Breast milk and subsequent intelligence quotient in children born preterm. *Lancet* 339(8788): 261–264.

13. Meier PP. 1988. Bottle- and breast-feeding: Effects on transcutaneous oxygen pressure and temperature in preterm infants. *Nursing Research* 37(1): 36–41.

14. Short RV. 1993. Lactational infertility in family planning. *Annals of Medicine* 25(2): 175–180.

15. Kramer FM, et al. 1993. Breast-feeding reduces maternal lower-body fat. *Journal of the American Dietetic Association* 93(4): 429–433.

16. Newcomb PA, et al. 1994. Lactation and a reduced risk of premenopausal breast cancer. *New England Journal of Medicine* 330(2): 81–87.

17. Ruff AJ. 1994. Breastmilk, breastfeeding, and transmission of viruses to the neonate. *Seminars in Perinatology* 18(6): 510–516.

18. Neifert M, and Seacat J. 1988. Practical aspects of breastfeeding the premature infant. *Perinatology-Neonatology* 12(1): 24–29, 31.

19. Meier PP, and Mangurten HH. 1993. Breastfeeding the pre-term infant. In *Breastfeeding and Human Lactation,* Riordan J, and Auerbach KG, eds. Boston: Jones & Bartlett, 253–278.

20. Lawrence R. 1994. Breastfeeding the infant with a problem. In *Breastfeeding: A Guide for the Medical Profession,* 4th ed. St. Louis: Mosby-Year Book, 405–472.

21. Huggins K. 1990. *The Nursing Mother's Companion.* Boston: The Harvard Common Press, 90–95.

22. Costa KM. 1989. A comparison of colony counts of breast milk using two methods of breast cleansing. *Journal of Obstetric, Gynecologic, and Neonatal Nursing* 18(3): 231–236.

23. Human Milk Banking Association of North America. 1993. *Recommendations for Collection, Storage, and Handling of a Mother's Milk for Her Own Infant in the Hospital Setting.* PO Box 370464, West Hartford, Connecticut 06137-0464: HMBANA, 1–23.

24. Sosa R, and Barness L. 1987. Bacterial growth in refrigerated human milk. *American Journal of Diseases of Children* 141(1): 111–112.

25. Meier PP, et al. 1994. A new scale for in-home test-weighing for mothers of preterm and high risk infants. *Journal of Human Lactation* 10(3): 163–168.

26. Walker M. 1990. Breastfeeding premature babies. In *Lactation Consultant Series,* Unit 14. Garden City Park, New York: Avery, 21–23.

27. Lang S. 1994. Cup-feeding: An alternative method. *Midwives Chronicle* 107(1276): 171–176.

28. McCain GC. 1992. Facilitating inactive awake states in preterm infants: A study of three interventions. *Nursing Research* 41(3): 157–160.

29. McEvoy GK, ed. 1995. *American Hospital Formulary Service Drug Information.* Bethesda, Maryland: American Society of Health-System Pharmacists, 2558–2562.

30. Mathew OP. 1990. Determinants of milk flow through nipple units: Role of hole size and nipple thickness. *American Journal of Diseases of Children* 144(2): 222–224.

31. McCain GC. 1995. Promotion of preterm infant nipple feeding with nonnutritive sucking. *Journal of Pediatric Nursing* 10(1): 3–8.

32. Shaker CS. 1990. Nipple feeding premature infants: A different perspective. *Neonatal Network* 8(5): 9–17.

33. VandenBerg KA. 1990. Nippling management of the sick neonate in the NICU: The disorganized feeder. *Neonatal Network* 9(1): 9–16.

Chapter 6

1. Novak JC. 1990. Facilitating nurturant fathering behavior in the NICU. *Journal of Perinatal and Neonatal Nursing* 4(2): 68–77.

2. Ladden M. 1990. The impact of preterm labor on the family and society, part 2: Transition to home. *Pediatric Nursing* 16(6): 620–622.

3. Gennaro S, Grisemer A, and Musci R. 1992. Expected versus actual life style changes in mothering of preterm, low birth weight infants. *Neonatal Network* 11(3): 39–45.

4. Kenner CA, et al. 1993. Transition from Hospital to Home: Across Three Levels of Care. Report of research funded by the University of Cincinnati Academic Challenge Grant and the National Association of Neonatal Nurses.

5. Shellabarger SG, and Thompson TL. 1993. The critical times: Meeting parental communication needs throughout the NICU experience. *Neonatal Network* 12(2): 39–44.

Chapter 8

1. Pursley DM, and Cloherty JP. 1991. Identifying the high-risk new-

References

born and evaluating gestational age, prematurity, postmaturity, large-for-gestational-age, and small-for-gestational-age infants. In *Manual of Neonatal Care*, 3rd ed., Cloherty JP, and Stark AR, eds. Boston: Little, Brown, 85–103.

2. Battaglia F, and Lubchenco L. 1967. A practical classification of newborn infants by weight and gestational age. *Journal of Pediatrics* 71(2): 159–163.

3. Sweet AY. 1986. Classification of the low-birth-weight infant. In *Care of the High Risk Neonate*, Klaus MH, and Fanaroff AA, eds. Philadelphia: WB Saunders, 69–95.

4. Endo AS, and Nishloka E. 1993. Neonatal assessment. In *Comprehensive Neonatal Nursing: A Physiologic Perspective*, Kenner C, Brueggemeyer A, and Gunderson LP, eds. Philadelphia: WB Saunders, 265–293.

5. Harmon JS. 1993. High-risk pregnancy. In *Comprehensive Neonatal Nursing: A Physiologic Perspective*, Kenner C, Brueggemeyer A, and Gunderson LP, eds. Philadelphia: WB Saunders, 157–170.

6. Bartram J, and Clewell WH. 1989. Prenatal environment: Impact on neonatal outcome. In *Handbook of Neonatal Intensive Care*, 2nd ed., Merenstein GB, and Gardner SL, eds. St. Louis: Mosby-Year Book, 31–50.

7. Cloherty JP, and Epstein MF. 1991. Maternal diabetes. In *Manual of Neonatal Care*, 3rd ed., Cloherty JP, and Stark AR, eds. Boston: Little, Brown, 3–16.

8. ACOG Technical Bulletin, Number 219. January, 1996. *Hypertension in Pregnancy*. Washington, DC: American College of Obstetricians and Gynecologists, 1.

9. Guerina NG. 1991. Viral infections in the newborn. In *Manual of Neonatal Care*, 3rd ed., Cloherty JP, and Stark AR, eds. Boston: Little, Brown, 114–146.

10. Shaw N. 1993. Assessment and management of hematologic dysfunction. In *Comprehensive Neonatal Nursing: A Physiologic Perspective*, Kenner C, Brueggemeyer A, and Gunderson LP, eds. Philadelphia: WB Saunders, 582–634.

11. Hall BD. 1988. Common multiple congenital anomaly syndromes in the neonate. In *Neonatology: Basic Management, On-Call Problems, Diseases, Drugs*, Gomella TL, Cunningham MD, and Eyal FG, eds. Norwalk, Connecticut: Appleton & Lange, 216–221.

12. Freeman RK, and Garite TJ. 1981. The physiologic basis of fetal monitoring. In *Fetal Heart Rate Monitoring*. Baltimore: Williams & Wilkins, 7–18.

13. Felblinger DM, and Weitkamp TL. 1993. Effects of labor and delivery on the fetus and neonate. In *Comprehensive Neonatal Nursing: A Physiologic Perspective*, Kenner C, Brueggemeyer A, and Gunderson LP, eds. Philadelphia: WB Saunders, 215–230.

14. Bradley BS. 1991. Birth trauma. In *Manual of Neonatal Care*, 3rd ed., Cloherty JP, and Stark AR, eds. Boston: Little, Brown, 420–426.

15. Minarcik CJ, and Beachy P. 1989. Neurologic disorders. In *Handbook of Neonatal Intensive Care*, 2nd ed., Merenstein GB, and Gardner SL, eds. St. Louis: Mosby-Year Book, 501–530.

Chapter 9

1. Hagedorn MI, Gardner SL, and Abman SH. 1993. Respiratory diseases. In *Handbook of Neonatal Intensive Care*, 3rd ed., Merenstein GB, and Gardner SL, eds. St. Louis: Mosby-Year Book, 316.

2. Miller MJ, Fanaroff AA, and Martin RJ. 1992. The respiratory system. In *Neonatal-Perinatal Medicine: Diseases of the Fetus and Infant*, 5th ed., Fanaroff AA, and Martin RJ, eds. St. Louis: Mosby-Year Book, 853.

3. Dransfield D. 1993. Breathing disorders in the newborn infant. In *Workbook in Practical Neonatology*, Polin RA, Yoder MC, and Burg FD, eds. Philadelphia: WB Saunders, 222.

4. Blackburn ST, and Loper DL. 1992. The integumentary system. In *Maternal, Fetal, and Neonatal Physiology: A Clinical Perspective*. Philadelphia: WB Saunders, 511.

5. American Academy of Pediatrics and American College of Obstetricians and Gynecologists. 1992. Maternal and newborn nutrition. In *Guidelines for Perinatal Care*, 3rd ed., Freeman RK, and Poland RL, eds. Elk Grove Village, Illinois: American Academy of Pediatrics, 181.

6. Pereira GR, and Barbosa NM. 1986. Controversies in neonatal nutrition. *Pediatric Clinics of North America* 33(1): 65.

Chapter 10 Information Compiled From

Ballweg DD. 1991. Neonatal seizures. *Neonatal Network* 10(1): 15–22.

Beachy P, and Deacon J, eds. 1993. *Core Curriculum for Neonatal Intensive Care Nursing*. Philadelphia: WB Saunders.

Bernbaum JC, and Hoffman-Williamson M. 1991. *Primary Care of the Preterm Infant*. St. Louis: Mosby-Year Book.

Blackburn S. 1992. Alterations of the respiratory system in the neonate: Implications for clinical practice. *Journal of Perinatal and Neonatal Nursing* 6(2): 46–58.

Blackburn ST, and Loper DL. 1992. *Maternal, Fetal and Neonatal Physiology: A Clinical Perspective*. Philadelphia: WB Saunders.

Bloom RS, and Cropley C. 1995. *Textbook of Neonatal Resuscitation*. Elk Grove Village, Illinois: American Heart Association and American Academy of Pediatrics, 1–10.

Carroll P. 1991. Pneumothorax in the newborn. *Neonatal Network* 10(2): 27–34.

Cloherty JP, and Stark AR, eds. 1992. *Manual of Neonatal Care*. Boston: Little, Brown.

Composto R. 1992. Congenital diaphragmatic hernia. *Neonatal Network* 11(6): 57–62.

Dietch JS. 1993. Periventricular-intraventricular hemorrhage in the very low birth weight infant. *Neonatal Network* 12(1): 7–16.

Doyle DK. 1986. Teratology: A primer. *Neonatal Network* 4(4): 24–28.

Goldsmith JP, and Karotken EH, eds. 1988. *Assisted Ventilation of the Neonate*. Philadelphia: WB Saunders.

Gomella TL, Cunningham M, and Eyal FG, eds. 1992. *Neonatology: Management, Procedures, On-Call Problems, Diseases, Drugs*. Norwalk, Connecticut: Appleton & Lange, 379.

Gracey KM, McLaughlin KL, and Smiley MJ. 1991. Caring for the infant with retinopathy of prematurity undergoing cryotherapy. *Neonatal Network* 9(7): 7–12.

Harrison H. 1983. *The Premature Baby Book*. New York: St. Martin's Press.

Kenner C, Brueggemeyer A, and Gunderson LP, eds. 1993. *Comprehensive Neonatal Nursing: A Physiologic Perspective*. Philadelphia: WB Saunders.

Lapido M. 1989. Respiratory distress revisited. *Neonatal Network* 8(3): 9–16.

Lemmons PK. 1990. Prenatal diagnosis and congenital disease. *Neonatal Network* 9(3): 15–22.

London ML. 1993. Resuscitation and stabilization of the neonate. In *Comprehensive Neonatal Nursing: A Physiologic Perspective*, Kenner C, Brueggemeyer A, and Gunderson LP, eds. Philadelphia: WB Saunders, 236–237.

Nugent J, ed. 1991. *Acute Respiratory Care of the Neonate*. Petaluma, California: NICU INK.

Robertson NRC, ed. 1992. *Textbook of Neonatology*. New York: Churchill Livingstone.

Rowe M. 1990. Asphyxiated infants. *Neonatal Network* 9(4): 7–10.

Chapter 11

1. Spear RM. 1992. Anesthesia for premature and term infants: Perioperative implications. *Journal of Pediatrics* 120(2): 165–176.

2. Emhardt JD, and Vasko MR. 1990. Do neonates need anesthesia? In *Advances in Anesthesia,* vol. 7, Stoelting RK, Barash PG, and Gallagher TJ, eds. Chicago: Year Book Medical Publishers, 45–81.

3. American Academy of Pediatrics, Committee on Fetus and Newborn and Committee on Drugs. 1987. Neonatal anesthesia. *Pediatrics* 80(3): 446.

4. Steward DJ. 1993. Eutectic mixture of local anesthetics (EMLA): What is it? What does it do? *Journal of Pediatrics* 122(5 part 2): S21–S23.

5. Williamson PS, and Williamson ML. 1983. Physiologic stress reduction by a local anesthetic during newborn circumcision. *Pediatrics* 71(1): 36–40.

6. Stang HJ, et al. 1988. Local anesthesia for neonatal circumcision: Effects on distress and cortisol response. *Journal of the American Medical Association* 259(10): 1507–1511.

7. Broadman LM, et al. 1987. Post-circumcision analgesia: A prospective evaluation of subcutaneous ring block of the penis. *Anesthesiology* 67(3): 399–402.

8. Robinson S, and Gregory GA. 1981. Fentanyl-air-oxygen anesthesia for ligation of patent ductus arteriosus in preterm infants. *Anesthesia and Analgesia* 60(5): 331–334.

9. Hickey PR, et al. 1985. Pulmonary and systemic hemodynamic responses to fentanyl in infants. *Anesthesia and Analgesia* 64(5): 483–486.

10. Hansen DD, and Hickey PR. 1986. Anesthesia for hypoplastic left heart syndrome: Use of high dose fentanyl in 30 minutes. *Anesthesia and Analgesia* 65(2): 127–132.

11. Gregory GA. 1989. Anesthesia for premature infants. In *Pediatric Anesthesia,* vol. 2, 2nd ed., Gregory GA, ed. New York: Churchill Livingstone, 803–831.

12. Wellborn LG. 1991. Perioperative apnea in the preterm infant. *Anesthesiology Clinics of North America* 9(4): 885–897.

13. Steward DJ. 1982. Preterm infants are more prone to complications following minor surgery than are term infants. *Anesthesiology* 56(4): 304–306.

14. Sweetwyne K. 1993. Neonatal sedation and analgesia. *Neonatal Pharmacology Quarterly* 2(1): 5–11.

15. Mainous RO. 1995. Research utilization: Pharmacologic management of neonatal pain. *Neonatal Network* 14(4): 71–74.

16. Beaver PK. 1987. Premature infants' response to touch and pain: Can nurses make a difference? *Neonatal Network* 6(3): 13–17.

Chapter 12

1. Coulter DM. 1992. The current status of replacement therapy with exogenous pulmonary surfactant for hyaline membrane disease. *Neonatal Pharmacology Quarterly* 1(1): 5–18.

2. Loper DL. 1991. Physiologic principles of the respiratory system. In *Acute Respiratory Care of the Neonate,* Nugent J, ed. Petaluma, California: NICU INK, 2.

3. Donovan EF, and Spangler LL. 1993. New technologies applied to the management of respiratory dysfunction. In *Comprehensive Neonatal Nursing*, Kenner C, Brueggemeyer A, and Gunderson L eds. Philadelphia: WB Saunders, 313–336.

4. Harris T, and Wood BR. 1996. Physiological principles. In *Assisted Ventilation of the Neonate*, 3rd ed., Goldsmith J, and Karotkin E, eds. Philadelphia: WB Saunders, 33.

5. Rodden DJ. 1993. Surfactant replacement therapy. In *Core Curriculum for Neonatal Intensive Care Nursing*, Beachy P, and Deacon J, eds. Philadelphia: WB Saunders, 136–147.

6. Pandit PB, et al. 1994. Evidence for surfactant inactivation in early neonatal chronic lung disease. *Pediatric Research* 35(abstract): 245A.

7. Pandit PB, et al. 1995. Surfactant therapy in neonates with respiratory deterioration due to pulmonary hemorrhage. *Pediatrics* 95(1): 32–36.

8. Karp TB. 1991. High frequency jet ventilation: Impact on neonatal nursing. In *Acute Respiratory Care of the Neonate,* Nugent J, ed. Petaluma, California: NICU INK, 147–170.

9. Gordin PC. 1993. High frequency ventilation. In *Core Curriculum for Neonatal Intensive Care Nursing,* Beachy P, and Deacon J, eds. Philadelphia: WB Saunders, 170–176.

10. Mamnel M, and Boros S. 1996. High frequency ventilation. In *Assisted Ventilation of the Neonate*, 3rd ed., Goldsmith J, and Karotkin E, eds. Philadelphia: WB Saunders, 199–214.

11. Avila K, et al. 1994. High-frequency oscillatory ventilation: A nursing approach to bedside care. *Neonatal Network* 13(5): 23–30.

12. Carter JM, et al. 1990. High frequency oscillatory ventilation and extracorporeal membrane oxygenation for the treatment of acute neonatal respiratory failure. *Pediatrics* 85(2): 159–164.

13. Kohelet DK, et al. 1988. High frequency oscillation in the rescue of infants with persistent pulmonary hypertension. *Critical Care Medicine* 16(5): 510–516.

14. Frose AB, and Bryon AC. 1981. Ventilation by high frequency oscillation—A preliminary report. In *Intensive Care of the Newborn*, Stern L, Salle B, and Friis-Hanson B, eds. New York: Masson, 271–273.

15. Hagedorn MI, Gardner S, and Abman SH. 1993. Respiratory diseases. In *Handbook of Neonatal Intensive Care*, 3rd ed., Merenstein GB, and Gardner SL, eds. St. Louis: Mosby-Year Book, 332.

16. Nugent J. 1993. Extracorporeal membrane oxygenation in the neonate. In *Core Curriculum for Neonatal Intensive Care Nursing*, Beachy P, and Deacon J, eds. Philadelphia: WB Saunders, 177–189.

17. Neonatal ECMO Registry Report of the Extracorporeal Life Support Organization. January 1995. Ann Arbor, Michigan: Extracorporeal Life Support Organization.

18. Glass P, Miller M, and Short B. 1989. Morbidity for survivors of extracorporeal membrane oxygenation: Neurodevelopmental outcome at one year of age. *Pediatrics* 83(1): 72–78.

19. Hofkosh D, et al. 1991. Ten years of extracorporeal membrane oxygenation: Neurodevelopmental outcome. *Pediatrics* 87(4): 549–555.

20. Schumacher RE, et al. 1991. Follow-up of infants treated with extracorporeal membrane oxygenation for newborn respiratory failure. *Pediatrics* 87(4): 451–457.

21. Lott IT, et al. 1990. Long-term neurophysiologic outcome after neonatal extracorporeal membrane oxygenation. *Journal of Pediatrics* 116(3): 343–349.

22. Ignarro L, Ross G, and Tillisch J. 1991. Pharmacology of endothelium-derived nitric oxide and nitrovasodilators. *Western Journal of Medicine* 154(1): 51–62.

References

23. Pepke-Zaba J, et al. 1991. Inhaled nitric oxide as a cause of selective pulmonary vasodilatation in pulmonary hypertension. *Lancet* 338(8776): 1173–1174.

24. Roberts JD, et al. 1992. Inhaled nitric oxide in persistent pulmonary hypertension of the newborn. *Lancet* 340(8823): 818–819.

25. Kinsella JP, et al. 1992. Low-dose inhalational nitric oxide in persistent pulmonary hypertension of the newborn. *Lancet* 340(8823): 819–820.

26. Kinsella JP, et al. 1995. Inhaled nitric oxide treatment for stabilization and emergency medical transport of critically ill newborns and infants. *Pediatrics* 95(5): 773–776.

27. Morrison SC, Fletcher BD, and Yulish BS. 1992. Diagnostic imaging. In *Neonatal-Perinatal Medicine: Diseases of the Fetus and Infant*, 5th ed., Fanaroff AA, and Martin RJ, eds. St. Louis: Mosby-Year Book, 565–571.

28. Levene MI. 1987. *Neonatal Neurology*. New York: Churchill Livingstone, 60–65.

29. Fawer CL, and Calame A. 1991. Ultrasound. In *Imaging Techniques of the CNS of the Neonate,* Haddad J, Christmann D, and Messer J, eds. New York: Springer-Verlag, 79–106.

30. Theorell CJ. 1993. Diagnostic imaging. In *Comprehensive Neonatal Nursing*, Kenner C, Brueggemeyer A, and Gunderson LP, eds. Philadelphia: WB Saunders, 846–871.

Chapter 13

1. Moskop JC, and Saldanha RL. 1986. The Baby Doe Rule: Still a threat. *Hastings Center Report* 16(2): 8–14.

2. Scully T, and Scully C. 1987. The Baby Doe dilemma: To treat or not to treat. In *Playing God: The New World of Medical Choices*. New York: Simon & Schuster, 194–229.

3. Bailey NA, Lay P, and the Loma Linda University Infant Heart Transplant Group. 1989. New horizons: Infant cardiac transplantation. *Heart and Lung* 18(2): 172–178.

4. Ashwal S, and Schneider S. 1989. Brain death in the newborn. *Pediatrics* 84(3): 429–437.

5. Scully T, and Scully C. 1987. Transplanting human organs and tissues—A new lease on life. In *Playing God: The New World of Medical Choices*. New York: Simon & Schuster, 124–151.

6. Loma Linda University Medical Center, Cardiac Transplant Center. 1987. *A Time for Sharing*. Loma Linda, California: Adventist Health Systems.

7. Garland KR. 1986. Grief: The transitional process. *Neonatal Network* 5(3): 7–10.

8. Gardner SL, and Merenstein GB. 1986. Perinatal grief and loss: An overview. *Neonatal Network* 5(2): 7–15.

9. Kübler-Ross E. 1969. *On Death and Dying*. New York: Collier.

10. Garland KR. 1986. Unresolved grief. *Neonatal Network* 5(3): 29–37.

11. Cumming ST, et al. 1966. Effects of the child's deficiency on the mother: A study of mothers of mentally retarded, chronically ill and neurotic children. *American Journal of Orthopsychiatry* 36(4): 595.

12. Cumming ST, et al. 1976. The impact of the child's deficiency on the father. *American Journal of Orthopsychiatry* 46(2): 246.

13. Eikner S. 1986. Dealing with long-term problems: A parent's perspective. *Neonatal Network* 5(2): 45–49.

14. Limbo RK, and Wheeler SR. 1986. *When a Baby Dies: A Handbook for Healing and Helping*. La Crosse, Wisconsin: RTS Bereavement Services, 14, 56, 59, 74.

15. Mehren E. 1991. *Born Too Soon*. New York: Doubleday.

16. Stinson R, and Stinson P. 1983. *The Long Dying of Baby Andrew*. Boston: Little, Brown.

17. Trouy MB, and Ward Larson C. 1987. Sibling grief. *Neonatal Network* 5(4): 35–40.

18. Fitzgerald H. 1992. Dealing with your child's emotional responses. In *The Grieving Child: A Parent's Guide*. New York: Simon & Schuster (Fireside), 112–113.

19. Marris P. 1974. *Loss and Change*. New York: Pantheon.

20. Hobbs N, Perrin JM, and Ireys HT. 1985. Severe and chronic illness in childhood. In *Chronically Ill Children and Their Families*. San Francisco: Jossey Bass.

21. Colgrove M, Bloomfield HH, and McWilliams P. 1991. When you might want counseling or therapy. In *How to Survive the Loss of a Love*. Los Angeles: Prelude Press, 98.

Chapter 14

1. Courtway-Myers C. 1986. The developmental needs of the high-risk infant. In *High-Risk Neonatal Care,* Streeter SN, ed. Rockville, Maryland: Aspen, 356.

2. Coen RW, and Koffler H. 1987. *Primary Care of the Newborn*. Boston: Little, Brown, 25–26.

3. Meier P, and Pugh EJ. 1985. Breastfeeding behavior of small preterm infants. *MCN: American Journal of Maternal Child Nursing* 10(6): 396–401.

4. VandenBerg KA. 1990. Nippling management of the sick neonate in the NICU: The disorganized feeder. *Neonatal Network* 9(1): 9–16.

5. McClure V. 1989. *Infant Massage: A Handbook for Loving Parents*. New York: Bantam, 141–157.

6. Shelov SP, and Hannemann RE, eds. 1991. Basic infant care. In *The American Academy of Pediatrics: Caring for Your Baby and Young Child—Birth to Age 5—The Complete and Authoritative Guide*. New York: Bantam, 48.

7. Seidel HM, Rosenstein BJ, and Pathak A. 1993. Newborn nursery policy statements. In *Primary Care of the Newborn*. St. Louis: Mosby-Year Book, 585.

8. Parker L, and Richardson C, eds. 1990. Illness. In *Ochsner NICU Babybook*. New Orleans: Alton Ochsner Medical Foundation, 1.

9. Shelov SP, and Hannemann RE, eds. 1991. The first month. In *The American Academy of Pediatrics: Caring for Your Baby and Young Child—Birth to Age 5—The Complete and Authoritative Guide*. New York: Bantam, 161.

10. Merenstein GB, Gardner SL, and Blake WW. 1989. Heat balance. In *Handbook of Neonatal Intensive Care*, 2nd ed., Merenstein GB, and Gardner SL, eds. St. Louis: Mosby-Year Book, 114.

11. Ahmann E. 1986. *Home Care for the High Risk Infant*. Rockville, Maryland: Aspen, 133–142.

12. Parker L, and Richardson C, eds. 1990. Mycostatin. In *Ochsner NICU Babybook*. New Orleans: Alton Ochsner Medical Foundation, 1–3.

13. Shelov SP, and Hannemann RE, eds. 1991. Abdominal/gastrointestinal tract. In *The American Academy of Pediatrics: Caring for Your Baby and Young Child—Birth to Age 5—The Complete and Authoritative Guide*. New York: Bantam, 485–486.

14. Shelov SP, and Hannemann RE, eds. 1991. Your baby's first days. In *The American Academy of Pediatrics: Caring for Your Baby and Young Child—Birth to Age 5—The Complete and Authoritative Guide*. New York: Bantam, 131–132.

15. McCollum LL, and Thigpen JL. 1993. Assessment and management of gastrointestinal dysfunction. In *Comprehensive Neonatal Nursing:*

A Physiologic Perspective, Kenner CA, Brueggemeyer A, and Gunderson LP, eds. Philadelphia: WB Saunders, 451–453.

16. Shaw N. 1993. Assessment and management of hematologic dysfunction. In *Comprehensive Neonatal Nursing: A Physiologic Perspective,* Kenner CA, Brueggemeyer A, and Gunderson LP, eds. Philadelphia: WB Saunders, 617–618.

Chapter 15

1. Amiel-Tison C, and Larroche JC. 1988. Brain development and neurological survey during the neonatal period. In *Neonatal Medicine,* Stern L, and Vert P, eds. New York: Masson, 245–267.

2. Lansdown R, and Walker M. 1991. Toward independence. In *Your Child's Development from Birth through Adolescence: A Complete Guide for Parents.* New York: Alfred A. Knopf, 92–93.

3. Seidel HM, Rosenstein BJ, and Pathak A. 1993. Newborn nursery policy statements. In *Primary Care of the Newborn.* St. Louis: Mosby-Year Book, 585.

4. Parker L, and Richardson C. 1990. Illness. In *Ochsner NICU Babybook.* New Orleans: Alton Ochsner Medical Foundation, 1.

5. Shelov SP, and Hannemann RE, eds. 1991. The first month. In *The American Academy of Pediatrics: Caring for Your Baby and Young Child—Birth to Age 5—The Complete and Authoritative Guide.* New York: Bantam, 133–164.

6. Shelov SP, and Hannemann RE, eds. 1991. Preparing for a new baby. In *The American Academy of Pediatrics: Caring for Your Baby and Young Child—Birth to Age 5—The Complete and Authoritative Guide.* New York: Bantam, 3–22.

7. American Academy of Pediatrics and American College of Obstetricians and Gynecologists. 1993. Postpartum and follow-up care. In *Guidelines for Perinatal Care,* 3rd ed., Freeman RK, and Poland RL, eds. Elk Grove Village, Illinois: American Academy of Pediatrics, 110.

8. Wood SL. 1991. Starting life under a cloud: The risks of passive smoking. *American Baby,* November: 44.

Chapter 16

1. Gorski PA. 1988. Fostering family development after preterm hospitalization. In *Pediatric Care of the ICN Graduate,* Ballard RA, ed. Philadelphia: WB Saunders, 27–32.

2. Harrison H. 1983. The first year. In *The Premature Baby Book: A Parent's Guide to Coping and Caring in the First Years.* New York: St. Martin's Press, 175–201.

3. Bernbaum JC, and Hoffman-Williamson M. 1991. *Primary Care of the Preterm Infant.* St. Louis: Mosby-Year Book, 87–133,181.

4. Block C, et al. 1989. Home care for high-tech infants: The first year. *Caring* 8(5): 11–17.

5. Embon CM. 1991. Discharge planning for infants with bronchopulmonary dysplasia. *Journal of Perinatal and Neonatal Nursing* 5(1): 54–63.

6. Ladden M. 1990. The impact of preterm birth on the family and society, part 2: Transition to home. *Pediatric Nursing* 16(6): 620–622.

7. Katz KS, Baker C, and Osborn D. 1991. Home-based care for children with chronic illness. *Journal of Perinatal and Neonatal Nursing* 5(1): 71–79.

8. Arenson J. 1988. Discharge teaching in the NICU: The changing needs of NICU graduates and their families. *Neonatal Network* 6(4): 29–30, 47–52.

9. Kenner C, and Bagwell GA. 1991. Assessment and management of the transition to home. In *Comprehensive Neonatal Nursing: A Physiologic Perspective,* Kenner C, Brueggemeyer A, and Gunderson LP, eds. Philadelphia: WB Saunders, 1134–1147.

10. Klein M, and Stern L. 1971. Low birth weight and battered child syndrome. *American Journal of Diseases of Children* 122(1): 15–18.

11. Perry MA, and Hayes NM. 1988. Bronchopulmonary dysplasia: Discharge planning and complex home care. *Neonatal Network* 7(3): 13–17.

12. Finston P. 1990. Identify the problem. In *Parenting Plus: Raising Children with Special Health Needs.* New York: Dutton, 63.

13. Craig S. 1988. Bringing Greg home: A case study in high-tech home care. *Caring* 7(9): 29–31.

14. Butts PA, et al. 1988. Concerns of parents of low birth weight infants following hospital discharge: A report of parent-initiated telephone calls. *Neonatal Network* 7(2): 37–42.

15. Hanson MJ, and VandenBerg KA. 1993. Homecoming: Transition from the hospital to the home. In *Homecoming for Babies After the Intensive Care Nursery: A Guide for Parents in Supporting Their Baby's Early Development.* Austin, Texas: Pro-Ed, 4–10.

16. Ebert, PR. 1994. *Bringing Your Baby Home: A Guide to Discharge Planning from Neonatal Intensive Care.* Indianapolis: Parent Care and Care Visions Corp., 3–9.

17. Parker L, and Richardson C. 1990. *Ochsner NICU Babybook.* New Orleans: Alton Ochsner Medical Foundation.

18. Shelov SP, and Hannemann RE, eds. 1991. The first month. In *The American Academy of Pediatrics: Caring for Your Baby and Young Child—Birth to Age 5—The Complete and Authoritative Guide.* New York: Bantam, 146–147.

19. Als H. 1982. Toward a synactive theory of development: Promise for the assessment and support of infant individuality. *Infant Mental Health Journal* 3(4): 229–243.

20. Lawhon G, and Melzar A. 1988. Developmental care of the very low birth weight infant. *Journal of Perinatal and Neonatal Nursing* 2(1): 56–65.

21. Cole JG, et al. 1990. Changing the NICU environment: The Boston City Hospital model. *Neonatal Network* 9(2): 15–23.

22. Wyly VM, and Allen J. 1990. Behavior of premature infants. In *Stress and Coping in the Neonatal Intensive Care Unit: The Health Professional in the NICU, the Infant in the NICU, the Family in the NICU.* Tucson, Arizona: Communication Skill Builders, 25–29.

23. Brazelton TB. 1992. *Touchpoints: The Essential Reference—Your Child's Emotional and Behavioral Development.* Reading, Massachusetts: Addison-Wesley, 60–64, 92–94, 231–238.

24. Eisenberg A, Murkoff HE, and Hathaway SE. 1989. *What to Expect the First Year.* New York: Workman, 186–187, 122–131.

25. Sears W, and Sears M. 1993. *The Baby Book: Everything You Need to Know about Your Baby—From Birth to Age Two.* Boston: Little, Brown, 309–327, 348–349.

26. Neifert M, Price A, and Dana N. 1986. Basic baby care. In *Dr. Mom: A Guide to Baby and Child Care.* New York: Penguin, 105–136.

27. Shelov SP, and Hannemann RE, eds. 1991. Basic infant care. In *The American Academy of Pediatrics: Caring for Your Baby and Young Child—Birth to Age 5—The Complete and Authoritative Guide.* New York: Bantam, 34–37.

28. Meier PP, and Mangurten HH. 1993. Breastfeeding the pre-term infant. In *Breastfeeding and Human Lactation,* Riordan J, and Averbach KG, eds. Boston: Jones & Bartlett, 262–276.

29. Huggins K. 1990. *The Nursing Mother's Companion,* rev. ed. Boston: The Harvard Common Press, 41, 90–95.

30. McCoy R, et al. 1988. Nursing management of breastfeeding for preterm infants. *Journal of Perinatal and Neonatal Nursing* 2(1): 42–55.

31. Meier PP, and Anderson GC. 1987. Responses of small preterm infants to bottle and breast-feeding. *MCN: American Journal of Maternal Child Nursing* 12(2): 97–105.

32. Hoffman HJ, and Hillman LS. 1992. Epidemiology of the sudden infant death syndrome: Maternal, neonatal, and postnatal risk factors. *Clinics in Perinatology: Apnea and SIDS* (Carl E. Hunt, guest ed.) 19(4): 717–737.

33. Guntheroth WG, and Spiers PS. 1992. Sleeping prone and the risk of sudden infant death syndrome. *Journal of the American Medical Association* 267(17): 2359–2362.

34. American Academy of Pediatrics, Task Force on Infant Positioning and SIDS. 1992. Positioning and SIDS. *Pediatrics* 89(6): 1120–1126. Published erratum appears in *Pediatrics* 90(2, part 1): 264.

35. Ponsonby AL, et al. 1993. Factors potentiating the risk of sudden infant death syndrome associated with the prone position. *New England Journal of Medicine* 329(6): 377–382.

36. Hunt CE, and Shannon DC. 1992. Sudden infant death syndrome and sleeping position. *Pediatrics* 90(1 part 1): 115–118.

37. Shelov SP, and Hannemann RE, eds. 1991. The first month. In *The American Academy of Pediatrics: Caring for Your Baby and Young Child—Birth to Age 5—The Complete and Authoritative Guide.* New York: Bantam, 159–161.

38. AWHONN Practice Resource. 1993. *Preparation for Home Care of Technology-Dependent Infants.* Washington, DC: Association of Women's Health, Obstetric, and Neonatal Nurses, 2–8.

39. Gennaro S, and Bakewell-Sachs S. 1991. Discharge planning and home care for low-birth-weight infants. *NAACOG'S Clinical Issues* 3(1): 129–145.

40. Ahmann E. 1986. *Home Care for the High Risk Infant: A Holistic Guide to Using Technology.* Rockville, Maryland: Aspen, 155–157, 195–204.

41. Platzker ACG. 1988. Chronic lung disease in infancy. In *Pediatric Care of the ICN Graduate*, Ballard RA, ed. Philadelphia: WB Saunders, 129–156.

42. Abman SH, et al. 1985. Pulmonary vascular response to oxygen in infants with severe BPD. *Pediatrics* 75(1): 80–85.

43. Howell LJ. 1988. Home ostomy care. In *Pediatric Care of the ICN Graduate*, Ballard RA, ed. Philadelphia: WB Saunders, 306–316.

44. Huddleston KC, and Ferraro AR. 1991. Preparing families of children with gastrostomies. *Pediatric Nursing* 17(2): 153–158.

45. 1987. *Care of the Percutaneous Endoscopic Gastrostomy (PEG) and the Button Replacement Gastrostomy.* Billerica, Massachusetts: CR Bard, 3–12.

46. Platzker ACG, et al. 1988. Home care of infants with chronic lung disease. In *Pediatric Care of the ICN Graduate*, Ballard RA, ed. Philadelphia: WB Saunders, 289–294.

47. Buzz-Kelly L, and Gordin P. 1993. Teaching CPR to parents of children with tracheostomies. *MCN: American Journal of Maternal Child Nursing* 18(3): 158–163.

48. Davidson Ward SL, and Keens TG. 1988. Ventilator management at home. In *Pediatric Care of the ICN Graduate*, Ballard RA, ed. Philadelphia: WB Saunders, 166–176.

Chapter 17

1. Bernbaum JC, and Hoffman-Williamson M. 1991. *Primary Care of the Preterm Infant.* St. Louis: Mosby-Year Book, 3–36, 249–280.

2. Ichord R. 1986. Developmental issues in care of the high risk infant. In *Homecare for the High Risk Infant: A Holistic Guide to Using Technology*, Ahmann E, ed. Rockville, Maryland: Aspen, 281–292.

3. Leonard CH. 1988. Developmental and behavioral assessment. In *Pediatric Care of the ICN Graduate*, Ballard RA, ed. Philadelphia: WB Saunders, 94–110.

4. McCormick MC. 1989. Long-term follow-up of infants discharged from neonatal intensive care units. *Journal of the American Medical Association* 261(12): 1767–1772.

5. Oehler JM, et al. 1993. How to target infants at risk for developmental delay. *MCN: American Journal of Maternal Child Nursing* 18(1): 20–23.

6. Goldberg S, and Divitto BA. 1983. *Born Too Soon: Preterm Birth and Early Development.* San Francisco: WH Freeman, 39–66.

7. Fischel JE, and Imbruglio LR. 1989. Developmental evaluation of the newborn intensive care graduate: The lost-to-follow-up problem. *Neonatal Network* 8(1): 23–27.

8. Zahr L, et al. 1989. Follow-up of premature infants of low socioeconomic status. *Nursing Research* 38(4): 246–247.

9. Harrison H. 1983. *The Premature Baby Book: A Parent's Guide to Coping and Caring in the First Years.* New York: St. Martin's Press, 202–219, 226.

10. Gorski PA. 1988. Fostering family development after preterm hospitalization. In *Pediatric Care of the ICN Graduate*, Ballard RA, ed. Philadelphia: WB Saunders, 27–32.

11. Hanson MJ, and VandenBerg KA. 1993. *Homecoming for Babies After the Intensive Care Nursery: A Guide for Parents in Supporting Their Baby's Early Development.* Austin, Texas: Pro-Ed, 19–25.

12. Belcher HME. 1991. Developmental screening. In *Developmental Disabilities in Infancy and Childhood*, Capute AJ, and Accardo PJ, eds. Baltimore: Paul H. Brookes Co., 113–131.

13. Katz KS, Baker C, and Osborn D. 1991. Home-based care for children with chronic illness. *Journal of Perinatal and Neonatal Nursing* 5(1): 71–79.

14. 1991. *Educating Children with Disabilities: A Guide to PL 94-142 and PL 99-457.* South Deerfield, Massachusetts: Channing L. Bete Co., 1–15.

15. Parker L. 1991. Discharge planning and follow-up care: The asphyxiated infant. *NAACOG'S Clinical Issues* 2(1): 111–163.

16. Arnold LS, and Bakewell-Sachs S. 1991. Models of perinatal home follow-up. *Journal of Perinatal and Neonatal Nursing* 5(1): 18–26.

17. Sumner G, and Spietz A, eds. 1994. *NCAST Caregiver/Parent-Child Interaction Teaching Manual.* Seattle: NCAST Publications, University of Washington, School of Nursing, 3.

18. Arenson J. 1988. Discharge teaching in the NICU: The changing needs of NICU graduates and their families. *Neonatal Network* 6(4): 29–30, 47–52.

19. Brooten D, et al. 1988. Early discharge and specialist transitional care. *Image: Journal of Nursing Scholarship* 20(2): 64–68.

20. Gennaro S, and Bakewell-Sachs S. 1991. Discharge planning and home care for low-birth weight infants. *NAACOG'S Clinical Issues* 3(1): 129–145.

21. Perry MA, and Hayes NM. 1988. Bronchopulmonary dysplasia: Discharge planning and complex home care. *Neonatal Network* 7(3): 13–17.

22. Arnold LS, and Grad RK. 1992. Low birth weight and infant mortality: A health policy perspective. *NAACOG'S Clinical Issues* 3(1): 1–12.

23. Embon CM. 1991. Discharge planning for infants with bronchopulmonary dysplasia. *Journal of Perinatal and Neonatal Nursing* 5(1): 54–63.

24. Ahmann E. 1986. *Home Care for the High Risk Infant: A Holistic Guide to Using Technology.* Rockville, Maryland: Aspen, 281–292.

25. Meissner HC. 1994. Prophylaxis and treatment of respiratory syncytial virus infection in high-risk infants. *Tufts University School of Medicine and Floating Hospital for Children Reports on Neonatal Respiratory Disease* 4(4): 1–4, 9–10.

26. Parker L, and Richardson C. 1990. Growth and development. In *Ochsner NICU Babybook.* New Orleans: Alton Ochsner Medical Foundation, 1–8.

27. Vessey JA, and Ritchie SR. 1993. The who, what, and when of pediatric immunization. *RN* 56(9): 42–48.

28. American Academy of Pediatrics, Committee on Infectious Diseases. 1988. *Report of the Committee on Infectious Diseases,* 21st ed. Elk Grove Village, Illinois: American Academy of Pediatrics.

29. American Academy of Pediatrics. 1992. *Policy Statement: Universal Hepatitis B Immunization.* Elk Grove Village, Illinois: American Academy of Pediatrics.

30. 1991. Hepatitis B virus: A comprehensive strategy for eliminating transmission in the United States through universal childhood vaccination. Recommendations of the Advisory Committee on Immunization Practices (ACIP). *Morbidity and Mortality Weekly Report* 40(RR-13): 1–25.

31. Centers for Disease Control. 1992. *Diphtheria, Tetanus, and Pertussis: What You Need to Know.* Atlanta: U.S. Department of Health and Human Services, Public Health Service, Centers for Disease Control.

32. Centers for Disease Control. 1992. *Polio: What You Need to Know.* Atlanta: U.S. Department of Health and Human Services, Public Health Service, Centers for Disease Control.

33. Connaught Laboratories. 1988. *Vaccine Facts: Immunizing Your Child Against Haemophilus B Disease at an Early Age.* Swiftwater, Pennsylvania: Connaught Laboratories.

34. Centers for Disease Control. 1992. *Measles, Mumps, and Rubella: What You Need to Know.* Atlanta: U.S. Department of Health and Human Services, Public Health Service, Centers for Disease Control.

35. Finston P. 1990. *Parenting Plus: Raising Children with Special Health Needs.* New York: Dutton, 193–200.

36. Block C. 1989. Home care for high-tech infants: The first year. *Caring* 8(5): 11–17.

37. Ladden M. 1990. The impact of preterm birth on the family and society, part 2: Transition to home. *Pediatric Nursing* 16(6): 620–622.

38. Craig S. 1988. Bringing Greg home: A case study in high-tech home care. *Caring* 7(9): 29–31.

39. Butts PA, et al. 1988. Concerns of parents of low birth weight infants following hospital discharge: A report of parent-initiated telephone calls. *Neonatal Network* 7(2): 37–42.

40. Green M, and Solnit A. 1964. Reactions to the threatened loss of a child: A vulnerable child syndrome. *Pediatrics* 34(1): 58–66.

Appendix B Information Compiled from:

American Medical Association. 1986. *Drug Evaluations,* 6th ed. Chicago: American Medical Association.

Gomella TL, Cunningham M, and Eyal FG. 1994. *Neonatology: Management, Procedures, On-call Problems, Diseases and Drugs,* 3rd ed. Norwalk, Connecticut: Appleton & Lange, 468–469.

Gregory G, ed. 1994. *Pediatric Anesthesia,* 3rd ed. New York: Churchill Livingstone.

Isaacs E, ed. 1992. *Pediatric Drug Dosage Handbook.* Winnipeg, Manitoba, Canada: Health Sciences Centre.

McCracken GH, and Nelson JD. 1983. *Antimicrobial Therapy for Newborns.* New York: Grune & Stratton.

Pawlak RP, and Herfert LT. 1990. *Drug Administration in the NICU: A Handbook for Nurses.* Petaluma, California: NICU INK.

Physician's Desk Reference. 1994. Montvale, New Jersey: Medical Economics Data Production Co.

Roberts RJ. 1984. *Drug Therapy in Infants.* Philadelphia: WB Saunders.

Shannon MT, and Wilson BA. 1992. *Drugs and Nursing Implications.* Norwalk, Connecticut: Appleton & Lange.

Sweetwyne S. 1993. Neonatal sedation and analgesia. *Neonatal Pharmacology Quarterly* 2(1): 5–11.

Young TE, and Mangum OB. 1994. *NeoFax: A Manual of Drugs Used in Neonatal Care,* 4th ed. Columbus, Ohio: Ross Products Division, Abbott Laboratories.

Table of Abbreviations

ABG:	Arterial blood gas
a.m.a.:	Against medical advice; also advanced maternal age
b.i.d.:	Two times per day
BPD:	Bronchopulmonary dysplasia
Ca:	Calcium
CBC:	Complete blood count
CBG:	Capillary blood gas
CDC:	Centers for Disease Control
CHF:	Congestive heart failure
Cl:	Chloride
cm:	Centimeter
CMV:	Cytomegalovirus; also conventional mechanical ventilator
CO_2:	Carbon dioxide
CP:	Cerebral palsy
CPAP:	Continuous positive airway pressure
CPT:	Chest physiotherapy
C&S:	Culture and sensitivity
CSF:	Cerebrospinal fluid
DIC:	Disseminated intravascular coagulopathy
diff:	Differential blood count
DNR:	Do not resuscitate
ECG:	Electrocardiogram
echo:	Echocardiogram
ECMO:	Extracorporeal membrane oxygenation
EDC:	Estimated date of confinement (due date)
EDD:	Estimated date of delivery (due date)
EEG:	Electroencephalogram
EFM:	Electronic fetal monitoring
EKG:	Electrocardiogram
ENT:	Ears, nose, and throat
ETT:	Endotracheal tube
Fe:	Iron
FiO_2:	Percentage of oxygen
FUO:	Fever of unknown origin
GI:	Gastrointestinal
gm:	Gram

Grav I, II, III:	Gravida (pregnancy) one, two, three, etc.
gtt:	Drops
GU:	Genitourinary
Hgb:	Hemoglobin
hct:	hematocrit
HMD:	Hyaline membrane disease
HFFI:	High frequency flow interruption
HFJV:	High frequency jet ventilation
HFOV:	High frequency oscillatory ventilation
HFPPV:	High frequency positive pressure ventilation
HFV:	High frequency ventilation
ICP:	Intracranial pressure
IDM:	Infant of diabetic mother
IFSP:	Individualized family service plan
IM:	Intramuscular
I&O:	Intake and output
IRDS:	Idiopathic respiratory distress syndrome
IUGR:	Intrauterine growth retardation
IUPC:	Intrauterine pressure catheter
IV:	Intravenous
K:	Potassium
K-care:	Kangaroo care
LBW:	Low birth weight
LGA:	Large for gestational age
LMP:	Last menstrual period
LP:	Lumbar puncture
lytes:	Electrolytes
MAP:	Mean arterial pressure; also mean airway pressure
MAS:	Meconium aspiration syndrome
mg:	Milligram
ml:	Milliliter
MRI:	Magnetic resonance imaging
MS:	Morphine sulfate
Na:	Sodium
NaCl:	Sodium chloride
NEC:	Necrotizing enterocolitis
NG:	Nasogastric
NNP:	Neonatal nurse practitioner
NO:	Nitric oxide

NPO:	Nothing by mouth
NS:	Nutritive sucking; also normal saline
O_2:	Oxygen
OG:	Orogastric
OT:	Occupational therapy
PDA:	Patent ductus arteriosus
PIE:	Pulmonary interstitial emphysema
PIH:	Pregnancy induced hypertension
PKU:	Phenylketonuria
p.o.:	Orally
PPHN:	Persistent pulmonary hypertension of the newborn
PPV:	Positive pressure ventilation
prn:	When required
PROM:	Premature rupture of membranes
PT:	Physical therapy; also preterm
PTL:	Preterm labor
q.d.:	Every day
q.n.s.:	Quantity not sufficient
RBC:	Red blood cell
RDS:	Respiratory distress syndrome
R/O:	Rule out
ROP:	Retinopathy of prematurity
SGA:	Small for gestational age
stat:	Immediately
STD:	Sexually transmitted disease
sz:	Seizure
TCM:	Transcutaneous monitor
TEF:	Tracheoesophageal fistula
TPN:	Total parenteral nutrition
TPR:	Temperature, pulse, respirations
TTN:	Transient tachypnea of the newborn
UA:	Urinalysis
UAC:	Umbilical arterial catheter
umbi:	Umbilical
US:	Ultrasound
UVC:	Umbilical venous catheter
VLBW:	Very low birth weight
VS:	Vital signs
WBC:	White blood cell
wt:	Weight

Glossary

A

ABG: See **Blood gas, arterial.**

Account manager: An individual, employed by the hospital treating your baby, who is assigned to handle the financial details of your baby's case.

Acetaminophen: Medication for relief of pain and lowering of body temperature that does not contain aspirin. Tylenol and Tempra are two of the brand names for acetaminophen.

Acrocyanosis: A bluish color to the skin of the hands and feet, caused by decreased circulation (especially if the infant's hands or feet are cool). A normal occurrence in newborns.

Acuity, visual: Sharpness of sight.

Acute care: Care given in an emergency or life-threatening situation.

Acquired immune deficiency syndrome: See **AIDS.**

Admitting privileges: Authorization (or authority) of a health care provider to have patients cared for at a given hospital.

ADN: Associate degree in nursing. A two-year community college nursing training program. Denotes educational level, not professional nursing licensure.

Adoption: The voluntary taking on of legal responsibility for a child who is not one's own.

Advanced registered nurse practitioner: See **ARNP.**

Advocate: Someone who speaks for and actively promotes another's best interests.

AIDS: Acquired immune deficiency syndrome. Caused by infection with the human immunodeficiency virus (HIV), which impairs the body's immune response. Increases the body's susceptibility to one or more secondary (opportunistic) infections that characterize the syndrome.

Air leak, pulmonary: Caused when air tears one or more breathing sacs (alveoli) in the lungs and leaks into spaces around the lung tissue.

Airway: The route by which air passes from the nose or mouth to the lungs; the breathing passages. Also, a tube or oral appliance used to provide a route for air to the lungs.

Albumin: The protein portion of the blood serum. Important for maintenance of blood volume.

Alveoli: Small air sacs in the lung.

Ambu-bag: The trade name for an anesthesia bag or oxygen bag. Used for delivery of air/oxygen mixture to the infant. When the bag is inflated with compressed air/oxygen, it is squeezed and delivers air/oxygen to the infant's lungs through a face mask or breathing tube.

Amino acid: The protein component essential to body cells.

Amniotic fluid: Liquid that surrounds the fetus inside the mother's uterus.

Amniotic membrane: The sac that surrounds the fetus inside the mother's uterus. Breaks before or during labor, allowing the amniotic fluid inside to escape (often referred to as when "the mother's water breaks").

Amniotomy: See **Artificial rupture of membranes.**

Anal atresia: See **Imperforate anus.**

Analgesia: Pain medication that relieves or decreases awareness of pain. Analgesia does not cause unconsciousness or loss of sensation (numbness).

Anemia: A condition marked by lower-than-normal hemoglobin and hematocrit levels in the blood.

Anesthesia: A medication that reduces or eliminates the sensation of pain or that produces loss of consciousness and, as a result, inability to feel pain.

Anesthesia, epidural: A type of regional anesthesia used during labor or cesarean birth to make a patient unable to feel pain from the navel to the midthigh; body coverage can be extended depending on the patient's anesthesia needs. An epidural block is injected through a catheter into the space outside the covering of the spinal cord.

Anesthesia, general: A drug given through an intravenous (IV) line and/or through inhalation. Produces unconsciousness and, as a result, blocks any sensation of pain.

Anesthesia, local: A type of nerve block that makes a patient unable to feel pain in a small specific area of the body. Does not cause loss of consciousness.

Anesthesia, regional: A type of nerve block that makes a patient unable to feel pain in a specifically targeted area of the body. Does not cause unconsciousness. Epidural block and spinal anesthesia are examples of regional anesthesia.

Anesthesiologist: A physician with specialized training in giving medications that reduce or abolish pain and/or cause unconsciousness.

Ankyloglossia: A physical characteristic in which a shorter-than-normal connection exists between the tongue and the floor of the mouth and interferes with free protrusion of the tongue. Commonly called "tongue-tied."

Anomaly, congenital: A defect existing at birth; an external or internal abnormality of an organ or structure. Commonly called a birth defect. See also **Malformation, congenital.**

Anterior: Located in the front or forward section of a body part or organ.

Antibiotic: A drug that kills bacteria or reduces their growth. Used to treat infection.

Antibiotic ointment: Medication applied to the skin surface to fight infectious bacteria.

Antibody: A disease-fighting substance in the blood; antibodies attack foreign substances in the body.

Anticonvulsant: Medication that stops or reduces involuntary muscle contractions (seizures).

Aorta: A large, branched artery that carries blood from the heart to the main arteries of the body.

Aortic arch: The part of the aortic artery that extends upward over the heart, through which blood passes as it flows to the body.

Aortic stenosis: A narrowing of the valve between the left ventricle of the heart and the aorta; reduces blood flow to the body. Can result from a birth defect.

Apgar score: The numerical result of a newborn assessment generally done at 1 minute and again at 5 minutes after birth; assesses heart rate, breathing, color, tone, and reflexes. A maximum of two points for each sign is given. A ten, the highest score, indicates an infant in optimum condition; lower scores (commonly seen in preterm infants) indicate less responsiveness. Apgar scoring may be continued every 5 minutes for up to 20 minutes or until two successive scores are eight or more.

APIB: See **Assessment of preterm infant behavior.**

Apnea: Pauses in breathing of 20 seconds or longer, or pauses of any length accompanied by cyanosis and bradycardia.

Apnea monitor: A mechanical device that is usually set to alarm if apnea occurs and/or if the heart rate slows or speeds up abnormally. This term usually refers to the monitor used by selected babies who require monitoring at home after discharge.

Apneic: A term for a baby who is experiencing apnea.

Appropriate for gestational age (AGA): A term for a newborn whose weight (and possibly length, and head circumference) falls between the 10th and 90th percentiles on a standard intrauterine growth chart; indicates appropriate growth for the length of time the baby was in the uterus. An AGA baby can be preterm, term, or postterm.

Areola: The brownish or pink circular area around the nipple of the breast.

ARNP: Advanced registered nurse practitioner. A legal term for professional licensure; may be used by a neonatal nurse practitioner.

Arrhythmia: A change in the regularity of the heartbeat.

Arterial line: A tube inserted into a major artery; used for administration of fluids and/or medications and sometimes for monitoring blood pressure. Some types can be used to withdraw blood for laboratory work.

Arterioles: A small branch of an artery, leading into many small vessels.

Artificial rupture of membranes (AROM): A procedure in which the physician or midwife "breaks" the bag of waters surrounding the fetus; used to augment labor. Also called an amniotomy.

Asphyxia: The result of insufficient oxygen reaching the body cells. The term denotes progressive hypoxia and an accumulation of carbon dioxide and acid waste products in the blood. If left uncorrected, asphyxia can result in permanent brain and organ damage or in death.

Aspirate/Aspiration: Breathing of a substance other than air (for example, regurgitated stomach contents, meconium, milk, or formula) into the trachea or lungs. Also, the removal of fluids from the body by suctioning.

Assessment: An evaluation of a baby's general condition and anything that differs from the baby's usual status. Nursing and medical actions are based on continuous assessment of the baby's condition.

Assessment of preterm infant behavior (APIB): A formal evaluation of a preterm baby's unique responses to and interaction with stimuli. Provides information on the baby's development and tolerance to handling. The APIB is useful for generating individual developmental care plans.

Asthma: A condition in which breathing (especially exhalation) is difficult and often accompanied by wheezing and tightness in the chest.

Associate Degree in Nursing: See **ADN.**

Asymmetry: A lack of balance, equality, or sameness on opposite sides of a dividing line (such as the left and right sides of the body); affects corresponding parts differently.

Atelectasis: The collapse of groups of alveoli (air sacs) in the lungs.

Atresia: A birth defect in which a passage (such as a valve, a vein, or an artery) is completely blocked or is absent.

Atretic: Having to do with an atresia.

Atrial: Having to do with the atrium (one of the two upper chambers of the heart).

Atrial septal defect (ASD): A birth defect in which a hole is present in the wall (septum) between the two upper chambers (atria) of the heart.

Atrium: One of the two upper chambers of the heart (plural: atria).

Attending physician: The physician who oversees your baby's treatment; may or may not perform all procedures.

Audiologist: A physician who specializes in diagnosing and treating hearing difficulties.

Audiology screening: A hearing test.

Auditory: Having to do with hearing.

Augmentation, labor: A method used to promote more effective uterine contractions when labor has already begun or contractions have stopped.

Autopsy: An examination by a pathologist of a body after death to determine the cause.

Aversion, oral: A negative association with or response to anything placed in or near the mouth.

Axillary: Having to do with the armpit.

Axillary temperature: A body temperature taken by placing a thermometer snugly between the skin of the chest and the inner upper arm.

B

Baby Doe Regulations: The results of a federal administrative ruling in 1983 that declared it a violation to withhold food or medical care from an infant on the basis of a handicapping condition. Ultimately, the ruling was revised to include provisions that place the primary responsibility for decision making about a handicapped or severely ill child with the parents, as long as their decisions are in the child's best interests; also places the responsibility for child protection with the states and instructs the state to intervene if parents do not act in the child's best interest.

Bachelor of Science in Nursing: See **BSN.**

Back transport: The return of a baby from the hospital of current treatment to the hospital where the pregnant woman or newborn was originally admitted and previously treated or to a local hospital for further care when the problems that required transport have resolved. Also called return transport.

Bacteria: Single-cell microorganisms that can cause infection in humans; can also be protective or helpful, however.

Bagging: Gently pumping oxygen into the lungs using an oxygen bag and a face mask or endotracheal tube. Also called hand-bagging. See also **Bag-mask ventilation.**

Bag-mask ventilation: A method used to "breathe" for a baby; the oxygen mask is placed firmly over the nose and mouth of the baby, and oxygen from the oxygen bag is puffed into the baby's lungs. This method is also called "bagging the baby."

Balloon atrial septostomy: A procedure used during heart catheterization to enlarge the hole in the wall between the two upper chambers of the heart.

Balloon valvuloplasty: A procedure used to enlarge a constricted heart valve. A balloon is fed into the heart inside a catheter and then inflated inside the valve.

Barrier property: The protective function of the skin; insulates and protects from infection.

Behavioral disorganization: Unpredictable activity patterns. Usually refers to the preterm infant's inability to organize endogenous rhythms, physiologic functions, and behavior to respond appropriately to the environment.

Bile: Green-colored liquid secreted by the liver and stored in the gallbladder. Intermittently ejected into the duodenum (upper portion of the small intestine).

Bilirubin ("bili"): The substance released when the body breaks down red blood cells; converted by the liver and disposed of mainly in the stool. Buildup of bilirubin in the blood may cause jaundice.

Birth defect: See **Anomaly, congenital.**

Bleed, a: Medical jargon for an intracranial or intraventricular hemorrhage.

Bleeding time: A laboratory test in which the time required for a sample of blood to clot is measured.

Blood culture: A laboratory test in which blood is placed on a special dish and microscopically monitored to see if harmful microorganisms grow. The purpose is to determine the presence and type of infectious agent.

Blood gas, arterial (ABG): A laboratory test performed on blood taken from an artery to determine levels of oxygen, carbon dioxide, and acid. The oxygen level of an ABG is more reliable than the oxygen level from veins or capillaries in helping to evaluate the baby's respiratory status.

Blood gas, capillary (CBG): A laboratory test performed on blood taken from a capillary (generally by pricking the baby's heel) to determine levels of oxygen, carbon dioxide, and acid. An important test for evaluating a baby's respiratory status.

Blood gas, venous (VBG): A laboratory test performed on blood taken from a vein to determine levels of oxygen, carbon dioxide, and acid. An important test for evaluating a baby's respiratory status.

Blood glucose: The concentration of glucose (sugar) in the blood.

Blue: A term denoting poor tissue oxygenation. See also **Cyanosis, color.**

Board certified: A term for a doctor who has taken and passed a standardized examination specific to a given medical specialty. Not required for medical licensure; denotes professional excellence in the specialty.

Bolus: A volume of fluid given all at once, instead of over a long period of time.

Booster: A dose of vaccine given sometime after the original vaccine is given to maintain or increase the effectiveness of an immunization.

Boundaries: Physical things (such as blankets, special buntings, or a hand) used to encircle or contain a baby or to create a sort of nest and to help the baby bring and keep the arms and legs close to the body; provide a feeling of security and promote behavioral organization.

Bradycardia: A significant slowing of the heart rate below the individual's normal rate. Generally, bradycardia for a newborn may be defined as a heart rate of less than 100 beats per minute. May accompany apnea and/or cyanosis, or occur independently.

Brain stem: One of three primary divisions of the brain; the stalk of the brain. All nerve fibers relaying signals between the spinal cord and the higher brain centers pass through the brain stem.

Breast milk: Milk produced by the breasts of a woman. Contains components that promote the baby's growth, enhance digestion, and protect from infection.

Breast pump: A mechanical device used to remove milk from the breasts.

Breathing, periodic: A cyclic pattern of brief (about five- to ten-second) pauses in breathing in babies, without any change in heart rate or skin color. A common pattern in preterm infants; also seen in some healthy term infants in the first few days of life.

Breech presentation: The birth position in which a baby's buttocks or feet approach the opening to the birth canal before the head.

Bromocriptine: A drug that suppresses milk production in the postpartum woman; rarely prescribed today because of potentially dangerous side effects.

Bronchioles: Small airways in the lungs; a subdivision of the bronchial tree.

Bronchitis: Inflammation or infection of the tubes leading to the lungs (the bronchial tubes).

Bronchopulmonary dysplasia (BPD): A chronic lung disease primarily affecting premature infants who have been mechanically ventilated; involves air sac damage, scarring of the lung tissue, and areas of atelectasis.

Bronchospasm: A contraction of the smooth muscle and a narrowing of the large air passages that lead to the lungs. Seen in asthma and bronchopulmonary dysplasia.

Brown adipose tissue (BAT): A special kind of fat around the shoulders, the base of the neck, the chest bone, and some organs in newborns. Newborns use BAT to produce heat because it breaks down more easily and makes heat more quickly than white fat does. Preterm babies have only small amounts.

BSN: Bachelor of Science in Nursing. A four-year college nursing training program. Denotes educational level, not professional licensure.

Bulb syringe: A tool used to apply suction by hand to remove secretions from the nose and the mouth of an infant.

Button gastrostomy: A modification of a gastrostomy with a valve on the abdominal wall. Usually done when an infant with long-term feeding problems reaches about 10 pounds or two to three months of age. Permits removal of the gastrostomy tube after each feeding and closure of the abdominal opening.

C

C-section: See **Cesarean section.**

Caffeine: A medication that stimulates the central nervous system; can be given to infants to reduce occurrences of apnea of prematurity.

Calorie: A measure of the energy value of food.

Cannula, nasal: A soft plastic tubing that wraps around a baby's face and has openings under the baby's nose. Used to deliver humidified oxygen.

Cannulation: A surgical procedure performed to place catheters into the body, as in extracorporeal membrane oxygenation (ECMO) therapy.

Capillaries: Extremely tiny blood vessels that form networks in most tissues, supply cells with oxygen and nutrients, and remove wastes.

Carbon dioxide (CO_2): A waste product of energy production in the body. Removed from the blood as it passes through the lungs and is exhaled.

Cardiac: Having to do with the heart.

Cardiac output: The amount of blood that the heart pumps out in a given period of time.

Cardiologist: A physician who specializes in diagnosing and treating problems associated with the heart.

Cardiopulmonary resuscitation (CPR): A technique for reviving someone whose breathing has stopped (or has slowed greatly) or whose heart is not beating (or is beating very slowly). Cardiopulmonary resuscitation involves artificial respirations and cardiac compressions.

Cardiorespiratory monitor: An electronic device attached to babies in NICUs to monitor heart rate and rate of breathing; sounds an alarm if either falls below or exceeds a desirable level.

Cardiorespiratory system: The body system made up of the heart, blood vessels, and lungs.

Cardiovascular: Having to do with the heart and blood vessels.

Care conference: A scheduled meeting at which members of a baby's health care team update parents on baby's health status, changes in the care plan, and expectations for improvement; questions are answered; parental involvement in care is sought if possible.

Care map: See **Clinical pathway.**

Care plan: An individualized outline that guides medical and nursing activities for a baby; revised as the baby's condition changes. Helps provide consistent methods of caregiving to meet the individual needs of the baby.

Carotid arteries: Large arteries in the neck that carry oxygenated blood from the heart to the brain. Internal and external carotid arteries are located on each side of the neck.

Case manager: A patient advocate who coordinates formal and informal health services during hospitalization. Also, insurance companies may utilize a case manager to oversee the financial aspects of hospitalization and/or home care.

Catastrophic illness: In connection with health care coverage, a major illness involving a lengthy hospital stay (usually) and high medical bills. If an insurance carrier provides catastrophic coverage, it pays 100 percent of the bills above a stated dollar amount of costs.

Catheter: A thin, flexible tube through which fluids are given to or removed from the body.

Catheter, umbilical arterial (UAC): A thin, flexible tube inserted into one of the two arteries (blood vessels) in the umbilical cord of the newborn. Can be used to provide fluids and medications, to remove blood for testing, and to monitor blood pressure. Also called an "umbi line."

Catheter, umbilical venous (UVC): A thin, flexible tube inserted into a vein in the umbilical cord of a newborn to facilitate administration of medications and/or fluids into the baby's bloodstream and to monitor blood pressure.

Catheterization: A procedure in which a thin, flexible tube (a catheter) is inserted into a body. In cardiac catheterization, the tube is fed (slowly advanced) into arteries or veins of the arms or legs and into the heart and may contain an inflatable balloon to enlarge or open a constricted heart passage.

CBG: See **Blood gas, capillary.**

CCRN: A certification designation for nurses denoting professional excellence. Voluntary standardized testing for neonatal, adult, or pediatric critical care; not required for legal licensure.

Central Line: See **Central venous line.**

Central nervous system (CNS): The body system made up of the brain and spinal cord.

Central venous line: An intravenous (IV) line fed through a vein to a location close to the heart. Also called a central line.

Cephalhematoma: A localized swelling on the head of a newborn caused by a collection of blood between one of the skull bones and its membranous covering.

Cerebellum: The rounded portion of the hindbrain. Serves to coordinate movement, posture, and balance.

Cerebral: Having to do with the brain.

Cerebral cortex: The outer layer (and nerve center) of the brain.

Cerebral palsy (CP): A condition in which posture or movement is abnormal because of a malformation of the brain or damage to the brain at or before birth, or after birth resulting from infection, faulty development, or lack of oxygen. The cause of CP is often unknown.

Cerebrospinal fluid: Fluid surrounding the brain and spinal cord. Acts as a cushion for those organs.

Certified registered nurse: See **RNC.**

Certified registered nurse anesthetist: See **CRNA.**

Cervix: The narrow passage at the end of the uterus closest to the vagina (birth canal). The passage dilates (expands) as labor progresses.

Cesarean section: A surgical procedure in which an incision is made through the abdomen into the uterus to deliver the baby. Also called a C-section.

Chest PT: See **Physiotherapy, chest.**

Child restraint system (CRS): A term for a car seat, or child safety seat. Used to contain an infant or child in a moving vehicle.

Chorioamnionitis: An infection of the membranes that contain the amniotic fluid in the uterus.

Chromosome: One of 46 threadlike structures (23 coming from the mother and 23 from the father) that make up the center of each cell in the human body. Chromosomes carry genetic information in the form of genes.

Chromosome defect: See **Genetic defect.**

Chronic: Lasting for a long period of time; long term.

Chronic-care facility: A facility that cares for patients with severe physical or mental disabilities or with fatal conditions. Also called a long-term care facility.

Chronic sorrow: An ongoing, unresolved feeling of sadness (sometimes intense; other times barely recognizable) in response to a negative situation that cannot be made right or resolved.

Chronic stress: Ongoing, long-term stress, often resulting from an unresolvable situation.

Circulatory system: The body system made up of the vessels through which blood and other fluids move.

Circumcision: The surgical procedure in which the foreskin covering the tip of the penis is removed.

Cleft lip: A birth defect marked by internal and external malformations of the mouth and nose areas. Usually involves an opening or slit from the upper lip to one or both nostrils. Sometimes accompanied by cleft palate.

Cleft palate: A birth defect marked by an opening in the roof of the mouth connecting the oral and nasal cavities. Sometimes accompanied by cleft lip.

Clinical nurse specialist: See **CNS.**

Clinical pathway: The normal, expected pattern or progression of a disease or a developmental sequence over a specific period of time in the majority of patients; not specific to an individual patient. Also called a care map or a critical pathway.

CNS: Clinical nurse specialist. A registered nurse with a master's degree who provides clinical expertise and information to the nursing staff; may be involved in teaching, research, consultation, and program development, as well as in patient care. Also, an abbreviation for central nervous system.

Coarctation of the aorta: A birth defect in which the main artery from the heart to the body (the aorta) is constricted, obstructing blood flow to the body.

Cold stress: Physiologic responses to a lower than normal body temperature such as increased metabolism and increased oxygen consumption; cold stress can lead to weight loss or failure to gain weight and respiratory distress.

Color: In reference to a baby, the look of the skin denoting general health, especially oxygenation. Normal color of the mucous membranes (inner lips, tongue, and gums) is a healthy pink, regardless of ethnicity. A pale, dusky (bluish pink), or blue color of the mucous membranes or a yellowish skin color may indicate medical problems.

Colostomy: A surgical opening made in the abdominal wall so that part of the large intestine can be attached to the abdominal wall surface; stool then drains from the bowel into a collecting bag or pouch placed over the opening. Often performed after surgical removal of part of the intestine because of disease (most commonly necrotizing enterocolitis) or malformation.

Colostrum: The thick, clear or yellowish secretion produced by the breasts of pregnant women beginning about week 16 of pregnancy; changes to a thinner, whiter substance called mature milk within a few days after the birth of a baby. Colostrum is rich in protein and immune factors.

Community hospital: A local hospital. Usually has an obstetrics and newborn area equipped to care for healthy mothers and newborn babies, to evaluate and stabilize patients for transport, and in some cases, to care for mildly ill and convalescing mothers and babies. See also **Level I nursery and Level II nursery.**

Complete blood count (CBC): A laboratory test that measures the cellular components—red blood cells (RBCs), white blood cells (WBCs), and platelets—in the blood. Often done as one of a series of tests to detect infection.

Compliance: When referring to the lung, the degree of flexibility.

Complication: A setback or physical difficulty related to (and resulting from) a medical condition, disease, or problem or to the treatment for that problem.

Compression, chest: Application of pressure to the chest, squeezing the heart between the breastbone and the spine to artificially pump the heart.

Computed tomography (CT) scan: A diagnostic imaging technique that uses a narrow beam of radiation (x-ray) rotated around the body and a computer to construct two-dimensional cross-sectional pictures of internal body structures. Among other uses, aids in diagnosis of bleeding or excess fluid in the brain.

Conditioned response: A learned action that occurs uncontrollably in reaction to a specific stimulus.

Congenital: Existing at birth.

Congenital heart defect: A malformation of the heart or of the blood vessels near it that exists at birth. Caused by abnormal development of the organ or vessels during gestation. Can be minor or life-threatening.

Congestive heart failure (CHF): A condition in which the heart has trouble meeting the body's energy needs. Not a disease itself, but the result of an underlying condition such as a congenital heart defect, severe anemia, or a patent ductus arteriosus.

Consent: Written permission granted for a specific medical procedure, often a surgery. "Giving informed consent" means that you understand what you are agreeing to and that all of your questions have been answered.

Constrict: To narrow or compress.

Containment, body: The encircling or nesting of a baby using boundaries (rolled blankets, special buntings, or a hand) to help the baby bring and keep the arms and legs close to the body. Provides a feeling of security and promotes behavioral organization. See also **Nest.**

Continuity, patient: For a health care provider (especially a nurse), a system that promotes familiarity with patients through consistency in patient care assignments.

Continuous positive airway pressure (CPAP): Air or an air–oxygen mixture mechanically pushed into a baby's lungs to keep the air sacs open after each breath, reducing the effort the baby must make to breathe; usually delivered through short tubes placed in the nose (nasal CPAP) or through an endotracheal (ET) tube.

Contracture: A tightness or stiffness (resistance to stretching) of a muscle or joint.

Contraindication: A reason a patient may not receive a medication or a treatment.

Contrast enhancement: A dye or some other material injected into the body to produce a difference between the appearance of two types of body structures on the images produced by radiography (conventional x-ray or CT scan).

Coping mechanism: A way or ways in which individuals deal with difficult situations and the stress they produce. Also called a coping strategy.

Corrected age: The number of weeks or months since a baby's birth, minus the number of weeks or months the baby was born before the due date. An important consideration when assessing the developmental level of the preterm infant.

Cot death: See **Sudden infant death syndrome.**

CPAP: See **Continuous positive airway pressure.**

CPR: See **Cardiopulmonary resuscitation.**

Crib death: See **Sudden infant death syndrome.**

CRNA: Certified registered nurse anesthetist. A registered nurse with advanced practice education who, under the supervision of and in collaboration with an anesthesiologist, is qualified to give medications that reduce or abolish pain and/or cause unconsciousness.

Critical pathway: See **Clinical pathway.**

Cryotherapy: A treatment involving use of liquid nitrogen to freeze tissues, as in treatment of retinopathy of prematurity (ROP).

CT scan: See **Computed tomography scan.**

Cue: An action or behavior that can indicate a baby's readiness for and reaction to stimulation; one means of infant communication.

Culture: A laboratory test in which blood or another body fluid is placed on a special dish and watched to see if microorganisms grow. The purpose of a culture is to determine presence of infection.

Cutdown: A surgical incision made into a blood vessel. Sometimes used for placement of a central line.

Cyanosis: A condition in which the skin and mucous membranes have a bluish color, caused by lack of oxygen in the tissues.

Cyanosis, circumoral: A condition in which the skin around the mouth has a bluish color, caused by lack of oxygen to the cells.

Cyanosis, generalized: A condition in which the skin over the entire body and of the mucous membranes has a bluish color, caused by lack of oxygen in the tissues. Also called central cyanosis.

Cyanotic defect: A heart defect that causes blood going to the body to contain a lower-than-normal amount of oxygen.

Cyst: A membrane-covered sac (often filled with liquid or a semisolid material) that develops abnormally in a body cavity or structure.

Cytomegalovirus (CMV): A virus that causes cellular enlargement and that often infects those with suppressed immune systems (such as in AIDS).

D

Decannulation: The removal of a tube, such as a catheter used in extracorporeal membrane oxygenation therapy or a tracheostomy tube.

Deductible: In connection with health care coverage, the amount you must pay before the insurance carrier begins to cover the bills.

Defense mechanism: One of the factors in the human body that protect it from infection.

Dehydrate: To lose body fluids or water.

Dehydration: The loss of water or fluids from the body.

Dependence, drug: The state of having grown accustomed to a drug's effects. Characterized by withdrawal symptoms experienced when the drug is stopped.

Depression: A mental and emotional state marked by fatigue, sadness, reduced activity, difficulty thinking, changes in eating and sleeping patterns, feelings of hopelessness, and sometimes thoughts of suicide.

Desaturation, oxygen: Too little oxygen bound to hemoglobin molecules in the bloodstream; causes lack of oxygen in the tissues.

Developmental delay: A slowness in mastering motor coordination skills (such as lifting the head, rolling over, or sitting), behavioral skills (such as self-calming or controlling anger), and living skills (such as learning simple tasks or mastering more complex schoolwork).

Developmental milestone: One of the many important basic skills an average baby masters at a specific age—for example, sitting with support by six months of age.

Developmental outcome: A baby's ability, as he or she grows, to master physical, behavioral, and emotional skills of living.

Developmental specialist: A health care provider who has special training in diagnosing and treating delays in a child's mastery of motor coordination and behavioral and learning skills.

Diagnosis: A conclusion about the cause of a medical problem.

Diagnostic imaging: Producing "pictures" of the inside of the body without opening it up, to identify the cause(s) and to help in the treatment of medical problems. Types of diagnostic imaging include the computed tomography (CT) scan, ultrasound, and magnetic resonance imaging (MRI).

Diagnostic testing: Laboratory and other tests (such as imaging techniques that produce "pictures" of the inside of the body) performed to help medical caregivers determine what is wrong with a patient.

Diaphragm: The dome-shaped muscle just below the lungs and above the stomach that separates the chest cavity from the abdominal cavity. Plays an important role in breathing.

Diaphragmatic hernia: A life-threatening birth defect caused by the fetal bowel pushing up into the chest cavity through an abnormal hole in the muscle separating the chest from the abdomen (the diaphragm).

Diarrhea: Frequent watery or liquid stools (feces); often foul smelling.

Digital: Something that shows results in numbers—for example, a thermometer that displays the number 98.6°F when reporting temperature.

Dilate: To enlarge, stretch, or widen.

Diploma program: A two- or three-year hospital training program for nursing. Denotes educational preparation, not nursing licensure.

Disability: A physical or mental abnormality or restriction.

Discharge coordinator: See **Discharge planner.**

Discharge planner: A nurse or other trained individual on the hospital's staff who makes all arrangements for a baby's release from the hospital and for any special care the baby may need after discharge. Also called a discharge coordinator.

Discharge planning: The process carried out by trained hospital staff to ensure that all designated medical care activities, tests, and parent teaching are completed before a baby's release from the hospital and that arrangements are made for any needed follow-up or special care.

Discharge summary: A written report of a baby's prenatal history and events of labor, birth, and hospitalization.

Disseminated intravascular coagulation (DIC): Bleeding at more than one location in the body because of toxins in the bloodstream released by infectious microorganisms.

Distention: An enlargement or swelling, especially caused by pressure from the inside.

Diuretic: A medication that removes excess fluid from the body by increasing urine production.

Do Not Resuscitate (DNR) order: A medical order written when a terminally ill or severely disabled patient is to be permitted to die peacefully, without futile attempts at revival.

Doppler ultrasound: An enhancement to a regular ultrasound scan. Detects blood flow disturbances caused by abnormalities in internal body structure. Used for an echocardiogram.

Down syndrome: A birth defect characterized by specific physical features and caused by an extra 21st chromosome. Also called trisomy 21.

DPT: Diphtheria-pertussis-tetanus vaccine.

Ductus arteriosus: A short vessel connecting the pulmonary artery with the aorta in the fetus. Before birth, sends most of the blood directly from the right ventricle of the heart to the aorta, bypassing the lungs; normally closes shortly after birth.

Duodenal atresia: A birth defect marked by a blockage in the upper portion (duodenum) of the small bowel.

Durable medical equipment (DME) company: A private firm that supplies medical equipment prescribed by a physician for home use, trains users in its operation and maintenance, and deals with equipment problems.

Dusky: A descriptive term for the bluish-pink color of skin and mucous membranes of babies who are cyanotic (whose cells lack oxygen).

Dynamics: The ways in which individuals interact; include such aspects as who leads and who follows and whether members share thoughts and feelings openly.

E

Early-intervention program: A public program designed to prevent developmental delays in at-risk children and to aid children already showing delays.

ECG: See **Electrocardiogram.**

Echocardiogram: An ultrasound of the heart.

Echocardiography: A diagnostic imaging technique in which an ultrasound of the heart is made.

Eclampsia: A term used to denote neurologic involvement that results in a seizure as a result of pregnancy-induced hypertension. A woman with this condition is said to be eclamptic.

ECMO: See **Extracorporeal membrane oxygenation.**

ECMO specialist: A trained medical caregiver (usually a specially trained nurse or respiratory therapist) who monitors and maintains an extracorporeal membrane oxygenation circuit at all times while it is operating.

Edema: An accumulation of excess fluid in body tissues, generally causing swelling.

EEG: See **Electroencephalogram.**

EFM: See **Electronic fetal monitoring.**

EKG: See **Electrocardiogram.**

Electrocardiogram (ECG or EKG): A diagnostic test that records the electrical activity of the heart and helps caregivers determine how well it is functioning.

Electrode: See **Lead.**

Electroencephalogram (EEG): A diagnostic test that records the electrical impulses of the brain; helps caregivers determine how well it is functioning.

Electrolytes ("lytes"): Basic body chemicals in the blood; essential for proper cell functioning. Include sodium (Na), potassium (K), chloride (Cl), calcium (Ca), and magnesium (Mg). Also, a laboratory test that measures the balance of these elements in the blood.

Electronic fetal monitoring (EFM): Using an electronic device to track an unborn baby's heart rate and monitor maternal uterine contractions, often during labor.

Embolus, air: A bubble of air obstructing blood flow through a blood vessel (plural: emboli).

Endothelial-derived relaxing factor (EDRF): A natural substance released by the body that helps relax and therefore open the arterioles (blood vessels near the breathing sacs in the lungs) after birth. Nitric oxide is an EDRF.

Endotracheal (ET) tube: A tube placed into the windpipe (trachea) through the nose or mouth to assist babies with breathing difficulties. Insertion of the tube is called intubation; removal, extubation. A baby with an ET tube is assisted with continuous positive airway pressure (CPAP) or a ventilator.

Engorgement, postpartum: A condition caused by increased blood flow and overfilling of the breasts with milk, often two to three days after delivery. Breasts become hard, painful, and warm; the skin covering them may feel tight; and swelling may extend into the armpits.

Enterohepatic shunt: A mechanism by which bilirubin (that has been processed by the liver [hepatic]) is unprocessed in the intestine (entero). In the first week of life there is a high concentration of the enzyme that initiates this conversion.

Enzyme: A complex protein produced by body cells. Makes possible certain necessary chemical reactions in the body.

Episiotomy: A surgical incision to enlarge a woman's vaginal opening shortly before the birth of a baby.

Erythropoietin: A hormone that controls red blood cell production.

Esophageal atresia: A birth defect marked by blockage or malformation of the esophagus (food pipe).

Esophagus: The passage from the mouth to the stomach. Also called the food pipe.

Estrogen: A hormone produced mainly by the ovaries; controls female sexual development.

Ethics: An area of study that involves moral principles or practice.

ET tube: See **Endotracheal tube.**

Exogenous: Not produced by the body.

Expiration, active: The mechanical pulling of gas out of the lung during the exhalation part of a breath; used in high-frequency oscillatory ventilation.

Expiration, passive: An exhalation portion of a breath that is allowed to occur naturally through relaxation (automatic recoil) of the breathing muscles of the chest wall and diaphragm; used in conventional ventilation, high-frequency positive pressure ventilation, high-frequency jet ventilation, and high-frequency flow interruption ventilation, and unassisted breathing.

Extracorporeal membrane oxygenation (ECMO): A mechanical technique for supporting both the heart and lung functions of critically ill term or near-term babies with severe lung failure; used when the baby does not respond to conventional ventilation and/or medication therapy. Equipment is a modified version of the heart-lung bypass machine used during open-heart surgery.

Extrauterine: Outside the uterus.

Extubate: To remove an endotracheal (ET) tube.

Eye patches: Soft coverings placed over a baby's eyes during phototherapy treatment to prevent possible injury to the eyes from bright light.

F

Failure to thrive: A term used to describe the condition of a baby or young child who, although there are no identifiable physical reasons for it, does not grow and develop normally.

Feeding on demand: Letting the baby decide when and how much to eat.

Feeding pump: A device attached to a feeding tube and used to feed babies who cannot handle large amounts of food at one time. Meters a tiny amount of breast milk or formula into the feeding tube and allows for continuous tube feeding.

Feeding tube: A narrow, flexible tube inserted through the infant's nose (nasogastric) or mouth (orogastric) and on into the stomach to provide a route for breast milk or formula. Also called a gavage tube.

Fellow, neonatal: In a teaching hospital, a physician who has completed medical school and pediatric residency and is in training to become a neonatologist.

Fetal: Having to do with an unborn baby (a fetus).

Fetal circulation: The movement of blood through a fetus's body before birth, specifically through the fetal heart and lungs. Much of the blood bypasses the fetus's lungs because of two open fetal shunts, the foramen ovale and the ductus arteriosus.

Fetus: An unborn baby of at least 8 weeks gestation.

Fever: In an infant, a body temperature higher than 99°F (37.2°C) axillary or 100°F (37.8°C) rectally.

Fever strip: A temperature-sensitive material applied to the forehead to estimate skin temperature.

Fiberoptic blanket: A flat, flexible wrapping covered with fiberoptic lights and used for phototherapy treatment; a baby can lie on it, or the blanket can be wrapped around the baby's torso to provide phototherapy treatment.

Finger feeding: A nursery technique for feeding a breastfeeding baby whose mother is not present in order to avoid use of a bottle and nipple; caregiver places a clean, gloved finger in the baby's mouth with a feeding tube filled with milk beside it. When the baby sucks on the finger, milk is drawn from the feeding tube.

Fistula: An abnormal passage or connection between two parts of the body.

Flaring, nasal: A condition that accompanies respiratory distress in an infant; the nostrils open widely during each inspiration in order to take in as much air as possible with each breath.

Flex: To bend, especially at a joint.

Fontanel: The soft spot on the top of a baby's head; a normal opening between the bones of the skull of a fetus or young infant where skull development is incomplete.

Foramen ovale: An opening in the wall between the two upper chambers (atria) of the fetal heart; normally closes at birth.

Forceps: Curved metal tongs used by medical personnel to help deliver a baby's head during the final stages of birth.

Foremilk: Breast milk produced at the beginning of a feeding; lower in fat and calories than the milk produced toward the end of the feeding (hindmilk).

Formula: A manufactured substitute for breast milk; often made from cow's milk or soybeans.

Foster care: Care given to a child (usually for a temporary period) by one or more individuals who are not related to the child by blood or under law; foster care providers generally must follow government regulations and usually receive some financial compensation for their services.

Frenulum: Fold of mucous membrane under the tongue; a short frenulum refers to a shorter than normal band of tissue that anchors the tongue to the bottom of the mouth.

Fundoplication: Surgical treatment for gastroesophageal reflux. Tightens the valve between the esophagus (food pipe) and the stomach; prevents food from moving back up into the baby's esophagus.

Fungus: A microorganism that can cause infection; yeast (Candida) is a common fungus.

G

Gas exchange: In the lungs, addition of oxygen to the blood with removal of carbon dioxide.

Gastroenteritis: An inflammation in the bowel, usually due to infection.

Gastrointestinal: Having to do with the stomach and intestines.

Gastrointestinal (GI) system: The body system made up of the stomach and intestines.

Gastrointestinal (GI) tract: The stomach and intestines. Also called the gut.

Gastroschisis: A birth defect in which abdominal organs push outside the baby's body through an opening in the wall of the abdomen usually just to the right of the navel.

Gastrostomy: A surgical opening in the abdominal wall through which part of the stomach can be attached to the abdominal skin; a feeding tube can be inserted into the opening. Usually used only in babies expected to have long-term feeding problems.

Gastrostomy (GT) tube: A feeding tube inserted into a surgically created opening in the abdominal wall to which a portion of the stomach is attached (a gastrostomy). During feeding, a measured amount of breast milk or formula flows through the tube by gravity into the baby's stomach.

Gavage feeding: Feeding a baby through a tube inserted through the mouth (orogastric) or nose (nasogastric) into the stomach (or occasionally, the intestine). Also called tube feeding.

Gavage tube: See **Feeding tube.**

GBS pneumonia: A type of pneumonia in babies caused by Group B β-hemolytic Streptococcus (GBS).

Gene: A unit of heredity. Found in the chromosomes in each cell of the body. Determines certain traits and physical characteristics (such as eye color) of a baby.

Generic: General. In reference to a drug, one that is not proprietary—that is, is not manufactured or controlled by a single company and does not have a trademarked (brand) name. For example, acetaminophen is a generic drug; Tylenol is an acetaminophen-containing medication manufactured and sold by a company called McNeil Consumer Products.

Genetic: Having to do with the genes; something one is born with or inherits.

Genetic defect: An abnormality caused by improper development of the chromosome pairs when the egg is fertilized. Also called a chromosome defect.

Gestation: The time period required for a fertilized egg cell to develop into a baby ready for birth. Human gestation averages 266 days (or 280 days from the first day of the last menstrual period).

Gestational age: The number of completed weeks that have elapsed between the first day of the last menstrual period (not the presumed time of conception) and the date of birth.

Glucose: A simple sugar used by the body for energy.

Glucose polymers: Additives for breast milk or formula that provide sugars in a form that immature newborns can digest and absorb easily.

Glycogen: A form of glucose (sugar) that a fetus stores for use during the energy-consuming process of birth and transition to extrauterine life.

Group B β-hemolytic Streptococcus: See **Streptococcus, Group B β-hemolytic.** See also **GBS pneumonia.**

Growth factor: A substance that promotes growth, especially of the cells of the body.

Grunting: The audible sound made by an infant at exhalation that indicates a breathing problem. A compensatory mechanism that prevents the small air sacs of the lungs from completely deflating after every breath.

Gut: See **Gastrointestinal tract.**

H

Hand-bagging: See **Bagging.**

Heart murmur: A characteristic swishing sound made as blood flows through the heart. Many heart murmurs are not associated with problems.

Heelstick: A prick of a baby's heel to obtain a small amount of capillary blood for testing.

Hematocrit ("crit"): The percentage of red blood cells in the blood. Also, a laboratory test that measures the percentage; results help show a baby's ability to supply oxygen to the body tissues.

Hematologic system: The body system made up of the blood and its components: plasma (the liquid portion), red blood cells, white blood cells, and platelets (the cellular portion).

Hemoglobin (Hgb): The substance in red blood cells that carries oxygen to body cells. Also, a laboratory test that measures the amount of this substance in the cells.

Hemolysis: Destruction of red blood cells.

Hemorrhage: Heavy or uncontrollable bleeding.

Hemorrhage, postpartum: The loss of more than 500 milliliters of blood through the vagina by a mother following the birth of a baby.

Heparin: A substance that keeps blood from clotting.

Heparin lock: A cap applied to the end of the insertion site of an intravenous line so that the long tubing can be disconnected and reconnected as needed while keeping the IV patent (open and unclotted); lets the patient move more freely between administration of medication and fluids. Also called a heparin well.

Heparin well: See **Heparin lock.**

Hepatitis: A disease that causes inflammation of the liver; different types (A, B, and so on) are caused by different viruses and are transmitted by different means (water, fecal contamination, or blood and blood products).

Hernia: A protrusion of part of an internal organ through a tissue that normally contains it.

Heroic measures: "Extraordinary" medical treatments or mechanical supports provided to a patient who has uncertain likelihood of survival; refers to treatments that may be futile and/or that are a burden to the patient.

Herpes: An inflammatory disease of the skin or mucous membranes caused by a virus that reproduces in the nuclei of body cells.

Glossary

Herpes simplex virus: A microorganism that reproduces in the nuclei of body cells and causes herpes.

Hindmilk: Breast milk produced at the end of a feeding; higher in fat and calories than the first milk produced (the foremilk).

Hirschsprung's disease: A congenital problem in which the rectum and sometimes the lower colon have failed to develop a normal nerve network. Contents of the bowel accumulate and distend the upper colon. Treatment requires surgery.

HIV: Human immunodeficiency virus, the virus that causes acquired immune deficiency syndrome (AIDS).

Home care: Care for a sick or disabled individual in the individual's home instead of at a hospital or care facility.

Home health agency: A health care organization that provides skilled nursing and/or rehabilitation services in the home or place of residence.

Home visit: A visit to your home by a nurse after your baby's discharge from the hospital where your baby was treated or from a community health agency to assess your baby's well-being and progress, review care procedures, and answer your questions.

Hood: See **Oxygen hood.**

Hormone: A substance produced by body cells; circulates in body fluids and stimulates the activity of other body cells.

Human immunodeficiency virus: See **HIV.**

Humidifier: A mechanical device that adds moisture to the air.

Hyaline membrane disease (HMD): See **Respiratory distress syndrome.**

Hydrocephalus: Literally, "water on the brain"; backup of cerebrospinal fluid in the ventricles (chambers) of the brain, producing pressure that causes head enlargement and can damage brain tissue. Spina bifida is associated with hydrocephalus.

Hyperactivity: Greater-than-normal movement or activity.

Hyperalimentation: See **Total parenteral nutrition.**

Hyperbilirubinemia: A higher-than-normal level or faster-than-normal rise in the level of bilirubin in the blood.

Hyperglycemia: A higher-than-normal level of glucose (sugar) in the blood.

Hypertension: High blood pressure; specifically defined in an adult as 140 mmHg systolic over 90 mmHg diastolic ("140 over 90").

Hyperventilation: Faster-than-normal breathing at rest.

Hypervigilance: A state of being excessively watchful or concerned.

Hypocalcemia: A lower-than-normal level of calcium in the blood.

Hypoplastic left heart syndrome (HLHS): A congenital heart defect that is fatal without treatment. Includes a small aorta, heart valve narrowing or absence, and a small left atrium and ventricle. Previously treated only somewhat successfully through a series of surgeries, but improved surgical techniques and heart transplants may eventually increase the survival rate.

Hypotension: A lower-than-normal blood pressure.

Hypothermia: A lower-than-normal body temperature. In infants, can lead to breathing problems, low blood sugar, and weight loss.

Hypovolemia: A lower-than-normal blood volume (amount circulating in the body).

Hypoxia: Insufficient oxygen in the tissues.

I

I&O: Intake and output. A method of measuring and recording all fluids that go into and come out of the baby's body to ensure correct fluid balance.

Idiopathic: A term for a condition for which no cause can be identified.

Ileostomy: A surgical opening in the abdominal wall made so that part of the small intestine can be attached to the abdominal wall surface. Stool then drains from the bowel into a collecting bag or pouch placed over the opening. Often performed after surgical removal of part of the intestine because of disease or malformation.

Immaturity: A state of incomplete growth or development.

Immune: Having resistance, antibodies, or lack of susceptibility to something—generally, to infectious agents such as bacteria or viruses.

Immunization: A vaccination given to eliminate or reduce a person's likelihood of getting a specific disease.

Immunoglobulin: A protein molecule that acts as an antibody, a disease-fighting substance in the blood. Some types of immunoglobulins can cross the placenta from mother to fetus during the final three months of pregnancy. Breast milk also contains immunoglobulins. Some types of immunoglobulins can be given to high-risk infants through an intravenous line as a preventive measure.

Imperforate anus: A birth defect in which the anal canal and/or opening is absent. Also called anal atresia.

Incarcerated hernia: A hernia in which the protruding body organ becomes trapped in the space it has invaded.

Incision: The cut made into tissue with a knife or scalpel for a surgical procedure.

Incubator: A transparent, boxlike enclosure in which sick or preterm babies are placed. Allows control of the temperature around the baby and provides limited protection of the baby from infectious agents. See also **Isolette.**

Individualized family service plan (IFSP): An outline for action prepared by a team of professionals participating in a state-sponsored early-intervention program who have assessed a developmentally delayed baby's needs, along with those of the family.

Induction, labor: Refers to deliberate initiation of uterine contractions with medication before labor begins on its own. Used only when medically indicated.

Infant of a diabetic mother (IDM): A baby, often preterm and large for gestational age, born to a diabetic mother.

Infection: An invasion of body cells and/or tissues by harmful microorganisms (bacteria, viruses, fungi, or protozoa) that generally multiply once established. Also, the body's response to the invasion.

Infection, acquired: Infection passed to a baby after birth.

Infection, congenital: See **Infection, intrauterine.**

Infection, intrauterine: Infection contracted by a fetus across the placenta (vertical transmission). Also called a congenital infection. For types, see **TORCH.**

Infection, perinatal: Infection passed to the fetus through the birth canal during development (especially if the amniotic membranes are ruptured) or contracted by the baby as he or she passes through the birth canal.

Infiltrated IV: An intravenous line that has become obstructed or dislodged from the vein, causing IV fluid to leak out of the vein and into the surrounding tissue.

Infusion, IV: Continuous instillation of a solution into a vein. Usually metered by a pump.

Inguinal hernia: A protrusion, in males, of part of the intestine into the scrotum through a gap in the muscle wall. In females, part of the intestine can slide into the groin. More commonly seen in males than in females.

Inhalatory: A term used to describe something (usually a medication) taken by breathing it in.

Insulin: A hormone produced by the pancreas. Helps move glucose from the blood into the cells.

Insurance case manager: An individual employed by your insurance carrier and assigned to handle the financial aspects of your baby's case.

Intensive care nursery: See **Level III nursery.**

Intermediate care: The level of care for sick and convalescing babies who do not require intensive care but do require medical and nursing supervision and caregiving; the form of care focused on preparing recovering babies for hospital discharge.

Intern: A physician who has graduated from medical school and is in the first year of a hospital-based program of specialized training; works under the close supervision of residents.

Intervention: A medical or nursing action or procedure.

Intracranial hemorrhage: A bleeding in or around the brain. Also called a bleed.

Intramuscular (IM): A term for a medication route into the muscle by needle. In lay terms, a "shot" is administration of an intramuscular medication.

Intraparenchymal: Within the functional tissue of an organ.

Intravenous (IV) catheter/line: A thin tube inserted into a vein by means of a needle (the needle is removed after the catheter is in the vein). Supplies medications, fluids, or nutrients directly into the bloodstream. Also called a peripheral line.

Intraventricular hemorrhage (IVH): Usually, bleeding in the brain tissue that may extend into the chambers (ventricles) of the brain. A type of intracranial hemorrhage. Severity is indicated by a Roman numeral, ranging from Grade I (least severe) to Grade IV (ventricular enlargement and bleeding into surrounding brain tissue). Also called a bleed.

Intubation: Insertion of an endotracheal (ET) tube.

Invasive: A term that describes a diagnostic or treatment procedure involving cutting into the skin or inserting something (an instrument or device; a foreign substance) into the body.

Inverted nipples: Nipples that do not protrude from the areola of the breast but that are recessed (sunken) into it.

IQ: The abbreviation for intelligence quotient. A person's IQ score is the result of a standardized test that expresses an individual's intellectual ability relative to the rest of the population. The best known for children are the Wechsler Intelligence Scale for Children (WISC) and the Stanford-Binet Intelligence Scale.

Isolette: A trade name for an incubator. Often used as a common term for an incubator.

IV: See **Intravenous.**

J

Jaundice, pathologic: Jaundice (buildup of bilirubin in the fatty tissues that results in yellow skin color) that occurs within the first 24 hours of life; or visible persistent jaundice after 1 week of age in term infants (2 weeks in preterm infants); or bilirubin values that exceed defined norms. Usually a result of increased production of bilirubin caused by hemolysis, as in Rh or blood type incompatibility.

Jaundice, physiologic: A condition in which the skin color in newborns is yellowish because of a buildup of bilirubin in the fatty tissues. A common condition caused by immature liver function.

Jet: See **Ventilator, jet.**

K

Kangaroo care: The practice of holding an NICU infant skin-to-skin (often between the mother's breasts) to provide close human contact between parent and baby and to facilitate parent-infant attachment. Additional benefits usually include stable vital signs, more time in sleep and quiet alert states, increased weight gain, and improved feeding.

Keratinization: The formation of keratin (a fibrous protein) in the outer layer (epidermis) of the skin. Responsible for dry, flaky skin as the baby's skin matures by two or three weeks of age.

Kernicterus: A rare complication of hyperbilirubinemia. Occurs with very high levels of bilirubin, when bilirubin passes into the brain. Can cause permanent brain damage.

Kidney: A bean-shaped body organ that disposes of the waste products of metabolism as urine. Humans have two kidneys, one on either side of the spine.

L

Lactation: Milk production in the breasts of a woman. Also, broadly, breastfeeding.

Lactation consultant/specialist: A nurse or other health care provider with special training and expertise related to breastfeeding. A nurse lactation specialist with advanced education is most often used to manage the complex problems of breastfeeding mothers and babies in the NICU and in the community after hospital discharge; a lay person may be used in the community to offer support and education to breastfeeding mothers of healthy babies.

Lanugo: The soft, downy hair covering a preterm infant. Most evident on the upper back and shoulders. Disappears with maturation.

Large for gestational age (LGA): A term for a newborn whose weight (and possibly length and head circumference) falls above the 90th percentile on a standard intrauterine growth chart; indicates a larger-than-expected baby for the length of time the baby was in the uterus. An LGA baby can be preterm, term, or postterm.

Laser therapy: A treatment that uses high energy concentrated in the form of a beam of light to destroy problem tissue.

Glossary

Lead: An adhesive patch placed on a baby's chest or abdomen that connects the baby to the cardiorespiratory monitor. Also called an electrode.

Learning disability: A disorder that interferes with one's learning processes.

Lesion: Any break in normal tissue or change in the structure of an organ because of disease or injury.

Let-down reflex: Contractions (caused by the hormone oxytocin) that squeeze a mother's breast milk into the holding reservoirs just behind the nipples. May be experienced as a gripping sensation or as "pins and needles" in the breasts. Milk may drip from the nipples as the milk "lets down." Also called a milk-ejection reflex.

Lethargy: Lack of energy; sluggishness.

Level I nursery: A hospital classification of perinatal care indicating obstetric and neonatal units equipped to manage healthy mothers and babies and to stabilize and initiate transport of ill and/or complex mothers and newborns.

Level II nursery: A hospital classification of perinatal care indicating obstetric and neonatal units equipped to care for selected complicated pregnancies and neonatal problems and for infants convalescing after a stay in a Level III nursery.

Level III nursery: Identifies an obstetric unit/nursery, generally in a regional medical center and often affiliated with a university, that is equipped to diagnose and treat all perinatal problems; provides intensive care for infants requiring technological support or surgery. Also called a neonatal intensive care unit or an intensive care nursery.

Licensed practical nurse: A designation of state licensure; a nurse who provides basic bedside care under the supervision of an RN. Also called a licensed vocational nurse (LVN).

Licensed vocational nurse (LVN): See **Licensed practical nurse.**

Long-term care facility: See **Chronic-care facility.**

Low birth weight (LBW) infant: Any infant who weighs less than 2,500 grams (5 pounds, 8 ounces) at birth, regardless of gestational age.

LPN: See **Licensed practical nurse.**

Lumbar puncture: Insertion of a needle into the lower back, through the membranous space covering the brain and spinal cord to withdraw spinal fluid; procedure is used in diagnosis and treatment. Also called a spinal tap.

LVN: Licensed vocational nurse. See **LPN.**

Lymphocyte: A type of white blood cell that fights invading microorganisms.

M

Magnetic resonance imaging (MRI): A diagnostic imaging technique involving interaction between a magnetic field and the atoms in the body; does not use radiation. Produces better images of soft tissue than does CT scanning or ultrasound, and dense bone and fatty tissue do not interfere with the image (as they can in ultrasound).

Malformation, congenital: An anatomical abnormality (external or internal) present in a baby at birth.

Master's degree in social work: See **MSW.**

Mastitis: Bacterial infection of the breast that shows itself as a hot, red, tender area on the breast and is usually accompanied by fever, chills, and flulike symptoms.

Maternal transport: The physical moving of a pregnant woman (by ground or air) from one medical facility to another for special care or delivery of a newborn expected to require neonatal intensive care.

Mature milk: Thin, whitish breast milk produced by a mother a few days after the birth of her baby. Follows production of colostrum.

Mean arterial pressure (MAP): One aspect of the blood pressure. Monitored by a transducer connected to an umbilical arterial catheter.

Mechanical ventilation: Use of a machine (called a respirator or ventilator) to supply a number of breaths per minute and a mixture of air, oxygen, and pressure with each breath. The machine is connected to an endotracheal tube or a tracheostomy tube.

Meconium: Dark green to blackish material present in the large intestine of the fetus before birth. Usually passed during the first few days of life.

Meconium aspiration: "Breathing" into the trachea or lungs of meconium (a stool-like material that a fetus may excrete from its intestine into the amniotic fluid) by a fetus before or in the first moments after birth. Can cause breathing difficulties.

Meconium aspiration syndrome (MAS): Severe breathing problems after birth caused by meconium "breathed" into the airways while a baby is in the uterus or in the first moments after birth.

Medium-chain triglyceride (MCT) oil: An additive for breast milk or formula that contains fats that can be digested and absorbed by immature newborns who are not yet producing certain enzymes and bile salts.

Memory cell: An infection-fighting blood cell that, after once contacting a specific microorganism, remembers the microorganism and immediately begins to destroy it if it appears again.

Meningitis: Inflammation of the membranes lining the brain and spinal column; usually caused by a bacterium or a virus.

Metabolic: Having to do with metabolism.

Metabolic activity: Chemical reactions in which the body changes the nutrients in food into substances it needs to function or to build cells and tissues.

Metabolism: All the processes carried out by and chemical reactions that occur in the cells of the body as energy is produced and used.

Metoclopramide hydrochloride: A drug that may increase milk supply in lactating women.

Micrognathia: A birth defect marked by an abnormally small jaw.

Milk ejection reflex: See **Let-down reflex.**

Motor development: The learning of skills having to do with muscle movement and coordination.

Mottled: A marbled or blotched appearance; a term used to describe skin color.

MSW: Master's degree in social work.

Multidisciplinary: Having many different areas of expertise or specialization; in a hospital setting, may refer to medicine, nursing, social work, respiratory care, etc.

Murmur: A characteristic swishing sound made by blood flowing through the heart. Many heart murmurs are not associated with problems.

Myelomeningocele: See **Spina bifida.**

N

Narcotic: A medication that dulls the senses (thereby relieving pain)—for example, morphine.

Nasal cannula: See **Cannula, nasal.**

Nasogastric (NG) tube: A feeding tube inserted through a baby's nostril into the esophagus (food pipe) and on to the stomach. Formula or breast milk flows through the tube into the baby's stomach. An NG tube is usually left in place for a number of feedings after insertion.

Nebulizer: A device for giving medication that must be breathed into the airway; administers a liquid in the form of a fine spray. A type of inhaler, a "puffer".

Necrotizing enterocolitis (NEC): A serious inflammatory bowel disease, most common in preterm babies.

Neonatal: Having to do with a newborn baby, from birth to 28 days of age.

Neonatal intensive care: Special care provided, usually at a regional medical center, to newborns with major health problems.

Neonatal intensive care unit (NICU): A nursery, usually located in a regional medical facility, equipped to treat newborns who have serious health problems; staffed with pediatricians, anesthesiologists, surgeons, and nurses with special training and experience in the care of sick newborns. See **Level III nursery.**

Neonatal nurse: A registered nurse with special training in the care of newborn babies.

Neonatal nurse practitioner: See **NNP.**

Neonatal team: A group of health care professionals who care for a newborn baby in a hospital setting.

Neonatal transport: The moving of a newborn who requires special care or surgery from one hospital (often a community facility) to another (usually a Level III nursery).

Neonatologist: A physician who specializes in care and development, diagnosis, and treatment of ill newborn babies; has one or two years of training beyond that required to treat well newborns.

Neonatology: A branch of medicine that deals with the diagnosis, care, and treatment of disorders of newborn babies.

Nerve block: A type of anesthesia that makes the patient unable to feel pain—"blocks" the sensation—either locally (in a limited area of the body) or regionally (over a larger area of the body). See also **Anesthesia, local** and **Anesthesia, regional.**

Nerves: Bandlike tissues that transmit impulses from the brain or spinal cord to motor and sensory nerves in a particular body region.

Nervous system: The body system designed to carry information to and from all parts of the body in the form of nerve impulses; made up of the brain and spinal cord (central nervous system), and the remaining nerves and ganglia outside the brain and spinal cord (peripheral nervous system).

Nest: To surround a baby with rolled blankets or other things (even the hands) that act as boundaries. Promotes behavioral organization and a feeling of security. See also **Containment, body.**

Neurochemical: Having to do with the chemistry of the nervous system.

Neurologist: A physician who specializes in the structure, function, diagnosis, and treatment of nervous system disorders.

Neuromuscular: Having to do with both the nerves and the muscles.

Neuron: A nerve cell specialized to transmit electrical nerve impulses and so carry information from one part of the body to another.

NICU: See **Neonatal intensive care unit; Level III nursery.**

Nitric oxide (NO) therapy: Experimental rescue therapy commonly used for treatment of persistent pulmonary hypertension of the newborn (PPHN), a serious condition in infants that causes high blood pressure in the arteries supplying blood to the lungs. When breathed into the lungs, NO relaxes the walls of the blood vessels near the breathing sacs, opening or enlarging those vessels and improving oxygen and carbon dioxide exchange.

NNP: Neonatal nurse practitioner. A registered nurse who has advanced education (often a master's degree) and training in the development, care, and treatment of babies and their families. Examines, diagnoses, plans care, and performs procedures. Works under the direction of and in collaboration with a neonatologist or an attending physician.

Nonnutritive sucking: Sucking on a pacifier or a finger (the baby's own finger or a caregiver's). Aids motor skill development. May enhance digestion and absorption of food and improve weight gain and oxygenation. Does not supply nutrition.

Nonpharmacologic: Without the use of drugs or medications.

Nonspecific sign: A change in body function that may be caused by any one of many disorders or illnesses.

NPO: Abbreviation of the Latin for a medical order meaning "nothing by mouth"; indicates that a patient should be given neither food nor fluids orally.

Nursery monitor: A listening device (transmitter) placed in a baby's room to allow caregivers in another room to hear (through the receiver) any equipment alarms or sounds the baby makes. The device is not attached to the baby and is not considered medical equipment.

Nursing supplementer: A device consisting of a bag or bottle to hold breast milk or formula and a tube that is taped beside a woman's nipple. Provides extra milk or supplemental nutrients to a nursing baby during the breastfeeding session.

Nutrients: Proteins, carbohydrates, fats, vitamins, and minerals that humans need for life.

O

Obstetrician: A physician trained to meet the special health care needs of women during pregnancy, labor, delivery, and the postpartum period.

Occupational therapist: A specially trained health care provider who uses structured activity to promote recovery or rehabilitation. In infants, may focus on developmental and behavioral tasks (such as feeding or positioning).

Oligohydramnios: A condition in which less amnionic fluid than normal surrounds the unborn baby in the uterus.

Omphalocele: A birth defect in which some or all of the intestine (or another abdominal organ) pushes out through the abdominal wall at the base of the umbilical cord.

Ophthalmologist: A physician who specializes in diagnosing and treating problems of the eye.

Opiate: A drug made from opium. Relieves pain, calms, and produces restfulness, lack of action, and often sleep. Sometimes used to refer to any narcotic.

Optic nerve: A nerve that controls sharpness of vision and ability to focus on and follow objects.

OR: Operating room.

Oral: Having to do with the mouth.

Oral feeding: Feeding a baby breast milk or formula; methods include, among others, gavage, bottle, and breast.

Oral-motor development: Having to do with the mouth and with movement. Ability to coordinate movements involving the muscles and nerves of the mouth—for example, the sucking movements used in feeding.

Organ: A body structure that performs a specific function. The heart, lungs, kidneys, liver, and brain are all organs.

Orogastric (OG) tube: A feeding tube inserted through a baby's mouth into the esophagus (food pipe) and on to the stomach. Formula or breast milk flows through the tube into the baby's stomach. Usually inserted at each feeding and removed afterward.

Orthopedic: Having to do with correction of problems in the bones and joints.

Orthopedist: A physician with specialized training in preventing, diagnosing, and treating problems with the bones (skeleton) and connective tissues.

Ostomy: A surgical opening into an organ or body part. See also **colostomy, gastrostomy, ileostomy, tracheostomy.**

Otolaryngologist: A physician with specialized training in diagnosing and treating problems of the ear, nose, and throat.

Ototoxic: A term for a medication with side effects that can cause hearing loss.

Outpatient clinic: A medical facility, staffed by a team of health care providers, at which individuals with medical problems are examined and treated without staying overnight.

Oxygen (O_2): A substance contained in air. Necessary for proper functioning of body cells. Absorbed into the blood from air breathed into the lungs (called oxygenation).

Oxygen, blow-by: A stream of oxygen that flows from a tube placed near a baby's nose and mouth to provide a breathing baby with supplemental oxygen.

Oxygenation: The level of oxygen in the blood. Also, supplying oxygen to the blood.

Oxygen hood: A clear plastic box or hood placed over a baby's head to hold supplemental oxygen. Also called an oxyhood or a "hood."

Oxygen saturation monitor: See **Pulse oximeter.**

Oxygen, supplemental: An air/oxygen mixture provided to an infant who, because of prematurity or illness, requires a higher concentration of oxygen than the 21 percent found in room air.

Oxygen tent: A plastic apparatus placed around a baby's upper body to contain supplemental oxygen.

Oxyhood: See **Oxygen hood.**

Oxytocin: A hormone that causes contractions (of the uterus during labor and of the muscles surrounding the milk glands in women who have just given birth). Produces the let-down (or milk ejection) reflex.

P

Pacifier: A nipple-shaped device on which a baby can suck; provides no nutrition.

Palate: The roof of the mouth.

Pale: A term denoting a deficiency of skin color, usually caused by reduced blood flow through the skin.

Palliative: A term for a treatment that provides relief from a condition but does not cure it.

Paramedic: A specially trained medical technician who provides emergency services before or during transport to a hospital.

Patent: Open.

Patent ductus arteriosus (PDA): A ductus arteriosus that has not closed shortly after birth as it normally would. See also **Ductus arteriosus.**

Pathologist: A physician with specialized training in interpreting and identifying changes in the body caused by disease.

Pediatric developmentalist: a health care provider specially trained to evaluate and treat babies who are at risk or have problems mastering developmental skills, commonly because of preterm birth or a long hospital stay.

Pediatrician: A physician specially trained to diagnose and treat children from birth to age 18.

Pediatric neurologist: A physician who specializes in the structure, function, diagnosis, and treatment of nervous system disorders in babies and children.

Pediatric nurse: A registered nurse with special training in the care of children from birth to age 18.

Percutaneous endoscopic gastrostomy (PEG) tube: A type of gastrostomy tube that can be inserted without surgery. An endoscope (a floppy tube with a light on the end) guides placement of the tube as it is passed through the mouth, into the stomach, and out through a small hole made through the skin of the abdomen.

Perforate: To tear or rupture.

Perfusion: The passage of fluid through a tissue; especially refers to blood passing through the lungs to pick up oxygen.

Perinatal: The period before and after birth; a broad definition is from week 20 of pregnancy until one month after birth.

Perinatal center: The maternal-fetal-neonatal components of a regional medical center.

Perinatologist: A physician specially trained in diagnosing and treating problems of the pregnant woman and the fetus, during pregnancy, labor, delivery, and postpartum.

Peripheral line: See **Intravenous (IV) line.**

Peritonitis: An infection of the abdominal cavity.

Periventricular leukomalacia (PVL): Damaged brain tissue resulting in brain cysts, usually as a result of brain hemorrhage.

Permeability, skin: In newborns, refers to the ability of the skin to absorb substances such as applied lotions and oils and to the skin's susceptibility to water loss and heat loss. Has to do with the ability of liquids or gases to pass through (penetrate) tiny openings in the skin.

Persistent pulmonary hypertension of the newborn (PPHN): A serious condition in which high blood pressure (hypertension) in the arteries supplying blood to the lungs forces blood away from the lungs, decreasing the amount of oxygen in the blood going to the body.

Phototherapy: Light treatment for hyperbilirubinemia. Light waves break down indirect bilirubin so that the baby's system can eliminate it in urine.

Physical therapist: A specially trained health care provider who uses physical and mechanical methods (such as exercise; electric current treatment; massage; and water, light, and heat treatments) to promote recovery or rehabilitation. Also known as a physiotherapist.

Physio: See **Physiotherapy, chest.**

Physiologic: Having to do with normal body processes.

Physiotherapy, chest: Gentle percussions of the chest to loosen and remove lung secretions. Also called physio or chest PT.

Pierre Robin syndrome: Birth defects involving the skull and face: micrognathia (abnormally small jaw) in association with cleft palate and glossoptosis (displacement of the tongue). Causes breathing difficulty because of a blocked upper airway.

PIH: See **Pregnancy-induced hypertension.**

Placenta: An organ inside the uterus that attaches the developing baby to the wall of the uterus. Provides the fetus with nutrients, eliminates wastes, and exchanges respiratory gases. Commonly called the afterbirth, because it is expelled after the birth of the baby.

Placental abruption: Separation of the placenta from the uterine wall before delivery of a baby. Causes bleeding that can be life threatening for an unborn baby and his mother.

Placenta previa: A placenta that is positioned low in the uterus and partly or completely covers the opening of the uterus. Potentially dangerous to mother and baby because of a risk of bleeding before or during delivery.

Platelet: A component of the blood involved in clotting. Also called a thrombocyte.

Pneumocardiogram (PCG): A test that may help determine the cause of apnea and bradycardia, often given overnight. Test equipment is similar to the cardiorespiratory monitor but has channels to record heart rate, respirations, air flow through the nose, and oxygen saturation. Also called a sleep study or a pneumogram.

Pneumomediastinum: Leakage of air into the space in the center of the chest containing the heart and major blood vessels.

Pneumonia: Inflammation or infection of the lungs.

Pneumopericardium: Collection of air in the sac around the heart; life-threatening.

Pneumothorax: Air trapped between the lung and the chest wall. Also called a pulmonary air leak.

Polyhydramnios: A condition in which more amniotic fluid than normal is present in the mother's uterus during pregnancy. Sometimes a sign of a fetal anomaly.

Postnatal: Taking place after birth.

Postoperative: The period of time after surgery.

Postpartum: Taking place after delivery of a baby.

Precipitous birth: An unusually fast vaginal delivery; by strict definition, a labor and birth that takes three hours or less.

Preeclampsia: A term used to denote renal involvement caused by pregnancy-induced hypertension. A woman with this condition is said to be preeclamptic.

Pregnancy-induced hypertension (PIH): A multiorgan disease process involving high blood pressure as an important symptom; onset is usually after 20 weeks gestation. Renal, neurologic, liver, and hematologic involvement is possible during the course of the disease.

Premature: A term for a baby born before week 38 of gestation. Also called preterm.

Premature rupture of membranes (PROM): Term used when the amniotic sac breaks ("water breaks") prior to the onset of labor. If the amniotic sac breaks prior to the onset of labor contractions and before the 38th week of gestation, the condition is called preterm premature rupture of membranes.

Prematurity: The condition of being born early, before week 38 of gestation.

Premie: A preterm or premature baby, or used to describe something used by a preterm baby.

Premie nipple: A small, soft, pliable nipple designed for bottle feeding a baby with a weak or immature suck. Provides more formula with less sucking effort.

Prenatal: Having to do with the period before birth.

Preterm: See **Premature.**

Primary apnea: See **Apnea of prematurity.**

Primary nurse: A nurse who works with a baby and his/her family throughout the hospitalization to coordinate care, and teach and support the family.

Progesterone: The hormone that stimulates growth of the endometrium (lining of the uterus); needed for growth of a fertilized egg.

Prognosis: The outlook or forecast for a baby's recovery or future condition.

Prolactin: A hormone that causes the milk glands to begin secreting milk in the breasts of a woman who has just given birth. Released by the body whenever the nipples of a postpartum woman are stimulated.

Prolonged rupture of membranes: Term used when 12–24 hours or more hours pass after the amniotic sac breaks without delivery of the newborn. Because the amniotic sac provides a barrier to infection, the infant can be at risk for infection if labor and delivery do not occur for a prolonged period of time after the membranes rupture.

Prone: Lying on the stomach.

Prophylactic treatment: Treatment designed to prevent something from developing or occurring.

Protocol: A standard plan or standard instructions for a specific situation.

Psychologist: A care provider (not a physician) who specializes in diagnosing and treating mental and behavioral problems.

Public Law (PL) 94-142: Education for All Handicapped Children Act. A 1975 federal law requiring special education programs for all disabled children from 6 to 21 years of age.

Public Law (PL) 99-457, part H: Education of the Handicapped Amendments. A 1986 federal law providing early-intervention programs for disabled or at-risk babies (from birth to age 2) and offering incentives for states to expand services for disabled children between ages 3 and 5.

Pulmonary: Having to do with the lungs.

Pulmonary atresia: A cyanotic heart defect in which the valve that allows blood to flow from the right ventricle of the heart to the lungs (the pulmonary valve) is absent.

Pulmonary edema: Leakage of fluid into the tissues of the lungs.

Pulmonary interstitial emphysema (PIE): Leakage of air from torn breathing sacs (alveoli) in the lungs into spaces around the lung tissue.

Pulmonary stenosis: A birth defect in which the valve that allows blood to flow from the heart to the lungs is narrowed, reducing blood flow through the pulmonary artery to the lungs. May be isolated or combined with other heart defects.

Pulmonary valve: A heart valve that opens to allow blood to flow from the right ventricle through the pulmonary artery and to the lungs.

Pulmonologist: A physician who specializes in the structure and function of the lungs and diagnosis and treatment of breathing difficulties and problems of the lungs.

Pulse: A measurement of the rate at which the heart is beating; the heart rate.

Pulse oximeter: A device that wraps around the hand or foot of an infant and uses a light sensor to determine the amount of oxygen bound to the hemoglobin molecules in the blood. A general indicator of a baby's oxygenation. Also called an oxygen saturation monitor.

R

R-2: A resident in the second year of a physician training program.

R-3: A resident in the third year of a physician training program.

Radiant warmer: An open mattress, usually on a mobile cart, with a heat source above it. Used to stabilize and warm a baby immediately after delivery, for easy access to the baby during caregiving in the NICU, and in other situations (during in-hospital transport and during surgery, for example). The baby is said to be "on a warmer."

Radiation: A type of energy involved in x-rays. Large amounts can damage body tissues and cells.

Radiology: The branch of medicine that performs and interprets radiographic (x-ray) and ultrasound procedures.

Recovery: A restoration period when a patient is to regain health or strength.

Rectal: Having to do with the rectum, the lower part of the intestine just inside the anus.

Rectal temperature: The body temperature taken by inserting a blunt-end thermometer into the lower part of the intestine just inside the anus (the rectum).

Rectal thermometer: A device inserted into the rectum to measure body temperature.

Rectum: The lower part of the intestine just inside the anus.

Red blood cell (RBC): A part of the blood that contains hemoglobin which carries oxygen to the tissues of the body.

Referral: A recommendation for a care provider.

Reflexes, feeding: Unconscious, automatic responses of the nerves to certain kinds of stimuli. Includes gagging, sucking, swallowing, and rooting reflexes.

Reflux, gastroesophageal: The backward flow of stomach contents into the esophagus (food pipe); in infants, may trigger apnea and/or bradycardia.

Regional medical center: A hospital facility, often associated with a university, staffed with medical specialists. Provides patient care, research, and regional education and consultation. Also called a tertiary care center.

Registered nurse: See **RN.**

Regressive behavior: A return to past ways of acting, often to less mature approaches. May be seen in children under stress or who want attention—for example, bed-wetting may be regressive behavior in a toilet-trained preschooler.

Rehabilitation facility: See **Transitional care facility.**

Renal: Having to do with the kidneys.

Rescue therapy: Treatment given for an existing medical problem (as opposed to prophylactic therapy, which is given to treat an anticipated problem). For example, surfactant replacement therapy can be given as a prophylactic therapy (immediately following delivery) or as rescue therapy (after respiratory distress syndrome is diagnosed).

Resident: A physician who has graduated from medical school and has progressed beyond the first year of a residency program (a hospital-based program of specialized training). A physician in his second year of training (R-2) or third year of training (R-3) usually instructs interns and works with senior residents and/or attending physicians. Many residents in NICUs are enrolled in pediatric residencies.

Residual: Food remaining in the stomach from the previous feeding at the time of the next feeding. Large residuals indicate feeding intolerance.

Respirations: Breaths.

Respirator: See **Ventilator.**

Respiratory: Having to do with breathing.

Respiratory depression: A reduction in or lack of breathing effort.

Respiratory distress syndrome (RDS): A condition that affects the lungs of preterm newborns, making it difficult for them to breathe. Caused by a lack of surfactant. Sometimes called hyaline membrane disease.

Respiratory syncytial virus (RSV): A virus that commonly causes infections of the upper and lower respiratory tract. The major cause of bronchiolitis and pneumonia in young children.

Respiratory therapist (RT): A health care provider who specializes in treating problems of the respiratory (breathing) system.

Respite care: The assumption of total care for an ill or disabled individual by an outside facility or individual for a short period of time, to permit the regular caregiver(s) to rest, relax, and re-energize.

Resuscitate/Resuscitation: To restore breathing and/or heart and circulatory function when either or both are functioning insufficiently to support life.

Reticulocyte ("retic") count: A laboratory test that shows how many red blood cells the body is producing. A reticulocyte is an immature red blood cell.

Retina: The light-sensitive lining of the interior of an eye. Receives visual images.

Retinopathy of prematurity (ROP): A disease affecting the retina of a preterm baby's eye. Involves rapid, irregular growth of blood vessels that can lead to bleeding, and scarring of the retina. Can cause retinal detachment and blindness if severe.

Retraction: The drawing in of the chest wall with each breath. Most visible at the breastbone, between the ribs, and above the collarbone. Generally indicates difficulty breathing.

Return transport: See **Back transport.**

Risk factor: Something (usually some characteristic or physical condition) that makes it more likely that a baby may experience problems.

RN: Registered nurse. A designation of state licensure. A person can prepare for state licensure as an RN by graduating from a diploma program (hospital training), a 2 year college (associate degree) program, or a 4 year university program (bachelor's degree).

RNC: Certified registered nurse. An RN who has voluntarily taken and passed a standardized examination denoting professional excellence in her specialty.

Rooming-in: Staying overnight at the hospital with your baby shortly before discharge; a "trial run" when parents care for their baby independently and use nursing staff only if necessary.

Rooting reflex: A baby's response to stroking of the face: head turns in the direction of the stroking and mouth opens.

Rotation, physician: For residents, the changing of assignment from one patient care specialty area to another; often takes place about once a month. Attending physicians, fellows, and interns may also rotate.

Rounds: Daily patient visits during which members of the health care team discuss and review each patient's condition and medical plan.

S ─────────────

Saline, normal: A liquid solution containing 0.9 percent sodium chloride; used to dilute some drugs for injection; also used to flush fluid through an IV line and insure patency. Normal saline can also be used to increase plasma volume, and thereby increase blood pressure.

Saturation, oxygen: The degree to which oxygen is bound to hemoglobin (a substance in red blood cells). Expressed as a percentage.

Screening test: A structured examination or review by a health care professional to identify potential or existing physical, mental, behavioral, or emotional problems.

Scrotum: In males, the pouch between the legs that contains the testes.

Secretion: A substance (such as mucus) produced by a gland and released to an external or internal body surface.

Sedate: To medicate to calm excitement or agitation.

Seizure: Abnormal brain electrical activity often accompanied by involuntary muscle contraction and relaxation (spasms).

Self-comforting: A term for a behavioral skill in which a baby takes actions (brings the hands to the mouth; sucks on a finger, a fist, or a pacifier; or clasps the hands together) to make him- or herself feel better. Facilitates behavioral organization.

Sensory system: The body system made up of the organs used to see, hear, feel, taste, and touch.

Separation anxiety: Concern or anxiousness about what will happen when one leaves a familiar environment or familiar people for an unknown situation.

Sepsis: The presence of harmful microorganisms in the blood and their effects on the body; a general infection.

Sepsis workup: The collection and laboratory culture (growth) of blood, urine, and/or spinal fluid samples to determine whether microorganisms are present in them. Identifies the presence of infection.

Septal defect: A birth defect marked by a hole in the wall (the septum) separating the left and right sides of the heart. May be atrial or ventricular.

Septicemia: An infection in the blood.

Sequela: A consequence that results from a preceding disease, for example, visual impairment is a potential sequela of retinopathy of prematurity.

Servomechanism/Servocontrol: A thermostat mechanism for regulating the body temperature of an infant on a radiant warmer or in an incubator. A skin temperature probe senses the infant's skin temperature and decreases or increases the heat source when the skin temperature is above or below a preset level.

Sexually transmitted disease (STD): An infection passed from one person to another during sexual activity. Also referred to as venereal disease.

Shock: An unstable condition marked by circulatory collapse: inadequate blood flow, insufficient oxygen to the tissues, and inadequate removal of waste products from them. Can occur in the presence of sepsis, acute blood loss, heart problems, or allergic reaction.

Short bowel syndrome: Having only a small length of healthy bowel (potential sequela of a disease like necrotizing enterocolitis); limits the bowel's ability to absorb nutrients and water from the stool. Also called short gut.

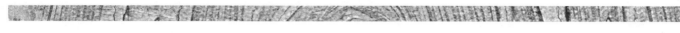

Short gut: See **Short bowel syndrome.**

Shunt: A thin tube used to drain fluid from one area of the body to another. Also, an abnormal connection between two areas of the body (as in a patent ductus arteriosus in a newborn).

Shunt, left-to-right: In newborns, a blood circulation pattern in which some of the blood leaving the heart flows back from the aorta into the lungs through a patent ductus arteriosus. Generally seen in a baby recovering from respiratory distress syndrome. The overabundance of blood entering the lungs can lead to signs and symptoms of a patent ductus arteriosus (for example, worsening respiratory problems).

Shunt, right-to-left: In newborns, a blood circulation pattern in which some of the blood entering the heart is directed away from the blood vessels in the lungs, which are narrowed by the effects of respiratory distress syndrome or pulmonary hypertension, causing oxygen-poor blood to be sent to the body.

Sibling: A brother or sister.

Side effect: A secondary effect of a medication or drug; can be undesirable.

SIDS: See **Sudden infant death syndrome.**

Sleep study: See **Pneumocardiogram.**

Small for gestational age (SGA): Term for a newborn whose weight (and possibly length, and head circumference) falls below the 10th percentile on a standard intrauterine growth chart; indicates small size for the length of time the baby was in the uterus. An SGA baby can be preterm, term, or postterm.

Social worker: An individual on the hospital staff who has training (and usually a master's degree) in helping patients and their families cope with stress, deal with financial concerns related to the hospitalization, utilize hospital and community resources, and prepare for discharge.

Socioeconomic status: In combination, the social and financial factors that determine a person's position in society relative to others.

Sonographer: A medical technician who performs ultrasounds.

Spastic diplegia: Stiffness and awkward movement of the limbs. A form of cerebral palsy.

Special-care nursery: A unit in a hospital that has staff trained to care for any baby requiring more than routine, well-born care. In some hospitals, the term may denote a unit for babies requiring intermediate or convalescent care.

Special-needs infant: A baby who requires technologic support or medications to live or who requires special intervention and attention to develop and grow normally.

Spina bifida: A birth defect in which the spinal column does not close completely and the covering of the spinal cord pushes out through the gap between the vertebrae, forming an external sac. Myelomeningocele is one type.

Spinal tap: See **Lumbar puncture.**

State, behavioral: Level of awareness. Babies experience these six states: deep sleep, light sleep, drowsy, quiet alert, active alert, and crying.

STD: See **Sexually transmitted disease.**

Stenosis: A birth defect in which a passage (such as a valve, a vein, or an artery) is narrowed. Flow through the passage is limited.

Stenotic: Having to do with a stenosis.

Stenotic lesion: An abnormal narrowing of a blood vessel or valve.

Step-down unit: A hospital nursery for recuperating babies that provides less intensive care than that given in an NICU; may be called an intermediate care unit (ICU), a Level II unit, or a special-care unit.

Steroid: A drug given to reduce swelling and inflammation.

Stimulation, oral: Sensory input (either positive or negative) to the area in and around the baby's mouth.

Stimulation, tactile: Gentle alerting of a baby by touching, stroking, rubbing, or flicking a body surface such as the soles of the feet. Used in this way to encourage breathing in an apneic infant.

Stimulus: Something that excites, alerts, or promotes activity (plural: stimuli).

Stoma: The artificial opening of a hollow organ. For a colostomy, the stoma is on the abdomen. For a tracheostomy, the stoma is on the neck.

Stool: Feces; the result of a bowel movement.

Streptococcus, Group B β-hemolytic: A type of bacteria sometimes found in the birth canal. Can cause pneumonia in newborns.

Stress: The body's response to disturbances in the environment (including emotional concerns), to pain, and often to infection. Signs include changes in heart rate, breathing patterns, blood pressure, and oxygen consumption. Also called physiologic stress.

Stress, environmental: Irritation caused by disturbance from light, sound, and temperature in the area around (environment of) a baby. Can produce physical (physiologic) changes in heart rate, breathing patterns, blood pressure, and/or oxygen consumption.

Stressor: Something that causes stress.

Subarachnoid: Located below the innermost membrane covering the brain.

Subdural: Located below the outermost membrane covering the brain.

Subependymal: Located beneath the lining of the brain chambers (the ventricles).

Subglottic stenosis: A narrowing of the trachea (windpipe); may be caused by prolonged mechanical ventilation or repeated intubations.

Substance abuse: Misuse or excessive use of a legal or illegal drug or a substance containing a drug.

Suction: Mechanical removal (drawing out) of air or fluid from the body.

Sudden infant death syndrome (SIDS): The death of an infant under one year of age during sleep with unidentifiable causes. Also called crib death or cot death.

Suffocation: An inability to breathe, as with drowning or smothering; can cause unconsciousness or death.

Support group: A group of individuals who meet to share a common concern or focus. Intended to promote sharing of information, feelings, and concerns.

Surfactant: A soaplike substance (made up mainly of fat) produced by lung cells. Coats inner surfaces of airways and air sacs in the lungs to keep those passages open between breaths. Absent or lacking in babies born preterm (production begins at about 24 weeks gestation but is not well developed until 36 weeks). Also, a manufactured substitute (exogenous surfactant) used to treat respiratory distress syndrome in preterm infants.

Surfactant replacement therapy: A treatment in which a preterm infant with expected or confirmed respiratory distress syndrome is given a natural or artificial substance (called an exogenous surfactant) through a tube placed in the windpipe (trachea) to replace the natural surfactant the baby lacks because of early birth.

Suture: The material used to sew up a surgical wound or close an incision. Can also refer to the thin line of connective tissue between 2 bones, as in cranial suture.

Syndrome: A pattern of signs and/or symptoms occurring together that form a clinical picture indicative of a specific disorder.

Syringe: A device for injecting fluids into or withdrawing them from the body or for washing out a body cavity.

System, body: The series of interdependent body parts (organs, vessels, muscles, nerves, and so on) that work together to accomplish something; the heart and the blood vessels, for example, make up the cardiovascular system, through which blood moves to every part of the body.

Systemic: Having to do with or affecting the whole body.

T ───────────────────

Tachycardia: A faster-than-normal heart rate.

Tachycardic: A term for a baby whose heart rate is faster than normal.

Tachypnea: A faster-than-normal breathing.

Tachypneic: A term for a baby who is breathing faster than normal.

Teaching hospital: A hospital associated with a university; offers programs designed to accommodate learning needs of students in health care related fields of study.

Technician: A trained hospital staff member who performs a specific function, often related to a diagnostic procedure.

Technology: An application of knowledge to achieve a desired outcome. In the NICU, technology includes state-of-the-art equipment and therapy used to treat infants.

Technology dependent: Needing mechanical equipment to survive.

Teratogen: An environmental agent (such as a drug, chemical, or toxin) that can cause birth defects if the fetus is exposed to it during development, especially during the first three months.

Term: A word for a baby born between the beginning of week 38 and the end of week 42 of gestation.

Tertiary care center: See **Regional medical center.**

Tetralogy of Fallot: A cyanotic heart defect involving four abnormalities of the heart and its vessels: a ventricular septal defect (VSD), pulmonary stenosis, an overly muscular right ventricle, and positioning of the aorta over the VSD.

Theophylline: A medication that stimulates the central nervous system. Given to reduce occurrences of apnea in selected babies.

Thermal stress: Undesirable changes in the body's vital signs caused by high or low environmental temperatures.

Thoracic: Having to do with the chest.

Thrombocyte: See **Platelet.**

Thrombocytopenia: A term for a low platelet count.

Thrush: A yeast (fungal) infection common in babies who have been on antibiotics; appears as a patchy white coating on the tongue and gums or as a persistent, pebbly, diaper rash.

Tidal volume: The amount of air breathed in (inhaled) and breathed out (exhaled) with one normal breath.

Time-out: A method used to calm an infant and facilitate behavioral organization; involves decreasing sound, light, and movement for a period of time.

Titrate: To adjust the dose of a drug to use the smallest amount that will produce a desire effect.

Tocotransducer ("toco"): The component of external electronic fetal monitoring that senses pressure changes on the pregnant woman's abdomen. Used to monitor frequency and duration of uterine contractions.

Tolerance: In reference to a drug, the need over time for an increasingly higher dose to achieve the same effect.

Tolerate: In reference to a baby receiving breast milk or formula, to retain, digest, and absorb the feeding.

Tongue-tied: See **Ankyloglossia.**

Topical: Applied to a limited surface area of the skin and affecting only that area.

Topical anesthetic: A preparation applied to the skin surface to numb it, temporarily blocking feeling in the area to which it is applied.

TORCH: A term that stands for the names of intrauterine, or congenital, infections that can cross the placenta to the fetus: **T**oxoplasmosis, **O**ther viruses, **R**ubella virus, **C**ytomegalovirus, and **H**erpes simplex virus.

Total anomalous pulmonary venous connection or return (TAPVR): A cyanotic heart defect in which the veins that return oxygenated blood from the lungs to the heart are not connected to the left atrium as they should be, but instead the blood drains through abnormal connections to the right atrium, mixes with unoxygenated blood, passes through an atrial septal defect into the left atrium and out to the body.

Total parenteral nutrition (TPN): The provision of essential nutrients (proteins, fats, sugar, vitamins, and minerals) and water through an intravenous line to replace or supplement a baby's intake by mouth. Also called hyperalimentation.

Trach ("trach" pronounced "trake"): See **Tracheostomy.**

Trachea: The windpipe.

Tracheoesophageal (T-E) fistula: A birth defect marked by an abnormal connection between the trachea (windpipe) and the esophagus (food pipe).

Tracheomalacia: A condition in which the airway is soft and collapses during breathing.

Tracheostomy: A surgical opening through the neck and into the windpipe (trachea) through which a breathing tube is inserted.

Tracheostomy tube: A breathing tube inserted into the windpipe (trachea) through a surgical opening in the neck.

Transcutaneous monitor (TCM): A device placed on the skin that, when calibrated with a laboratory test called a blood gas, approximates the oxygen and carbon dioxide levels in the blood.

Transducer: A device that converts energy from one form to another.

Transfusion: The giving of fluid, such as whole blood or a blood component (such as red blood cells, to treat anemia) directly into the bloodstream through a catheter.

Transfusion, exchange: A method for replacing (exchanging) a portion of the blood volume through repeated removal of small amounts of blood and replacement with equal amounts of donor blood. Done to reduce the concentration of undesirable elements in the blood, such as excess bilirubin.

Transient tachypnea of the newborn (TTN): A respiratory condition caused by delay in the body's absorption after birth of the fluid that fills the fetal lungs.

Transillumination: An assessment/diagnostic technique that involves shining a bright light through body tissues.

Transitional care: The level of medical care that falls between what is provided in a hospital and what can be provided in the home.

Transitional care facility: A facility that provides care that falls between what is provided in a hospital and what can be provided in the home. The goal is independent caregiving and discharge home. Also called a rehabilitation hospital.

Transposition of the great arteries: A cyanotic heart defect in which the pulmonary artery (which normally carries unoxygenated blood to the lungs) and the aorta (which carries oxygenated blood to the body) are reversed, resulting in oxygen-poor blood being sent to the body.

Transpyloric feeding: Feeding through a tube that descends beyond the stomach and is placed in the upper intestine.

Tricuspid atresia: A cyanotic heart defect in which the valve that allows blood to flow from the right atrium of the heart to the right ventricle (the tricuspid valve) is absent.

Trisomy 21: See **Down syndrome.**

Truncus arteriosus: A complex heart defect in which only one artery (a combination of the aorta and the pulmonary artery) leaves the heart.

Tube feeding: See **Gavage feeding.**

Tuberculosis: A communicable disease affecting the lungs. Caused by a bacterium.

Tympanic thermometer: A device that measures body temperature through a probe inserted a short distance into the ear.

U

Ultrasonography: A diagnostic imaging technique that uses reflections of high-frequency sound waves (called echoes) to make two-dimensional images of internal body structures, tissues, and blood flow; often used to scan the brain. Does not involve radiation. Often can be done at the baby's bedside.

Umbilical cord: A cord connecting the fetus with the placenta. Contains two arteries and one vein. Is clamped and cut at birth. The location at which it attaches to the infant becomes the navel.

Umbilical hernia: A skin-covered protrusion of part of the intestine through a weakness in the abdominal wall at the navel (the umbilicus).

Umbilicus: The navel or belly button.

Uterus: In a woman, the organ that surrounds and protects the unborn baby (fetus) during development and until birth; the womb.

V

Vaccine: A killed or less-powerful version of a bacterium or a virus given to stimulate the development of antibodies (blood protein that attacks any foreign substance) and thus give immunity (resistance to infection) to disease.

Vacuum extraction: A method of birth assistance in which a suction cup is applied to the top of the unborn baby's head in the final pushing stage of labor; working with uterine contractions, the physician applies gentle traction to assist with delivery of the baby's head.

Validate: To ensure that someone understands what has been said, perhaps by asking the person to repeat the information in his or her own words.

Vasoconstriction: The narrowing, tightening, or partial closure of blood vessels, reducing blood flow through them and producing more resistance to flow.

Vasodilate: To widen or open blood vessels. Produces less resistance to flow.

Vasodilator: A drug that widens or opens blood vessels, reducing resistance to flow.

Venereal disease: See **Sexually transmitted disease.**

Venoarterial (VA) bypass: A technique used to start extracorporeal membrane oxygenation therapy. Involves inserting parallel catheters into the right side of the neck: one, placed in a vein, is threaded into the upper right chamber of the heart; the other, placed in the carotid artery, is threaded to the aortic arch. Insertion of the catheters is called cannulation.

Venoarterial extracorporeal membrane oxygenation therapy (VA ECMO): A therapy used to treat babies who have both lung and heart function or blood pressure problems; requires insertion of two catheters, one in a vein and the other in an artery. Blood is drained from the upper right chamber of the infant's heart by gravity through the catheter in the vein, carbon dioxide is removed, oxygen is added, and the blood is then warmed and pumped back to the aortic arch and into the baby's body through the catheter in the artery. The ECMO equipment circuit includes a membrane oxygenator (artificial lung) and a pump. See also **Extracorporeal membrane oxygenation.**

Venovenous (VV) bypass: A technique used to start extracorporeal membrane oxygenation therapy; involves inserting a double lumen catheter into a large vein in the right side of the neck and threading it into the upper right chamber of the heart. Insertion of the catheter is called cannulation.

Venovenous extracorporeal membrane oxygenation therapy (VV ECMO): A therapy used to treat babies who have lung problems but whose heart function and blood pressure are normal; requires insertion of a split catheter into a vein in the neck. Blood is drained from the upper right chamber of the heart by gravity through one side of the tube, carbon dioxide is removed, oxygen is added, and the blood is then warmed and pumped back into the baby's heart through the other side of the catheter. The ECMO equipment circuit includes a membrane oxygenator (artificial lung) and a pump. See also **Extracorporeal membrane oxygenation.**

Ventilation: Mechanical breathing assistance; passage of air in and out of the airways.

Ventilator: A mechanical device that assists breathing and supplies an air/oxygen mixture under pressure. Used with an endotracheal tube or tracheostomy tube. Also called a respirator.

Ventilator, jet: A mechanical device that delivers short bursts of air into the windpipe at high rates of flow. Used to provide high-frequency jet ventilation. Sometimes called a jet.

Ventricle: A small chamber; one of the central chambers in the brain or one of the two lower chambers of the heart.

Ventricular septal defect (VSD): A birth defect marked by a hole in the wall (septum) between the two lower chambers (ventricles) of the heart.

Vernix caseosa: Greasy white or yellow, cheeselike material from fetal oil glands; made up of skin cells and fine hairs that cover the skin of the fetus. Protects the fetal skin from abrasions, chapping, and hardening before birth.

Very low birth weight (VLBW) infant: Any infant who weighs less than 1,500 grams (3 lbs, 5 oz) at birth, regardless of gestational age.

Virus: An infectious microorganism that can live and multiply in the cells of the body.

Visual: Having to do with sight.

Vital signs: Body temperature, pulse (heart) rate, and rate of respirations (breathing), and, if clinically indicated, blood pressure.

Vulnerable child syndrome: A tendency to continue to see a child who was once sick or physically disabled as still sickly or very susceptible to disease or injury despite normal findings on physical examination.

W

Warmer: See **Radiant warmer.**

Wean: To gradually stop one method of doing something and accustom the baby to another method; commonly used in reference to removal of a baby from technologic support, such as weaning from the ventilator to independent breathing. To slowly decrease the use of an intervention, such as a medication.

White blood cell (WBC): The part of the blood that plays a role in defending against infection.

X

X-ray: An electromagnetic wave that produces an image of internal body parts. Used in diagnosis.

Y

Yeast infection: Infection with a fungus such as Candida. An oral yeast infection, called thrush, is common in babies who have been treated with antibiotics. Babies may get this type of infection in their mouths; nursing mothers may get it on their nipples. A systemic yeast infection (inside the body) can be life-threatening for NICU babies.

Bibliography

ACOG Technical Bulletin Number 219. January 1996. *Hypertension in pregnancy.* Washington, DC: American College of Obstetricians and Gynecologists, 1.

The Bantam Medical Dictionary, rev. ed. 1990. Prepared by the editors of Market House Books, Ltd. New York: Bantam Books.

Blackburn ST, and Loper DL. 1992. *Maternal, Fetal, and Neonatal Physiology: A Clinical Perspective.* Philadelphia: WB Saunders.

Bloom RS, and Cropley C. 1993. *Textbook of Neonatal Resuscitation.* Elk Grove Village, Illinois: American Heart Association/American Academy of Pediatrics.

Dorland's Illustrated Medical Dictionary, 28th ed. 1994. Philadelphia: WB Saunders.

Freeman RK, and Poland RL, eds. 1992. *Guidelines for Perinatal Care,* 3rd ed. Elk Grove Village, Illinois: American Academy of Pediatrics.

Korones SB. 1986. *High-Risk Newborn Infants: The Basis for Intensive Nursing Care,* 4th ed. Philadelphia: Mosby-Year Book.

Merriam-Webster's Collegiate Dictionary, 10th ed. 1995. Springfield, Massachusetts: Merriam-Webster.

Shelov SP, and Hannemann RE, eds. 1991. In *The American Academy of Pediatrics: Caring for Your Baby and Young Child—Birth to Age 5—The Complete and Authoritative Guide.* New York: Bantam.

Sherwen LN, Scoloveno MA, and Weingarten CT, eds. 1991. *Nursing Care of the Childbearing Family.* Norwalk, Connecticut: Appleton & Lange.

Stedman's Medical Dictionary, 26th ed. 1995. Baltimore: Williams & Wilkins.

Index

Index

Index

O

Index

Allie Eight Weeks Old

Allie's hand is like a little flower;
fisted, a soft closed bud
that holds the promise of what
she will become.

Open, a pink and white rose,
lovely in full bloom
reaching out to touch
sunshine, sky and moon.

Dewy soft and smelling sweet
baby hands and baby feet.

Baby Holder

My hand cradles the silken globe
of the baby's head.
His warm weight satisfies my arms.

On my shoulder I sniff his fragrant cheek
and feel soft puffs of feathery breath
on my neck.

His hand grasps my finger
with surprising strength
and the small, steady breathing of his sleep
is a mantra that brings
peace to both of us.

These are only two poems from the spectacular book

Baby Hands & Baby Feet

Poems and Drawings from the Nursery
written by Nancy Kennedy, RN, with Drawings by David Pegher

*This book reveals to us the true source of healing—the relationships between children
with enormous courage and wisdom, their parents (including those who are yet children
themselves), their grandparents, their siblings, their nurses and therapists, and their doctors.*

*This magnificent gift book will speak to anyone who has worked with newborn infants
and their families. To get your copy, call the toll free number listed below.
This is truly a book that speaks to your heart.*
